Benign Childhood Partial Seizures and Related Epileptic Syndromes

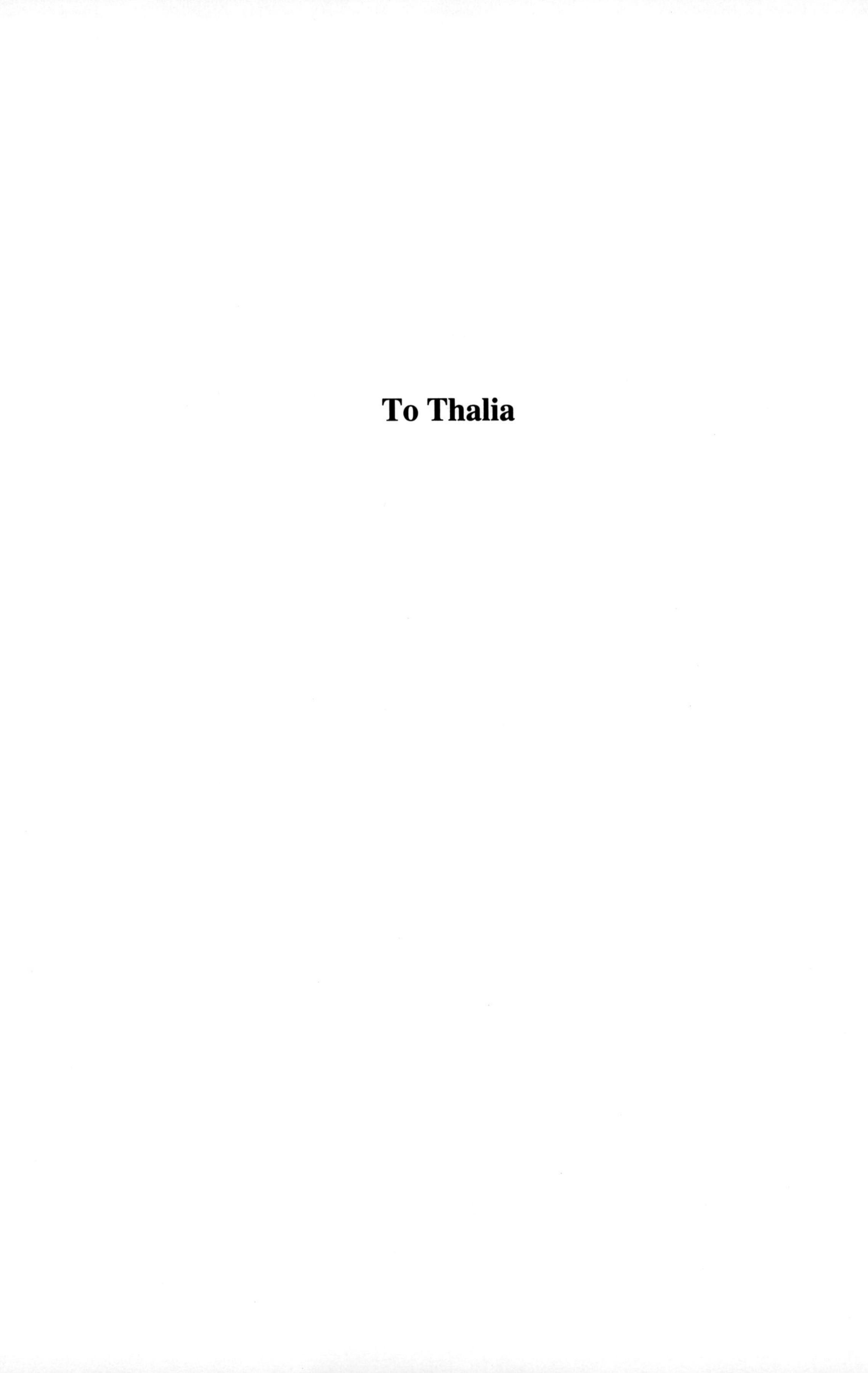

To Thalia

Benign Childhood Partial Seizures and Related Epileptic Syndromes

C P Panayiotopoulos MD PhD FRCP

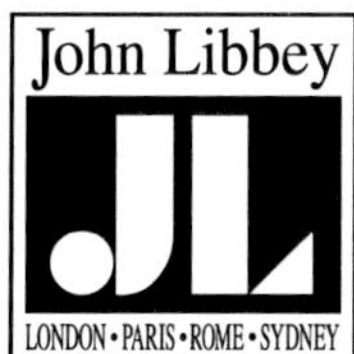

British Library Cataloguing in Publication Data

Panayiotopoulos, C.P. (Chrysostomos P.)

Benign childhood partial seizures and related epileptic syndromes

(Current problems in epilepsy series; 15)
1. Epilepsy in children 2. Convulsions in children
I. Title
618.9'2853

ISSN: 0959 4591 (Current Problems in Epilepsy: 15)
ISBN: 0 86196 577 9

Published by

John Libbey & Company Ltd, 13 Smiths Yard, Summerley Street,
London SW18 4HR, England
Telephone: 081–947 2777; Fax: 081–947 2664; e-mail johnlibbey@aol.com

John Libbey & Company Pty Ltd, 15–17 Young Street, Sydney, NSW 2000, Australia
John Libbey Eurotext Ltd, 127 avenue de la République, 92120 Montrouge, France
John Libbey at C.I.C. Edizioni s.r.l., via Lazzaro Spallanzani 11, 00161 Rome, Italy

Printed in Malaysia by Kum-Vivar Printing Sdn Bhd, Rawang, Selangor.

Contents

Preface

Benign childhood partial seizures and related epileptic syndromes are the commonest and probably the most fascinating and rewarding topic in paediatric epileptology. They form a significant part of the everyday practice of paediatricians, neurologists and clinical neurophysiologists who care for children with seizures. Yet, despite significant progress in their clinico-EEG recognition in the last four to five decades, only Rolandic seizures are widely known and identified with an excellent prognosis. However, even for Rolandic seizures expert opinions are still divided regarding genetics, neuropsychological consequences, possible progression to more severe diseases such as Landau–Kleffner syndrome, treatment and relations to other syndromes of generalised and partial epilepsies. Chapter 4 details the clinical aspects of Rolandic seizures. The centrotemporal spikes, the EEG marker of Rolandic seizures, peak at 8–9 years of age and may also occur in 2–3 per cent of normal children. Their characteristics and other EEG abnormalities are extensively reviewed and illustrated in Chapter 5.

Benign childhood occipital seizures, despite their sound clinico-EEG manifestations, are less well known and still debated. The official position of the Commission on Classification and Terminology of the International League Against Epilepsy[176,177] exemplifies the existing confusion. The Commission has recognised only one clinical phenotype, childhood epilepsy with occipital paroxysms, manifested with visual seizures at a mean age of onset of 7–9 years with an unpredictable prognosis. The relationship of this condition to migraine, with which it is often erroneously equated or misdiagnosed, has raised considerable interest and debate. Yet, benign childhood visual seizures are extremely rare and their clinical differentiation from migraine is relatively easy. Furthermore, occipital spikes are equally well known as centrotemporal spikes, also remitting with age. They are 2–3 times less frequent than centrotemporal spikes but occur at an earlier age with a peak at 5 years. We should have predicted that occipital spikes, like the centrotemporal ones, also have a clinical representative. This is what I have described through a 25 years prospective study. Early onset benign childhood occipital seizures, or Panayiotopoulos syndrome as some authors propose to name them, are now confirmed world-wide as the second commonest after Rolandic seizures, the clinical syndrome of benign childhood partial seizures with a peak onset at 5 years, manifested by infrequent (often solitary) mainly nocturnal fits with deviation of the eyes, vomiting or both, which are sometimes prolonged for hours, and with a predicable excellent prognosis. This, by virtue of a similar prevalence, age at onset and remission, is the 'natural' clinical counterpart of occipital spikes. Photosensitive occipital seizures are an interesting but still developing topic.

It is for all the above that I decided to devote the major part of this book to an exhaustive review of the literature regarding occipital seizures and occipital epilepsies in general (Chapters 6 and 7), early and late onset benign childhood seizures (Chapters 8 and 9), occipital spikes and occipital paroxysms (Chapter 10), an extensive historical and literature review (Chapter 11), photosensitive epilepsies and idiopathic photosensitive occipital seizures (Chapter 12) and my personal studies on relevant matters (Chapter 13). I have also detailed the differentiation of visual seizures from migraine with aura, basilar and acephalgic migraine (Chapter 14) and re-assessed basilar migraine through an extensive review (Chapter 15).

Benign childhood partial seizures may present with other than Rolandic or occipital clinical manifestations and spikes that are localisation related, such as benign partial seizures with affective symptoms, with parietal, extreme somatosensory evoked responses, frontal or midline spikes. These are all reviewed in Chapter 16.

Chapter 17 is devoted to severe syndromes of mainly linguistic and neuropsychological deficits, seizures or both, and marked EEG abnormalities from the Rolandic and neighbouring regions, such as Landau–Kleffner syndrome, epilepsy with continuous spikes and waves during slow sleep, autosomal dominant Rolandic epilepsy and speech dyspraxia, an atypical benign partial epilepsy of childhood.

It is likely and I propose that all these conditions are linked together due to a common, genetically determined, mild and reversible, functional derangement of the brain cortical maturational process (Chapters 3 and 18). This is often clinically silent, manifested in more than 90 per cent with EEG sharp and slow waves with an age-related localisation. In the remaining minority, there are infrequent partial seizures with symptoms, that are also localisation and age-related and dependent. It is possible that some of these children, with or without seizures, also have usually minor and fully reversible neuropsychological symptoms that are rarely clinically overt, requiring special neuropsychological testing for their detection. Finally, there may be a very small, less than 1 per cent, number of patients for whom this derangement of the brain maturation process may be derailed, resulting in a more aggressive condition of seizures, neuropsychological manifestations and EEG abnormalities of various combinations and various degrees of severity, such as in atypical benign partial epilepsy of childhood, Landau–Kleffner syndrome, and continuous spike and slow wave during sleep.

The main topics of this book are preceded by two chapters on the significance of the syndromic diagnosis of epilepsies and the contribution of the EEG. It is my conviction that this book would serve no useful purpose without emphasising that patients with epileptic seizures are endangered medically, socially or both by the inclusive diagnostic label 'epilepsy' instead of a precise seizure and syndrome categorisation. This is one of the main reasons that I decided to write *Benign Childhood Partial Seizures and Related Epileptic Syndromes.*

Repetitions are purposely made in order to secure relative autonomy of each chapter and to emphasise important matters. I have to realistically accept that despite all my efforts, omissions and errors are unavoidable. I regret if I have unintentionally undermined, omitted or misunderstood the work of some colleagues and I would be grateful if this is brought to my attention so that the appropriate corrections can be made in this or other relevant publications of mine.

I do hope that this book will serve to draw attention to these common conditions in children.

C P Panayiotopoulos MD, PhD, FRCP
Department of Clinical Neurophysiology and Epilepsies
St. Thomas' Hospital, London SE1 7EH
London September 1998

Acknowledgements

In the 25 years since I first started my prospective studies on benign childhood occipital seizures and the last 2 years that I devoted to writing this book, there are many colleagues and EEG technologists who made this work possible. Not all can be mentioned.

In Athens, many of the children were referred to me by Dr A. Goumas-Kartalas, Neuropsychiatrist, who also drew my attention to the ictal vomiting of children with early onset benign childhood occipital seizures. My friend P. Nastas, engineer, performed all the EEGs with dedication, scientific curiosity and care for the children.

In London, I enjoy the tremendous support and friendship of eminent colleagues in the departments of neurology and paediatrics of St. Thomas' Hospital. In Neurology, Dr R. Ross Russell, Professor M. Wiles and Professor H. Webb were fundamental in helping me to establish the clinic for the epilepsies. I consider myself extremely lucky that the new Consultants, Dr R. Howard and more recently Dr M. Sharief, match their high standards of scientific investigation with humour, understanding and patience. I am in debt to them.

I was equally lucky with the consultants in paediatrics. I am grateful to Professor J.W.Scopes, Dr C. Stern, Dr G. du Mont and Dr G. Clayden, who often share with me their thoughts regarding their patients with seizures and allow me direct access to their files and also to see the children and their parents if I wish.

Professor R.O. Robinson of paediatric neurology in Guy's Hospital honoured me by starting with me a joint clinic for children with epileptic disorders. I have enjoyed and learned a lot from this.

In the last 10 years I was privileged to have in my department some of the most talented, devoted and thoughtful younger colleagues who spent days and nights in ensuring the success of everyday routine and research programmes of the department. These collaborators chronologically are Dr E. Chroni, Dr S. Giannakodimos, Dr C. Ferrie, Dr M. Koutroumanidis, Dr A. Agathonikou, Dr A. Parker and Dr I. Ahmed-Sharoqi. Their contribution to this department and to my knowledge cannot be praised enough.

The technologists are the driving force of the department. Mr S. Rowlinson and Mrs S. Sanders are superb, not only in performing a legge artis EEG or video-EEG but also in providing us with crucial clinical information for patients who are not enrolled in our clinic for epilepsies. They are masters of their work. Mrs A. Baker, Mrs C. Carr and Mr P.Walsh, who now work elsewhere, provided me with equally high-standard work. I am grateful to all of them. Dr D. Sadoh, with his devotion and expertise in peripheral clinical neurophysiology, allows me time to explore my personal field of interest – epilepsies.

Nothing could work well without a good, dedicated, friendly and efficient secretary, who is Mrs D. Sharpe.

I wish also to acknowledge the Special Trustees of St. Thomas' Hospital, the British Telecom Charitable Organisation and the Epilepsy Research Foundation for their generous grants to support my studies on the syndromic diagnosis of epilepsies.

Those colleagues and the editors who allowed me to reproduce parts of their work for this book are duly acknowledged in the relevant parts of the book.

Dr W. Whitehouse, consultant in paediatric neurology, offered me valuable advice regarding the genetics of Rolandic seizures.

The children and their parents of my studies on benign childhood partial seizures have for years unquestionably trusted me, and are still giving me details over the phone or at interviews. It is so pleasing that they all do so.

This work would not have been possible without the help of all the people mentioned above. I also wish to acknowledge the financial risks undertaken by John Libbey and his team, the most expert and efficient publishers on Epilepsies.

Part I

General aspects

Chapter 1. The diagnosis of epilepsies

Chapter 2. The significance of the EEG in the diagnosis and management of epilepsies

Chapter 3. Benign childhood partial seizures
General aspects and nomenclature

Benign Childhood Partial Seizures and Related Epileptic Syndromes. C P Panayiotopoulos
©1999 John Libbey & Company Ltd., pp. 3–11.

Chapter 1

The diagnosis of epilepsies

Patients with epileptic seizures and their families are entitled to a diagnosis, prognosis and management that is specific and precise. The inclusive, monolectic diagnostic label 'epilepsy' is unsatisfactory to patient and physician alike and may result in avoidable morbidity and mortality. 'Epilepsy' is not a single disease entity. Epilepsies encompass many diseases. The fundamental rules of diagnosis, which apply to all other physical diseases, are often ignored in the epilepsies. The short- and long-term management of epilepsies is syndrome-related and often differs markedly between various disorders manifesting with seizures, emphasising the need for accurate diagnosis.

The epileptic syndromes

Introduction

The most important milestone in modern epileptology has been the recognition of epileptic syndromes and diseases, most of which are well-defined and easy to diagnose.[177] This achievement originated from a meeting of astute clinicians in the Centre Saint-Paul, Marseilles, France in July 1983 and the proceedings were edited by Roger *et al.*[683] in *Epileptic syndromes in infancy, childhood and adolescence* (John Libbey, 1985, published in French and English). It is not only for historical reasons that I feel that the views of the editors should be repeated in this book.[683]

> The last 20 years have seen substantial advances in knowledge concerning the diagnosis as well as the long-term evolution of epilepsies in infants and children. More accurate observation of seizures, using simultaneous video-recording of the patients and of their EEG tracings, has permitted classification of some epileptic seizures in childhood and their incorporation in the Kyoto International Classification of Epileptic Seizures (1981).[175] However, many gaps must yet be filled and video information concerning many seizure types is lacking.
>
> Above all, there is no general agreement among epileptologists on the framework of the epileptic syndromes. There is little unanimity concerning definitions and what may be included under individual syndromic rubrics. Thus, some authors consider that almost all severe epilepsies in infancy and childhood may be included in the West and Lennox–Gastaut syndromes, using in such cases a variable terminology (for example: 'minor motor epilepsy') while others demand more rigorous criteria. Several syndromes have recently been described, but this information has not been widely disseminated, and these entities remain arcane. This is the case in severe myoclonic epilepsy, benign neonatal convulsions, myoclonic absences, and epilepsy with continuous spike-waves during slow sleep, for example.
>
> For these reasons a number of specialists working in the field of childhood epilepsy convened in order to review the different types of the childhood epilepsies and to try to more rigorously

> define a number of epileptic syndromes in infants, children and adolescents. This volume presents the proceedings of the first Workshop on Childhood Epileptology held at the Centre Saint-Paul, Marseilles, France in July 1983. To realize the aim of elaborating a uniform terminology, it was felt to be important that such a definition of syndromes must be based on clinical, electroencephalographic, aetiological and evolution data, avoiding, in so far as possible, a consideration of those physiopathological concepts which are often purely hypothetical. It is essential for all researchers working in the field to use the same terminology and to know that if a case is classified as a West syndrome or as a Lennox–Gastaut syndrome by an author, it would not be classified elsewhere by other authors.
>
> However, a classification of syndromes cannot ignore the ultimate place of each syndrome in a classification of the epilepsies, which must take the physiopathological data into account. Thus it is not surprising to see that the reviewers and discussants of the following chapters have used different words pending future classification of epilepsies which is under consideration by the ILAE Committee on Classification and Terminology. Some authors speak of 'primary' epilepsy while others use the word 'idiopathic', and 'secondary' epilepsy when others say 'symptomatic' or 'lesional'.
>
> Because of the interaction between the syndrome classification activity and classification in progress, the members of the ILAE Committee on Classification and Terminology actively participated in the workshop.
>
> As most epileptic syndromes of childhood are age-dependent, the program of the meeting followed a chronological order (neonate, infant, child, adolescent), though some syndromes may cover a larger range of ages.
>
> In order to reduce the number of pages of the book, we have attempted to apportion the length of individual reports and discussions and keep these commensurate with the perceived importance of the topic in the scheme of things.
>
> Implicit in such workshops is the awareness that many problems remain in spite of a few answers. Only the gathering of further data together with the long-term studies of such populations will allow validation of the practical viability of the syndromic classification.
>
> There is no general agreement regarding some problems: what are the nosological limits between benign myoclonic epilepsy, severe myoclonic epilepsy, myoclonic astatic petit mal and the Lennox–Gastaut syndrome? Is it possible to define an idiopathic West syndrome clearly different from the symptomatic West syndrome and what would be its nosological place? What are the electroclinical forms of symptomatic partial epilepsies in neonates and infants? Is it feasible to make a definitive differentiation between simple febrile convulsions and complicated febrile convulsions nosologically? Is there a type of epilepsy with unilateral seizures only?
>
> All these problems will be discussed in further meetings on childhood epilepsy. However we do not pretend that all cases of childhood epilepsy can be subsumed under definite syndromes and recognize that a number of cases will, for the present, remain outside such a syndromic classification even if the elements can be identified and the individual seizures recorded.[683]

The classification and definitions from this meeting were adopted in 1985 by the Commission on Classification and Terminology of the International League Against Epilepsy, 1985)[176] and remained essentially the same in the revised proposal of 1989.[177] Therefore, the existing classification of epilepsies and epileptic syndromes is already 15 years old. Recent advances in the clinical-EEG manifestations of previously recognized and newly described syndromes, video-EEG information, functional and structural imaging, investigative procedures in neurosurgical series and genetics mandate a new thorough and realistic revision of this classification and the definitions of epileptic syndromes. Irrespective of this, a start has been made to move irreversibly away from the unsatisfactory situation where all these diverse conditions with epileptic seizures are diagnosed as 'epilepsy'.

Definition, classification and significance of epileptic syndromes

The definition of a medical syndrome is 'a distinct group of symptoms and signs which, associated together, form a characteristic clinical picture or entity', while 'a disease has common aetiology and prognosis despite individual modifications'.[166] Similarly, in the epilepsies, the recognition of non-fortuitous clustering of symptoms and signs requires the study of detailed clinical and laboratory data.[177]

Important clinical features include the type of seizures, their localization, frequency, sequence of events, circadian distribution, precipitating factors, response to treatment, age at onset, mode of inheritance, and physical or mental symptoms and signs. A routine EEG may be insufficient to contribute to diagnosis. Sleep deprivation or an EEG on awakening may reveal important information about a patient with nocturnal seizures or seizures on awakening. Video-EEG recordings of ictal events are often diagnostic for seizure categorization. High resolution structural and functional brain imaging, biochemical and haematological tests sometimes also requires tissue biopsy. Although some symptoms predominate and may indicate the underlying disease, no single symptom or sign can be considered entirely pathognomonic. The process of differential diagnosis requires close scrutiny of the clinical data before a list of possible diagnoses can be drawn up and the final diagnosis reached. It should be realized that some epilepsies are easy to diagnose and some more difficult, but this is not unusual in medicine. Molecular genetics are already making decisive discoveries in the identification of epilepsies.[98]

The proposed ILAE classification of epilepsies[177] is based on two major features: first, whether the predominant seizure type is focal, localized (localization-related syndromes) or generalized (generalized syndromes), and secondly whether the aetiology is idiopathic (with genetic predisposition), symptomatic (structural) or cryptogenic (supposedly but not demonstrably structural). These divisions shape the first two major groups of epileptic syndromes; a third group covers syndromes with seizures of uncertain type (often the case in nocturnal seizures) and a fourth seizures associated with a specific situation (fever, drugs, metabolic imbalance). It should be emphasized that the number of cryptogenic epilepsies is decreasing in favour of the symptomatic ones with the use of high resolution MRI which demonstrates structural cortical lesions previously undetected with CT brain scan and first generations of MRI scanners.

The significance of the syndromic diagnosis of epilepsies has been recently detailed by Grunewald and Panayiotopoulos[365] and Benbadis and Luders.[93] The results to be expected of syndromic diagnosis of epilepsies can be compared with the advances which have accrued from the widespread acceptance of syndromic diagnosis of connective tissue and neuromuscular diseases. If diagnosed on a few symptoms alone, distinction would often be impossible between rheumatoid disease, ankylosing spondylitis and psoriatic arthropathy, diseases with different (although unknown) aetiology, management, inheritance and prognosis. Similarly, most neuromuscular disorders are mainly characterized by muscle weakness and atrophy. Despite the occasional occurrence of 'overlap syndromes', syndromic classification allows the scientific analysis of the underlying disease processes and their specific clinicopathological features, genetics and provides a framework for clinical trials aimed at optimizing treatment.

Some parts of the ILAE classification[177]remain contentious; some syndromes are ill or broadly defined and require further clarification. There are patients whose clinical and EEG features do not appear to fit neatly into any recognized category or erroneously appear to evolve from one syndrome to another. Some may represent new or 'overlap' syndromes, others may be unusual forms of known syndromes or cases where clinical history is misleading. However, many syndromes are common, easily diagnosed and well-characterized. Syndromic diagnosis of epilepsies provides a firm foundation for short and long-term therapeutic decisions, and enables natural history, inheritance, treatment efficacy and prognosis of epilepsies to be studied scientifically. The benefits of syndromic diagnosis over seizure/symptom diagnosis or an inclusive diagnosis such as 'epilepsy' far outweigh any morbidity from miscategorization that may arise in difficult cases.

Attitudes in the diagnosis of epilepsies

The fundamental rules of diagnosis, which apply to all other physical diseases, are often ignored in epilepsies, resulting in avoidable morbidity and mortality. Vague and broad terms, such as 'epilepsy' or 'patient with seizures', are often accepted as a diagnosis irrespective of the aetiology, type of seizures, prognosis and appropriateness of treatment. Furthermore, the differential diagnosis is often limited to 'epilepsy', 'pseudoseizures' and progressive causes of 'seizures'.[365]

The distinction of 'fits' from 'faints and funny turns' is an issue familiar to all students of medicine. Traditionally, once the nature of the event has been established as epileptic, the next step is to exclude an underlying progressive brain lesion. For patients without a structural epileptogenic abnormality, there is little guidance on diagnosis, prognosis or treatment. Physicians are more capable and ambitious than this.

The inclusive term 'epilepsy', still almost universally used in social, psychological and medical studies, inadequately describes a highly heterogeneous population of patients with recurrent seizures. Such studies and opinions are often biased towards those more severely affected and extrapolation to common, but more benign, epileptic syndromes can be highly misleading. Results are incorporated into textbook recommendations on drug treatment and management, which perpetuate inappropriate generalizations.

A diagnosis of 'epilepsy' unjustly carries a serious social stigma, with implications of loss of self-control, mental disease, physical handicaps and even demonic possession. Dictionary definitions are unhelpful, inadequate and inaccurate, often equating 'epilepsy' with generalized tonic–clonic seizures; it is a diagnostic label unsatisfactory to patient and physician alike.

Epileptic seizures[175]are symptoms of many diseases of different aetiology, severity and prognosis, which are often self-limited and which may require minimum medication, if any.[177] However, the description of epileptic seizures is usually limited to the events surrounding generalized tonic–clonic seizures (GTCS), while less dramatic minor seizures, though more important than GTCS for diagnosis and management, are often not considered.

In other diseases, accurate diagnosis is considered important. For example, a neurologist is rightly required to know the symptoms and signs of neuromuscular disorders, and to be able to differentiate between Duchenne and Becker muscular dystrophy (though they are genetically linked), and between spinal muscular atrophy and limb girdle muscular dystrophy (though treatment is unavailable); terms such as 'dysdiadochokinesia' or 'biotin-responsive multiple carboxyl deficiency', which are difficult to remember or even pronounce, are frequently included in the medical dictionary and even in students textbooks. Conversely, in epilepsies, attempts to encourage differential diagnosis are met with criticism as controversial or unrealistic. A report advocating the proper diagnosis of epileptic syndromes and diseases (Grunewald and Panayiotopoulos, 1996)[365] was rejected by five neurological and medical journals prior to its final acceptance because of expert reviewers' comments such as 'they are all the same', 'they may be genetically linked', 'what difference does it make?', 'treatment is the same', 'physicians are reluctant to accept epileptic syndromes', 'the names are difficult to pronounce and remember' and the worse of all 'so what?'.

Such arguments are, however, unsubstantiated. The treatment of different epileptic seizures is not the same (vigabatrin, a highly effective anti-epileptic drug for partial seizures, exaggerates absences and may also induce absence status)[624] and long-term strategies are syndrome related (juvenile myoclonic epilepsy is a life-long liability to generalized seizures requiring continuous treatment while childhood absence epilepsy may be limited to childhood requiring ethosuximide or sodium valproate for a few years).[617] Simplistic rules and advice on a unitary treatment strategy for 'epilepsy', 'start with sodium valproate and if this does not work change it to carbamazepine', 'treatment is after the second seizure' (not even specifying the type of seizure and the need to specifically enquire for minor fits) and 'stop treatment after 2–3 years free of seizures', are often detrimental to the care of a large number of patients. Genetic heterogeneity has been documented even in a relatively phenotypically uniform and short-lived disease, such as benign familial neonatal convulsions[111,479,488,518,686,695,740] though additional phenotypic heterogeneity has been reported by other authors.[97] Prognosis of different syndromes is often entirely different, even if symptoms are similar, e.g. benign childhood partial epilepsies and symptomatic partial epilepsies of children.[177]

One explanation for such discrimination against the epilepsies is firstly our traditional approach and secondly seizures cannot be accurately qualified and quantified. Epileptic seizures are short, transient, largely unpredictable and exhibit difficult to demonstrate symptoms. This problem should be partly overcome by the use of video-EEG and home camcorders, which are particularly suited to the study of epilepsies with frequent seizures, and also absence seizures because of their frequency and precipitation by hyperventilation. Camcorders should be more widely used in the clinical evaluation of epilepsies, as they provide the only practical means of demonstrating the physical symptoms of the disease.

Differential diagnosis, the most fundamental process in medicine, is seldom undertaken for epilepsies. Indeed, those who try to apply such an approach to the epilepsies are derogatorily labelled spliters instead of the appropriate term diagnosticians which is the analogous name in other medical specialities.[612,613]

I often have to argue against generally applauded statements, such as 'patients with absences have been reported in symptomatic epilepsies and therefore they are all the same', 'a patient with one seizure may not need treatment and therefore an EEG is not needed', 'an individual with epileptic seizures may not fit a particular epileptic syndrome', 'the EEG is not useful as it may be normal or show non-specific abnormalities', and 'I do not ask for an EEG after the first seizure because I will not treat the patient'.[612,613] Such unfounded arguments are never raised in the field of neuromuscular diseases, where limb-girdle muscular dystrophy may imitate spinal muscular atrophy, Guillain–Barre syndrome usually presents with proximal muscle weakness characteristic of myopathies, and the electromyographic features of all myopathies are similar. There is a basic defect in our traditional thinking and education about 'epilepsy' compared with that in all other medical diseases and this is the main problem that the next generation has to deal with.

A change in emphasis from epilepsy to epilepsies may stress that epilepsy is not a single disease entity, and that accurate prognosis, genetic analysis and improvement of management largely depend on a precise diagnosis of the epileptic syndrome.

Attitudes to the diagnosis and management of epilepsies often differ from those applied in other medical conditions. For example, a physician, who is rightly anxious to reproduce muscle fatiguability in a patient with a clear-cut history of myasthenia gravis, rarely asks to see video recordings of frequent seizures which can be easily captured with camcorders. Another physician, who rightly emphasizes the differential diagnosis between spinal muscular dystrophy and limb-girdle muscular dystrophy, may give little significance to the differentiation between absences of juvenile myoclonic epilepsy and complex partial seizures of temporal lobe epilepsy. A paediatrician, who may be concerned that the diagnosis of a rare metabolic disease is often missed, may not be concerned that 40 per cent of children with typical absences are inappropriately treated with carbamazepine if valproate fails.[642] Vigabatrin, which is contraindicated in typical absences, may also be erroneously prescribed.[624]

There are numerous studies on the prognosis of 'epilepsy' and the effect of withdrawn medication after a few years of freedom from 'seizures' or the initiation of medication after the first 'seizure', ignoring the fact that these are syndrome related. Many of these patients have minor seizures (absences, myoclonic jerks, partial seizures) many years after their last and many years before their first generalized tonic–clonic seizure. What have we learned from these studies? No more than one would expect to learn from a general study on the prognosis of febrile illnesses (irrespective of whether the fever is due to viruses, bacteria or malignancies) and their response to antibiotics.

A patient with idiopathic reading epilepsy who may never suffer generalized tonic–clonic seizures or loss of consciousness is not allowed to drive under the present legislation in the United Kingdom because of 'active seizures' (jaw myoclonus on reading) although the risk for accident is less than for other patients, with symptomatic epilepsies, who after being free of seizures for more than a year on anti-epileptic polypharmacy may be allowed to drive. The law does not discriminate between different types of seizures and syndromes because the importance of such a distinction has not been stressed by the expert physicians.

Despite significant progress in the diagnosis and management of epilepsies, there are many reports in influential Medical and Neurological Journals in which patients with 'epilepsy or seizures' are erroneously classified together irrespective of the underlying disease.

'Not all childhood seizures develop into progressive disease. Epilepsy is commonly considered a progressive disease' were the introductory comments in 1997 of a major Medical Journal referring to a study of a mixed population of children who had generalized tonic–clonic seizures due to a variety of epileptic syndromes. As expected in such a heterogeneous population, the results was that seizures were either remitting and decelerating or accelerating. That more than one third of childhood seizures are of excellent prognosis and that many epilepsies decline with age has been well known for centuries. It is not just a matter of diagnostic precision.

'Epilepsy: a fatal disease?' was the scaring title of a lecture on the increased mortality of patients with epileptic seizures in a well advertised and well attended meeting. A lecture on 'Epilepsy: a benign disease?' based on benign childhood partial seizures could have achieved some balance.

Seizure/symptom diagnosis

Since the principal, and often sole, clinical feature is the seizure itself, traditional diagnosis and management of epilepsies has emphasized the importance of events occurring during the seizure, which may be classified as generalized (tonic, tonic–clonic, myoclonic, typical or atypical absences) or partial (simple or complex).[175]

Under such a diagnostic system, all clinically generalized tonic–clonic seizures, whether the result of a static or progressive brain lesion, metabolic derangement, drug effect or inherited predisposition, are classified together; treatment is symptomatic and no aetiologic or prognostic significance is conveyed. Avoidable morbidity is the result.

Importance of accurate diagnosis

The danger from a unified diagnosis of 'epilepsy' or a symptom diagnosis of 'seizures' is exemplified by three common epileptic syndromes.

Benign childhood partial seizures, juvenile myoclonic epilepsy and temporal lobe epilepsy comprise more than 40 per cent of all epilepsies. They are entirely different in presentation, cause and genetics, investigative procedures, short- and long-term treatment strategies and prognosis.

Unfortunately, current textbooks and other publications pay scant attention to these syndromes, often considering childhood seizures under the heading 'epilepsy' without considering the aetiology and prognosis.

Benign childhood partial seizures, like febrile convulsions, are age-related, show genetic predisposition, may be manifested by a single seizure, remit within a few years of onset, and may or may not require a short course of anti-epileptic medication. The risk of recurrent seizures in adult life (1–2 per cent) is less than in febrile convulsions (4 per cent).[609] Recognition of the characteristic clinical and EEG features of benign childhood partial epilepsies will enable the parents to be re-assured of the invariably benign prognosis with spontaneous resolution of the disorder by the middle teens. The prognostic implications are such that in a recent editorial I suggested removing the label 'epilepsy' from these patients, as has already been done with febrile convulsions,[609] and this is my proposition in this book.

Juvenile myoclonic epilepsy, an idiopathic epileptic syndrome with myoclonic jerks on awakening, generalized tonic–clonic seizures (GTCS) and, more rarely, absences, has a prevalence of 8–10 per cent among adult patients with seizures.[364,614] The management of juvenile myoclonic epilepsy differs from standard medical practice for the treatment of seizures in several important respects.[364,614] Recommendations not to treat after the first seizure are usually inappropriate, not only because affected patients have usually experienced other epileptic events (e.g. myoclonic jerks, absences) for many months or years before the first GTCS, but also because juvenile myoclonic epilepsy is a life-long disease with a high risk of major and minor seizures, particularly after sleep deprivation, fatigue and alcohol indulgence. Emphasizing avoidance of precipitating factors in juvenile myoclonic epilepsy is part of the management strategy. Withdrawal of medication after 2–3 seizure-free years and substitution of carbamazepine instead of sodium valproate are also inappropriate, because relapses are inevitable.

In our studies,[363,610,634,637] the avoidable consequences of misdiagnosing juvenile myoclonic epilepsy, in addition to the psychological and social effects of poor seizure control, included loss of driving licence, loss of employment, status epilepticus, recurrence of seizures after long remission, and injury to self or child. Common diagnostic errors in juvenile myoclonic epilepsy include: failure to elicit a history of myoclonic jerks; absences mistaken for complex partial seizures; predominantly unilateral jerks mistaken for motor partial seizures; GTCS or early morning shaking diagnosed as alcohol-induced events; and focal EEG abnormalities used to support an erroneous clinical diagnosis of partial seizures.

Temporal lobe epilepsy, comprising more than 30 per cent of epilepsies, is mostly due to progressive or non-progressive structural lesions of the temporal lobe, such as mesial temporal sclerosis, benign tumours, migrational disorders and others shown mainly with high resolution MRI which should be preferred to CT brain scan. Temporal lobe epilepsy can begin at any time between infancy and old age but usually in mid-teens. The diagnosis is often easy on clinico-EEG grounds. Complex partial seizures is the commonest type of fits; 75 per cent of patients experience simple partial seizures and approximately 50 per cent of patients also have secondarily generalized tonic–clonic seizures. Remission may occur in 30 per cent of the patients but 20 per cent may become medically intractable.

Even the most sceptical physicians, including those who doubt the clinical or practical significance of the syndromic diagnosis of epilepsies, have to accept that benign childhood partial epilepsies, juvenile myoclonic epilepsy and symptomatic temporal lobe epilepsy have nothing in common other than the fact that they may all be complicated by GTCS, which are primary in juvenile myoclonic epilepsy, and secondary in benign childhood partial epilepsies and symptomatic temporal lobe epilepsy. Furthermore, the short- and long-term treatment strategies are entirely different for each disorder: benign childhood partial epilepsies may or may not require drug treatment, mainly with carbamazepine, for a few years; sodium valproate is the drug of choice in juvenile myoclonic epilepsy and treatment is life-long; and cryptogenic/symptomatic temporal lobe epilepsy may be resistant to the drugs of choice, such as carbamazepine, phenytoin, phenobarbitone, vigabatrin or topiramate, and may require neurosurgical resection of the affected area of the temporal lobe.

It should not be difficult to distinguish an intelligent child with benign partial seizures or childhood absence epilepsy from a child with Rasmussen's, Down's or Sturge–Weber syndromes, or a child with severe post-traumatic cerebral damage, brain anoxia, trisomy and deletion of chromosome 4p or Baltic myoclonic epilepsy. Describing all these children as simply having epilepsy just because they have seizures offers no more benefit than a diagnosis of muscle atrophy, irrespective of whether it is localized or generalized, post-traumatic or genetically determined, static, reversible or progressive, or whether the underlying cause is in the muscle, nerve or spinal cord, and is treatable or untreatable.

Epileptic syndromes may have superficial similarities

Though phenotypic heterogeneity of the same genetic disease is well recognized, it is also well known that many medical syndromes may appear to be superficially the same (e.g. myopathies and spinal muscular atrophies manifest with proximal muscle weakness and atrophy). In the epilepsies, however, such similarities have unfortunately been used as proof of a similar aetiology and prognosis.

A triad of typical absences, myoclonic jerks and GTCS may occur in juvenile myoclonic epilepsy, juvenile absence epilepsy and eyelid myoclonia with absences. Superficially, these disorders could be considered as the same disease.[612,617] Closer analysis, however, reveals three distinctly different syndromes.

The hallmark of juvenile myoclonic epilepsy is myoclonic jerks on awakening, with GTCS as the next most common type of seizure (often heralded by clusters of myoclonic jerks). Absences are simple and mild without myoclonic components.

In contrast, the predominant features of juvenile absence epilepsy are absences of relatively long duration with severe impairment of consciousness and frequent automatisms. GTCS are uncommon and may be heralded by absences rather than jerks. Myoclonic jerks, if present, are mild and random.

The hallmark of eyelid myoclonia with absences is eyelid myoclonia associated with brief absences involving mild or moderate impairment of consciousness, which may persist without absences, but absences do not occur without eyelid myoclonia. All patients are photosensitive and have pronounced EEG abnormalities associated with eye-closure, which are eliminated by darkness. GTCS and myoclonic jerks of the limbs are uncommon, and may be provoked by flickering lights.[256, 323]

Treatment

Common epileptic conditions, such as benign childhood partial epilepsies, juvenile myoclonic epilepsy and temporal lobe epilepsy, in which treatment differs markedly, have already been described. Even among idiopathic generalized epilepsies, specific treatment regimens may be necessary. Clonazepam, though useful in the treatment of myoclonic jerks, should not be used alone in juvenile myoclonic epilepsy as it may not control GTCS. It is, however, the drug of choice in idiopathic reading epilepsy. Eyelid myoclonia with absences is resistant to treatment, and a combination of sodium valproate and ethosuximide may be required. In childhood absence epilepsy, monotherapy with sodium valproate or ethosuximide is often sufficient and withdrawal should be planned after a period of 2–3 years without absences. Small doses of lamotrigine may be highly beneficial as add-on treatment with sodium valproate in patients with childhood or juvenile absence epilepsy, but may not be effective in others.[280]

Most treatment recommendations are based on clinical impression, and there is an urgent need for controlled trials to investigate the syndrome-specificity of drugs and to establish treatment regimens. The need for such trials has become even greater with the introduction of five new drugs for 'epilepsy' in the last 5 years, with many more undergoing experimentation. In the 5 years since vigabatrin and lamotrigine were licensed as add-on treatment in refractory partial seizures, they have been shown to have entirely different indications and, probably, seizure-specificity and profile. Vigabatrin is usually effective in partial seizures, infantile spasms and symptomatic seizures of tuberous sclerosis, while lamotrigine is usually effective in idiopathic generalized epilepsies, particularly in combination with sodium valproate. This profile was revealed mainly through the observations of astute clinicians rather than through sponsored drug trials.

Over one hundred years ago, Hughes Bennett, in 1884[94] after studying the effect of bromides on 117 patients with 'epilepsy' for 5 years, concluded:

(1) in 12.1 per cent of patients, bromide completely arrested attacks throughout the whole period of treatment;

(2) in 83.3 per cent of patients, the attacks were greatly diminished both in number and severity;

(3) in 2.3 per cent of patients, the treatment had no apparent effect;

(4) in 2.3 per cent of patients, the number of attacks increased during the period of treatment.

These results are very similar to those obtained with the new and very expensive drugs for 'epilepsy' today. This does not mean that we should return to the bromide treatment but rather that we should exercise some caution towards the new anti-epileptic drugs. There is no doubt that the new anti-epileptic drugs are a major advance as they present a new challenge and opportunity for physicians to improve the management of epilepsies. However, they also introduce a new problem: patients who have been free of seizures for many years may relapse when their 'old' medication is changed to a new and 'more effective and free of side effects' drug. We still have to learn about the new drugs and their short- and mainly long-term adverse effects, which may be predicted for some and unexpected for others. We cannot ignore the 'old' ones. There is a great need for the physician to know what drug to prescribe, for how long, the dose and for what type of epilepsy.

Long-term treatment planning is syndrome related and therefore depends upon diagnostic decisions: Are these epileptic seizures? What type of epileptic seizures? Are there any other epileptic seizures (myoclonic jerks, partial seizures, absences)? What are the precipitating factors? What type of epilepsy is this?

Improving the diagnosis of epilepsies

The diagnosis of epilepsies could be improved by adopting a number of simple measures.

(1) The proper medical diagnosis should be used for the particular epileptic syndrome/disease. A seizure categorization may be sufficient when a syndromic classification is not possible. Categorizing the patient to one or another syndrome if data are unavailable or symptoms do not fit a particular condition should be avoided.

(2) The terms 'epilepsy' or 'seizures' should never be used as a diagnostic label.

(3) The precise diagnosis, genetics, precipitating factors, short- and long-term treatment strategies should be explained to the patient/family and the family practitioner. Appropriate literature should also be provided.

In order to achieve a proper diagnosis, I find it useful to ask the patient to fill in a specially designed and detailed questionnaire regarding their seizures and their family and personal history. Home-made videos of the seizures, when practical, are part of my diagnostic procedure.

Conclusions

The issues of when to start anti-epileptic therapy and when to stop treatment are clearly influenced by the type of epileptic syndrome. Although there is general agreement that the choice of anti-epileptic drug that is prescribed is defined primarily by the seizure type, there is controversy as to the relative importance of the type of epileptic syndrome in this decision-making process. To make the final diagnosis, it is necessary to be aware of all the symptoms that a patient is experiencing, but it is also important to make clinicians (e.g. paediatricians, general practitioners, paediatric neurologists and neurologists) understand that epilepsies are sometimes difficult to diagnose fully and that it is not sufficient to define solely the seizure type.

Dramatic progress in the management of epilepsies can be expected if more time and emphasis are given on 'how to diagnose epilepsies' rather than the current theme of 'how to treat epilepsy'.

Benign Childhood Partial Seizures and Related Epileptic Syndromes. C P Panayiotopoulos
©1999 John Libbey & Company Ltd., pp. 13–20.

Chapter 2

The significance of the EEG in the diagnosis and management of epilepsies

The electroencephalogram (EEG), entirely harmless and relatively inexpensive, is a most important investigation in the diagnosis and management of epilepsies provided that it is properly performed by experienced technicians, carefully studied and interpreted in the context of a well described clinical setting by experienced physicians.

The EEG is an integral part of the diagnostic process in epilepsies and this should not be underrated.

Introduction

The EEG is a recording of cerebral electrical activity by electrodes on the scalp. There are many recent reviews and books on the EEG.[118,570,824] The purpose of this chapter is to outline the significance of the EEG in the diagnosis and management of epilepsies. The factors of error often involved are noted and possible means of improving the contribution of the EEG in epilepsies are proposed.

In the seven decades of use of the EEG since the first human scalp recordings by Berger in 1929, it has been associated with great achievements, particularly in the field of epilepsies, and great disappointments particularly in the field of mental disorders and structural lesions of the brain. The disrepute of the EEG amongst clinicians was due to the frequent false positive and false negative findings mainly related to structural lesions of the brain. This was in a period when the EEG was the only non-invasive investigative method of brain disorders. Advances in neuroimaging have now reliably taken away this responsibility from the EEG and clinical neurophysiologists should concentrate on diseases where the EEG is indispensable, such as in the diagnosis and management of epilepsies. More than half of children and adults presently referred for a routine EEG are suspected of having or suffer from epilepsies. The EEG is indispensable for the correct syndromic diagnosis of these patients.

The value of the routine interictal or ictal extracranial EEG in epilepsies should neither be underestimated nor overrated

The EEG in epilepsies is overrated by some and undervalued by others. The reality lies somewhere in between.

Those who underestimate the EEG should remember that:

(a) The EEG is the only available investigation that is able to record and evaluate the paroxysmal discharges which cause seizures. The appropriate evaluation of patients with epileptic disorders is often impossible without an EEG. In the majority of the cases the clinical diagnosis is concordant with the EEG findings. However, it is often with the help of the EEG that the correct diagnosis is established, particularly if the clinical information is inadequate or misleading. On other occasions, the clinical data are more sound than the EEG, particularly if this is non-specific or in chronic cases of treated epilepsies.

(b) The present seizure and epileptic syndrome classifications are based on combined clinico-EEG manifestations. Epileptic syndromes, the most important advance of recent epileptology, were mainly identified because of their EEG manifestations.[176,177]

(c) Partial and generalized epilepsies are often difficult to differentiate without an EEG, even by the most experienced epileptologists.[627,633]

(d) It is the EEG which will often demonstrate beyond any doubt that the 'day dreaming' of a child is due to absence seizures, long lasting episodes of behavioural changes are due to non-convulsive status epilepticus, 'eyelid ticks' are due to eyelid myoclonia with photosensitivity, clumsiness on awakening is due to myoclonic jerks and periodic bed wetting is due to nocturnal seizures.

Those who overestimate the EEG should remember that:

(a) The EEG may be oversensitive to some conditions such as the benign childhood seizure susceptibility syndromes detailed in this book, and sightless to others, such as frontal or temporal lobe epilepsies. Rarely, even ictal events may not be detected with a surface EEG. Patients mainly with partial epilepsies may have a series of normal EEGs, and the EEG localization is not always concordant with ictal intracranial recordings. More than 40 per cent of patients with epileptic disorders may have one normal interictal EEG, although this percentage falls dramatically to 8 per cent with a series of EEGs and appropriate activating procedures, particularly sleep.[118]

(b) The frequency of seizures is not proportional to the EEG paroxysmal 'epileptogenic' discharges. Severely 'epileptogenic' EEGs may be recorded from patients with infrequent or controlled clinical seizures and vice versa. The EEG abnormalities do not reflect the severity of the epileptic disorder.

(c) More than 10 per cent of normal people may have non-specific EEG abnormalities and around 1 per cent may have 'epileptiform paroxysmal activity' without seizures. The prevalence of these abnormalities is higher in children, with 2–4 per cent having functional centrotemporal or occipital spikes.

(d) Paroxysmal epileptiform activity is high in patients with non-epileptic, neurological or medical disorders or with neurological deficits. Children, with congenital visual deficits, for example, frequently have occipital spikes and patients with migraine have a high incidence of sharp paroxysmal activity.

Factors of error

Even the most reliable investigative tools in medicine cannot escape severe errors either because of poor technical quality (equipment, personnel or both), interpretation by poorly qualified physicians, or both. A competent report should not only accurately spot the EEG abnormality but also provide its significance and meaning in accordance with a well described clinical setting. Failure to achieve this leads to severe errors which are responsible for comments such as 'Routine interictal EEG is one of the most abused investigations in clinical medicine and is unquestionably responsible for great human suffering'.[160,161]

Provided that the EEG is technically correct, the following are in my opinion the most important factors of error, listed in order of significance:

(a) The single most significant source of error is that the EEG is often interpreted out of the clinical context. There are two reasons for this. Firstly, the referring physician provides inadequate information regarding the events ('patient with loss of consciousness or grand mal seizures', 'Black-outs. Epilepsy?', 'Unexplained aggressiveness. Temporal lobe epilepsy?') and often fails to mention other medical conditions or drugs which may or may not be related to the EEG. Secondly, the reporting clinical neurophysiologist prefers a convenient but rather unhelpful and uncommitted approach ('normal EEG', 'an abnormal EEG with active spike in the occipital regions', 'focal episodic left temporal slowing without genuine epileptiform activity'). In St. Thomas' Hospital, I am in the advantageous position to be the referring and the reporting physician and this practice may expand to other clinics for epilepsies.

(b) Non-specific EEG abnormalities are overemphasized without suggesting means of clarifying their significance, with a sleep-deprived EEG, for example, or after obtaining more clinical data. Episodic focal slow waves are non-specific and may occur in a normal person, a patient with migraine, or in a mild cerebrovascular disease or even cerebral tumours. They may be of lateralizing significance, even if they are infrequent and of small amplitude in a patient with a well established clinical history of temporal lobe seizures.[451a]

(c) EEGs during hyperventilation, drowsiness and sleep may produce significant changes which are often difficult to interpret even by experienced neurophysiologists. An EEG in babies and children is even more complex and demanding. Non-epileptic episodic transients, such as benign epileptiform transients of sleep, 6 and 14 per second positive spikes and rhythmic mid-temporal discharge, may often be misinterpreted as evidence of 'epilepsy'.

(d) Previous EEG records and results are lost, destroyed or not sought. This is significant in the re-evaluation of patients with long standing epilepsy because the EEGs recorded at the initial stages of the disease and particularly before treatment are usually diagnostic. These patients are mainly referred for treatment modifications because they are free of seizures and still on medication, they have had a recent convulsion after a long seizure-free period, seizures are not controlled with long standing medication, there are adverse reactions to their medication or appropriateness to change to new anti-epileptic drugs, or anticipated pregnancy in women. The resolution of these cases is difficult, often requiring a thorough clinical evaluation, review of previous medical and EEG records and the establishment of the appropriate epileptic syndrome. It does not depend on the findings of a new EEG, which may be misleading as it might be, for example, normal for a patient with idiopathic generalized epilepsy who is on sodium valproate, or might show focal slow wave paroxysms in patients with well documented generalized spike and polyspike discharges in early EEG. However, on other occasions a recent EEG may prompt the correct advice, documenting mild epileptic seizures such as myoclonic jerks or absences in a patient 'free of seizures' or of 'continuing focal seizures' inadequately treated with carbamazepine. Generalized discharges of patients 'free of seizures' indicate a high proportion of relapses after treatment withdrawal.

(e) Alteration of the EEG by drugs (such as neuroleptics or anti-epileptics) or co-existing medical conditions (cerebrovascular disease, electrolyte disturbances, previous head injury).

That a patient with a brain tumour may not have clinical signs does not invalidate the clinical examination and the same is true for the EEG. The main cause of concern and suffering is that patients with 'epileptic seizures' are erroneously unified together under the inclusive term 'epilepsy' which inadequately describes the underlying condition. The usefulness of the EEG can be highly appreciated by those who attempt a proper differentiation amongst the epilepsies.

Activating procedures

These attempt to improve the EEG diagnostic yield by inducing or enhancing epileptogenic paroxysms. Hyperventilation (HV) and intermittent photic stimulation (IPS) are the only activating procedures applied in routine waking EEG. Drowsiness, sleep and awakening are also important activating procedures.

HV often induces physiological changes such as diffuse and paroxysmal slow activity, particularly in healthy young persons who overbreath well. They do not last for more than 60 s after cessation of HV and they should not be confused with abnormal epileptogenic disturbances which are also activated by HV. The 3–4 Hz generalized spike and slow wave which is the electrical accompaniment of typical absences is almost invariably (for more than 80 per cent of the patients) induced or enhanced by HV. Cognition during generalized discharges can be practically evaluated in routine EEGs by asking the patient to count their breaths during HV.[322,633] Using this method and video-EEG recordings we frequently detected patients supposedly 'free of seizures' who stop or hesitate, make errors, or have localized or generalized myoclonic jerks during these discharges. These patients are not free of seizures. Activation of focal spikes may need more prolonged and vigorous HV.

IPS is significant for the detection of photosensitive patients who show photoparoxysmal discharges which are often initiated from the occipital regions.[616] These discharges indicate a genetically determined photosensitivity and may occur in more than 1 per cent of healthy subjects. Other forms of appropriate activation should be used and they are both fascinating and rewarding in patients with reflex seizures such as reading, pattern, musicogenic, proprioceptive and noogenic epilepsy.[616] Their detection is of significance regarding diagnosis and management. Avoidance of precipitating factors may be all that is needed in certain patients.

Drowsiness, sleep and awakening are important studies in patients with epileptic disorders, particularly those who produce a normal routine awake EEG, and their seizures are consistently associated with these physiological stages. However, drowsiness and sleep are associated with dramatic physiological EEG changes which may imitate epileptogenic paroxysms; their interpretation should be left to highly experienced clinical neurophysiologists otherwise significant errors are inevitable. Sleep recording should always include the awakening stage as it is well known that in certain epileptic syndromes, such as idiopathic generalized epilepsies, seizures and EEG paroxysms may only occur at this stage.

All-night sleep deprivation is a well known activating procedure in epilepsies but it may also jeopardize the diagnosis because it is associated with a higher incidence of EEG abnormalities in normal people and may unnecessarily induce seizures to a susceptible individual. We have adopted a rather practical, more natural, less disturbing and equally rewarding approach. We ask the patient to go to sleep 1–2 h later and wake 1–2 h earlier than their routine practice. The EEG is usually recorded after lunch, the patient is allowed to sleep for an hour and the recording is then continuous for another 30 min after awakening, when HV and IPS are also performed.

Technicians

The role of the technician should not be limited to achieving a competent recording but should extend to history taking, which may provide crucial information for the performance and interpretation of the EEG. The 15–20 minutes spent in preparing the patient before and after the EEG, may be valuably used to obtain information about minor seizures, precipitating factors, circadian distribution and other aspects of the particular individual. A well qualified EEG technician is expected and should be trained to have thorough knowledge of seizures and epileptic syndromes. In my department, technicians often provide me with the correct syndromic diagnosis of our patients based on such a dual approach.

The EEG should be tailored to the specific circumstances of the individual patient

A routine EEG may be sufficient to confirm the clinical diagnosis of an epileptic syndrome in newly diagnosed patients with seizures such as idiopathic, cryptogenic or symptomatic generalized epilepsies, benign childhood partial seizures, temporal lobe or other focal epilepsy. A routine EEG may also provide the correct answer or give clues to the correct diagnosis in certain reflex epilepsies such as photosensitive epilepsy with photoparoxysmal discharges elicited during intermittent photic stimulation. On other occasions, the technician should be alerted to apply the appropriate stimulus, such as in reading epilepsy, proprioceptive or fixation-off sensitivity.[616]

However, this is not always the case. Patients with idiopathic generalized epilepsies having generalized convulsions after awakening may have a normal or non-specific routine EEG. An EEG after partial sleep deprivation with video-EEG recording during sleep and awakening frequently reveals clinical and EEG ictal events which are important for diagnosis and treatment. The same applies to patients with nocturnal seizures who may have a normal EEG while awake.

Video-EEG should be made routine practice

Video-EEG machines are relatively inexpensive today and their use should be mandatory in the evaluation of patients suspected of or having seizures. An EEG discharge is of great diagnostic and

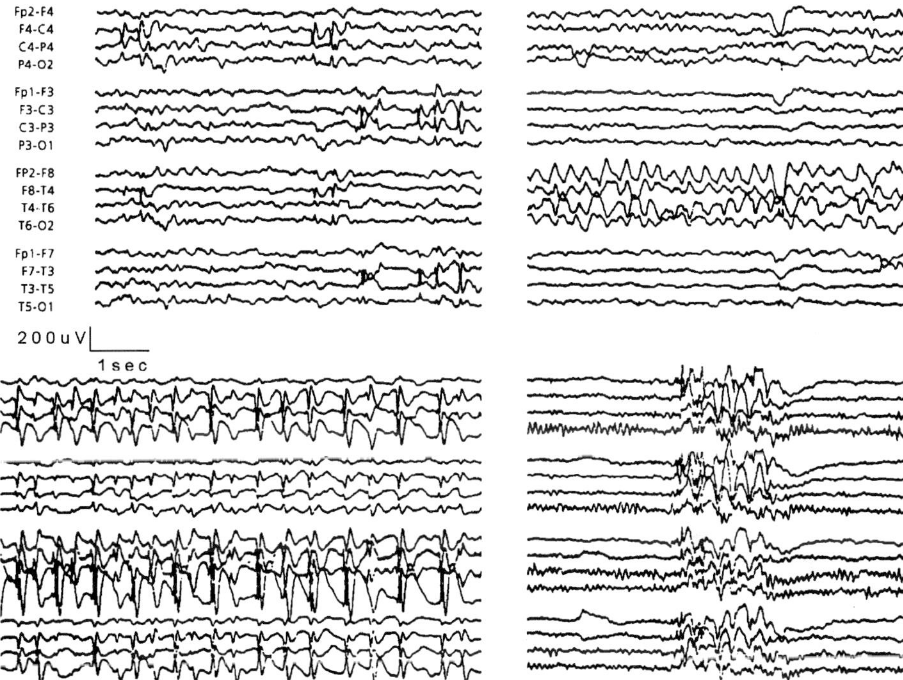

Fig. 2.1. EEG of four patients with epileptic diseases.
Upper left. Centrotemporal spikes are abundant during sleep in a 7-year-old child who had a nocturnal convulsive seizure. This finding enabled the paediatrician to make an accurate diagnosis and predict an excellent prognosis, which would be impossible without the EEG.
Lower left. Electrical status epilepticus during slow sleep in a 5-year-old child referred for 'learning difficulties and absence seizures'. On the basis of the EEG findings, the child was appropriately assessed and found to suffer from Landau–Kleffner syndrome.
Upper right. Ictal EEG of a 4-year-old boy who had frequent brief episodes of 'panic' without impairment of consciousness or convulsive features. The resting EEG was normal but a 'panic' attack was video-EEG recorded with ictal EEG changes of 2 min on the right, mainly involving the right temporal regions. The child accurately answered all questions and communicated well with the technician during the ictus. This EEG unequivocally established the diagnosis and dictated the appropriate treatment.
Lower right. A brief generalized discharge of 3–4 Hz spike-multiple spikes and slow waves in a 32-year-old man with 3–4 GTCS every year from age 16. All GTCS were preceded by absence status diagnosed as 'prodrome' or 'temporal lobe aura'. Treatment included inappropriate use of phenytoin, even vigabatrin. During the video-EEG discharge there were brief rhythmic myoclonic jerks of the eyelids, which would be impossible to detect without video. This enabled us to establish beyond doubt the correct diagnosis of idiopathic generalized epilepsy with brief mild absences (phantom absences), absence status and generalized tonic–clonic seizures.[633]

therapeutic significance if it is associated with a minor jerk or impairment of consciousness which often escape recognition in routine EEG without video recordings (Fig. 2.1).

Video-EEGs are particularly important in the identification and categorization of absences that are easily elicited by hyperventilation, myoclonic jerks that may be inconspicuous, pseudoseizures (particularly those of the hyperventilation syndrome) partial seizures or other convulsive seizures that may incidentally occur during the EEG or may predictably be recorded based on their circadian distribution and the precipitating factors. Video-EEG should probably be mandatory during hyperventilation, photic stimulation, sleep and awakening.

Seizures or other paroxysmal events may occur at any stage during the EEG (Fig. 2.1). Therefore, it is advisable to start and continue video recording during the whole process of EEG preparation. Vasovagal attacks often occur during the EEG electrode placement, and fraudulent or other pseudoseizures during the disconnection period, particularly when the patient is reassured that the EEG is normal. Other types of paroxysmal disorders may also be captured with video-EEG, as was recently the case in our department for a child with previously unrecognized paroxysmal kinesiogenic choreoathetosis diagnosed as partial seizures.

A request for an EEG should describe adequately the clinical problem

The EEG is not a substitute for a clinical examination. It is part of it. The diagnosis of an epileptic disorder is primarily based on clinical information. The events before, during and after an episode of loss of consciousness and convulsions should be intelligently and patiently gathered from the patient and witnesses. A major convulsive seizure that usually prompts the medical referral is often not the only epileptic seizure in the patient's life. Other seizures, such as absences or myoclonic jerks, less dramatic than generalized convulsions, may be missed by the physician or not be disclosed by the patient. Minor seizures, such as simple or complex partial seizures, myoclonic jerks and absences, are more important than the major ones for an appropriate diagnosis and management. Precipitating factors (flickering lights, sleep deprivation, alcohol indulgence, stress, reading) as well as a particular circadian distribution (on awakening, nocturnal, diurnal) may give invaluable clues to the correct diagnosis and may also prompt for the appropriate EEG procedure.

For chronic cases, obtaining previous medical and EEG reports is essential. In this respect I often refer[610,614] to the example of a successful businessman who was correctly diagnosed in 1949 in a district hospital as suffering from 'constitutional (idiopathic, juvenile) myoclonic epilepsy' but was repeatedly misdiagnosed recently in major teaching hospitals in London as 'temporal lobe epilepsy', 'epilepsy' or 'grand mal seizures'. The diagnostic errors inevitably lead to treatment failures.

The diagnosis of epilepsies may be facilitated with home video recording of the epileptic seizures; camcorders are widely available and seizures are often frequent and predictable.

The role of the EEG is to help the physician to establish an accurate diagnosis. In most conditions (infantile spasms, myoclonic epilepsies, symptomatic generalized epilepsies, idiopathic generalized epilepsies (IGE), temporal lobe epilepsy, Landau–Kleffner syndrome, benign childhood partial seizures, photosensitive and other reflex epilepsies) the EEG may specifically confirm or may specifically direct towards such a diagnosis if this is clinically missed (Fig. 2.1). In other situations it may not be helpful, if such situations involve normal rhythms or some non-specific diffuse or paroxysmal slow activity. These cases may need an EEG during sleep, awakening, or both, and again it may not reveal specific changes in approximately 10 per cent of the patients. However, even a normal EEG in an untreated patient may be useful as it may exclude some of the above conditions where EEG abnormalities are expected to be high (generalized epilepsies, benign childhood partial epilepsies).

Epilepsies are usually easy to diagnose. However, as with any other medical conditions, they are sometimes difficult and challenging. I use the EEG as an integral part of the diagnostic process. In this sense, there is more than enough justification to have an EEG after the first generalized convulsion. That the patient may not be treated is not a convincing argument against such a practice; the prime aim in medicine is the diagnosis which determines treatment strategies. The EEG may be the only means of an incontrovertible syndromic diagnosis in cases with a single seizure, such as in benign partial or video-game induced seizures. This, amongst others, may have genetic implications which will not be implemented if an EEG is not requested after the first seizure.

An EEG report should be helpful and committed, not an abbreviated factual report

I have emphasized above that an important factor of error, adding to the disrepute of the EEG, is that the reporting clinical neurophysiologist prefers a convenient but rather unhelpful and uncommitted approach which is often an abbreviation of the factual technical report: 'normal EEG', 'an abnormal EEG with active spike in the occipital regions', 'focal episodic left temporal slowing without genuine epileptiform activity', 'an abnormal EEG with normal background and generalized discharges of spike wave with a frontal onset'. This is inadequate and sometimes misleading. The receiving physician may not be familiar with these EEG terms and their significance. My approach is to provide as much information as possible, supplementing the traditional conclusion with an opinion and often a comment which improves the EEG contribution. Let me take an example of an EEG with occipital paroxysms for a 6-year-old child referred because of 'an episode of loss of consciousness with convulsions':

> **Conclusion.** The EEG is of good organization with well formed alpha rhythm which is often interrupted by abnormal clusters of high amplitude bi-occipital sharp and slow waves. The occipital paroxysms occur mainly when the eyes are closed and show fixation-off sensitivity tested in darkness and Ganzfield stimulation.
>
> **Opinion.** The EEG abnormality of this type of occipital spikes is often associated with a benign condition in this age group that is called early onset benign childhood partial seizures. These are of excellent prognosis, often solitary or infrequent as you will see from the enclosed paper (I enclose a brief report if the referring physician is not aware of the condition). However, occipital paroxysms may also occur in 1 per cent of normal children or more in children with congenital visual abnormalities (strabismus, amblyopia) and other conditions with or without seizures.
>
> **Comment** This EEG should be interpreted in accordance with the clinical manifestations of this child. In particular, was the event nocturnal or diurnal? what were the symptoms that precede the loss of consciousness and what was their duration? did he have autonomic disturbances, eye deviation or vomiting? is this a normal child with normal vision and development? Please, let me know as treatment may not even be needed.

This report as a rule generates a positive response from the referring paediatrician and often a correct diagnosis is made.

For an EEG with small random occipital spikes with a similar referral I also emphasize the need for a sleep EEG. Conversely, if the clinical description is characteristic of early onset benign childhood or Rolandic seizures but the routine EEG is normal, I supplement the conclusion of a normal EEG as follows:

> **Opinion.** Despite the EEG being normal, the clinical manifestations are such that Rolandic seizures are possible. Ten per cent or more routine EEGs in these cases may be normal. A sleep EEG may reveal expected EEG abnormalities in these cases and this has been arranged (or please let me know if you want us to arrange this).

There are numerous similar examples that this type of communication between electroencephalographer and clinician is essential for a better diagnosis and management of patients with epilepsies.

The significance of the EEG after the first afebrile seizure

In the UK, physicians are discouraged from requesting an EEG after the first afebrile seizure, a practice that may have significant adverse implications in the correct diagnosis and management.[619]

The first seizure

Most of the epilepsies are manifested with primarily or secondarily generalized tonic–clonic seizures (GTCS) which may herald the onset or occur long after the beginning of the disease. Studies on the prognosis and treatment of the 'first seizure' mainly refer to a GTCS although this may not be the first seizure in the patient's life.[95,379,380,400,553,722,723] Myoclonic jerks, absences and partial seizures are less dramatic but more important than a GTCS for diagnosis. In one study, 74 per cent of patients with newly identified unprovoked seizures had experienced multiple seizure episodes prior to their first medical contact.[380] The recurrence rate after a first convulsive seizure varied from 27 to 81 per cent reflecting significant differences in selection, treatment and methodological criteria. [95,379,380,722,723]

An abnormal EEG, particularly, for generalized spike wave discharges, has been reported as a consistent predictor of recurrence in all[95,379,380,722,723] but one study[400] which was for adults. In a meta-analysis of 16 publications on the risk of recurrence after a first fit, seizure aetiology and EEG were the stronger predictors of recurrence.[95] This was confirmed in a more recent study of 407 children with a first unprovoked afebrile seizure.[722] In idiopathic and cryptogenic seizures the EEG was the most important predictor of outcome with 52 per cent risk of recurrence at 2 years in those with abnormal versus 28 per cent in those with a normal EEG.[722] The EEG showed specific abnormalities of focal spikes or generalized discharges in 32.5 per cent of 268 children after their first idiopathic seizure.[723]

In other studies of patients with a syndromic classification, it was possible to predict an excellent prognosis in children with benign childhood partial epilepsies, with more than 98 per cent remission within one year from onset for those in their late teens, as detailed later in this book. In other syndromes such as juvenile myoclonic epilepsy, there is a life-long liability to seizures.[364,614]

Why an EEG after the first afebrile seizure?

That an epileptiform EEG is associated with a 2–3 times higher risk for recurrence than a normal EEG is well established.[95,379,380,722,723] However, the most significant reasons to have an EEG after a single afebrile convulsion are fourfold. Firstly, it is possible to recognize children with the features of specific epileptic syndromes.[177,365] Ten to forty per cent of children with benign childhood partial seizures may not have more than a single fit, thus depriving them of a precise diagnosis and prognosis under the current practice.[609] On other occasions, a symptomatic generalized epilepsy may be established requesting early attention. Secondly, minor seizures such as absences and myoclonic jerks may be recorded, also having significant diagnostic and treatment implications. Thirdly, the EEG is imperative in establishing seizure precipitating factors such as video-games or television, thus leading to early and appropriate advice. Fourthly, an EEG in an untreated stage of an epileptic syndrome is imperative. This is most likely to happen if the EEG is requested after the first seizure. Many paediatricians would be reluctant to withhold treatment after a second or possibly further seizure, which are expected to occur in a quarter of children within 3 months after their first fit.[95,379,380,722,723] Requesting an EEG at that stage may be too late. Masking or altering the EEG with anti-epileptic drugs may be detrimental even for a seizure diagnosis of an epilepsy condition that may need long-term and expensive medication which is often seizure-specific.

A convulsive seizure is a dramatic event in the life and family of a child.[395] As in all other fields of medicine, they are entitled to a diagnosis, prognosis and management which is specific and precise. Even if this would benefit only a few, an EEG should be requested after the first seizure.

In conclusion, the contribution of the EEG to the diagnosis and management of epilepsies is immense but significant improvements of the service are needed and this is our responsibility. The EEG is an integral part of the diagnostic process in epilepsies and this should not be underrated.

Benign Childhood Partial Seizures and Related Epileptic Syndromes. C P Panayiotopoulos
©1999 John Libbey & Company Ltd., pp. 21–29.

Chapter 3

Benign childhood partial seizures: General aspects and nomenclature

The benign childhood partial epilepsies or benign childhood partial seizures (BCPS) as I would prefer, exemplify the importance of the syndromic classification of epilepsies.[176,177,609] They are common, comprising about one quarter of all epilepsies with onset between 2 and 13 years of age, and have an excellent prognosis.[609] According to the Commission on Classification and Terminology of the International League Against Epilepsy[176,177] BCPS are classified among 'age and localization-related idiopathic epilepsies'.[176,177,609] This is because the epileptic seizures and the EEG abnormalities are focal *(localization-related)*. They only occur in *children (age-related)*. Physical, mental and laboratory examinations other than EEG are normal *(idiopathic)*.

Abbreviations

BCPS =	Benign childhood partial seizures
CTS =	Centrotemporal spikes
EBOS =	Early onset benign childhood occipital seizures (Panayiotopoulos syndrome)
LBOS =	Late onset benign childhood occipital seizures (Gastaut type of childhood occipital epilepsy)
CEOP =	Childhood epilepsy with occipital paroxysms

The combination of a normal child with infrequent seizures and an EEG with disproportionately severe focal epileptogenic activity is highly suggestive of benign childhood partial seizures. The prevalent practice of not requesting an EEG after a first seizure may result in underestimation of the prevalence of BCPS, as 10–40 per cent of children with BCPS may have only a single fit.

Two syndromes of BCPS are currently recognized by the ILEA:[177] benign childhood epilepsy with centrotemporal spikes, also better known as Rolandic seizures, and childhood epilepsy with occipital paroxysms (CEOP). Rolandic seizures are well described but the clinical variants of CEOP are still unnecessarily controversial. There are also phenotypic clinical variations of benign childhood partial seizures with EEG spikes in other cortical regions, such as benign childhood epilepsy with parietal spikes, somatosensory evoked spikes, fronto-parietal-temporal spikes and affective symptomatology, frontal, or midline spikes (Fig. 3.1).

Benign childhood epilepsy with centrotemporal spikes or Rolandic seizures

Rolandic are the most frequent amongst benign childhood partial seizures, probably two-thirds of them, and they are characterized by striking ictal clinical manifestations (Chapter 4) and interictal EEG abnormalities of centrotemporal spikes (Chapter 5).

Seizures usually remit within 1–3 years from onset and no later than 13–16 years of age. The benign

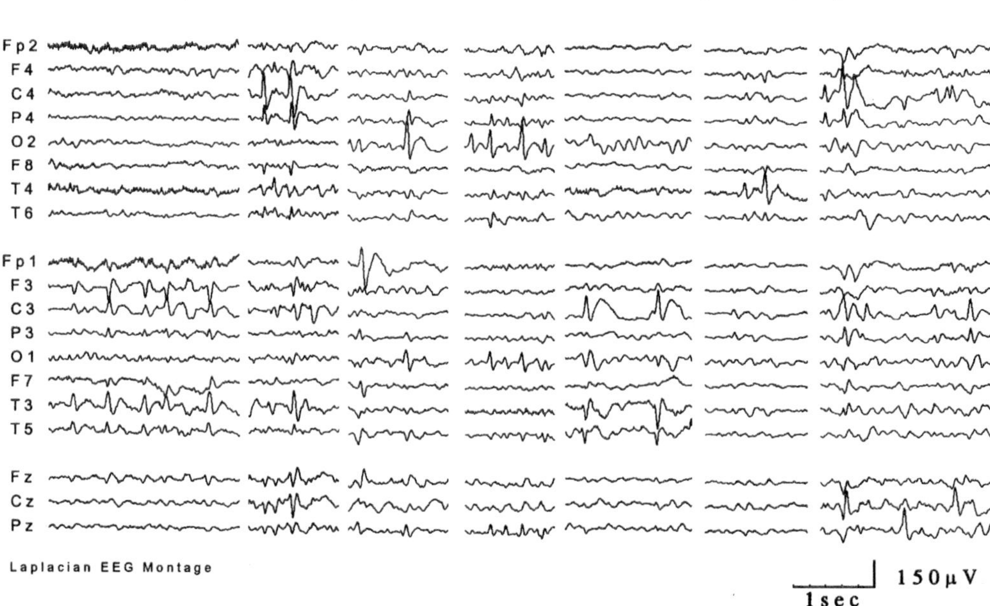

Fig. 3.1. EEG from seven children with benign childhood partial seizures. Note the morphological similarities of the functional spikes despite their different locations. Upward deflection denotes negativity.

character of this syndrome has been demonstrated in long follow-up studies. Ten to 25 years after the last seizure only around 2 per cent of the patients over the age of 16 had solitary or infrequent mainly generalized seizures. Thus, the prognosis of Rolandic seizures is better than for febrile convulsions where afebrile seizures may occur in around 4 per cent of the cases.

The interictal EEG shows frequent centrotemporal spikes (CTS) which are of very high amplitude sharp and slow wave complexes, unilateral or independently bilateral in the central and midtemporal areas exaggerated by sleep. The morphological characteristics of CTS and the dipolar topography of their electrical field (focal negativity in the centrotemporal regions with simultaneous positivity in the frontal regions) are more frequently associated with Rolandic than symptomatic seizures. Ten to 20 per cent of patients with CTS may also have sharp slow wave complexes in other cortical locations. Centrotemporal spikes also occurring in 2–3 per cent of normal school age children are in more than 90 per cent of the cases clinically silent without seizures.

Childhood epilepsy with occipital paroxysms. The early and late onset benign childhood occipital seizures

It would be surprising if an age-related epileptogenic susceptibility was confined only to the centrotemporal area of the cortex. Evidence predating the documentation of Rolandic seizures as the clinical representative of CTS indicated that occipital spikes are also frequent in children, 2–3 times less frequent than CTS, with an earlier peak onset at 5 years, occurring in children with or without seizures and disappearing with age. Their clinical representative, which should be suspected and predicted by virtue of their remarkable similarities with CTS, eluded expert physicians until Panayiotopoulos[600–603,605,606,608,609,615,621,636] described and defined the early onset benign childhood occipital seizures as detailed in Chapter 8. Early onset benign childhood occipital seizures (Panayiotopoulos syndrome) are like the occipital spikes, 2–3 times less frequent than the Rolandic seizures; they peak at an earlier age of 5 years and are of an excellent prognosis with solitary or infrequent mainly nocturnal seizures. The ictal clinical manifestations consist of mainly prolonged tonic deviation of the eyes, vomiting and autonomic symptoms with or without impairment of consciousness usually ending with secondarily hemi or generalized convulsions. Remission occurs within 1–2 years from onset and one third of the children have only a single seizure.

Despite several publications of Panayiotopoulos dating from 1980,[600–603,605,606,608,609,615,621,636] early onset benign childhood occipital seizures were denied by 'epilepsy' expert opinions until overwhelming world-wide confirmation[150,192,270–272,274,275,277,367,443,517,793,797] forced their recognition. Instead, the Commission on Classification and Terminology of the International League Against Epilepsy[176,177] preferred and adopted a rare, probably 2 per cent of the BCPS, clinical phenotypic variant associated with occipital paroxysms as described and proposed by Gastaut from 1981[302–306,308] and detailed by Gastaut and Zifkin in 1987.[313] The retrospective studies of Gastaut were prompted by a publication of Camfield *et al.*, 1978[146] who described four patients who they thought suffered from basilar migraine causing occipital spikes and seizures, an association which Panayiotopoulos questioned as early as in 1980.[599] Childhood epilepsy with occipital paroxysms of Gastaut occurs in older children with a peak onset at 7–9 years and may be misinterpreted as basilar migraine. The seizures are frequent, mainly diurnal and brief, lasting between a few seconds to 2–3 min. They are characterized by visual hallucinations, blindness or both, often followed by post-ictal headache. Consciousness is usually preserved but episodes of loss of consciousness may occur with hemi-, generalized seizures or without convulsions. Prognosis was considered generally good but often uncertain.[176,177] Late onset childhood occipital seizures with mainly visual symptoms are detailed in Chapter 9. My view is that though benign visual seizures undoubtedly exist these cannot be the natural clinical counterpart of the occipital spikes because seizures are very frequent, peak age at onset is later, prevalence is small and active seizure duration is longer than that of their EEG markers which are the occipital spikes. However, benign visual seizures are very interesting because they often imitate migraine with aura, basilar and acephalgic migraine though their true epileptic nature cannot escape clinical scrutiny.[602,608] Furthermore, the post-ictal headache raises the possibility of seizure triggered migraine rather than the traditional concept of migraine triggered seizures.[602,618]

Photosensitive occipital seizure is an interesting but still developing topic that I detail in Chapter 12B. Idiopathic occipital seizures induced by television, video-games and intermittent photic stimulation are well documented. Onset is between 5 and 17 years. Seizures are photically triggered and manifest with multi-coloured circular visual hallucinations often associated with blindness. Tonic deviation of the eyes, epigastric discomfort and vomiting, headache and generalized convulsions may follow. Duration varies from 2–5 min up to 2 h. Prognosis is uncertain. Some children may have only 1–2 seizures but others may not remit. Interictal EEG shows spontaneous and photically induced occipital spikes. Centrotemporal spikes may co-exist. Ictal EEGs documented the occipital origin and the spreading of the discharges to the temporal regions.[369,370]

Other clinical phenotypes of benign childhood partial seizures associated with functional spikes in other than the centrotemporal and occipital regions

EEG studies in children have convincingly documented that functional spikes may infrequently occur in other than the centrotemporal and occipital brain locations such as frontal, parietal or midline. They are morphologically similar to the CTS, are age dependent, disappearing after a few years of active presence, and may or may not be associated with seizures.[327] Ictal symptomatology is often dictated by localization.

Benign childhood seizures with affective symptoms is probably one of these examples with multiple, brief fits of terror and screaming, autonomic disturbances (pallor, sweating, abdominal pain, salivation), chewing and other automatisms, arrest of speech and mild impairment of consciousness. Generalized seizures do not occur, response to treatment is excellent and remission is reported to occur within 1–2 years. At the active stage of the disease, behavioural problems may be prominent but these subside with the seizures.[191]

The interictal EEG shows high amplitude sharp and slow wave complexes, morphologically similar to CTS, which are located around the frontotemporal and parietotemporal electrodes. In common with the other benign childhood partial seizures, EEG abnormalities are exaggerated by sleep and may be associated with generalized discharges.[191]

Benign childhood epilepsy with parietal spikes and frequent somatosensory evoked potentials may also be another clinical variant of benign childhood partial seizures. Based on a literature review and my experience I concluded that somatosensory evoked potentials are not specific for any such syndrome as they also occur in 10–20 per cent of children with Rolandic seizures. Functional parietal spikes with or without somatosensory evoked spikes are most likely expressed clinically with mainly diurnal, infrequent, versive seizures of the head and body, often without impairment of consciousness. Rare cases of multiple daily episodes and partial status epilepticus have been described. Remission usually occurs within one year from seizure onset but EEG abnormalities may persist for longer.[205,759]

Benign childhood partial seizures associated with frontal[85] *and midline spikes* have been described and long follow-up reports have confirmed a benign course, but no systematic studies have been published.

These clinical phenotypes of benign childhood partial seizures associated with functional spikes in other than the centrotemporal and occipital regions are detailed in Chapter 16.

Unified concept for the benign childhood partial seizures

Benign childhood epilepsies with partial seizures and focal EEG sharp – slow wave complexes are a group of syndromes of probably one disease, which, in my opinion, share common clinical and EEG characteristics. Seizures are infrequent, usually nocturnal and remit within 1–3 years from onset. Brief or prolonged seizures, even status epilepticus, may be the only clinical event of the patient's lifetime. Ictal hypersalivation, vomiting, headache, pallor or sweating, unusual in other epileptic syndromes, are frequent and may occasionally appear in isolation. Children with the clinical and EEG characteristics of one may evolve into or simultaneously develop features of another form of benign childhood partial seizures. Febrile convulsions are common. Neurological examination and intellect are normal, but some children may experience mild and reversible neuropsychological problems at the active stage of the disorder. Brain imaging is normal. There are severe EEG abnormalities which are disproportionate to seizure infrequency. Epileptogenic foci, irrespective of their location, manifest abundant, high amplitude sharp – slow wave complexes, mainly in clusters. They are often bilateral, independent or synchronous, frequently combined with foci from other cortical areas or brief generalized discharges, and are exaggerated in stages I – IV of sleep. A normal EEG is exceptional and should provoke a sleep EEG study. Similar EEG features resolving with age are frequently found in normal school age children (2–3 per cent), and children having an EEG for reasons other than seizures.

There is no reason to believe that all these syndromes differ from each other merely because an 'epileptogenic' focus is a little anterior or posterior, lateral or medial to the centrotemporal regions. A unified concept of benign childhood partial seizures is also suggested by the frequency of more than one type of benign childhood partial seizures in an affected child, sibling or both.

It is likely and I propose that all these conditions are linked together due to a common, genetically determined, mild and reversible, functional derangement of the brain cortical maturational process. This is often clinically silent, manifested in more than 90 per cent with EEG sharp and slow waves with an age-related localization. In the remaining minority, there are infrequent partial seizures having symptoms that are also localization and age related and dependent. It is possible that a few of these children, with or without seizures, also have usually minor and fully reversible neuropsychological symptoms that are rarely clinically overt requiring special neuropsychological testing for their

Schematic Presentation

Childhood Seizure Susceptibility Syndrome

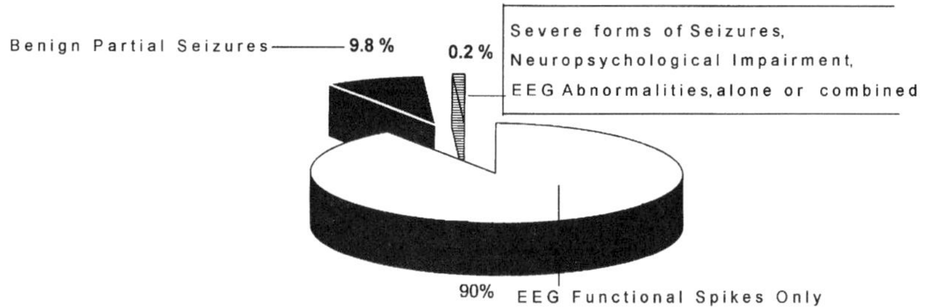

Prevalence of Spikes by Location

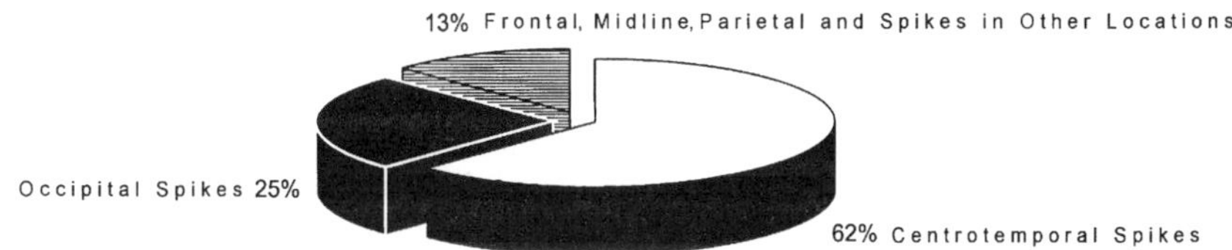

Prevalence of Partial Seizures

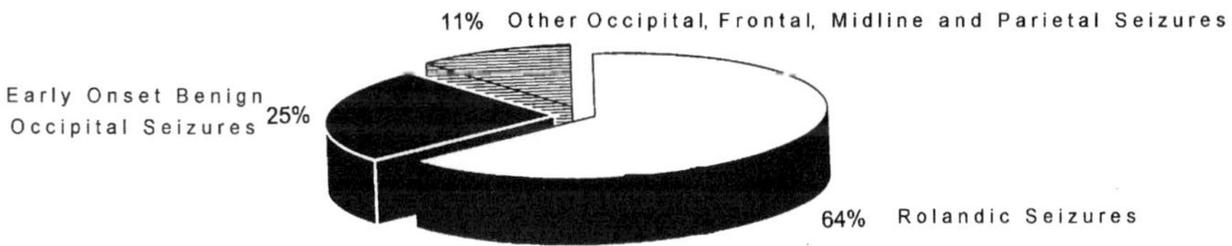

Fig 3.2. Schematic presentation of the benign childhood partial seizure susceptibility syndrome.

detection. Finally, there may be a very small, less than 1 per cent, number of patients in which this derangement of the brain maturation process may be derailed, resulting in a more aggressive condition of seizures, neuropsychological manifestations and EEG abnormalities of various combinations and various degree of severity such as in atypical benign partial epilepsy of childhood, Landau–Kleffner syndrome, continuous spike and slow wave during sleep. These severe syndromes of mainly linguistic and neuropsychological deficits with seizures and EEG abnormalities from the Rolandic and neighbouring regions are detailed in Chapter 17 together with the 'autosomal dominant Rolandic epilepsy and speech dyspraxia: a new syndrome with anticipation', a rare hereditary condition newly described by Scheffer *et al.*, 1995.[708]

Figure 3.2 depicts my concept of the benign childhood partial seizure susceptibility syndrome. The percentages are by approximation, depicted from available relevant data detailed in the various chapters of this book.

Treatment

There is no consensus on whether to treat benign childhood partial seizures with anti-epileptic drugs. Most authors recommend a 1–2 or a few more years' treatment, mainly with carbamazepine, after a second documented seizure, but treatment may not be needed. All major anti-epileptic drugs have been reported successful even in small doses though carbamazepine appears to be preferred. Epileptogenesis secondary to kindling has been feared by some authors; but the benign course of benign childhood partial seizures is reassuring.

Nomenclature

The Commission on Classification and Terminology of the International League Against Epilepsy[176,177] proposed the name 'benign childhood epilepsy with centrotemporal spikes' instead of Rolandic seizures and 'childhood epilepsy with occipital paroxysms' is the corresponding name for the syndrome established by Gastaut. These and other synonyms are given in Table 3.1.

This proposed nomenclature of the Commission[177] may not be entirely appropriate. Many children with 'benign childhood epilepsy with centrotemporal spikes' have only one seizure which by definition is not 'epilepsy' and in others EEG centrotemporal spikes may not be detected. Similar is the situation regarding the early onset benign childhood occipital seizures, with one third of the children having a solitary fit or with others not having EEG occipital paroxysms. 'Epilepsy', even in its strict definition of two unprovoked seizures, is inappropriate for 30 per cent of the children with EBOS or Rolandic seizures with only one fit. The other 70 per cent of these children should not be discriminated and labelled with 'epilepsy' just because they have two or more seizures.

It is also important to remember that idiopathic is not synonymous with benign.

Idiopathic comes from the Greek words *idios* (meaning self, own, personal) and *pathic* (suffer, compare also pathology, pathological). The history of the term idiopathic has been masterly detailed by P. Wolf.[815] *Benign* does not need translation. There are idiopathic epilepsies with bad prognosis or life-long duration and conversely there are symptomatic epilepsies with a few seizures that may not even need treatment.

The Commission on Classification and Terminology of the International League Against Epilepsy[176,177] explains that in idiopathic epilepsies 'there is no underlying cause other than a possible hereditary predisposition. Idiopathic epilepsies are defined by age-related onset, clinical and EEG characteristics, and a presumed genetic aetiology'. Idiopathic epilepsies are divided into localization-related and generalized and some of them may be undetermined as to whether they are focal, partial or generalized. Furthermore, there are many examples of an idiopathic situation-related predisposition to seizures.

Table 3.1.

Synonyms of Rolandic seizures
Benign childhood epilepsy with centrotemporal spikes
Rolandic epilepsy
Sylvian epilepsy
Rulandic epilepsy
Benign childhood centrogyral seizures

Synonyms of the early onset benign childhood occipital seizures
Early onset benign childhood epilepsy with occipital paroxysms[605]
Benign nocturnal childhood occipital epilepsy[606]
Panayiotopoulos type of benign childhood occipital epilepsy [150,270,271,272,274]
Panayiotopoulos syndrome[12]

Synonyms of the late onset benign childhood occipital seizures
Childhood epilepsy with occipital paroxysms[177]
Benign partial epilepsy of childhood with occipital spike-waves[304]
Benign epilepsy of childhood with occipital paroxysms[310]
Basilar migraine, seizures and severe epileptiform EEG abnormalities[146]
Childhood epilepsy with migrainous phenomena and occipital paroxysms[602]
Migraine and epilepsy with infantile onset and EEG findings of occipital spike-wave complexes[213]
Infantile epilepsy with occipital focus and good prognosis[74]
Late onset benign childhood epilepsy with occipital paroxysms[605]
Gastaut type of benign childhood occipital epilepsy[270,271]

All agree that benign childhood partial seizures or, at least, Rolandic and early onset benign occipital seizures (the major representatives of the group) have a benign course with remission within a few years of onset and no later than 16 years of age. Unfortunately, current textbooks and even journals of paediatrics, medicine and neurology pay scant attention to these syndromes, often considering childhood seizures under the heading 'epilepsy' without considering aetiology and prognosis. There is still a considerable social stigma attached to the diagnosis of epilepsy, and such seizures currently exclude patients from life-long employment in certain fields. Benign childhood partial epilepsies, like febrile convulsions, are age related, show genetic predisposition, may be manifested by a single seizure only, remit within a few years of onset, and may or may not require a short course of anti-epileptic medication. The risk of recurrent seizures in adult life is less (1–2 per cent) than in febrile convulsions (4 per cent). Although the use of the term 'benign childhood convulsions' would draw the parallel with febrile convulsions better, some of these children never convulse, others may have only one seizure occurrence in their life and the majority may have the EEG marker of benign childhood partial seizures without the companion fits. It is for all these reasons that I proposed the term benign childhood partial seizure susceptibility syndromes (BCSSS) or 'benign childhood partial seizures' for simplification to denote exactly what these children have, which is an idiopathic and benign propensity to focal seizures, EEG manifestations, or both, that is limited to childhood.

In accordance with this proposition individual clinical seizure phenotypes could be identified by localization 'benign childhood (occipital, centrotemporal, frontal, parietal) seizure susceptibility syndrome'. However, though benign childhood centrotemporal seizures would be consistent with the EEG nomenclature and localization of spikes in this syndrome, the word 'temporal' may be misleading as these children have no symptoms associated with the temporal lobes. These are centrogyral seizures.

van Huffelen (1989)[786] suggested that the name Rolandic epilepsy (from the sulcus of Rolando) is inappropriate and proposed instead Rulandic epilepsy. van Huffelen[786] argued that the description of the Central or Rolandic sulcus was erroneously attributed by Leuret to the Italian anatomist Luigi Rolando (1773–1881). It was first described by the French anatomist Vicq d'Azy but Leuret was mislead by an edition of the works of Vicq d'Azyr that 'had been mutilated and falsified by an unscrupulous editor'. van Huffelen (1989)[786] further rightly debated that Rolando has made no contribution in relation to benign childhood seizures with centrotemporal spikes and epileptic symptoms do not come from the Rolandic (central) fissure but from the pre- and post-central gyrus.[786] Though all these arguments are correct, Rolandic fissure is a well established anatomical name that cannot change. Though the appropriate anatomical name for the Rolandic seizures could probably be benign childhood centrogyral seizures/epilepsy, Rolandic epilepsy is very well established and well identified by neurologists, neurophysiologists and paediatricians with this form of benign childhood partial seizures that have an excellent prognosis. Realistically, I have no other option but to comply with the name Rolandic seizures in this book. All understand it as a benign seizure syndrome of children with ictal symptoms originating from a well known anatomical region of the brain, the inferior part of the pre-and post-Rolandic gyrus.

Childhood epilepsy with occipital paroxysms is the name proposed by the Commission[177] for the clinical variant established by Gastaut. The term 'benign', 'seizure susceptibility' or 'seizures' instead of 'epilepsy' may be entirely suitable for patients who have a good prognosis and respond to treatment with cessation of seizures, such as for EBOS. However, other patients may manifest with daily visual fits and may have a relatively long seizure life span, sometimes expanding into adulthood, and the term LBOS may not be entirely appropriate. Late onset idiopathic childhood occipital epilepsy may be an alternative in order to encompass the entire population of patients with an idiopathic disorder starting mainly with visual seizures in late childhood. However, for uniformity and until the prognosis of LBOS is better established I use the term late onset benign childhood occipital seizures in this book.

The Commission on Classification and Terminology of the International League Against Epilepsy[176,177] does not have a name for early onset benign childhood occipital seizures because this was never considered in this classification.

Fejerman,[270–272] Ferraro and colleagues,[274,275] Caraballo *et al.*[150] and Ahmed Sharoqi and collaborators[12] honoured me by proposing that early onset benign childhood occipital seizures should be named Panayiotopoulos syndrome or Panayiotopoulos type of benign occipital seizures.

A personal note on Panayiotopoulos syndrome. I gave a great deal of thought to the use of the term 'Panayiotopoulos syndrome'. My considerations reflected the conflict between scientific modesty and public recognition of a lifetime of hard work against many odds. I also considered the response of many eminent physicians whose names have similar associations with syndromes and diseases: Aicardi syndrome, Lennox–Gastaut syndrome, Landau–Kleffner syndrome, Rasmussen encephalopathy, Kennedy (or Kennedy–Alter–Sunk or Kennedy–Stefanis) syndrome, Shy–Dragger syndrome and so forth. Finally, I felt that it would be hypocritical on my part not to accept such an honour of having one of the most benign and common childhood seizure condition associated with my name. In reaching this decision of acceptance I also considered if my contribution deserves such a recognition.

My reports were based on a prospective study of occipital seizures and occipital spikes that I started in 1973 and continue today. I first reported the reactivity of occipital paroxysms in terms of fixation-off sensitivity in *Neurology* in 1980[599] and 1981.[600] I questioned the proposition of basilar migraine of Camfield *et al.*[146] and I described the clinical manifestations of two cases with early onset benign childhood occipital seizures with prolonged nocturnal seizures. Of an additional two patients with occipital paroxysms, one had LBOS and the other had symptomatic occipital epilepsy, illustrating the wider spectrum of clinical conditions associated with occipital paroxysms.[600] These reports escaped the attention of Gastaut, this great French epileptologist, who subsequently described LBOS in 1981,[302] 1982[303–306] and 1985[308] as 'benign partial epilepsy of childhood with occipital spike-waves' which dominated the literature and the definition of the Commission.[176,177] It was in 1987 that Gastaut with Zifkin[313] stated that: 'Before benign epilepsy with occipital paroxysms has been fully described Panayiotopoulos (1980,1981) showed that this interictal activity is not suppressed with the eyes open in darkness but that subsequent fixation on a very small light source abolishes it'. Later, in 1987,[602] 1988[603] and 1989[605,606] I reported in detail the clinical manifestations, the EEG findings and the invariably excellent prognosis of the early onset benign childhood seizures after 15 years of follow-up of 16 children with this condition. In particular, I emphasized that seizures were mainly nocturnal, often singular, frequently of long duration lasting for hours, the peak age at onset was at 5 years, and remission occurred within 1 year after the first seizure. Prominent ictal manifestations were ictal vomiting and tonic deviation of the eyes. EEG occipital paroxysms could persist for years after seizure remission. Centrotemporal spikes and Rolandic seizures could occur later in some patients. Publication of my results was not easy. Ictal vomiting was not a traditional seizure symptom to report, partial status epilepticus with a good prognosis was not easy to support, and the established concept of visual seizures of childhood epilepsy with occipital paroxysms (LBOS) of Gastaut was not easy to compete. In addition, the fact that this work was coming from a developing country was not helpful. It took 4 years from the first submission of one of my reports[606] in 1985 before it was finally published in 1989.[606] Even when confirmation of my conclusions and definition of EBOS started accumulating, expert opinions doubted,[36] and EBOS still remains unrecognized by the Commission on Classification and Terminology of the International League Against Epilepsy.[176,177]

Finally, Panayiotopoulos syndrome may serve as a reminder and reassurance for young colleagues in developing countries that their work may finally be recognized despite initial resistance and difficulties. Medicine and sickness do not and should not have national barriers.

However, I would have the same wish as Landau in 1992[467] which I quote: 'Just as Schilder's disease has become a more intellectually gratifying illness called adrenoleukodystrophy, Frank Kleffner and I hope that an organized research effort may spare the next generation of paediatric neurologists from the useless chore of recalling our names'.

Part II

Rolandic seizures and centrotemporal spikes

Benign Childhood Partial Seizures and Related Epileptic Syndromes. C P Panayiotopoulos
©1999 John Libbey & Company Ltd., pp. 33–70.

Chapter 4

Benign childhood epilepsy with centrotemporal spikes or Rolandic seizures

Definition

Rolandic seizures (RS) or Rolandic epilepsy is the commonest manifestation of a childhood seizure susceptibility syndrome that is age related and genetically determined. The cardinal features of RS are infrequent, often single, partial seizures consisting of unilateral facial sensory motor symptoms, oropharyngolaryngeal (OPL) manifestations, speech arrest and hypersalivation. Facial seizures may be only sensory or motor but often these combine together with speech arrest and hypersalivation.

Oropharyngolaryngeal manifestations are unilateral numbness and dysaesthesia inside the mouth, cheek, teeth and tongue alone or usually with motor phenomena producing strange sounds such as death rattle, gargling, grunting, guttural sounds and their combinations. Oropharyngolaryngeal but mainly facial seizures usually are simple partial without impairment of consciousness though they may progress to hemi- or generalized convulsions. The seizures are usually brief for 1–2 min unless they progress to convulsions which may last longer. Three quarters of the seizures are nocturnal and there is a 1.5 male preponderance. Onset is between 1 and 13 years, three quarters start between 7 and 10 and there is a peak at 8–9 years. Remission occurs within 2–4 years from onset and before the age of 16 years. The total number of seizures is low, 10–20 per cent of patients have a single seizure, most have less than 10 and 10–20 per cent may have frequent seizures which also remit. Prognosis is invariably excellent with a less than 2 per cent risk of developing infrequent generalized seizures in adult life.

Febrile convulsions prior to RS are common (10–20 per cent).

The EEG shows centrotemporal spikes (CTS) that are high amplitude sharp and slow wave complexes localized in a 10/20 EEG electrode placement system in the central or mid-temporal electrodes (Fig. 4.1). These may be unilateral but more often they are bilateral and abundant, 4–20 per min, and usually occurring in clusters. They show marked accentuation during sleep by a factor 2–5 and in 10–20 per cent these may also be evoked by somatosensory stimuli of the fingers or toes. Rarely, children with RS may have CTS only during sleep and it is even more rare to have a normal awake and sleep EEG. Centrotemporal spikes may occur simultaneously in the same EEG with morphologically similar sharp and slow waves in other locations such as midline, parietal, frontal and occipital. These multi-focal sharp waves are more frequently seen in serial EEG where occipital spikes are usually first to appear. Frequency, location and persistence of centrotemporal spikes do not determine clinical manifestations, severity and frequency of seizures or prognosis. Centrotemporal spikes occur in 2–3 per cent of normal school age children with less than 10 per cent of them developing Rolandic seizures. They are age dependent appearing at a peak age of 7–10 years, often persisting despite clinical remission and usually disappearing before the age of 16 years. They are common amongst relatives of children with RS with a proposed, not certain, autosomal dominant with age-dependent penetrance. Age-dependent centrotemporal spikes frequently occur in a variety of organic brain diseases with or without seizures.

A typical case of nocturnal RS is a 9-year-old normal boy who half an hour after he goes to sleep makes guttural, death rattle noises, eyes are opened, rivers of saliva are pouring out of his mouth and he is unresponsive. Mouth is pulled to one side and within 1–2 min this is followed by hemiconvulsions. An EEG show frequent high amplitude independently bilateral centrotemporal spikes that multiplied during sleep. No treatment was initiated. A similar nocturnal seizure occurred 6 months later but this time he woke up with feelings of numbness inside his mouth and strangulation; he tried unsuccessfully to speak, feeling as though his tongue was tangled, and within a minute, unilateral clonic jerks of the right side of the mouth followed. The whole seizure lasted for 2 min and there was no impairment of consciousness. EEG again demonstrated abundant centrotemporal spikes. No further seizures occurred in the next 10 years. Annual EEG showed persistence of CTS but this normalized at age 16 years.

A typical case of diurnal RS is a 9-year-old boy who had five hemifacial seizures within a month. These consisted of clonic convulsions limited to one side of the corner of the mouth associated with dysaesthesia in the same side, inability to speak and hypersalivation without impairment of consciousness. 'I felt that air was forced into my mouth and my tongue was tight. I could not speak but I could understand well everything said to me'. These lasted for a minute with no post-ictal symptoms. Similar brief episodes occurred in the next few months and on one occasion clonic convulsions spread to the ipsilateral side of the face and hand. EEG showed frequent centrotemporal spikes. Treatment with carbamazepine resulted in complete cessation of seizures. EEG normalized at age 15 years and treatment was withdrawn. No further seizures occurred in the next 10 years.

Abbreviations

RS =	Rolandic seizures
BCPS =	Benign childhood partial seizures or Benign childhood partial seizure susceptibility syndrome
OPL =	Oropharyngolaryngeal symptoms
CTS =	Centrotemporal spikes
GTCS =	Generalized tonic–clonic seizures
LOC =	Loss of consciousness

Introduction

Benign childhood epilepsy with centrotemporal spikes is the name proposed by the Commission of the ILAE[177] for Rolandic seizures/epilepsy and it is defined as follows:

> Benign childhood epilepsy with centrotemporal spikes is a syndrome of brief, simple, partial, hemifacial motor seizures, frequently having associated somatosensory symptoms which have a tendency to evolve into GTCS. Both seizure types are often related to sleep. Onset occurs between the ages of 3 and 13 years (peak 9–10 years) and recovery occurs before the age of 15–16 years. Genetic predisposition is frequent, and there is male predominance. The EEG has blunt high-voltage centrotemporal spikes, often followed by slow waves that are activated by sleep and tend to shift or spread from side to side.

The description of the syndrome of Rolandic seizures can now be found in all textbooks of neurology

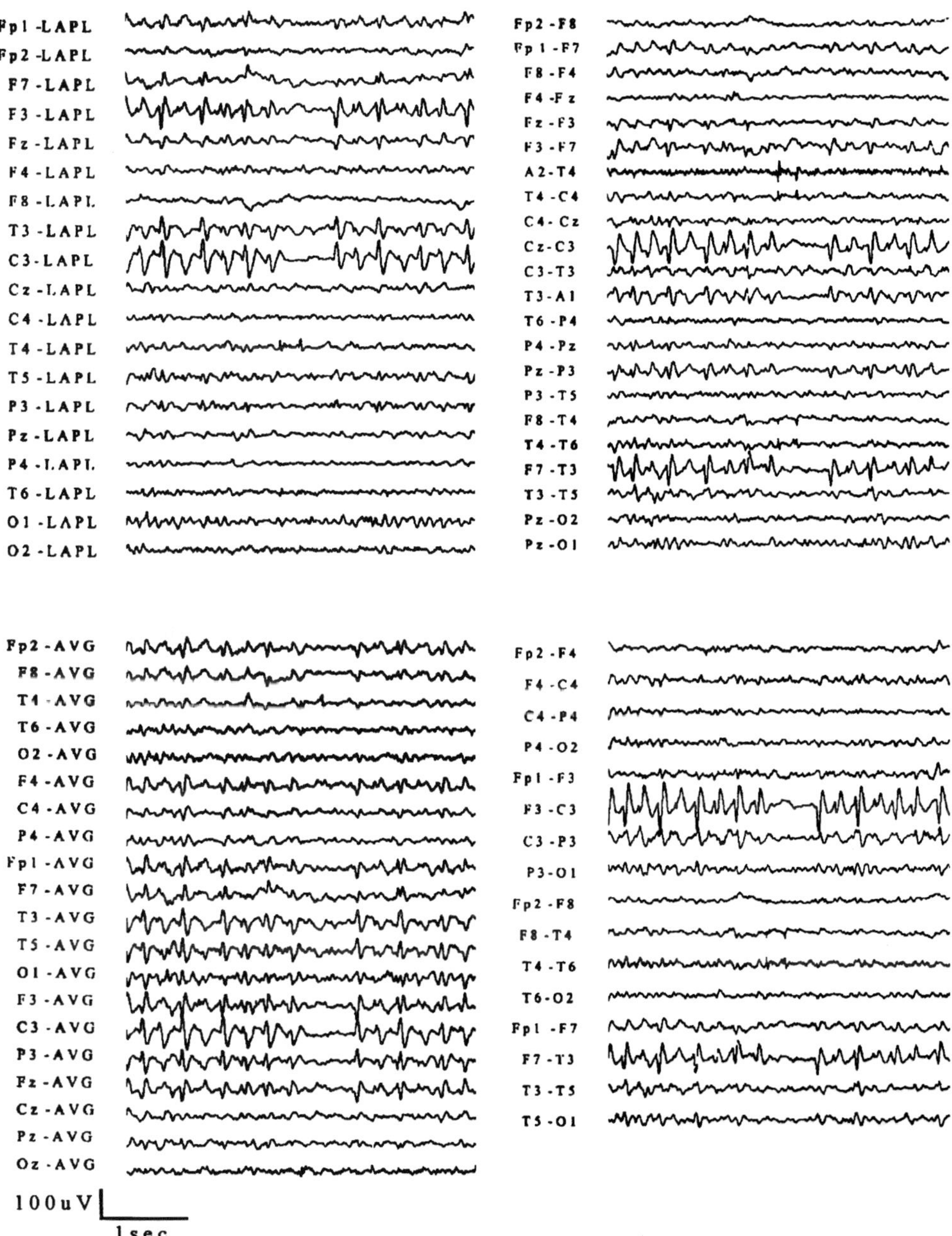

Fig. 4.1. Centrotemporal spikes of case 4.2 (page 62) using various EEG montages for the same EEG sample. The spikes are mainly localized around the C3 electrode. LAPL = laplacian; AVG = common average montage.

and epilepsy. Excellent reviews have been provided mainly by authors with sound experience and contributions to the recognition of RS such as Aicardi,[14,15] Holmes,[397,398] Lerman,[481,482] Loiseau,[496]

Loiseau and Duche,[500–502] Luders and colleagues,[512] Roger *et al.*,[682] Dravet [248], Watanabe,[797] and Wirrell.[812] A recent meta-analysis of 13 cohorts, comprising a total of 794 patients, has been published by Bouma *et al.*, 1997.[136]

Nomenclature

This has been discussed in Chapter 3. Briefly, the proposed nomenclature 'benign childhood epilepsy with centrotemporal spikes' for the Rolandic seizures by the Commission of the ILAE[177] may not be entirely appropriate. Many children with 'benign childhood epilepsy with centrotemporal spikes' have only one seizure which by definition is not 'epilepsy' and in others EEG centrotemporal spikes may not be detected.

Synonyms for the Rolandic seizures

Benign childhood epilepsy with centrotemporal spikes
Rolandic epilepsy
Sylvian epilepsy
Rulandic epilepsy
Benign childhood centrogyral seizures

Panayiotopoulos[609] proposed the name benign childhood (occipital, centrotemporal, frontal) seizure susceptibility syndrome to denote precisely what these children have, that is a benign propensity to focal seizures, EEG manifestations or both, limited to childhood. Though benign childhood centrotemporal seizures would be consistent with the EEG nomenclature and localization of spikes in this syndrome, the word 'temporal' may be misleading as these children have no symptoms from the temporal lobes. Benign childhood centrogyral seizures/epilepsy would probably be the appropriate anatomical name. van Huffelen (1989)[786] proposed the name Rulandic epilepsy to acknowledge that it was Martinus Rulandus who in 1597 possibly described the first case of Rolandic seizures.

However, Rolandic epilepsy/seizure is well established and well identified by neurologists, neurophysiologists and paediatricians with this form of benign childhood partial seizures and realistically we have to comply with this name. They all understand that Rolandic seizures occur in childhood, ictal symptoms originate from a well known anatomical region, the pre-and post-Rolandic (central) gyrus and the prognosis is excellent.

Historical aspects of the syndrome

Prior to the EEG era and the recognition of RS there are some reports of children who may have suffered from this benign condition. Thus van Huffelen (1989)[786] detailed the contribution of a famous Bavarian physician Martinus Rulandus who published a series of booklets each consisting of 100 case histories. The following case translated by van Huffelen,1989[786] was published in 1597 in the 9th book of Martinus Rulandus:

> Ninety-ninth treatment of a case of epilepsy, of falling sickness. That treatment has well been tested and proven in Oberbechinga where the 10-year-old son of Burgl Mairin was seized on very often, both at day and at night, by a horrible epileptic disorder. During the seizure the left eye, the mouth, and the left hand convulsed, he lost speech. and his left arm became paralysed. The seizure, however, passed off quickly and the boy came round without having fallen as occurs in more serious forms of epilepsy. The following treatment was attempted in the boy. *Diet:* During one month he drunk a concoction of lime tree blossom. *Purgation:* On half ounce of brandy from Aloe (1 oz equals 30.76 g). After ingestion of this purge he lost very much fetid and very solid extrement with phlegm and soon he started speaking again and improved further. After two days I gave him a second time from the same brandy 2 drachms during four days (1 drachm was 1/8 oz). Due to this he was well purged and cured. Praise be alone to the Lord of Lords, for ever. Amen.

Karbowski and Donati, 1992[434] cited that Maissonneuve in 1803 reported that a woman in the care of a French doctor named Freteau had from the age of five epileptic seizures always at 4 o'clock in the morning. The fits resulted in facial spasms, foaming at the mouth and fixed stares, and they vanished once the patient reached the age of 14, four months before her first menstruation, and did not recur during the next 11 years of observation.

Rolandic seizures were described in the 1950's thanks to the work of astute electroencephalographers, clinicians or both. These are discussed in Gibbs and Gibbs, 1952,[327] 1954,[326] 1960,[328] from the USA; all others are from France – Gastaut,Y,1952,[314] Nayrac and Beaussart,1958,[562] Bancaud *et al.*, 1958,[65] Courjon and Cotte, 1959[181], and Faure and Loiseau, 1960[267]. It is mainly Gibbs and Gibbs,[326–332] and Beaussart[87–91,498] and Loiseau[498–502,504,506,507] who continued their works for decades, publishing their results and insisting that this is a benign form of childhood partial seizures deserving special attention and categorization. Bray and Wiser, 1965[*140–142] Blom with Brorson, 1966[125] and later with Heijbel,[126–128,382–385] Lombroso,1967[508**] and later Lermann and Kivity[480,483,484] are amongst the leading authorities that made us know RS. Their frequent frustration of the attitude of the expert opinions or epilepsy policy makers is probably best expressed by Gibbs and Gibbs:[332]

> 'For reasons that are hard to explain some of the most striking correlations and the most useful distinctions remain unrecognized by leading authorities. Even though there is marked difference between the correlates of spike focus in the mid-temporal area and one in the anterior-temporal area, the distinction is more often disregarded than regarded. They added as a comment: 'Bei Nacht sind alle Katzen grau' which is the same as the English proverb: All cats are grey in the dark (All cattes are grey in the darke, 1596).

These concerns are still shared by many of us today and are expressed in this book on many occasions. There are still those who lump these children with more severe forms of epilepsies for the study and prognosis of the 'first seizure' (often erroneously equating seizure with epileptic convulsion), and even worse there are still those who categorize them under the inclusive term 'epilepsy' (see Chapter 2). In this respect the words of Blom and Heijbel[127] from Sweden regarding the long-term sequences of RS may be a good lesson:

> The only major problem for these patients is obtaining and retaining their drivers' licences. We have found repeatedly that they were requested by authorities to obtain medical testimonials and EEG investigations many years after their last seizure.[127]

The authorities do not recognise RS because they were not properly advised by us, the physicians.

Gibbs and Gibbs[326–328] gave excellent illustrations of the mid-temporal spikes as they called them: they established their prevalence in children with a peak at age of 9 years,[326,327] they studied them extensively in normal children and for children with or without seizures,[326–328] they emphasized the need for sleep EEG[326,327] and they established with long-term follow-up their disappearance with age, which was often associated with remission of seizures.[326]

Gibbs *et al.*, 1954[326] restudied after the age of 15 years 98 children who were known to have a 'mid-temporal focus of seizure activity'. In 53 per cent the EEG had become normal and seizures remitted. Nine per cent still had the focus and one third of them were seizure-free. In 15 per cent the focus had shifted to the anterior temporal area and all continued having seizures. In 23 per cent the mid-temporal focus was replaced by 14 and 6 per s positive spikes and half of them were seizure free. That seizures in these patients were predominantly facial is adequately emphasized in their reports and the illustrative cases.

The brief report by Y. Gastaut[314] is widely cited as the first to demonstrate focal functional spikes

* *Though of interest, the reports by Bray and Wiser[140–142] cannot be considered as representative of RS because they included adult patients.*

** *There should be no doubt that this report by Lombroso,1967[508] has been very influential in establishing RS particularly in the USA. However, it is interesting that in this report Lombroso makes no reference to European authors who already, 10 years prior to his report, had established the clinical and EEG characteristics of RS, and it is even more surprising that there is also no reference to the reports of Bray and Wiser from the USA.[140–142]* (prerolandic spikes) in patients without seizures. This is translated in Appendix 1 (Chapter 5, page 100).

The history of the 'discovery of benign Rolandic epilepsy' has been recently vividly described by two of the main French protagonists, Marc Beaussart and Pierre Loiseau,[92] as follows:

> Let us come back to the fifties. In 1951, Ms. Gastaut presented to the French EEG Society a paper called 'Un elément deroutant de la semeiologie électroencéphalographique, les pointes prérolandiques sans signification focale'.[314] Her notion might be summarized as follows: a confusing EEG sign is to find epileptiform abnormalities clearly localized in a premotor area without any cortical lesion in this area. Her patients were children with various static conditions, but without epilepsy. This presentation did not alert neurologists and electroencephalographers.
>
> When considered from an electroencephalographic viewpoint alone, central (Rolandic) epileptiform abnormalities look like a very heterogeneous condition ...
>
> However, in 1952, the Gibbses demonstrated the existence of functional and transitory EEG spike foci in midtemporal area.[327] The children were followed up, and the Gibbses' paper from 1959[328] is the first American description of a benign focal epileptic syndrome. However, they used the misleading term of temporal epilepsy. Furthermore, this paper came from an EEG laboratory, and gave no detail on the clinical features. Lastly, it was not a pure series of childhood benign epilepsy, since the mandatory spontaneous remission lacked in quite a few patients.
>
> Two years earlier, in December 1957, Marc Beaussart[562] presented to the French EEG Society the first European description of the EEG pattern. The analysis of the EEG characteristics was quite accurate: description of a slow spike, i.e. of a sharp wave, followed by a slow wave, or not; shifting of these abnormalities from one hemisphere to the other; and their possible disappearance. The pattern was exclusively seen in children, with various clinical conditions. As Ms. Gastaut had done, the author considered the pattern as functional, without any structural Rolandic lesion. Six months later, in a presentation at the meeting of the same Society, Beaussart's number of cases was more than doubled. Most patients had seizures, but not all of them, and neither deficit nor epilepsy was present in six children.
>
> Once described, the EEG pattern was easily recognized. Interesting details were given in 1959 by authors from Lyon.[181] They reported more variable location than that of Nayrac and Beaussart.[562] As clearly appeared many years later, the morphology of the sharp waves is more important than their precise location. Enhancement by sleep, already noted by Marc Beaussart, was confirmed. A retrospective study, done in the main EEG hospital department of a large city, was convenient to find some patients followed up for several years, and to ascertain the favourable outcome of the condition. However, these functional foci observed in children and disappearing after puberty were not correlated with a particular type of epilepsy.
>
> Pierre Loiseau was trained in clinical neurology, but started in 1955 a private practice as an electroencephalographer. As he recorded many children with epilepsy, he accumulated in a short time a small series of benign partial epilepsy with centrotemporal sharp waves. The first report was presented at the annual meeting of the French EEG Society in December 1959.[267] The series included 15 otherwise healthy children, with an onset of rare nocturnal seizures between 4 and 10 years of age. In keeping with Beaussart's findings, the EEG foci were under electrodes C5/C6, and not F7/F8. Their description was not flawless: in 13 children the seizures were diagnosed as generalized seizures. A favourable outcome was suggested. However, the follow-up period was short. In subsequent papers the existence of a particular form of childhood epilepsy with Rolandic paroxysms was stressed. The syndrome appeared to have a real autonomy, and had to be removed from the heterogeneous group of functional Rolandic spikes.[506] Based upon a series of 122 patients, ... a more accurate symptomatology was delineated.[498] Partial seizures were found in 75 per cent of the children and peculiar features were described. Oropharyngeal manifestations, speech impairment and hypersalivation were noted in at least one-third of the cases. As the first patients grew older, a more documented outcome was possible. Forty patients were seizure-free for 5 years or more, with no medication, and a normal EEG.
>
> In 1967 also, Cesare Lombroso published an outstanding paper,[508] with an accurate description of sylvian seizures and their EEG correlate. He concluded: 'Their age incidence, the peripheral manifestations, the clinical and electrographic correlates, the mode of propagation, prognosis are sufficiently homogenous to justify a special subgrouping'.
>
> Over the years, additional features of the syndrome were published, thanks to the identification of more

> and more numerous cases in France. In 1973, 275 seizures observed in 190 patients were analysed.[87] In Europe, Blom and Brorson,[125] and then Pinchas Lerman[480] admitted the reality of a benign partial epilepsy of childhood with Rolandic (or centrotemporal, term used by the Scandinavian authors) spikes or sharp waves. Very, very slowly, other groups in various countries 'discovered' benign idiopathic epilepsies of childhood.
>
> As for our own discovery, we were helped by an identical EEG training, and our private practice. We both had attended Antoine Remond's EEG department, at the Hopital de la Salpetriere. Antoine Remond did not use the international 10–20 disposition of electrodes. He placed low Rolandic electrodes, corresponding to electrodes C5 and C6, and had very personal montages. Consequently, Rolandic foci were clearly distinguished from temporal foci. Doctors in private practice have to listen to patients and patients' parents. They establish a personal relationship with them. So it was, that our new conviction, that not all partial epilepsies have a dismal outcome, was accompanied by deep personal feelings of relief.[92]

I also quote for comparison an American view, that of Lombroso[508] regarding the work of Gibbs and Gibbs1952,[327]1954,[326]1960:[328]

> The distinct electrographic pattern of a midtemporal spike focus was recognized long ago by F A Gibbs and E L Gibbs; these authors in 1960 also mentioned that 'children with mid-temporal lobe spike foci have a far better prognosis that those with anterior temporal lobe spike'. In their clinical correlations, these authors have associated such foci with 'generalized or focal convulsions' without further description. Further, they were the first to point out 'the generally good prognosis for children with mid-temporal epilepsy' and to caution on the need of qualification of the term 'Temporal lobe epilepsy'. At the same time, they postulated that a midtemporal focus may develop as the result of the forward migration of an occipital one and, further, that it might become replaced by 14 and 6 per s positive spikes or 'move into the anterior temporal region'.

Lombroso[508]further states:

> My experience has not been similar to theirs in this respect. I have not been impressed by such migration or evolution of foci in the same patient, and I prefer to stress the difference in origin and significance between the midtemporal–central spike foci, characterized by rather elementary partial epilepsies, on the one hand, and the anterior temporal spike foci, characterized by the well known complex symptomatology, on the other. Further, I consider it unwise to equate interictal discharges such as spikes at midtemporal or anterior leads with '14 and 6/s positive spikes' (clenoids), which are without significant correlation with either epilepsy or other neurological disorders.'[508]

That Gibbs and Gibbs 1952,[327]1954,[326]1960,[328]overemphasized 'the 14 and 6/s positive spikes' (clenoids) and the migration of midtemporal spikes to the anterior temporal spikes cannot undermine their tremendous contribution to our present knowledge of RS.

A detailed and fair historical review of Rolandic seizures was also made by Karbowski and Donati, 1992.[434]

Today, the syndrome of RS has been established through more than 500 publications from all over the world.[136]

Incidence and prevalence

The syndrome of RS is the commonest amongst other forms of epilepsies in the age group in which they occur with a peak onset mainly at 7–10 years. Table 4.1 shows incidence and prevalence of RS in various studies.

The prevalence and incidence of epileptic disorders in children with a particular emphasis on RS are well studied in a county of Northern Sweden from 1972 by Blom, Heijbel, Bergfords, Rasmuson, Blomquist, Sidenvall and Forsgren.[128,383,725,726] The population of this county is around 250,000 with approximately 50,000 children aged 0–15 years. In the initial study of Heijbel *et al.*, 1975[383] the incidence of epileptic seizures for children 0–15 years was 134/100,000. The incidence of RS was 21/100,000 and these represented about 16 per cent of all epileptic seizures excluding febrile convulsions. RS were four times more common than typical absence epilepsy with 3 Hz spike and wave discharges. In a subsequent study in the same region, Sidenvall *et al.*, 1993[725] during a 20-month period attempted to find all children with unprovoked non-febrile seizures. The first attendance and incidence rates were 95 and 89/100,000, respectively, in the age group 0–15 years. The highest incidence was during the first year of life where generalized seizures dominated. There was a higher proportion of girls (male:female ratio 1:1.4), the incidence of partial seizures increased with age up to the age of 10 years and 10 per cent of these children had a history of febrile convulsions. RS had an incidence of 10.7/100,000 and were the commonest epilepsy syndrome.

Table 4.1. Prevalence and incidence of Rolandic seizures

Age range (years)	Incidence	Prevalence in epilepsies	Authors	Prevalence in my studies[605,608]
0–15	21/100,000	16%	Heijbel *et al.*[383]	15.3%
0–15	10.7/100,000		Sidenvall *et al.*[725]	
0–16		17.4%	Sidenvall *et al.*[726]	14.6%
5–14		23.9%	Cavazzuti[153]	24.6%
0–8	5.6/100,000	8%	Doose and Sitepu[246]	10.5%
0–15	8.63/100,000		Loiseau *et al.*[495,496]	
2–13				19.8%

In their more recent study Sidenvall *et al.* 1996[726] assessed 'active epilepsy' in all children aged 0–16 years in the same area. One hundred and fifty-five children had 'active epilepsy' giving a prevalence rate of 4.2/1000. The proportion of boys to girls was 1:1.1. Partial seizures were more common than generalized seizures. RS occurred in 17.4 per cent, absence epilepsy in 6.5 per cent and Lennox–Gastaut syndrome in 5.8 per cent.

Cavazzuti, 1980[153] performed an epidemiological study of epilepsy in school age children, 5 to 14 years, in Modena, Italy, during the period 1968 to 1973. The prevalence of 'epilepsy' was 3.98 per cent and 4.91 per cent and the incidence varied between 60/100,000 and 98/100,000. Prevalence of Rolandic seizures was 23.9 per cent of all epilepsies, idiopathic generalized epilepsies 30.8 per cent, other types of partial epilepsy 42.1 per cent, and Lennox–Gastaut syndrome 3.2 per cent. Of the 178 children with seizures diagnosed during school age, 159 were followed-up for at least 4 years, with recovery in 55 per cent of the cases and tendency to improve in 24 per cent.

Doose and Sitepu 1983[246] calculated the incidence of epilepsy in children between 0 to 8 years in Kiel, Northern Germany. The mean cumulative risk for a single or recurrent epileptic seizures through the age of 8 was 7.27 per cent for boys and 5.12 per cent for girls. The incidence rate for children below the age of 9 was 71.9/100,000 in 1965 and 72.4/100,000 in 1966 and this was 201.6/100,000 in the first year of life. The prevalence, estimated by summation of the cumulative incidence, was 4.5 per cent. Generalized tonic–clonic seizures dominated (68 per cent), followed by partial seizures with complex (17 per cent) and elementary symptomatology (16 per cent), nonconvulsive generalized seizures (13 per cent) and infantile spasms (8 per cent). RS comprised 8 per cent of the total group giving an incidence of 5.6/100,000.

Loiseau *et al.*, 1990[495] reported the results of a one year (1984) epidemiological survey in Gironde, Southern France with 1,128,164 residents in 1982. All neurologists and electroencephalographers obtained information by questionnaire from all persons who had experienced an epileptic seizure for the first time in their lives. Recurrent, isolated, and situation-related seizures were included. Febrile convulsions and neonatal seizures were excluded. The global incidence rate of diagnosed epileptic seizures was 71.3/100,000. The incidence rates per year and per 100,000 persons by type of epileptic syndrome were 1.7 for idiopathic and 13.6 for symptomatic localization-related epilepsies, 5.6 for idiopathic and 1.1 for symptomatic generalized epilepsies, 1.9 for undermined epilepsies, 29.0 for situation-related seizures, 18.3 for isolated seizures and 0.3 for television epilepsies. The annual incidence rate of benign focal childhood epilepsies was 8.63/100,000 children below the age of 15 years (8.3 for age 0–4 years, 13.3 for 5–9 years and 4.7 for 10–14 years).[495,496]

In another study, Loiseau *et al.*, 1991[505] attempted to classify, according to the Classification and Terminology of the International League Against Epilepsy[176,177] 986 patients consecutively examined during a 13-month period either in a specialized private practice ($n = 642$) or in an adult neurology unit in a university hospital ($n = 344$). They were able 'without major difficulty to classify 97 per cent of patients in more or less clearly defined syndromes. Benign frontal and benign psychomotor epilepsies of childhood were represented in this sample of patients. In either partial or generalized idiopathic epilepsies, a diagnosis of epilepsy appears justified even after a single epileptic event when sufficient electroclinical characteristics were present. Patients with symptomatic generalized epilepsies often had to be classified under two or three headings. Many children with a symptomatic generalized epilepsy also experienced partial seizures. Alcoholic epilepsy was described as a true epileptic syndrome. The distribution of epileptic syndromes was clearly different in the two samples, 'casting doubt on the value of some epidemiological surveys based on selected groups of patients'. Of 300 patients aged less than 15 years, 29 per cent had idiopathic partial epilepsy.

Deonna *et al.*, 1986[225] in a clinico-EEG study of 107 neurologically normal children with onset of partial seizures between 6 weeks to 15.5 years found 38 cases (35.5 per cent) of RS. Only one child had 'benign epilepsy with occipital spike-waves'.

Table 4.2 is from my studies on benign partial epilepsies in Athens.[603,605] The prevalence of RS is 17.2 per cent amongst 418 patients with onset of seizures earlier than 13 years. In the same group idiopathic syndromes with mainly typical absence seizures was 11 per cent and photosensitive epilepsy 3.1 per cent. As shown in Table 4.1 the prevalence of RS was increased to 19.8 per cent amongst children with onset of seizures between age 2–13 years and reached 24.6 per cent for those between 5 14 years which is similar to the 23.9 per cent reported by Cavazzuti[153] for a similar age group. Conversely, prevalence was reduced to 10.5 per cent for the age group 0–8 years and 14.6 per cent for 0–16 years (Table 4.2).

Table 4.2. Classification of seizures/syndromes with onset before the age of 13 years[603]

	Number of patients	%
Generalized seizures/syndromes	177	42.3
Infantile spasms	9	2.2
Febrile convulsions	23	5.5
Typical absences	46	11.0
Lennox–Gastaut syndrome	25	6.0
Myoclonic progressive epilepsy	11	2.6
Generalized tonic–clonic seizures	44	10.5
Photosensitive epilepsy	13	3.1
Juvenile myoclonic epilepsy	6	1.4
Partial seizures/syndromes	241	57.7
Complex partial seizures (excluding BCPS)	70	16.7
Simple partial seizures (excluding BCPS)	77	18.4
Benign childhood partial epilepsies	94	22.5
Total	418	100
Benign childhood partial epilepsies	94	22.5
Rolandic seizures	72	17.2
Early onset benign childhood occipital seizures	16	3.8
Late onset benign childhood occipital seizures	2	0.5
Other benign childhood partial seizures (two had midline and two frontal spikes)	4	1.0

Blume[129] estimated that only 1.75 per cent of children with CTS develop Rolandic seizures. He reached this number based on the incidence of RS, 21/100,000 reported by Heijbel *et al.*[383] in relation to the finding by Eeg-Olofsson *et al.*[260] that 1.2 per cent of normal children have central spikes. Luders *et al.*[512] estimated that only 8.8 per cent of children with EEG CTS will develop seizures. This estimation was based on a 1.6 per cent prevalence of centrotemporal spikes in normal children aged 1–15 years[260] and 0.107 per cent of RS in similar age groups.[128]

Rolandic seizures: The symptoms

There are only a few Rolandic seizures recorded with EEG[23,25,135,155,178,195,196,249,372,401,538,682,797,801,812] (see ictal EEG in Chapter 5). Therefore, the ictal semiology of RS is mainly based on descriptions by the patients and witnesses. This together with the fact that RS are mainly nocturnal explains variations amongst authors regarding the prevalence of the various types of ictal symptoms. However, there is unanimous world-wide agreement[3,14,48,78,134,155,216,235,249,315,397,428,445,452,455,456,477,492,512,523,549,575,576,580,721,744,748,784,822] regarding the main ictal features of RS and these are well described by Lombroso,[508] Loiseau and Beaussart,[498] and Lermann and Kivity.[483] Rolandic seizures are partial, mainly simple orofacial, with or without secondary generalization. The cardinal ictal manifestations involve hemifacial and oropharyngolaryngeal (OPL) muscles, frequently with sensory symptoms in the same regions that may precede, follow or co-exist with the motor manifestations. Hypersalivation and speech arrest alone or in combination are prominent ictal symptoms of RS.

These ictal manifestations of RS are well in agreement with the symptoms described by Penfield and Rasmussen[651] during electrical stimulation of the lower part of the precentral and postcentral gyrus in man which are reproduced in Appendix 1 of this chapter (page 67).

Motor and sensory hemifacial seizures

Hemifacial seizures, mainly motor, occur in approximately one third of the patients. These may be entirely localized in the lower lip manifesting with sudden, continuous or bursts of clonic contractions, lasting usually seconds to 1 min. Involvement of the ipsilateral eye lids is not unusual in my experience but I do not recall any case where the clonic hemiconvulsions were limited only to the eye although RS of the mouth corner only are abundant. Hemifacial motor seizures may be the only ictal manifestation but often this is associated with inability to speak and hypersalivation. More rarely, ictal symptoms of clonic convulsions may appear nearly simultaneously or spread to the ipsilateral upper extremity. Involvement of the leg is rare. What may be common is tonic contraction of the mouth to one side which may progress or appear synchronously with OPL and other buchal symptoms of RS. Also, I do not consider it unusual that the child complains also of the mouth pulling to one side with or followed by ipsilateral clonic contractions. Any combination of these symptoms is possible but I should emphasize that motor hemifacial seizures may occur alone and also be the only seizure type in the life of a child.

Hemifacial symptoms of numbness in the corner of the mouth preceding or together with motor hemifacial seizures are less common. More common is numbness but mainly paraesthesias (tingling, prickling, freezing and their variations) inside the mouth, tongue, inner cheek, gums, teeth and pharyngo-laryngeal regions. These are usually unilaterally diffuse or exceptionally highly localized even in one tooth. Ludders *et al.*[512] give particular importance to the 'freezing' sensation which they consider as a negative motor phenomenon, Lombroso[508] illustrated the case of a girl who constantly had ictal pain at one of her lower premolars and O'Donohoe refers to a similar case in his book on epilepsies of childhood.[582] I have never encountered such an isolated symptom in my patients.

Oropharyngolaryngeal symptoms (OPL)

These are the most characteristic of all other ictal symptoms of RS and are often difficult to describe by the patient, witnesses and physicians. They are common, occurring in more than half of the seizures (53 per cent). The OPL ictal symptoms are mainly motor but sensory disturbances may co-exist and these are difficult to differentiate. It is mainly the strange sounds from these symptoms that attract the attention of the parents during a nocturnal seizure. These are described as guttural sounds, moaning, gurgling, gargling, gasping, grunting, chattering, death rattle, roaring, barking, chuckling or glugging, as if choking and their variations (see illustrative cases). Other descriptions given by Loiseau and Beaussart[498] are: 'jerky respiration', 'inspiration with closed glottis', 'wheezing' and 'as if to vomit'. Usually, at this stage the child is unconscious. However, on other occasions and mainly in diurnal seizures, incomprehensible conscious laryngeal rather than mouth sounds like 'aaa, brru brru, grrru' come from a fully conscious child in an unsuccessful effort to speak and explain his problem. Frustrated and scared (because of what is happening and not of a temporal seizure manifestation of fear) the child often points with the index finger to the one side of the throat or mouth to explain that something is wrong there and looks desperate for some help and reassurance. A sensation that the tongue and throat are tightening in a knot or stiff, the tongue feels big, swollen or is moving to the top or one side of the mouth; unilateral bucchal (tongue, lips, gums, inner cheek) parasthesia of dryness, prickling, electricity or numbness, the chin, tongue and lips trembling or contracting to one side and teeth chattering – all are amongst the characteristic descriptions in mainly diurnal RS or nocturnal simple partial seizures. Some children may describe a feeling of suffocation or strangulation. These often occur together with excessive drooling and hypersalivation. The combination of these symptoms in a child are typical of RS.

For description from my patients and their relatives see illustrative cases and Tables 4.3, 4.4 and 4.5.

Arrest of speech

Arrest of speech is another common and also characteristic ictal symptom of RS as it is almost invariably associated with OPL manifestations or simple partial hemifacial seizures. It occurs in more than 40 per cent of seizures.[129,483,498,508] The child is inarticulate and attempts to communicate with gestures. A few mainly laryngeal sounds, not words, may be uttered, particularly at the beginning. There is no impairment of the cortical language mechanisms. The child is perfectly able to understand what is heard but unable to utter a single intelligible word. Some authors call it aphonia or aphemia. Aphemia is a name given by Bastian to motor aphasia[183] or pure word mutism and does not appear to be correct. Aphonia is the inability to produce sounds by laryngeal mechanisms[183] which also does not appear to be the case in RS. The arrest of speech in RS is more akin to anarthria, that is loss of the power and co-ordination to articulate words. This is the predominant view[129,483,498,508] also to explain that ictal arrest of speech is equally common in left or right sided RS seizures.[498] I have also seen cases with RS where children are purely dysarthric, that is they are able to pronounce with difficulty some words but these are distorted as 'there are stones in his mouth' one mother said. Luders *et al.*[512] expressed the view that though ictal arrest of speech in RS is mainly due to a positive motor seizure, a negative motor effect may also be responsible and interference with the language process may be a causative factor in children having RS arising from the dominant hemisphere. They based this hypothesis on stimulation studies of the low Rolandic region in man, demonstrating that arrest of speech, without impairment of consciousness, can be elicited by three mechanisms: a positive or negative motor effect elicited from the right or left hemisphere, or interference with the language process elicited only from the dominant hemisphere. Luders *et al.*[512] may be theoretically correct but their conclusions are not justified by the descriptions of the patients and witnesses of a purely anarthric/dysarthric impairment. Two of my patients clearly had post-ictal dysarthria that lasted for a few minutes after the end of the seizures (see illustrative cases, page 61).

Speech arrest from the classical electrical studies of Penfield and Rasmussen are detailed in Appendix 1, pages 67–70.

Hypersalivation

Hypersalivation, not just frothing, 'my mouth becomes full of saliva', 'rivers of saliva' as my patients have vividly explained, is one of the most characteristic ictal symptom of RS, probably occurring in as many as one third of them. This is often associated with OPL symptoms but also with pure hemifacial seizures and may be a pronounced ictal manifestation. Hypersalivation is difficult to explain on neurophysiological evidence as it is extremely rare in adults. In the experience of Luders *et al.*[512] of cortical low Rolandic stimulation of 'more than 50 patients', there was only one patient where this produced hypersalivation. In this case a 5-s stimulation of a subdural electrode in the low Rolandic, immediately suprasylvian region produced profound salivation. According to these authors,[512] this meant 'that similar to the secondary sensory area, a salivatory centre is usually located in the superior bank of the sylvian fissure and only exceptionally on the suprasylvian convexity. In other words, the frequent observation of salivation in patients with benign focal facial seizures is most probably due to involvement of the superior bank of the sylvian fissure. However, drooling could also be due to post-ictal facial paresis with swallowing difficulties.' Though this may be theoretically correct, it does not explain the almost exclusive appearance of hypersalivation in RS of children and that drooling may occur in the contralateral side of the hemifacial convulsions. In my opinion, hypersalivation of RS is a similar situation to the ictal vomiting of EBOS. Both are ictal autonomic manifestations, mainly shown in children as the most common symptoms of benign childhood partial seizures while only exceptionally occurring in adults. Simple rules of localization are not sufficient for their interpretation.

Consciousness

The majority of the seizures (58 per cent) are simple partial, that is consciousness is fully retained and the patient is able to describe well the events after the fits. In others (13 per cent of the seizures) consciousness is initially preserved but becomes impaired during the ictus (simple progressing to complex partial seizures). However, in one third of the seizures there is no recollection of ictal events. These are usually nocturnal seizures progressing to GTCS. On other occasions, not emphasized in the literature, the child may become unconscious without generalized convulsions. 'After this (OPL movements and noise), she lies there, unconscious with no movements, no convulsions, like wax, no life', as one very observant and reliable mother told me of her child.

Secondary generalized tonic–clonic seizures

Secondary GTCS are reported in one to two thirds of children with RS.[129,512] Primary GTCS are not part of the syndrome of RS. Only five of 72 children with RS in my series were found by witnesses in a stage of GTCS and these were all in nocturnal seizures. It is right to assume that the initial part of the partial seizure was missed in these few cases. Primary GTCS were never reported in diurnal seizures from carefully interviewed witnesses and patients. Furthermore, those with nocturnal GTCS may subsequently have GTCS witnessed from the beginning with a clear cut onset and with focal symptomatology (see illustrative cases, page 61). It is the 'anxious or overprotective' mothers who, despite firm advice against sleeping in the same room and monitoring their children during sleep, may stay up all night watching their children who provided me with this valuable information. Another argument that primary GTCS are not part of the syndrome of RS is that all of the EEG-recorded cases are partial seizures.[23,25,135,155,178,195,196,249,372,401,538,682,797,801] (See Chapter 5, page 95).

Table 4.3. Descriptions of nocturnal seizures from my records

Age/sex		EEG foci
10/B	Death rattle, found him unresponsive on his stomach, hypersalivation	Bilat. CTS
10/B	Mouth pulled to the right, he could not speak, as if he was chewing, LOC. post-ictal dysarthria	Bilat. CTS
10/B	Woke up as if in a dream, trying to speak 'mmmmou, mou', unresponsive for 10 min	Left CTS
11/B	Death rattle, stood up on his bed, raised his right hand, his mouth pulled to the left. Went back to sleep. One week later same episode followed by GTCS	Bilat. CTS
5/B	Opened eyes, looked vacant, hypersalivation, convulsions, right Todd's paralysis	Bilat. CTS
8/B	As if he was talking to himself, guttural noises, ataxic movements of hands, looked confused	Bilat. CTS

10/B	Raised his head from the pillow, his jaw moving up and down, eyes opened, moving right and left, loose and unresponsive for 10 minutes	Right CTS
10/B	Many episodes where he awakes with numbness of the tongue, an unpleasant taste in the mouth, hypersalivation, arrest of speech. Twice followed by GTCS	Bilat. CTS
9/B	A noise as if he was barking, found him standing in bed on four limbs, squint, unresponsive for 20 min. No convulsions	Left CTS
7/B	Moaning, bilateral convulsions	Right CTS
10/B	We heard a voice (aaa), convulsions of upper limbs	Bilat. CTS
8/G	She could not speak as her tongue was tied in a knot. Only noises came out of her mouth. Left hemifacial and arm convulsions followed	Bilat. CTS
12/G	I was scared, I had headache, my right hand was numb and stiff. My mouth opened and I could not speak. I wanted to say I cannot speak. At the same time it was as if somebody was strangulating me	Left CTS
6/G	Her parents heard her as if she was sucking milk shake. She woke up and tried unsuccessfully to speak. 'She was trying but her tongue was tied up in her mouth'. Right sided hemiconvulsions followed	Bilat. CTS
9/B	Roaring with or without right sided hemiconvulsions	Bilat. CTS
10/G	Left sided clonic convulsions of the mouth and arrest of speech	Right CTS
7/G	Opened eyes and had left clonic convulsions of the mouth	Right CTS
9/B	He suddenly opens his eyes, right sided clonic convulsions of eyelids and mouth, right hemiconvulsions of arm and leg followed by GTCS	Bilat. CTS
7/B	Hemiconvulsions followed by post-ictal hemiparesis	Bilat. CTS
11/B	Awakened by numbness in his mouth, tongue was tightened, arrest of speech	Right CTS
10/B	Awakened by numbness and clonic jerks of the right side of the mouth and right hand. Unable to speak and he sees double. Convulsions spread to the right leg	Left CTS
10/B	As if he had difficult breathing. Tried to wake him up but he was unconscious for 3 min. No convulsions	Bilat. CTS
7/B	Death rattle and chattering of teeth. Unresponsive. Eyes widely opened and rotated upwards. Smile in the face	Right CTS
12/B	Awakened by right hand moving upwards. Conscious. Unable to speak. Eyes deviated to the left followed by right hemiconvulsions	Bilat. CTS
7/B	Guttural noises, mouth pulled to the right, 'as if he was chewing his tongue'	Bilat. CTS

Table 4.4. Descriptions of diurnal seizures from my records

Onset/sex		EEG foci
6 /B	Tonic deviation of the mouth to the right for less than 30 s	Right CTS
10/B	Within 3 weeks two brief seizures with right sided mouth and eye clonic movements for less than 1 min	Bilat. CTS
7/B	Two clusters of 4–6, brief for seconds, left sided clonic movements of the corner of the mouth associated with speech arrest but no other symptoms	Right CTS
7/B	Mouth pulled tonically to the left, marked hypersalivation, scared and dysarthric. Subsequently, eyes became vacant followed by brief left sided hemiclonic convulsions for 1 min without losing consciousness. A second seizure had only the initial symptoms of the previous one	Left CTS

Table 4.5. Descriptions of nocturnal and diurnal seizures from my records

Onset/sex		EEG foci
6 /B	Stood on his knees, hands shaking, hypersalivation, jaw turned to the right. One week later, the same while watching TV	Bilat. CTS
5/B	A nocturnal seizure with jaw shaking, could not speak, hypersalivation. No convulsions, no treatment. At age 10 while awake, twice he felt his mouth moving, hypersalivation, dysarthria	Right CTS
8/B	Nocturnal. Roaring, found him on his stomach, could not awake him. Six months later while reading he had a secondary GTCS	Left CTS
5/B	While eating as if he choked then rigid for a minute. Three years later in sleep, noises as choking, as if talking to himself without talking, sitting on the bed, rigid, mouth pulled to one side	Right CTS
8/G	Parents heard her 'roaring' and found her unresponsive, head raised from the pillow, eyes widened open, rivers of saliva coming out of her mouth, rigid	Bilat. CTS
9/B	While watching TV. Frizzed, eyes opened, shaking of the jaw, hypersalivation, unresponsive for 1 min. Three months later just after he went to sleep, chattering of the mouth and spitting lots of saliva for a minute. No convulsions	Bilat. CTS

Other type of seizures

Febrile convulsions prior to the development of RS are common (10–20 per cent)[136,429,481,482] but other type of afebrile seizures do not usually occur. In particularly and despite my studies and interest in idiopathic generalized epilepsies, I never came across a child with RS also having myoclonic jerks or absences or the classical EEG 3 Hz spike and slow wave. I have seen a small number of patients with childhood absence epilepsy and CTS but these did not have Rolandic seizures. I have also seen generalized discharges in EEGs of children with RS but these were usually brief, never the classical 3 Hz spike and slow wave of typical absence seizures and never associated with clinical manifestations. However, the experience of other authors is different and this is detailed below.

Absences

Though children with RS may have brief generalized discharges in their EEG (see Chapter 5, page 89) it is only Beaumanoir *et al.*, 1974[78] who found a high incidence of absences amongst 26 children with RS. These were exhaustively investigated with all types of EEG during awake and sleep (see details in Chapter 5, page 89). Six patients had clinical and EEG evidence of typical absence seizures. In a patient an EEG performed shortly after a generalized nocturnal seizure revealed 'petit mal status' which was arrested with diazepam intravenously. In tele-EEG, 11 of 15 RS patients had brief 3–4 Hz synchronous and generalized spike and slow wave discharges which were mostly clinically silent but occasionally they were accompanied by mild clinical manifestations such as halting of speech or an involuntary, usually facial, twitch.[78]

In the same report of Beaumanoir *et al.*, 1974[78] 11 of 26 patients, adults and children with typical absence seizures alone (12 patients) or associated with GTCS (12 patients) and atypical absence epilepsy (two patients), had unilateral or bilateral CTS.

Of 72 children with RS that I followed for many years clinically and with annual EEG, only one patient developed phantom absences and infrequent GTCS but this was many years after remission of RS and relevant normalization of her EEG.[9] We also reported a woman with eyelid myoclonia with absences who had RS as a child.[323,362] However, these are exceptions and none of them had absences at the same time as RS.

Febrile convulsions

Children with RS have a high prevalence of febrile convulsions, 7–10 per cent according to Lermann,[481,482] 18.9 per cent according to a meta-analysis by Bouma *et al.*[136] and 18 per cent according to the systematic studies of Kajitani *et al.* 1992.[429] The latter authors[429] investigated the incidence of febrile convulsions in 100 children with RS in comparison with 100 non-epileptic controls matched for age and sex. The incidence of febrile convulsions in children with RS was 18 per cent as opposed to 8 per cent of the controls ($P < 0.05$). There was also an increased family history of febrile convulsions in children with RS (48 per cent within third degree relatives) compared with controls (21 per cent, $P < 0.05$). Furthermore, there were 14 pairs of siblings, one having RS and the other febrile convulsions. All of seven siblings with febrile convulsions that had an EEG examination exhibited CTS.[429]

Partial Status Epilepticus

Some children with RS may have prolonged seizures and possibly convulsive status.[225,498,813] Deonna *et al.*, 1986[225] reported that four of 38 cases with RS and good prognosis had status epilepticus. Similarly, Wirrell *et al.*[813] found that three of 42 children with RS had status epilepticus. The type of status epilepticus was not specified in these retrospective studies of specialized hospital paediatric neurology clinics.[225,813] Amongst 72 of my patients only one experienced hemifacial clonic status epilepticus (see case 4.16 of illustrative cases, page 65). The prognosis in a 20 years follow-up was excellent.

An association with RS and an interesting form of partial status epilepticus was first reported in two children by Fejerman and Di Blasi (1987).[273] The first was a boy who had at age 3 years an entirely atypical or exceptional for RS onset with 'atypical absences and partial motor seizures', later developing drug resistant seizures of 'hemifacial contractions with sialorrhea and speech arrest'. EEG had right CTS and brief generalized spike and wave discharges. At age 6 years, he had for one month almost continuous seizures with synchronous contractions of eyelids, left side of mouth, and tongue, dysarthria or anarthria, difficulties in swallowing and continuous sialorrhea. This was not modified by sleep. The child was somnolent with moderate behavioural and learning disturbances. EEG showed continuous generalized slow 2 Hz spikes and slow waves of higher amplitude in the central regions. At this time, he was on phenytoin and carbamazepine. Diazepam intravenously was not effective and this status epilepticus was terminated within 3 h after intravenous administration of dexamethasone. The child remained well in the next 2 years of follow-up with normal development and two brief Rolandic seizures.[273]

The second case of Fejerman and Di Blasi (1987)[273] was a boy with a history of febrile convulsions and onset of Rolandic seizures at age 3 years. Medication with phenobarbitone started at age 5 with good response but this was changed to phenytoin and carbamazepine after 'two partial seizures with Jacksonian march'. At age 7 years he had for 5 days 'continuous seizures of right hemifacial clonic contractions synchronous with tongue clonus, anarthria and sialorrhea' without impairment of consciousness. Ictal EEG had generalized slow 2 Hz spikes and waves, more prominent in the centrotemporal regions. The status epilepticus stopped with prednisolone and the child was well in the next year of follow-up.[273]

Roulet, Deonna and Despland (1989)[691] reported a child with prolonged but intermittent drooling, lingual dyspraxia, and other clinical and EEG features which the authors considered as compatible with RS. MRI was normal. The fluctuating course of the symptoms and their correlation with the intensity of the paroxysmal discharges on EEG were attributed to 'epileptic dysfunction located in the lower Rolandic fissure'.

Also, Deonna and colleagues (1993)[227] reported three children who suffered 'temporary oromotor or speech disturbances as focal epileptic manifestations within the frame of RS' and reviewed another six previously reported similar cases. These could occur as an initial symptom of the disorder without visible epileptic seizures and interfered in a variable way with simple voluntary oromotor functions or complex movements including speech production, depending on the exact location and spread of the discharging epileptic focus around the perisylvian region. The most severe deficit produced the anterior operculum syndrome. More subtle non-linguistic deficits such as intermittent drooling, oromotor apraxia or dysfluency, as well as linguistic ones involving phonologic production, could occur. The rapidity of onset, progression and recovery of the deficit was very variable as well as its duration, and presumably reflected the degree of epileptic activity. In some cases, rapid improvement with anti-epileptic medication occurred and coincidence between the paroxysmal EEG activity (which was usually bilateral) and the functional deficit was seen. According to the authors[227]this deficit could be explained by frequently recurring seizures with prolonged or repeated post-ictal deficits or sometimes true focal status epilepticus. Both mechanisms can probably occur. In the first of these three cases, these symptoms appeared 2 weeks after initiation of treatment with carbamazepine and improved within days on discontinuation of carbamazepine.

Colamaria *et al.* (1991)[173] reported partial status epilepticus manifesting as anterior operculum syndrome in a child with RS. These were long lasting attacks involving the mouth and pharynx, with speech arrest, sialorrhea and drooling. Both clinical and EEG data were considered compatible with the diagnosis of RS. Only during status epilepticus (SE) was the clinical picture similar to that observed in the operculum or Foix–Chavany–Marie syndrome. Remission of status epilepticus was obtained with anti-epileptic medication of diazepam, clobazam and sodium valproate. EEG showed CTS and continuous spike-waves during slow sleep. Interictal centrotemporal spikes were inhibited by mouth or tongue voluntary movements.

That carbamazepine may exceptionally cause deterioration of seizures and clinical conditions similar to the above is illustrated in the cases of Caraballo *et al.* (1989).[149] They reported carbamazepine induced atonic seizures and absences as well as continuous spikes and waves during slow sleep in children with Rolandic seizures. This may have been the cause of some of the reported cases (case 1 of Deonna *et al.*)[691] and I have such an example from my patients, though this was by no means a typical case of Rolandic seizures (see page 358 in atypical benign partial epilepsy of childhood).

Frequency of seizures

There is unanimous agreement that 10–20 per cent of RS patients may experience only one witnessed single seizure, 60–70 per cent may have infrequent 2–10 fits in their life time but in the other 10–20 per cent seizures may be frequent and resistant to treatment.[87,481–483,507,512,682,797] Clusters of fits may occur in one night only or in a brief period of weeks or months. However, in others, isolated seizures or clusters may occur randomly after brief or long intervals of suspected remission. The various patterns regarding frequency of RS are well illustrated amongst the examples provided from my patients on page 61.

Circadian distribution

In all studies, Rolandic seizures are more frequent during night or day sleep (approximately 75 per cent)[136] and in my experience it is not unusual that a seizure is first observed while the child is asleep in the back of the family car. In the latter occasions, also emphasized by Lerman[482] the seizure is usually brief, mild and mainly hemifacial, indicating that fits may be missed in these children with CTS (see illustrative cases). On average two thirds of children have seizures during sleep only (Table 4.6). In 10–15 per cent of cases seizures are exclusively during awake states and the remainder may have seizures both during sleep and awake (Table 4.6). Rolandic seizures can occur at any sleep stage but more likely at onset of sleep or before awakening. (see also illustrative cases, page 61). Frequently, the parents give a history of a previous bad day for the child regarding minor illnesses, fatigue and school problems. However, more commonly seizures come out of the blue with no precipitating factors.

Seizures during sleep are usually longer and may progress to generalized tonic–clonic seizures which are rare in diurnal seizures of an awake child. That RS occur mainly during sleep and often within the first hour from sleep onset is in accordance with the well documented finding of EEG activation of centrotemporal spikes during sleep (Chapter 5).

Table 4.6. Circadian distribution and main ictal manifestations at onset (seventy two patients with RS from my studies).

Ictal onset	Nocturnal only	Nocturnal and diurnal	Diurnal only	Total	%
Oropharyngolaryngeal	25	14	2	41	57%
Hemifacial	13	5	8	26	36%
GTCS*	5	0	0	5	7%
Total	43	19	10	72	100%
%	60%	26%	14%	100%	

*These were most likely secondary GTCS but the preceding symptoms were not witnessed (see text).

Age at onset and sex

Though reported age at onset ranges from 6 months to 14 years,[136] the consensus is that onset is mainly from 3 to 13 years with a peak at 7–10 for more than three quarters of patients (Fig. 4.2). Onset before the age of 3 or after the age of 13 years is exceptionally rare and in these cases the diagnosis of RS should be made with caution. Age at onset of 72 patients with RS from my studies in Athens[603,605] ranged from 3 to 13 years, the median age being 8 years, and mean ± SD = 8.1 ± 2.4 years. There were two peaks, one at 8 and another at 11 years.

In all studies there is a clear cut predominance of boys with a male to female ratio calculated as 1.5. Thus in a review of nine studies with RS, Luders *et al.*[512] found that 240 were boys and 159 were girls. In the meta-analysis by Bouma *et al.*[136] 58.2 per cent were boys (ratio boys/girls = 1.4). Of 72 patients with RS from my studies[603,605] 55 (76.4 per cent) were boys with a boys/girls ratio = 3.2. I have no explanation for this high male preponderance amongst my patients.

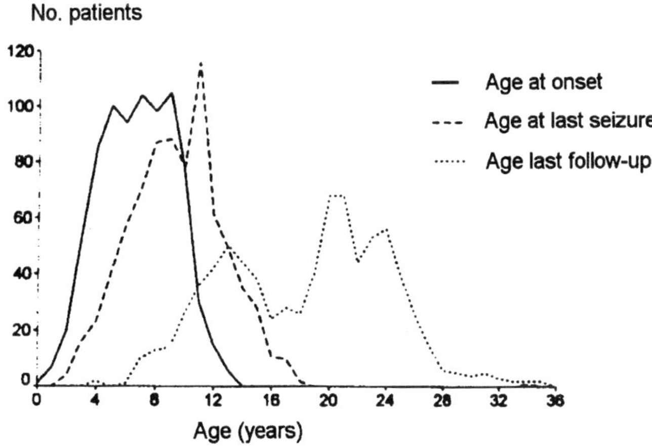

Fig 4.2. Course of Rolandic seizures: number of patients by age. Curves represent the number of patients by age at onset (range: 0–14 years), age at last seizures (range: 3–35 years), and age at the end of follow-up (range: 3–36 years).
[From Bouma et al., Neurology 1997;48: 430–437, with permission of the authors and the editor of Neurology.]

Genetics of the syndrome of Rolandic seizures or more accurate genetics of the EEG centrotemporal spikes

Rolandic seizures (RS) are genetically determined but the mode of inheritance is not yet known despite the fact that in handbooks and some reviews, RS are considered to be an autosomal dominant inheritance with age-dependent penetrance. This mode of inheritance refers to the EEG centrotemporal spikes, generalized discharges, or both, and not to Rolandic seizures. This view of the EEG trait is mainly based on reports by Bray and Wiser (1964, 1965)[140–142] from the USA and Heijbel, Blom and Rasmuson (1975)[384] from Sweden. A similar conclusion of an autosomal dominant inheritance was also more recently reached by Degen and Degen, 1990–92[217–219] from Germany. However, Okubo *et al.*, 1994[586] from Japan found that CTS occurred in only two (5.3 per cent) of 38 probands with EEG CTS and concluded that 'an autosomal-dominant genetic factor for centrotemporal spikes in waking EEGs of healthy children could not be confirmed'. Doose *et al.*, 1977–1997[237–241,243–245,321] from Germany support a multifactorial pathogenesis.

Furthermore, those studies of Bray and Wiser,[140–142] Heijbel *et al.*[384] and Degen and Degen[217–219] suggesting an autosomal dominant inheritance with age-dependent penetrance have conflicting results which do not allow definite conclusions. The subject should not be considered settled by any means. In the study of Bray and Wiser[140–142] adult probands were included who did not have RS and some of the provided EEG samples are not centrotemporal spikes. The report by Heijbel *et al.*,[384] who have also made significant contributions to our understanding of other clinical, EEG and prognostic aspects of RS,[125–127,382–385] is the more complete genetic study. However, this is the only study with such a high incidence of Rolandic seizures and centrotemporal spikes amongst first degree relatives of probands with RS. Furthermore, their hypothesis of an autosomal dominant inheritance with an age-dependent penetrance has not been confirmed by others.[217,218,586] Doose and Baier[240] expressed reservations regarding the validity of the theory of quasi-continuous trait as applied by Heijbel *et al.*[384] from their conclusion, and the authors have not excluded the possibility that 'the expression of the main gene is influenced by a few other genes or by a multitude of genetic and environmental factors'. Moreover, Degen and Degen[217,218] based their opinion of an autosomal dominant inheritance on EEG findings again but these were by far more generalized discharges (22 of 69 siblings) rather than centrotemporal spikes (two to three siblings). Finally, in the studies of Doose *et al.*[237–241,243–245,321] the main inclusion criterion is an EEG with 'well-structured sharp waves such as those that occur in Rolandic or another type of benign partial epilepsy'. Less than 24 per cent of their probands had RS, more than half of them had EEG sharp wave foci in other than the centrotemporal regions, and for one third of them seizures started between 1–3 years which is an unlikely age of onset for RS. Furthermore, by selecting their patients on the basis of an EEG 'sharp wave' only, Doose *et al.*[237–241,243–245,321] assume that this common EEG abnormality has the same pathogenetic significance in all patients and their families, or in other words underlines the same disease process with different phenotypic expressions. This is unlikely in view of the fact that EEG centrotemporal, occipital and sharp waves at other locations occur in diverse clinical idiopathic, symptomatic or cryptogenic brain diseases that may or may not be associated with seizures as we know from the work of Gibbses[327,329–331] and Kellaway.[438] This approach of Doose *et al.*[237–241,243–245,321] may be similar to undertaking a genetic study based on a myopathic EMG marker which would be the same in numerous genetically different myopathic disorders. It is probably because of this non-specific EEG criterion for selection that Doose *et al.*[237–241,243–245,321] found that 'the phenotypic expression of the genetic anomaly underlying focal sharp waves shows considerable variability' with 'very variable symptoms that included partial seizures and generalized seizures of partial onset, astatic and nodding fits, atypical absences, minor or subclinical status' even 'psychomental retardation and selective performance deficits'.[237,240] Benign centrotemporal spikes and associated seizures are age dependent while psychomental retardation is not. This alone would contradict these authors' assumption that all these conditions are a continuum of 'hereditary impairment of brain maturation'[237–241,244,245,321] simply because they have in common a sharp focus in their EEG which is non specific. In this sense fragile

X syndrome which frequently shows centrotemporal spikes and also manifests with seizures similar to those of RS,[276,444,556,674] should be the genetic prototype of RS, which is not the case.[673] Similarly, children with congenital visual deficits who often exhibit EEG occipital spikes[438]should be categorized in this 'hereditary impairment of brain maturation syndrome' together with normal and mentally handicapped children who may or may not have, benign or intractable, seizures. Are we also to include in this 'hereditary impairment of brain maturation syndrome' the severely brain damaged children of Fukuyama type congenital muscular dystrophy[823] or the girls with Rett syndrome[376,572] who may often have centrotemporal spikes and RS?[823] This challenging approach is interesting but does not appear to be correct. EEG sharp wave foci are non specific electrical manifestations of the brain which may or may not be associated with seizures. Centrotemporal and occipital sharp wave foci are frequently age dependent, have a low seizure potential, are often determined by different genetic backgrounds and may also be caused by structural, metabolic or other brain diseases. The brain does not have many options to express in surface EEGs the various electrical changes associated or caused by diverse genetic or acquired neural derangement. This may also be the case with a condition newly described by Scheffer *et al.* (1995),[708] as of 'autosomal dominant Rolandic epilepsy and speech dyspraxia: a new syndrome with anticipation'. This involves a family of nine affected individuals over three generations with age-related nocturnal oro-facio-brachial partial seizures, secondary generalized partial seizures, and centrotemporal epileptiform discharges, associated with permanent oral and speech dyspraxia and cognitive impairment. Though this is an extremely interesting but rare disease, I would not agree with Scheffer *et al.* (1995)[708] in their conclusion that 'The electroclinical features of this new syndrome of autosomal dominant Rolandic epilepsy resemble those of benign Rolandic epilepsy' and that 'molecular studies on this syndrome could also be relevant to identifying a gene for benign Rolandic epilepsy'.[708] The clinical presentation of these patients with permanent neurologic deficit, sometimes preceding the seizures, can hardly accord to the conclusion that it 'epitomized the archetypal benign Rolandic epileptic attack'.[708]

The following are details of the most cited references on the genetics of EEG traits in RS.

Bray and Wiser (1964)[140] reported the 'evidence for a genetic aetiology of temporal-central abnormalities in focal epilepsy'. Subjects were selected as index cases because of a seizure and the fact that their EEGs 'showed paroxysmal sharp waves or spikes in the vicinity of T3 and T4 electrodes'. Control subjects had no neurological complaints and were matched for age, sex and socio-economic status. EEGs were obtained while awake and during sleep with hyperventilation, and intermittent photic stimulation performed in all cases. There were 40 families of index cases with 30 per cent having at least one member with similar EEG abnormality, 36 per cent amongst siblings and children and 19 per cent amongst parents. Conversely, only 5 per cent of control families showed similar EEG abnormalities that were equally distributed between siblings (2 per cent) and parents (2 per cent). The authors also present EEG samples and clinical information of three types. The first is an unequivocal case of RS with also typical centrotemporal spikes in the other three of eight siblings, the parents having normal EEGs. The second is a woman who has had 'poorly controlled generalized seizures since middle childhood and later required institutionalization because of overt psychosis'. Though her daughter's EEG showed rather typical centrotemporal sharp waves, the patient's spikes mainly over the right midtemporal regions cannot be considered as characteristic CTS. The third illustrative case had from age 6 years generalized nocturnal seizures and obvious mental deficiency. His EEG also exhibited double spikes, an asymptomatic brother had centrotemporal sharp waves and a paternal uncle had temporal lobe epilepsy with complex partial seizures and an anterior temporal spike focus. Though emphasizing these genetic, mainly EEG links, between family members of these patients, Bray and Wiser[140] make no reference to possible mode of inheritance in this paper but later[142] concluded that this suggested that 'the disorder is transmitted by one or more autosomal dominant genes (i.e. either it is caused by a single dominant gene with variable penetrance, or it is a polygenic trait). Gene penetrance of this trait as measured by EEG is low in early childhood (14 per cent between birth and 5 years), reaches a peak in middle childhood (56 per cent between 6 and 10 years), and then tapers off to low levels in adult life.' Yet, they also concluded that 'this hereditary form of focal temporal lobe epilepsy can manifest itself in adults as a psychomotor seizure disorder with anterior temporal lobe EEG foci', a conclusion which cannot be accepted with the present knowledge for RS (see prognosis of RS on page 57). However, this was 35 years ago when Bray, a paediatric neurologist, and Wiser, a predoctoral student in genetics, made their significant contribution through hard work on genetic factors in centrotemporal EEG foci. In another report Bray and Wiser (1965)[141], using the same criteria as in their first study of a seizure and T3–T4 EEG foci of children and adults, emphasized the high occurrence (48 per cent of the 40 families) of generalized discharges in the patients and their relatives. These generalized discharges occurred in longitudinal EEG studies in 42 per cent of the index cases (8/19), 13 per cent of siblings and children (10/77), 16 per cent of parents (5/31), 20 per cent of uncles and aunts (4/20), 5 per cent of nieces and nephews (3/60) and 5 per cent of cousins (3/58). These EEG abnormalities for the majority of the cases were not associated with overt clinical epileptic seizures. Only 1 per cent of the control siblings and only 2 per cent of parents had similar EEG abnormalities. The authors rightly concluded that 'the EEG concept of idiopathic epilepsy should be broadened to include not only diffuse rhythmic 3 Hz spike-wave epileptiform discharges but also some cases of "focal" temporal or temporal-central abnormalities' and added 'these conclusions are not intended to reduce the physician's awareness of and vigilance for focal, structural lesions in or near the cerebral cortex'. The view of Bray and Wiser[142] regarding autosomal dominant inheritance was challenged by Loiseau and Beaussart, 1969.[497]

Heijbel, Blom and Rasmuson (1975)[384] reported a genetic study of 19 probands with RS and centrotemporal EEG foci, 36 their full parents, and 34 full siblings. All subjects had awake and sleep EEGs. However, of the 19 probands only six had partial seizures. Eleven had generalized seizures and in six of them these were diurnal. From the 34 siblings, 15 per cent (5/34) had generalized seizures and 'Rolandic discharges', and 19 per cent (6/32) had centrotemporal spikes alone. Of the 36 full parents, four (11 per cent) had seizures only in childhood but 'The seizure types in parents were largely unknown.... The parents' own descriptions were mostly vague and regarded as unreliable. Therefore, they were not analysed and classified in detail'. An additional parent, a father who did not have seizures, was the only one to show in EEG 'sporadic low amplitude spikes or sharp waves over central and temporal regions'. These five parents were considered as affected for the genetic analysis. The results were tested against different genetic hypotheses and indicated that an autosomal dominant mode of inheritance with age-dependent penetrance is most likely responsible for the EEG trait.

Degen and Degen (1990)[217,218] reported 'some genetic aspects of Rolandic epilepsy: waking and sleep EEGs in siblings'. Though their methods, inclusion criteria, EEG recordings and conclusion of an autosomal dominant inheritance of EEG abnormalities were similar to those of Heijbel *et al.*[384] their results regarding the prevalence of centrotemporal spikes amongst siblings were markedly different. Only four (5.8 per cent) of 69 siblings of 43 probands with 'Rolandic epilepsy and/or centrotemporal spikes' had EEG sharp waves. These were unilateral (one sibling) or bilateral (one sibling) centrotemporal spikes, unilateral occipital (one sibling) and unilateral frontal with spreading to the centrotemporal regions. Thus, in this study of Degen and Degen[217,218] only two (2.9 per cent) of 69 siblings had centrotemporal spikes which is close to what is found in normal children. The incidence also of occipital spikes is not greater than that of normal children. More analytically, in their study Degen and Degen[217,218] 'recorded waking and sleep EEGs in 69 siblings of 43 patients with Rolandic spikes. Thirty six had Rolandic epilepsy and seven with symptoms such as headaches, migraine and learning problems had no seizures. Epileptic activity was recorded in at least one sibling in 22 (51.16 per cent) of 43 patients. In 26 of 69 (37.68 per cent) siblings, epileptic discharges were observed. These were recorded only in waking in one subject (1.5 per cent), in waking and sleep in 13 (18.8 per cent), and in sleep only in 12 (17.4 per cent). The greatest number of epileptic discharges was noted in waking during hyperventilation (52.4 per cent) and in sleep stage III (88 per cent). Foci were recorded in only four (5.8 per cent) of the 26 cases with epileptic discharges, and generalized spike-wave complexes were recorded in 22 (31.9 per cent). One epileptic discharge was observed every 74.9 s in waking and every 150.9 s in sleep. Epileptic activity was greatest in the group between 5 and 12 years of age (54.3

per cent). The same activation rates were noted in siblings of patients with (47.2 per cent) and without seizures (42.9 per cent), and no differences were noted in siblings with (40 per cent) or without (37.5 per cent) seizures. Family history and sex of the siblings did not play a role in the rate of activation.' It is also interesting that only five siblings had seizures, but contrary to the results of Heijbel *et al.*[384] these were not RS. Three of these five seizure patients had normal EEG, one had bilateral centrotemporal spikes and the fifth patient had generalized 3–4 Hz spike-wave discharges and photosensitivity. The authors assumed an autosomal dominant inheritance, probably mainly for the generalized discharges observed in the siblings, but emphasized the need for further investigations. In another report by the same authors, Degen *et al.* (1991)[219] waking and sleep EEGs in 67 siblings of 52 patients with febrile seizures revealed a similar incidence of 'epileptic activity' as that of RS. Thus in siblings of children with febrile seizures, epileptic activity was noted in at least one sibling for 28 of the 52 patients (53.8 per cent). Epileptic discharges were noted in 33 (49.2 per cent) of the 67 siblings. Thirty-two siblings had 3–4 Hz spike wave complexes, in five these were IPS induced and one sibling had independent centrotemporal spike foci. Epileptic discharges were noted in 83.3 per cent of siblings with seizures, but in only 45.9 per cent of siblings without seizures.

Doose *et al.* have published an impressive number of reports on the genetics of childhood epilepsies. The most relevant to RS are from over 20 years of work.[237,238,240,241,243–245,321] In all these studies the primary criterion for selection is 'at least one EEG with focal sharp waves characteristic of benign partial epilepsies' irrespective of localization and clinical symptomatology with or without seizures. This could be the only selection criterion[244,321] or combined with 'at least another sibling having an EEG with typical focal sharp waves'[237,240,241] or 'at least one of their siblings investigated with EEG'.[243] Only waking EEGs were studied. In the initial reports[244,321] of '203 epileptic children who had at least once focal sharp waves in the EEG' seizures were multiform ranging from different types of partial, primary and secondary generalized seizures to infantile spasms. Organic brain lesions played an important role. In 23 per cent of cases there was a family history of seizures with mothers and maternal siblings more often affected than fathers and their siblings. In these reports[244,321]only 2.9 per cent of the siblings had focal sharp waves which is similar to the low incidence found by Degen and Degen.[217,218]

When probands and at least one of their siblings having an EEG sharp wave were studied,[237,240,241] Doose *et al.* found 'a broad spectrum of epileptic and non-epileptic conditions ranging from mild selective performance deficits to severe complex psychomental retardation, from simple Rolandic epilepsy to severe epilepsies with minor seizures or bioelectrical status.' Only a few cases were normal children with RS. Similarly, EEG findings were quite variable with centrotemporal spikes found in only 22 per cent of the probands. The remainder had foci in other regions (17 per cent) or multiple foci (61 per cent). Based on their results Doose and Baier[240] hypothesized 'a multifactorial pathogenesis with hereditary impairment of brain maturation in benign partial epilepsy and related conditions' and concluded 'The complexity of causal factors, which potentially include organic brain lesions, account for the wide spectrum of epileptic and non-epileptic conditions ranging from mild selective performance deficits to complex psychomental retardation, and from simple Rolandic epilepsy to severe epilepsies with minor seizures or bioelectrical status. These conditions are not "syndromes" in the stricter sense, but sets of variably weighted symptoms of a complex pathogenetic background. A genetic disposition to focal anomalies of brain function is of decisive importance. The biological background is as yet unknown. The marked age-dependency of symptoms and almost regular disappearance of seizures and EEG abnormalities at puberty justify the assumption of an hereditary impairment of brain maturation. The hypothesis of autosomal dominant inheritance awaits appraisal by studies of larger populations and quantitative genetic approaches.' This view was further expanded by Doose (1992)[238] in all epilepsies as a whole and concluded that 'from a neurobiological point of view, epilepsy is always a multifactorially determined disease. The nowadays usual separation of idiopathic and symptomatic types of epilepsy may be helpful for communication in daily practice, but represents a simplification under pathogenetic aspects.'

In their most recent report Doose *et al.*[243] investigated 147 children (134 with seizures, 13 without) with (a) at least one EEG with focal sharp waves characteristic of benign partial epilepsies, and (b) at least one sibling investigated by EEG. The families were questioned orally or in writing regarding the occurrence of seizures. Patients' records were evaluated by a standardized scheme'. Similar to their previous studies, Doose *et al.*[243] found 'multiform seizure types such as febrile convulsions, afebrile generalized tonic–clonic seizures, simple and (rarely) complex partial seizures; and Rolandic seizures in the strict sense'. Neonatal seizures were over-represented (6 per cent). Families of 32 patients with typical Rolandic seizures (24 per cent of the 134 probands with seizures) showed no aggregation of Rolandic epilepsy, but did show variable seizure types. In the entire sample, EEG investigations showed focal sharp waves in 11 per cent of siblings aged 2–10 years. No relation existed between clinical symptomatology and sharp wave findings in siblings. In 66 per cent of probands, the EEG disclosed generalized genetic patterns. Siblings with generalized spike-waves and/or theta rhythm had focal sharp waves more often than those without generalized spike-waves and/or theta rhythm. The authors concluded that 'the phenotypic expression of the genetic anomaly underlying focal sharp waves shows considerable variability. The clinical and EEG findings are in agreement with a multifactorial pathogenesis of epilepsies with "benign" focal epileptiform sharp waves.'

The lack of specificity of these EEG based studies may be indicated by the results of a careful PhD thesis of Eva Andermann (1972)[32] in Montreal (cited by Newmark and Penry).[567] She studied 315 relatives of 60 probands with intractable surgically treated temporal lobe epilepsy who had an anterior temporal focus. Generalized spike-wave discharges occurred in 35 (11 per cent) and focal epileptiform abnormality in 47 (15 per cent) of relatives. Five per cent of the relatives had seizures. There was a peak incidence of 33 per cent epileptiform discharges in relatives in the age group 5–15 years. However, a high incidence of epileptiform abnormalities and seizures was also found in the relatives of a control group (12 per cent) with 4 per cent of the control siblings also having seizures.

Kajitani *et al.* 1981,[430]1992[429] have stressed the frequent association of febrile convulsions and RS and suggested that there is a genetic link between them.

Finally, Eeg-Olofsson *et al.*[261] investigated the occurrence of human leukocyte (HLA) antigens and haplotypes in 21 children with RS and in their parents and siblings. In families with more than one affected child the distribution of shared haplotypes suggested a dominant inheritance. There was also a statistically significant low incidence of the haplotype Al,B8 in both probands and parents. This finding enabled Eeg-Olofsson[258] to hypothesize 'that a lack of HLA haplotype Al,B8 may be the expression of a genetically determined immune defect resulting hypothetically in a viral persistence'.[258] In another study of patients with intractable partial epilepsies, Eeg-Olofsson *et al.*[259] found that onset of seizures was frequently related to a history of febrile illness and that patients had low incidence or absence of haplotype Al,B8.[259] These findings together with some immunological findings led the authors to support the possibility that focal epilepsy (including RS) may be linked to a genetically dependent immune dysregulation which may in turn contribute to 'the variability underlying the multifactorial inheritance of the epilepsies'.[259] There may be too many assumptions in this theory.

In the molecular genetic front, Rees *et al.*[673] have excluded linkage to the fragile X region in six pedigrees with probands with RS, Whitehouse *et al.*[802] to the HLA region on chromosome 6p in 11 families of probands with RS and one or more first degree relatives with centrotemporal spikes, and Neubauer *et al.*[566] to EBN1 (chromosome 20) and EBN2 (chromosome 8) of benign neonatal familial convulsions in 12 families with RS probands having one or more relatives with CTS in the EEG with or without RS. The results of Neubauer *et al.*[565] with 'typical and atypical families' with RS are recently reported.[565a] (see next page 55).

In my clinical, not genetic, studies of 72 children with RS there were two siblings and a father/daughter pair suffering from the same clinical condition with RS. This accords with the experience of W. Whitehouse who was only able to ascertain two families each with a sibling pair with RS from over 400 families with probable or definite familial epilepsies (personal communication).

In conclusion, though it appears that relatives of children with RS have a high incidence of EEG 'epileptiform abnormalities, generalized, focal or both' (not necessarily centrotemporal spikes), and probably Rolandic seizures, the genetics of RS and the benign childhood seizure susceptibility syndrome are largely unknown.

Centrotemporal spikes in families with Rolandic epilepsy: linkage to chromosome 15q14

A major breakthrough in the genetics of centrotemporal spikes and Rolandic seizures was reported by Neubauer and associates in the December issue of *Neurology*[565a] while this book was in press. In a well performed study they found evidence of linkage to chromosome 15q14.

They studied 22 nuclear families with 54 members having centrotemporal spikes, 43 of these also with Rolandic seizures and 11 without seizures. They conducted a DNA linkage study screening all chromosomal regions known to harbour neuronal nicotinic acetylcholine receptors (ACHR) subunit genes. In an 'affected-only' study, best P values and lod scores were found in an 8-cM interval spanning D15S165, D15S1010 and D15S1007 on chromosome 15q14 encompassing the 7-cM region where the alpha 7 subunit gene of the ACHR is localized. The nonparametric linkage score calculated by GENEHUNTER, which does not allow for heterogeneity, produced a Z(all) score of 3.33 (nominal P value 0.0005). Best parametric results were obtained under an autosomal recessive model with heterogeneity (multipoint lod score 3.56 with 70 per cent of families linked to the locus). For autosomal dominant inheritance a maximum multipoint lod score with heterogeneity of 2.15 with 66 per cent of the families linked to the locus was obtained. In one family the affected siblings did not share a single haplotype and therefore they were unlinked to this locus regardless of the mode of inheritance, providing strong proof of heterogeneity.

It is interesting that in another recent study by Elmslie *et al.*, 1997[264a] linkage with heterogeneity was found for juvenile myoclonic epilepsy at a similar location 'encompassing the region in which the gene encoding the alpha 7 subunit of nAChR (CHRNA7) maps on chromosome 15q14 (HLOD = 4.4 at alpha = 0.65; Z(all) = 2.94, P = 0.0005)'.

In order to explain these similar results for a benign partial childhood seizure/EEG syndrome and a life long persisting idiopathic generalized epilepsy, Neubauer *et al.*[565a] stated: 'Data provided by both studies do not allow a precise localisation of the linked locus ... Amazingly, the alpha 7 ACHR subunit was mapped convincingly in individuals with a familial reduced inhibition of cortical responses to repeated auditory stimuli (P50 auditory evoked response) ... Although these results are currently difficult to interpret, it is remarkable that the same candidate approach results in the detection of linkage at the same chromosomal area in a generalized as well as in a partial common idiopathic epilepsy syndrome. Several possibilities are conceivable. Closely neighbouring but different genes could be responsible for either phenotype. Different disease-specific mutations in one gene might account for different phenotypes. Defects in the same gene not associated with a specific phenotype but influencing cortical excitability in a general sense seems a third possibility. Mutational analysis of the alpha 7 ACHR subunit gene in all three phenotypes is now required to clarify these questions. This might be of potential importance because this receptor type can be influenced by pharmacologic agents.'[565a]

Having contributed to the study of JME by Elmslie *et al.*, 1997[264a] with a large family that had three first cousins affected by JME, I am in a position to confirm that none of the JME or other members had Rolandic seizures.

Neuropsychological aspects of Rolandic seizures

The general view is that children with RS are no different from other normal children regarding intelligence, school performance, behaviour and development. This is also my view. However, special neuropsychological testing may show some mild EEG-related abnormalities. Their practical significance is presently unclear.

Piccirilli, D'Alessandro *et al.* from Perugia, Italy in a number of well performed and longitudinal studies[185,654,655] have found mild neuropsychological impairment in children with RS only during the active period of EEG centrotemporal spikes. In all their studies patients met strict criteria for idiopathic RS and were free of seizures and off medication for at least 6 months prior to the testing.

In their first report Piccirilli *et al.*,1988[655] used a dual task procedure to assess language lateralization in 22 right handed children with RS. Sample test selection included factors believed to influence both the mental capabilities and functional cerebral organization. RS patients with a right hemispheric focus showed left language lateralization as expected. Conversely, those with a left CTS focus showed a different pattern of functional representation (modified hemispheric specialization) suggesting right hemisphere involvement in their language mechanisms. These results of an interhemispheric prevalence pattern related to the focus site, suggested that focal epileptic activity can alter the cerebral mechanisms underlying cognitive functions.

D'Alessandro *et al.* (1990)[185]investigated with an extensive neuropsychological battery 44 children with RS and matched controls. Three subgroups of RS patients were assigned depending on EEG focus, right, left or bilateral. There were small differences in cognitive performance mainly on tests of attention and visuomotor skills between the whole group and the controls. Among the subgroups, those with bilateral CTS score worst; those with right did better than those with left CTS focus. A follow-up assessment of 13 patients showed that the neuropsychological abnormalities had disappeared as had the seizures and the EEG CTS. They concluded that the paroxysmal cortical activity of CTS was sufficient to cause cognitive dysfunction.[185]

Piccirilli and colleagues (1994)[654] assessed the impact of CTS lateralization on attention mechanisms and abilities in processing visuospatial information in 43 children with RS. Children with right sided CTS focus did not score well. There were no differences between those with left CTS and control subjects.

Binnie and co-workers, 1992[115] reported that children with RS show transitory cognitive impairment (TCI) during interictal CTS. This was a study of eight patients with CTS but as the authors admitted 'it cannot be claimed that the patients studied are a typical unselected sample of subjects with RS'. Behavioural or cognitive problems were reported in most of these children.

The psychological test employed to detect TCI was that described by Aarts *et al.* (1984)[2] and consisted of a test of short-term memory for spatial material presented in the form of a video game. All subjects with typical RS exhibited a trend, the error rate being substantially higher in those trials accompanied by EEG discharge. This association was significant in four instances (in two others a strong trend failed to reach significance, but the number of discharges captured was small). The two children who showed morphologically typical Rolandic spikes without the typical syndrome of RS manifested no such effect.

The authors[115]stated that 'The conclusions which can be drawn from this necessarily selected series are clearly limited. It is probable that in some patients psychosocial problems led to referral in the first instance, or were a factor determining the parents' willingness to allow their children to undergo further investigation. Obviously, one can adopt the position that patients with RS by definition do not exhibit cognitive deficits and therefore none of the present subjects exhibited that syndrome. This is not an approach likely to enhance understanding of the condition. These subjects in the present series regarded as having RS were typical in all respects except the presence, in some, of cognitive or behavioural problems. The present findings leave no doubt that Rolandic spikes in association with the typical seizure pattern and clinical evolution of RS may be accompanied by transient cognitive impairment. As the discharges of benign epilepsy with centrotemporal spikes occur so frequently, it might be expected that in this condition TCI would be likely to have an adverse effect on psychosocial function. It is therefore of interest that, although otherwise clinically typical, all those children in the present series who showed TCI did appear to have some form of behavioural or cognitive difficulties. Clearly, further investigations are required of a better unselected series of newly diagnosed children with RS.'[115]

In a more recent study of the same group[665] less typical cases of RS than in their previous report were tested for TCI during EEG recording using a short-time memory test (N-Grams). These were three children with RS, three with atypical benign partial epilepsy and two with epilepsy of childhood with occipital paroxysms. Their age was from 7 to 13 years with frequent subclinical epileptiform discharges. In addition psychosocial function was evaluated by means of the Conner rating scales and compared with eight matched children with idiopathic generalized epilepsy. TCI was diagnosed in a patient if error rate during discharges was significantly higher during trials with discharges compared to trials without discharges. They found TCI in two of the three patients with RS, three out of three with atypical benign partial epilepsy and one out of two with epilepsy of childhood with occipital paroxysms. They stated that: 'comparing the Conner rating scales of the two groups, children with benign partial epilepsy have significantly more behavioural problems than the group of children with idiopathic generalized epilepsy showing no or only few discharges. Our data suggests that TCI may have implications for the cognitive development and psychosocial function of children with benign partial epilepsy.' However, these eight children with three having atypical benign partial epilepsy can hardly be considered as representing the vast majority of RS and the comparison with 'idiopathic generalized epilepsy showing no or only few discharges' may be biased. Binnie[114,117] believes that 'it may be possible to treat TCI by antiepileptic drugs' but this view would need better documentation and consideration. It should also take into account the fact that both carbamazepine[149] and lamotrigine[152]can exaggerate seizures in children with RS in addition to other physical and neuropsychological adverse reactions that they may have. Furthermore, it is also known that if neuropsychological disturbances exist in children with CTS, these are mild, only detected with appropriate testing and they are fully reversible.

More recently, Weglage *et al.* (1997) reported that neuropsychological, intellectual and behavioural deficits in 40 children with CTS with or without seizures. Also, Staden *et al.* (1998) reported that 13 of 20 children with Rolandic seizures showed language dysfunction with difficulties in two or more of twelve standardized language tests.

Prognosis

Seizure prognosis

The prognosis of RS is unquestionably excellent as it is well documented in all relevant studies[48,89,127,216,225,328,455,483,503,504,507,541,542,652,721,748] with some authors having followed up their patients for 10–30 years. These include Beaussart[89] who reported on 154 subjects over 13 years of age, Blom and Heijbel[127] who re-investigated 37 of their 40 patients 13–27 years after their first seizure, De Romanis *et al.*[216] with 16 years follow-up of 150 children with RS and Loiseau *et al.*[504] with follow-up after the age of 20 years of 168 patients.

The consensus from these long-term studies is that 10–20 per cent of these children may have one seizure only and 60–70 per cent may have 2–10 RS only. In the remaining 10–20 per cent seizures may be more frequent but in all they remit usually within 1–3 years from onset and patients are free of seizures after the age of 15–16 years without medication.

Rolandic seizures do not relapse in adult life. There is only one case report for such an instance.[27] Less than 2 per cent of patients with RS may develop long after remission of RS infrequent generalized tonic–clonic seizures. Amongst my 72 patients with RS only a girl developed, long after remission of RS, phantom absences and infrequent GTCS which are entirely controlled with small doses of sodium valproate. These are isolated cases, not more than 2 per cent, which cannot cast doubt on the benign character of RS. Rolandic seizures are certainly of better prognosis than febrile convulsions where 4 per cent of the children will later develop afebrile seizures.

Beaussart (1981)[89] reported the outcome of 154 patients over 13 years of age; 87 were older that 20 years. Only five had seizures after remission of RS. Three had GTCS in their late teens without recurrences in the next 3–13 years. One had four GTCS between 17–19 years of age and the last patient

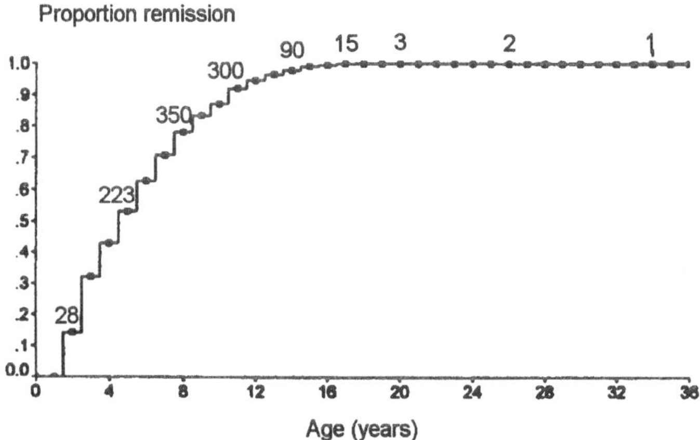

Fig 4.3. Remission from Rolandic seizures by age. Numbers in the figure represent the number of patients in the analysis. Life table calculation is described in the methods and results section of Bouma et al.[136] *The actuarial remission at 18 years was 0.9970.*
[From Bouma et al., Neurology 1997;48: 430–437 with permission of the authors and the editor].

had three secondary GTCS at age 17. Treatment was not resumed in three cases which had not had another seizure for 11, 13 and 2 years, respectively. All patients showed a good social adaptation.

Blom and Heijbel (1982)[127] re-investigated 37 of 40 patients with RS 10 years after their initial publication[128] and 13–27 years (mean, 21 years) after the first Rolandic seizure. Present age was 26–34 years (mean, 29 years). Thirty-six patients had been seizure free for 14–23 years (mean, 18.5 years) and 32 were off medication for 5–22 years (mean, 18.5 years). No epileptic discharges were found in 24 patients who had a new EEG. Only one patient, a 34-year-old man, reported two generalized seizures 'in connection with alcohol abuse'.

Loiseau *et al.* (1988)[504] re-investigated 168 of 268 patients with RS, born between 1941 and 1967. All but three patients were seizure-free with follow-up ranging from 7 to 30 years. Of the three patients with subsequent seizures, one had an isolated post-partum diurnal GTCS at age 34 years, another had an isolated GTCS at age 18 years and the last patient had at age 22 years 'two versive secondary GTCS on the same day during emotional stress' with 'diffuse and erratic EEG sharp waves'. The authors concluded that 'the occurrence of such seizures after recovery from RS is a rare event (approximately 2 per cent of cases) and a relapse with partial seizures is quite uncommon. These patients do not differ from patients remaining seizure-free'.

Partial seizures are extremely rare after remission of RS.[27,89,504] This highly exceptional situation can not be attributed to 'ischaemic cortical lesions sustained during a prolonged seizure in the past' which was hypothesized by Lerman.[482] The only case of Rolandic seizures re-appearing in adult life has been reported by Ambrosetto *et al.*, 1985.[27] This was a 30-year-old man who after an 8-year seizure-free period started having at age 21 partial motor seizures with or without secondary GTCS and an EEG centrotemporal focus.[27]

Bouma and colleagues (1997)[136] in a meta-analysis of 20 reports of 13 cohorts, comprising a total of 794 patients with RS, confirmed the extremely favourable outcome of RS (Fig. 4.3). They found that the mean duration of the active seizure disorder was less than 3 years. Remission occurs in 50 per cent by the age of 6 years, 92 per cent by the age of 12 and 99.8 per cent by age 18. There is a steep peak of remission (last seizure) at age 13 years. For most, the last seizure occurred at age 13 years. These authors[136] also stated that 'The clinical characteristics of the patients who had ongoing seizures at the end of the studies may suggest that the outcome of RS is always perfect – 100 per cent remission;

because 15 of the 18 patients who were still having seizures had mean ages of 10 to 11 years at the end of follow-up, and may have reached remission at an older age. This is reflected in the results of the Kurtzke survival analysis: this method implies correction for patients in whom follow-up ended while not being seizure free; hence, the proportion seizure free at older age is higher than the actual proportion. The other three patients may have suffered from seizures unrelated to RS; one patient had alcohol related seizures and two other patients had seizures at older age (one at the age of 34 in puerperium, another one had one isolated generalized seizure at the age of 18 years under circumstances of emotional stress), who remained seizure free afterward.'

Loiseau *et al.*[504] and other authors[541,721,748] have found that early onset RS, before the age of 4 years, herald significantly longer active disease periods and a RS at age 6 years may be a single one. This is contrary to the work of Nishiura and Miyazaki, 1975[580] who based on only 20 patients concluded that RS with onset between 4 and 9 years produced attacks for longer periods than those before three and after 10 years.

The presence of convulsive generalized seizures as the sole ictal manifestation is considered as a predictor of infrequent seizures in one[24] but not in another study.[504] Longer average interval between first and second seizure may also be associated with infrequent seizures.[24]

Developmental and social prognosis

Development, social adaptation and occupation of adults with a previous history of RS appears to be normal in the studies of Beaussart, 1981,[89] Blom and Heijbel,1982[127]and Loiseau *et al.*, 1988.[504] According to Blom and Heijbel,1982[127] the only problem was with five patients who had difficulties in obtaining their driving licence and one patient who despite a 15-year seizure-free period was still on phenytoin because of concerns of her physician regarding her driving licence. Loiseau *et al.*[504] found that 'for unknown reasons' social levels seems to be even higher than for non-epileptic control.

Treatment

Starting medication

Children with RS may not need anti-epileptic medication, particularly if the seizures are infrequent, mild, nocturnal or onset is close to the age of natural remission of this age-limited disorder.

In deciding management for a child with RS the following should be considered:

(a) Ten to twenty per cent of patients may have only a single seizure and in another 60–70 per cent seizures may be infrequent, usually 2–10. Some children may have only brief simple partial seizures without secondary generalized convulsions. Most of the fits are nocturnal and may not endanger the child. However, 10–20 per cent of patients may have frequent seizures, sometimes resistant to treatment.

(b) Remission of RS is expected in all patients.

(c) There is no evidence that untreated children have a worse long-term prognosis though they may be unprotected for seizure occurrences.

(d) Some children become frightened even by simple partial seizures and some parents despite firm re-assurances are unable to cope with the possibility of another fit.

(e) Persistence and frequency of EEG centrotemporal spikes are not predictive of clinical severity, frequency and degree of liability to seizures.

Short- and long-term treatment strategies of RS are empirical. I am not aware of any control drug trials or prospective treatment studies in RS. In the meta-analysis of Bouma *et al.* (1997)[136] 81.6 per cent of 794 children with RS received treatment: 'phenytoin, barbiturates, valproate, carbamazepine and clonazepam all had the same result; as in patients who never received medication, virtually all became seizure free. The indication to start medication seems not to have a firm basis; when seizures are infrequent and exclusively nocturnal, drugs are often not considered necessary. If the seizures are frequent, especially if they occur during waking hours, antiepileptic medication can be prescribed.' Relapses after drug withdrawal occurred in 14.2 per cent of patients.[128,136,216,541]

De Romanis *et al.* (1986)[216] followed-up for 16 years 150 children with RS. Anti-epileptic drugs were withdrawn after an initial 2 years' period of treatment. Only 29 patients relapsed within 6–12 months from drug withdrawal and these received treatment for a further 5 years. No seizures occurred after the age of 14 or in the 8 years following final discontinuation of drug therapy.

Ambrosetto and Tassinari (1990)[26] found that seizure frequency, seizure recurrence, active seizure period and social adjustment were similar in a small sample of 10 untreated and 20 treated patients with RS that were studied retrospectively.

In accordance with the present practice in paediatrics, treatment is not recommended after a first, convulsive or non convulsive, seizure. This is particularly sensible for RS, partial, with or without secondary generalization, as the first seizure may be an isolated event for 10–20 per cent of these children. Treatment may also not be needed after a second seizure as this also may be the last one irrespective of whether it occurred soon or long after the first one (see illustrative cases) though a shorter interval between them may be a predictor of more seizures.[662]

Though short- and long-term treatment practices vary amongst experts, they all agree on the following:

(a) There is no need for medication after the first seizure and probably the second. I would add that not only the number but also the type and timing of seizures are important regarding these decisions. Some children tend to have only brief simple partial seizures and these may cluster in a short period of time without secondary hemi or generalized convulsions.

(b) If treatment is considered necessary, either because of repeated seizures or the wish of the parents, this should be monotherapy with the least possible side-effects. Most patients respond well to a low dose of a single drug[797] and this should be taken after dinner in nocturnal seizures. It should be remembered that many children have their RS soon, within an hour, after going to sleep.

(c) The drug of choice for the majority of experts is carbamazepine but this is again empirical and anecdotal. Furthermore, all anti-epileptic drugs, phenobarbitone, phenytoin, sodium valproate, clobazam and clonazepam, appear to be equally effective. Ten per cent of children may not be able to withstand carbamazepine because of skin rash but otherwise this is well tolerated particularly if titration is slow and dose moderate. Known side-effects of other drugs, such as impairment of concentration and behavioural problems with phenobarbitone, cosmetic problems with phenytoin, problems of overweight with sodium valproate, and sedative effects with diazepines, may be avoided in RS which requires small doses and treatment for a few (usually two) years only. In the well cited and influential report by Lerman and Kivity, 1975[483] of 100 patients who all did well, most were treated with phenytoin or phenobarbitone and only one received carbamazepine. 'Complete seizure control was usually achieved with moderate doses of phenytoin' in a single bed time dose.[483] Doose *et al.*[242] and Lermann[482] have reported that resistant cases of RS may respond well to sulthiame. New anti-epileptic drugs may not be needed and there is a report of worsening of seizures after lamotrigine.[152] Physicians should be aware of the remote possibility that carbamazepine, in therapeutic target range, may induce in RS a new type of fit such as absences, absence status, atonic and myoclonic jerks with an exaggeration of EEG abnormalities that tend to become generalized.[149,230,406,752] These carbamazepine-induced clinico-EEG features imitate atypical benign childhood epilepsy.[149] I have seen a similar case and this is described in Chapter 17, case 17.3, page 358. Non-epileptic myoclonic jerks and tic-like movements (sniffing, coughing or sighing) are also induced by carbamazepine.[11,754] Also, the first of the three cases reported by Deonna *et al.*[227] with 'speech and oromotor deficits of epileptic origin' was probably due to carbamazepine.

(d) In all cases the parents and often the child, if old enough, should be involved in the treatment decision-process, having been informed thoroughly of all facts regarding RS and medication.

(e) The good old rule that drug treatment is for 'clinical and not EEG manifestations' equally applies to RS or normal children with EEG centrotemporal spikes. However and despite existing evidence to the contrary, I should confess that in the past, I was influenced by an EEG showing nearly continuous bilateral CTS which were also seen in other locations together with giant somatosensory evoked spikes. In these cases, I advised the use or continuation of anti-epileptic medication. In most of the cases I was wrong, as indicated by the good outcome of those who did not follow my recommendations, either at the initiative of their parents or of the referring paediatricians.

Stopping medication

Regarding withdrawal of medication, practices differ amongst experts, though they all agree that there is no need to continue medication after the age of 14 years when the majority of RS remit, or 16 years when RS practically do not exist. Thus, length of treatment depends on age at onset. Aicardi[15] and Lerman[482] recommend withdrawal of medication 1–2 years after the last seizure while Loiseau[496] and Luders *et al.*[512] are in favour of continuing medication until the age of 14–16 years 'at least in psychologically fragile patients'.[496] Luders *et al.*[512] are also of the view that 'patients who have been seizure-free for 3 years and have a normal awake and complete sleep EEG should have the anticonvulsants slowly discontinued' because centrotemporal spikes 'as a function of age follows closely the corresponding curve for seizure occurrence'. However, this view contradicts the fact that EEG abnormalities are not of predictive value in RS.

My practice is to start gradual withdrawal of medication 2 years after the last seizure, making sure that the child does not have any minor partial seizures of which the parents may be unaware. However, I do not adhere to fixed rules and may continue medication until the age of 13–15 years depending on the severity, frequency and age at onset of seizures. Thus, in a child who had frequent, severe and difficult to control convulsive fits in early childhood, I would not stop medication if there is a 2–3-year seizure-free period by age 7 years with AED. Conversely, for a child who had three to four nocturnal seizures at age 11 and 12 years I would certainly slowly discontinue medication after a 2-year seizure-free period. I advise very slow withdrawal at monthly steps of reduction so as the drug is completely discontinued approximately 6 months later. The reason for this is that I expect that possible seizure recurrence during the process of very slow drug discontinuation would manifest with mild, brief and simple partial seizures without secondary generalized convulsions. In the case of barbiturates and diazepines, slowly stopping medication is mandatory in order to avoid risking a possible withdrawal seizure.

Personal experience and illustrative cases

The following three cases are amongst the last patients with RS that I saw before completing this book. Younger colleagues may be interested in my approach and I quote from my medical reports.

The first patient illustrates the problems that such patients even today may experience because of mismanagement. This also illustrates that EEGs may become worse despite treatment and despite freedom of seizures.

Case 4.1. Z, born 2.4.1982, is a girl that I saw in 1995. 'She was born and developed normal. She is good at school and from what I can gather from my conversations with her, a very sensible, intelligent, well behaving and mature girl. She has a 19-year-old brother who is well.'

There is no family history of epileptic seizures but a maternal niece was having 'fainting tendencies' at around the age of 8 years.

Z had one single seizure in her life at age 8 years. She was asleep. Her father heard her as if she was crying and she was moving under the blanket. He lifted her in the sitting position. Z was trying to speak but only noises came out of her mouth 'as if her tongue was tied'. She was probably having oropharyngolaryngeal movements. There was little salivation. She was not unconscious. Left sided convulsions of the eyes, mouth and hand followed. She recovered within 3–4 min. She was well afterwards. Z has clear recollection of the first part of this event. She is adamantly clear that she was able to understand but could not speak.

She was seen by a neurologist who did an EEG and advised treatment with sodium valproate and phenobarbitone because 'the EEG was highly epileptogenic'. One year later, EEG got worse and sodium valproate was replaced with carbamazepine 600 mg added to phenobarbitone 50 mg nocte. This treatment continues today, 5 years after a single benign seizure.

All her annual EEGs are lost. In a recent report of a normal EEG there is a note saying: 'Previous EEG from 1990 showed paroxysmal epileptic-type abnormalities with left sided preponderance'.

There is no much doubt in my mind that Z's episode in 1990 was a Rolandic seizure. Her annual EEGs were worse and this is probably the reason for changing medication.

I explained all this to her and her parents. I told her that she is not epileptic. There are some children who have an age-related susceptibility to seizures. This is now past. Her chances of having seizures in the future is no more than 2 per cent. These are well established facts.

I told her to start gradual withdrawing of phenobarbitone 10 mg every month. Then Tegretol should stop at steps of 100 mg per month. I am overcautious because I do not wish to have a withdrawal seizure.

Z and her parents have to forget the event of 1990. She is an entirely normal child who will do well in her life.

Treatment was withdrawn, no further seizures occurred. She is now age 18, off medication and prepares for the University entry exams. She and her parents know that she does not have epilepsy.

The next case is a good description of RS; seizures may not be entirely stereotyped and there may be post-ictal dysarthria.

Case 4.2.: A was born 3.12.84 and developed well. She has a younger brother. Her father, a successful lower businessman, suffers from well controlled temporal lobe seizures due to a congenital cystic lesion of the right temporal lobe.

What was of concern to her parents is that on the 26 July 1996, she had a nocturnal episode described below. This occurred after a tiring day at school and for the whole day she was complaining of headaches, dizziness and pain in her stomach. In the night she watched on TV the funeral of a popular politician and she read a rather scary book by Jane Ayer.

Fifteen to 30 min after she went to sleep, she woke up: "I was scared, I had headache, my right hand was numb and stiff. My mouth opened and I could not speak although I knew what I wanted to say. I wanted to say I can not speak. At the same time it was as if somebody was strangulating me'. She went to her mother and lost consciousness without convulsions. The whole episode lasted for no more than 1 min. She was well but scared afterwards. She stayed awake for one to two hours before she went to bed again.

I was informed about this first episode by her parents over the phone. I thought that this was a Rolandic seizure. I asked them to have an EEG, which her parents told me over the phone was reported as normal. It was not. It was recorded on 27.7.66 and showed high amplitude sharp waves localized over the left centrotemporal regions. She also had an MRI which is of good quality and is normal.

The second episode occurred during a siesta on 5 August 1996. Again this happened within the first quarter of an hour after she went to sleep. Her mother was around and she was able to describe everything well. A opened her mouth but she could not speak. It was as if somebody was strangulating her. She then became stiff and started falling to one side. At this stage, she lost consciousness and she was crying 'ah ah ah' and jerked two or three times. She became blue. The whole episode lasted for approximately 2 min.

On both occasions, she was fine post ictally but her tongue felt tangled and her speech was slightly dysarthric. She was not dysphasic.

In both episodes, there was no excessive salivation but only slight dribbling.

Her parents called me the same day and I advised them to start medication with Tegretol 100 mg bd. Since then, A has been well.

Retrospectively in the last six months, she may have become slightly agitated.

Neurological examination was normal.

1997. Two more episodes occurred, September and December 1996 within the first 10 min of her sleep. The first one occurred in the car and was of short duration. The parents heard a voice like 'Ah, Ah, Ah', A is trying to speak but is unable to do so. Her eyes flutter and turn to one direction, probably to the right.

There is a little bit of saliva coming from one side of her mouth. She looks as if she is smiling and subsequently she may have lost consciousness for a few seconds. Immediately, after this, she is fine with the exception that her speech is still dysarthric. post-ictal dysarthria sometimes is so intense that the parents are not able to understand what she wants to say.

After the second episode Tegretol was increased to 5 ml (100 mg) mane and 10 ml (200 mg) nocte. Since then she has been well.

EEG demonstrated left sided centrotemporal spikes (Fig. 4.1).

I saw her again in July 1998. She had had no other seizures, she behaves well and she is top of her class. A's new EEG continues to show centrotemporal spikes but less frequently.

The next patient is presented because her father also had RS and she may be an example of a child needing medication.

Case 4.3. D was born 13.9.87. She has two older brothers and a sister who are well. Her father (case 4.4) had between age 10–12 years three nocturnal seizures. An EEG reported by Prof H Hopff in Vienna in 1956 demonstrated singular spikes in the 'left precentral regions'. No further seizures occurred after stopping phenobarbitone at age 15. A maternal sister had febrile convulsions.

D had her first seizure at age 6 years while asleep in the car. Her parents heard her 'as if she was sucking milk shake'. Simultaneously she woke up and tried unsuccessfully to speak. 'She was trying but her tongue was tied up in her mouth'. This was followed by right sided hemiconvulsions but within 2–3 min she was back to normal. Treatment was initiated with carbamazepine and phenobarbitone. Two similar nocturnal seizures occurred 10 months later when the mother stopped medication. EEG demonstrated bilateral centrotemporal spikes, left more active than the right, infrequent midline spikes (Cz,Pz), somatosensory evoked spikes by tapping fingers and toes (Figs 5.5 and 5.6). She continued treatment with carbamazepine alone. However, six months later medication was discontinued at the initiative of her parents and two days later D, 10 min after having a siesta, had another focal seizure with clonic movements in the right eye and mouth involving also the right hand. There was little salivation. It lasted for approximately 1 min. On recovery D said clearly that she was tired and she went to sleep again. Carbamazepine was re-established. However, two years later the dose was halved by her parents and she had a minor nocturnal focal seizure again. This occurred 10 min after she went to sleep and the seizure was witnessed from the beginning. She woke up and tried to tell her mother that she was shaking on the right side. Again, she was dysarthric and she was not able to say what she wanted. There was no excessive salivation. This lasted for seconds.

All the following cases are from 72 children that I saw in Athens mainly between 1973 and 1984 (see Chapter 13). Most of them have more than 5 years follow-up and some of them still communicate with me.

The next child is the only one in these series whose father also had RS. It also demonstrates that minor ictal events of oropharyngolaryngeal movements may occur alone and be dismissed as nightmares.

Case 4.5. This boy had two seizures in the same night at age 9 years. The first occurred at 2 a.m. The parents heard him making strange noises 'like roaring' but when they reached his bedroom they found him asleep. They thought that he had a nightmare. However, 6 h later they heard him making the same noises which progressed to right sided hemiconvulsions. EEG showed bilateral centrotemporal spikes. His father also had two similar nocturnal seizures at age 8–9 years old.

Two of the 72 patients with RS were siblings, brother and sister. They are also presented to demonstrate that the first awake EEG may not show CTS.

Case 4.6 and 4.7 are sister and brother. The girl had at age 7 a nocturnal probably secondary generalized convulsion. Another convulsive seizure preceded by arrest of speech occurred the next year before going to sleep. Her EEG showed consistently for 3 years high amplitude frequent clusters of centrotemporal spikes that were mainly or exclusively left sided. No further seizures occurred in the next 5 years of follow-up.

Her brother, 3 years younger, had at age 6 years two brief diurnal seizures in 2 days. These consisted of tonic deviation of the mouth to the right for less than 30 s. His first EEG 3 weeks after the seizures showed some non-specific slow waves but all three subsequent annual EEGs showed consistently high amplitude clusters of mid-temporal spikes on the right. No further seizures occurred in the next 3 years.

Hemifacial convulsions may be entirely localized in the corner of the mouth or eye and mouth, with or without progressing to hemiconvulsions of the upper and occasionally of the lower limb. They may be brief for seconds but may also be prolonged (partial status epilepticus) as demonstrated by the following cases.

The next case is to illustrate brief diurnal hemifacial clonic seizures.

Case 4.8. This boy had at age 10 years within 3 weeks two brief seizures while watching television. They were stereotyped with right sided mouth and eye clonic movements for less than 1 min. His first EEG showed rare left centrotemporal spikes. EEG in the next two years deteriorated with frequent clusters of high amplitude centrotemporal spikes, right more active than left. EEG normalized at age 13 years. He took carbamazepine for 3 years. No further seizures occurred in the next 6 years of follow-up.

Similar mild hemifacial convulsions may also occur during night sleep or a siesta. It is surprising how frequently the first Rolandic seizure is observed during short trips while the child is asleep in the family car as illustrated with the following case. This may also indicate that these children have had more seizures which were not observed.

Case 4.9. This 16-year-old girl had her first seizure while asleep in the family car at age 10. Her parents described her having clonic convulsions of the left side of the face lasting for 1 min. She did not awake from sleep. A similar brief episode occurred 3 months later in the hypnagogic phase of sleep. The first EEG showed centrotemporal spikes on the right. Subsequent annual EEG were either normal or showed small amplitude spikes or sharp waves in the central electrodes bilaterally. No further seizures occurred on cyclohexyl-2-methylamino-propranol-phenylethyl barbiturate 50 mg nocte for 3 years from onset.

Hemifacial seizures may come into infrequent clusters and initial EEG may be normal.

Case 4.10. This 11-year-old boy had at age 7 years, within 6 months, two clusters of four to six hemifacial seizures for two days each. These consisted of left sided clonic movements of the left corner of the mouth associated with speech arrest but no other symptoms. Their duration was seconds 'for as long as to walk 9 m' he said. All annual awake EEG from age 7 were normal except an EEG at age 9 years which showed right mid-temporal spikes. He was treated with carbamazepine for 3 years with no further seizures after drug discontinuation.

On other occasions hemifacial convulsions may occur alone or progress to hemiconvulsions of the upper and less frequently of the lower extremity.

Case 4.11. This 15-year-old daughter of a physician had her first seizure at age 7 while asleep. She opened her eyes and had clonic convulsions of the left side of the mouth for a minute. Three weeks later a similar nocturnal episode occurred and progressed to clonic convulsions of the left arm. This lasted for 2 min and she became incontinent. On recovery she had a right sided headache. She was treated with cyclohexyl-2-methylamino-propranol-phenylethyl barbiturate 50 mg daily but had another three rather minor left hemifacial convulsions occasionally also involving the arm in the next 2 years. Annual EEG consistently showed right centrotemporal spikes that disappeared at age 12 years.

Case 4.12. This 12-year-old girl had aged 8 years, 5 min after going to sleep, left sided convulsions of head, arm and leg lasting for 2 min. EEG showed frequent bilateral centrotemporal spikes with the left more active. EEG got worse in the next 2 years before normalizing at age 12. No further seizures occurred while on carbamazepine for 3 years.

Some children may always have the same sequence from hemiconvulsions to secondary GTCS.

Case 4.13. This 17-year-old boy had from age 9 to 13 years random nocturnal secondary GTCS. They all occurred within the first 5–10 min of sleep and are stereotyped. He suddenly opens his eyes with clonic convulsions of the right eyelid rapidly spreading to the ipsilateral corner of the mouth, right upper and lower limbs and within 1 min secondary GTCS. He was allergic to carbamazepine, phenytoin and phenobarbitone. The last four seizures occurred while on sodium valproate. No further seizures occurred after the age of 13 despite stopping medication at 15. EEG showed centrotemporal spikes that were on the right at age 9 and left at age 13. All subsequent EEG showed non specific abnormalities of slow waves and finally normalized at age 17.

The EEG lateralization may not be concordant with the seizure side.

Case 4.14. This 11-year-old boy had a seizure whilst watching television at age 7. Suddenly his mouth pulled tonically to the left and became full of saliva that was running out. He became very scared and asked his mother with a dysarthric speech 'what is wrong mummy?'. His eyes became vacant and he subsequently developed brief left sided hemiclonic convulsions. He did not lose consciousness. He recovered within 1 min. A similar event occurred 2 weeks later but this was brief manifesting only with initial symptoms of the previous seizure. An EEG had frequent high amplitude left centrotemporal spikes. He did not have any more seizures; he was an excellent student but he had developed a compulsive neurosis.

Hemiconvulsions may be followed by post-ictal Todd's hemiparesis.

Case 4.15. This 7-year-old boy had a nocturnal left hemiconvulsion lasting for 3 min and followed by post-ictal ipsilateral hemiparesis for 10–15 min. An EEG showed bilateral centrotemporal spikes. No treatment was prescribed. He did not return for review.

Hemifacial clonic status which is rare, is demonstrated by the next patient.

Case 4.16. This 30-year-old engineer had his first seizure aged 11. He had just fallen asleep when he was awakened by numbness in his mouth, his tongue was tightened and he was unable to speak for 1 min after which he went back to sleep. The next year he had two brief similar nocturnal seizures. In one of these episodes post-ictally and briefly he could not see his mother's head or a glass in front of him. Treatment with phenobarbitone 50 mg nocte was initiated. Six months later he had a prolonged diurnal seizure after some partial sleep deprivation. While skating, he felt that the left side of his tongue was numb and that he could not see well. This within seconds was followed by repetitive and continuous left sided clonic hemifacial spasms involving mouth and eye that ended 40 min later with left hemiconvulsions. There was post-ictal Todd's paralysis. In addition he had frequent right sided headaches. Brain scan was normal but EEG showed right mid-temporal spikes that appeared only in two EEGs when aged 12 and 13 years. His first EEG, 8 days post-ictally, had shown mainly right sided slow waves. He had treatment with carbamazepine for 4 years. No further seizures and no more serious headaches occurred in the next 18 years. He does not suffer from migraine.

Some children may have a cluster of hemiconvulsions with secondary GTCS for a very short time. The following case also illustrates ictal symptoms (diplopia in this case) which are difficult to attribute to seizure events.

Case 4.17. This 14-year-old boy had at age 10 and within a month three stereotyped nocturnal seizures. In all he wakes up from numbness and clonic jerks of the right side of the mouth and right hand, unable to speak; he sees doubleand hemiconvulsions spread to the right leg. This lasts for 2–3 min. An EEG showed rare left centrotemporal spikes that disappeared 2 years later. No further seizures occurred although he took medication only for 6 months.

Some children may have both diurnal and nocturnal seizures

Case 4.18. This girl had at age 8 years her first nocturnal seizure. Her parents were alerted by roaring noises and found her unresponsive with her head raised from the pillow, eyes widely opened, 'rivers of saliva coming out of her mouth' and rigid. This lasted for 1 min. Two nights later a similar but more violent seizure occurred. An EEG showed right sided frequent and of high amplitude mid-temporal spikes. She had skin rash with carbamazepine and was treated with sodium valproate. Frequent clusters of diurnal seizures occurred for 6 months. These were not always stereotyped though hypersalivation, oropharyngolaryngeal symptoms and speech arrest were the main seizure components. Some were very mild for 10–20 s: 'I felt that air was forced in my mouth, I could not speak and I could not close my mouth. I could understand well everything said to me'. 'Other times I feel that there is food in my mouth and there is also a lot of salivation. I can not speak'. On other occasions the main symptom was hypersalivation: 'suddenly my mouth is full of saliva, it runs out like a river and I can not speak'. Once such a diurnal episode was followed by a few mild clonic jerks of the right arm and leg. In the same year she also had three nocturnal seizures with secondary generalization. Seizures improved in frequency with primidone and stopped one year later. Medication was withdrawn at age 13 years. No further seizures occurred in the next 2 years of follow-up. EEG during the active stage of her seizures showed frequent, nearly continuous, bilateral centrotemporal spikes and on one occasion an 8 s generalized discharge of synchronously occurring sharp and slow wave complexes without clinical manifestations. EEG normalized at age 12 years.

Loss of consciousness may occur without convulsions. Initial awake EEG may show excess of slow waves without CTS.

Case 4.19. This 15-year-old boy had one seizure during a siesta at age 10. His parents who were in the room heard him making noises as if he was 'having difficult, copious breath'. They tried to wake him up but he was unconscious. There were no convulsions or other movements. He gained consciousness within

2–3 min and was subsequently well. CT brain scan was normal but annual EEGs from age 10 showed frequent centrotemporal spikes initially left, later bilateral and more frequent and finally normalized at age 13. He was treated with cyclohexyl-2-methylamino-propranol-phenylethyl barbiturate for 3 years. No further seizures occurred in the last follow-up at age 15.

Case 4.20. This boy had at age 7 years, within 2 weeks, two similar seizures, one in the middle of the night sleep, the other during a siesta. On both occasions the parents were alerted by death rattle noises and chattering of the teeth. They found him unresponsive, eyes widely opened and rotated upwards to the extreme. He recovered within a minute with a smile on his face though he explained that he was not laughing. First EEGs one month later showed a significant excess of slow waves. Second EEGs one year later had frequent high amplitude right sided centrotemporal spikes which had disappeared in another EEG 2 years later. This new EEG had frequent paroxysms of high amplitude generalized theta waves intermixed with small spikes. EEGs normalized at age 14 years and no further seizures occurred.

Sometimes seizures may cluster in one night without recurrence.

Case 4.21. This 18-year-old man had two seizures at the same night at age 12 years. The first one occurred at 2 a.m. and was a brief probably secondary generalized tonic–clonic seizure. He slept afterwards but at 6.30 a.m. he was awakened by his right hand moving upwards. He could not speak but was conscious of this right hand movement. Within a minute his eyes turned to the right and he had a brief hemiconvulsion. Treatment with cyclohexyl-2-methylamino-propranol-phenylethyl barbiturate was initiated for 3 years and no further seizures occurred with or without treatment. There were some schooling problems initially which subsequently subsided. His first EEG at age 12 years showed frequent high amplitude centrotemporal spikes right more active than left. All subsequent annual EEG up to the age of 18 years did not show any centrotemporal spikes but these were frequently abnormal because of significant amounts of high amplitude slow waves, mainly posteriorly.

Younger children may have only nocturnal, probably secondary generalized convulsions.

Case 4.22. This 11-year-old boy had during the same night two nocturnal generalized convulsions at age 5. His parents were not aware of any other symptoms preceding these fits. Treatment with cyclohexyl-2-methylamino-propranol-phenylethyl barbiturate was initiated for 3 years. In annual EEG only one at age 7 years showed bilateral centrotemporal spikes. No further seizures occurred in a 6 years follow-up.

The next patient is presented because of a diurnal secondary generalized tonic–clonic seizure which according to Lerman[481] may be extremely rare.

Case 4.23. A 16-year-old boy had only one diurnal seizure in his life aged 12. He felt that his tongue moved and stuck to the top of his mouth. He wanted to pull it out with his right hand but this also became stiff and adverted. Though fully aware of the situation, he was unable to speak, saliva was coming out of his mouth and within a minute he lost consciousness with generalized convulsions. post-ictally he was confused but he became back to normal within half an hour. He received no treatment and no more seizures occurred in the next 4 years of follow-up.

Resistant cases. It is apparent in the literature review and the above illustrated cases that RS may be single, well controlled and cause no serious problem to the child and family if properly managed. However, it is also known that some children, 10–20 per cent, may be difficult to control.

Case 4.24. This 16-year-old boy had his first nocturnal seizure at age 7. He was making guttural noises, his mouth was pulled to the right and the parents thought that he was chewing his tongue. Three similar nocturnal seizures occurred in the next year and treatment with phenytoin was initiated. One year later he had a diurnal hemifacial clonic seizure involving the right eye and the right corner of his mouth. Treatment was discontinued but in the next 2 months he had another three diurnal hemifacial seizures of 1–2 min duration. Despite treatment with carbamazepine, sodium valproate and phenobarbitone alone or in combination he had numerous, sometimes five times per day, brief right hemifacial seizures lasting for a few seconds to a minute and occasionally involving the right hand. This continued until age 16 years when he, understandably disappointed, had the last follow-up with me. Two CT brain scans were normal. Development was normal. EEG from age 7 to 16 years consistently showed high amplitude and frequent clusters of bilateral centrotemporal spikes.

Finally, clinical seizures may be unusual as in the following case whose Rolandic seizures, well witnessed on several occasions from the beginning, always started with bilateral eyelid fluttering:

Case 4.25. This physically and mentally normal girl was born in Jan. 1987. Her problems started at the end of September 1992 with approximately seven to eight nocturnal seizures within one week. They all occurred within the first half an hour of her going to sleep. They started with eyelid flickering which is rapid and lasts approximately ten to fifteen seconds. This is immediately followed by an upward deviation of the head while her eyes are open and fixed with terror. She says she is trying but is unable to speak and there is a little salivation. Her body remains rigid, her colour does not change and the whole episode does not last any longer than a minute and a half. It may vary in duration and intensity.

An EEG before treatment demonstrated centrotemporal spikes independently right and left with a tremendous increase during sleep (it looks like electrical status). CT brain scan and MRI are normal.

Despite treatment with carbamazepine, she continued having stereotyped nocturnal seizures always during the first half an hour of sleep. These occurred approximately every three to four months with an exaggeration regarding frequency at age 7 when she had six seizures within a week.

She does not like school very much and is a moderate performer.

A new video EEG during alert, 3 h of natural sleep and awakening states demonstrated again bilateral centrotemporal spikes independently right and left, also evoked by contralateral finger stimuli, which became bi-synchronous and occurred nearly continuously during sleep.

Her last seizure occurred at age 8. Since then she has been well. In her last follow-up at age 11 (September 1998) she was well. No further seizures occurred. She never had any intellectual, linguistic or behavioural problems. Her EEG is qualitatively similar to the previous ones. Despite exacerbation there is no continuous spikes and waves during slow sleep.

The only case from my Athens study of 72 patients with Rolandic seizures that later developed brief phantom absences and infrequent GTCS is detailed here.

Case 4.26. This woman, born in May 1972, had from age three and a half, infrequent and brief nocturnal hemifacial Rolandic seizures with speech arrest, sometimes also involving the hand. All her seizures occurred in the first hour of sleep and the last ever hemifacial seizure occurred at age 10 years upon withdrawal of phenobarbitone. All drugs were stopped at age 15 years. Her EEG showed high amplitude, frequent centrotemporal spikes mainly on the right (Fig. 5.10). Subsequently, she was well until age 19 to 20 years when she had, within a year, two brief GTCS on awakening that were precipitated by sleep deprivation. A video-EEG at age 20 showed brief, 2–4 s, phantom absences of generalized spike/polyspike and slow wave discharges, often associated with eyelid flickering but no cognitive impairment (Fig. 5.10). In addition, there were brief runs of single sharp and slow waves, independently in the left but more frequently the right mid-temporal electrodes. I last saw her in July 1998. She was well with no GTCS or other overt seizures on sodium valproate 500 mg mane.

Appendix 1

Clinical manifestations from electrical stimulation of the inferior precentral and postcentral gyrus in man

Extracts from Penfield and Rasmussen (1957) [651]

The motor and sensory responses to electrical stimulation of the precentral and postcentral gyrus are well known and the homonculus of Penfield is illustrated in all relevant textbooks. Therefore these are not presented here. Instead as I considered that 'Rolandic arrest' and 'Rolandic vocalization' may be less known, extracts from the book of Penfield and Rasmussen are cited below.[651]

Rolandic word arrest

Patients talk quite freely during cortical stimulation except when it is carried out in sensorimotor areas devoted to word articulation or in areas of cortex related to speech. Arrest of speech was recorded 74 times in the course of 35 operations.*

The effect of such stimulation is of interest both from a physiological and a psychological point of view. The usual practice was to carry out stimulation without the patient's knowledge either while he

* *This is exclusive of the arrest of speech produced by stimulation of the superior frontal (supplementary motor) areas.*

was talking or counting. In either case he was apt to volunteer the information, after the stimulation was over, that he had wanted to speak but could not.

Speech was arrested with equal frequency from the sensorimotor area of both the dominant and nondominant hemispheres. It occurred four times more often from stimulation of the precentral gyrus than from the postcentral gyrus.

The location of the points from which speech arrest was produced was between the representation of 'throat movement' below and 'upper face' above, but there seemed to be no discrete localization within this zone. The position and extent, therefore, correspond with that of vocalization.

The effect of stimulation in these areas was either to stop speech, interrupt counting, or to slow down the speaking. It occurred as an isolated phenomenon in two thirds of the stimulations, and was associated with some lip movement in one fifth. In the remaining cases, there was accompanying sensation of tongue, mouth, nose, etc., or swallowing, or movement of eye or brow.

The results of some of the responses are described below... When quotation-marks are used the patient's own words are being employed. Associated responses, or responses additional to the arrest, are placed in parentheses.

Speech arrest from Rolandic convolutions – right side

Arrest. 'Felt as though I couldn't speak.'

Unable to talk (lips drawn to contralateral side).

Unable to speak (mouth drawn to contralateral side).

Unable to speak (mouth puckered and contralateral eye turned to ipsilateral side).

Slight stutter, 'tongue seemed to be paralysed.'

Unable to speak (lips puckered).

Arrest. There was a slurred sound of the word 'five' and clonic movement of the mouth while continuing to try to say the word. Afterward she explained, 'I could not say five.'

Unable to speak (swallowing).

Difficult to speak.

Counting stopped (twitching of lips).

Continued to count during stimulation. Afterwards he said it had been difficult. 'Something was wrong,' he 'felt strained' and had 'an indescribable sensation.'

Arrest (mouth drawn to contralateral side).

Arrest (lifting of eyebrows).

Patient stuttered during the stimulation.

Arrest. 'I was not able to answer,' (twitching of contralateral angle of mouth).

Counting slowed; 'hard to count and funny feeling in my nose.'

Arrest; 'for a second I could not speak.'

Arrest. Patient tried to speak after withdrawal of electrode and finally said, 'My mouth was paralysed.'

Speech arrest from Rolandic convolutions – left side

Arrest; 'difficulty in making my lips say yes.'

Counting stopped; after 20 to 30 s he explained he had had a tingling sensation in his tongue.

Slowness and thickness of speech (postcentral).

'Couldn't get breath or words out.'

'Something happened to my speaking.'

Arrest; movement of lips and slight sound as though trying to speak; explained he was unable to speak.

Arrest; made a little sound, then said he had been unable to speak; difficulty in continuing to speak; some involuntary lip movement.

Thickness of speech. Repeated at nearby point – speech stopped; after interval he began from beginning as though he had forgotten.

Speech slowed. He explained he seemed to lose control of his lips.

Counting slowed and then continued into vowel sound of vocalization.

Stopped counting; vocalization produced; said he was unable to 'control his vocal cords.' Repeated-stimulation stopped counting again. Stimulation repeated a second time, and this time he only slowed down.'

Vocalization

Although words and speaking are not produced by stimulation, simple vocalization may be. With extended experience in simple galvanic and faradic stimulation of the human cortex, Foerster (also Penfield) encountered no examples of clear vocalization, although there were occasional grunts or growls from stimulation of the lower end of the sensorimotor strip.

Rolandic vocalization

In 1935, while using a thyratron stimulator* on the precentral gyrus of a conscious patient, one of us (W.P.) produced a well-sustained vowel cry as follows:

Case H.My. In this case the threshold was high. There was no face or mouth movement and no associated cortical sensation. After the electrode was withdrawn following the first stimulation, the patient observed that something had made him speak. By repeated trials it was found that if stimulation was carried out until his breath was exhausted the patient stopped vocalizing, took a breath, and then continued. When he was asked to try not to make a noise, he did his best but the cry followed stimulation just the same. After having made the effort and having failed to influence the cry, he observed humorously that if he could just come around to the other side of his head so that he could get his hands on the operator he would be able to stop it.

In the case of this patient two discrete areas were found on the precentral gyrus where vocalization was produced with stimuli of minimal intensity. Each area was no more than 2 mm in diameter. The pitch of the cry was consistently somewhat different when the one area was stimulated as compared with the other.

Such vocalization is a vowel sound, a cry without words. One might consider that it resembles the cry of the infant if allowance is made for the difference in structure of the larynx of the adult which produces a heavier tone. It also resembles the cry of some epileptics at the onset of a seizure. Compared with other motor responses which follow cortical stimulation, it is quite complicated as it includes innervation of abdominal muscles, larynx, pharynx and tongue. But there is none of the interruption of expiratory movement, and no co-ordinated alteration in position of tongue, lips and jaw such as are necessary for word utterance.

Out of 51 vocalization responses which were incidental findings in a series of 206 operations (1936–1947), about three quarters of the responses came from the precentral and one quarter from the postcentral gyrus. In half of the cases vocalization was associated with some involuntary lip movement. In one quarter, it was associated with some other sensory or motor neighbourhood response, such as movement of face, jaw or tongue, or sensation in mouth, tongue, etc., or swallowing. Once only there was sensation in arm, and once there was hand movement.

In one quarter of the responses, vocalization was not complicated by any other response that

* *Friedman (1934) did report barking of a dog as the result of stimulating the motor gyrus of the cortex.*

could be detected. But the difficulty of attempting to place vocalization within the motor series may be shown as follows: When lip movement localization was determined independently as well as vocalization, lips were found to be below vocalization in nine cases, while in 18 cases the relationship was found to be reversed. When tongue localization was determined independently, vocalization was found to be below it 11 times and above it 10 times.

It seems obvious, therefore, that although vocalization may occur as an isolated response to stimulation, and consequently might be expected to have a constant sequential position in relation to lips and tongue, we are forced to conclude that its representation really overlaps that of lips, jaw and tongue movement.

This overlap is less surprising when one considers the fact that, in the case of man, word articulation is such an important function calling for simultaneous employment of tongue, lips, jaw and vocalization. Vocalization occurs with equal frequency from stimulation of the dominant and the nondominant hemispheres.'[651]

Benign Childhood Partial Seizures and Related Epileptic Syndromes. C P Panayiotopoulos
©1999 John Libbey & Company Ltd., pp. 71–100.

Chapter 5

Centrotemporal spikes and other electroencephalographic findings in children with Rolandic seizures

Interictal EEG

Introduction

Centrotemporal spikes (CTS) are the hallmark of the syndrome of benign childhood epilepsy with centrotemporal spikes (BCECTS) or Rolandic seizures (RS). They can also be encountered in other symptomatic epilepsies such as cerebral tumours, the Rett syndrome, the fragile X syndrome and cortical congenital malformations. Furthermore, CTS may incidentally be found in non-epileptic children with various symptoms such as behavioural problems, headache, mental retardation, neurological deficits, speech disturbances and in normal, non-symptomatic children.

Definitions

According to the glossary of terms most commonly used by clinical electroencephalographers of the International Federation of Societies for Electroencephalography and Clinical Neurophysiology (IFSECN) (1974)[407] spikes and sharp waves are defined as follows:

> **Sharp wave:** A transient, clearly distinguished from background activity, with pointed peak at conventional paper speeds and duration of 70–200 ms, i.e. over 1/14–1/5 s approximately. The main component is generally negative relative to other areas. Amplitude is variable.
>
> **Spike:** A transient, clearly distinguished from background activity, with pointed peak at conventional paper speeds and duration of 20 to under 70 ms, i.e. over 1/50–1/14 s approximately. The main component is generally negative relative to other areas. Amplitude is variable.
>
> Spikes and sharp waves are closely related and both can be recorded in surface and depth recordings.[570] The rising phase of the sharp waves has the same time course as of spikes but the descending phase is prolonged. However, not all sharp waves have a steeper ascending phase.
>
> I would agree with Niedermeyer[570] that 'EEG spikes should be differentiated from sharp waves, i.e. transients having similar characteristics but longer duration. However it is well to keep in mind that this distinction is largely arbitrary and serves primarily descriptive purposes.' 'It is certainly not incorrect to use the term "spike" and "sharp wave" synonymously when a local paroxysmal event is discussed, although purists of nomenclature would regard this as a breach of etiquette.' (Niedermeyer, p. 220).[570]

According to the above definition what we call centrotemporal spikes are centrotemporal sharp waves because their duration is usually more than 70 ms (Figs. 5.1 and 5.2). However, I do not think that this is of any practical importance other than a breach of etiquette.

Abbreviations

CTS = Centrotemporal spikes
ESEP = Extreme somatosensory evoked potentials or giant somatosensory evoked spikes
RS = Rolandic seizures
BCECTS = Benign childhood epilepsy with centrotemporal spikes

Synonyms of Centrotemporal spikes (CTS)

Prerolandic sharp waves[314]
Midtemporal spikes[326–330]
Rolandic sharp waves[65]
Central sharp waves[732]
Temporal-central sharp waves[140,142]
Centrotemporal sharp waves[87]
Sylvian sharp waves[508]

Characteristics of centrotemporal spikes

Centrotemporal spikes (CTS) are characterized by their morphology, amplitude and duration, location and field distribution, frequency and pattern of occurrence, reactivity to external stimuli and sleep–wake cycle as well as age-dependence and evolution.[61,99,125,128,145,153–155,170,171,193,194,260,267,314,326,327,355,438,483,484,508,512,562,586,620,687,732,767] See Figs. 5.1, 5.2 and 5.3.

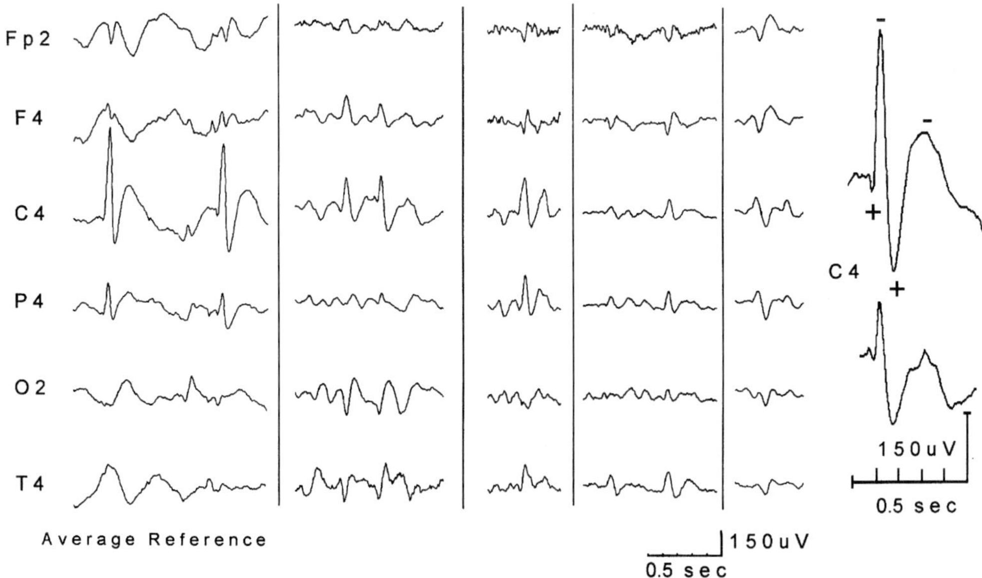

Fig. 5.1. Centrotemporal spikes of five different children who all had Rolandic seizures. Note that centrotemporal spikes are morphologically similar despite differences in amplitude, localization and dipole organization. On the right of the figure details of two amplified centrotemporal spikes from different cases are shown. Common average reference.

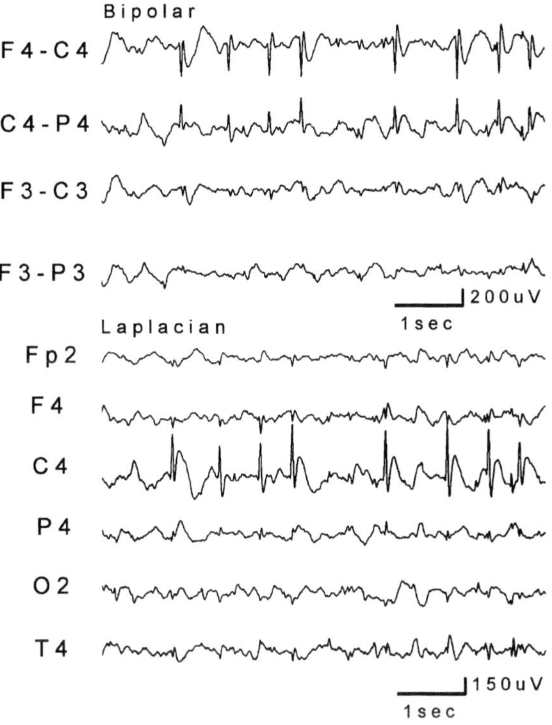

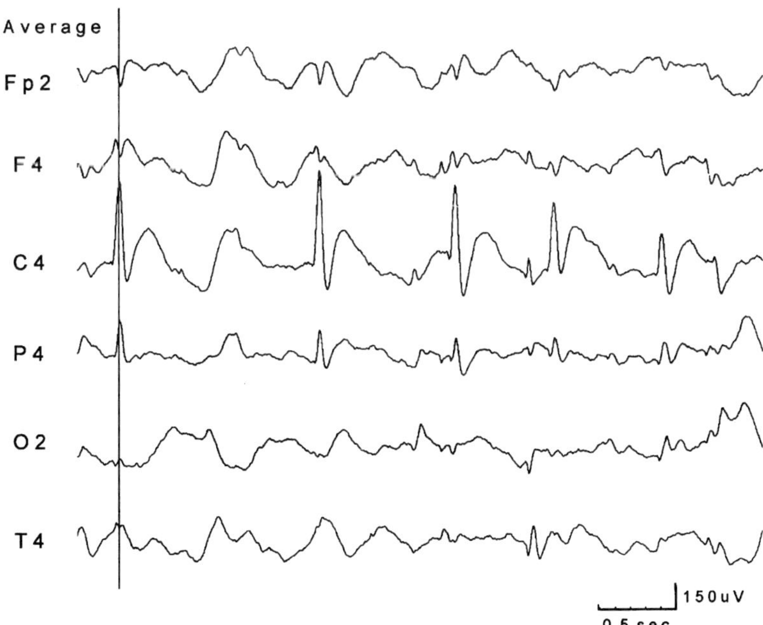

Fig. 5.2. Centrotemporal spikes of a child during sleep in bipolar, Laplacian and common average reference montage. Note that the spikes over 600 μV are highly localized in the right central C4 electrode. Midtemporal electrode is hardly affected.

Morphology

The waveform morphology is the most characteristic property of all 'benign, functional' spikes in childhood. This is consistent and well described mainly in the centrotemporal spikes which are the commonest of all. What we call 'centrotemporal spikes' (CTS) are mainly sharp and slow wave complexes (Figs. 5.1, 5.2 and 5.3).

The main spike (sharp wave) component is diphasic with a maximum surface negative rounded peak that is followed by a smaller positive peak. This is followed by a negative or negative–positive slow wave (Fig. 5.1). A relatively minute positive spike often precedes this spike–slow wave complex.[359]

Amplitude and duration

The amplitude of the main spike (or sharp wave) component often exceeds 200 μV though it may be smaller or much higher as illustrated in Fig. 5.2 where there is a peak to peak amplitude of 700–800 μV. The negative is higher than the positive phase of the spike and the preceding or following components of the spike–slow wave complex.

The rising is usually faster than the descending phase of the spike which has a variable duration from less but usually of more than 70 ms. The mean duration of the spike was 88 ms in one study.[784] The slow components that follow the spikes have a much longer duration, usually 100–300 ms, but may be longer: up to 500 ms (Figs. 5.1 and 5.2). The amplitude and duration of the spike and of its components show marked variations even in the same EEG and these are more evident with sleep facilitation and in bilateral localization.

Localization

By definition of a centrotemporal spike, main localization is in the central and midtemporal electrode in EEG recordings of the International 10/20 electrode placement system. Voltage gradient studies by Lombroso, 1967[508] using additional electrode positions found them in the midtemporal positions (T3-T4) 'often with spread to the central or Rolandic region. Less often the central or Rolandic spikes (C3 or C4) exhibit slightly higher voltages than the midtemporal in the scalp EEG'. This is at variance with recent studies of Legarda *et al.*,1994[477] evaluating interictal spikes in 33 patients with Rolandic seizures using closely spaced electrodes arranged over the perisylvian cortex. In particular, they also used C6 and C5 electrodes which are situated midway between the C4–T4 or C3–T5 electrodes. None of the 33 patients had spikes showing maximum negativity in the midtemporal regions (T3/T4). Instead, maximum negativity was evident in the high central region (C3/C4) in 10 children (30.3 per cent) and in the low central region (C5/C6) in 23 (69.7 per cent). This was also correlated with clinical symptoms. Hand involvement was significantly frequent (50 per cent) in the high central group, and drooling with oromotor involvement was a distinctive symptom (65.2 per cent) in the low central group. The authors concluded that 'the spikes in patients with Rolandic seizures are exclusively suprasylvian in origin and correlate with two electroclinical subgroups'.[477]

CTS may be unilateral or bilateral in the same or serial EEG. Unilateral CTS occur equally on the right or left and in subsequent EEGs may appear in the same or the opposite site. More than one third of the patients have bilateral CTS usually firing independently right or left, though bisynchronous CTS are not unusual.[508,512] In this respect Y. Gastaut's[314] initial descriptions reproduced in Appendix 1 (page 100) are confirmed: 'They are unilateral or bilateral and, in the latter case, asynchronous or synchronous, asymmetric or symmetric (asymmetry of amplitude and not of topography). They are sporadic but can be grouped in brief volleys assuming a pseudo-rhythmic appearance.'[314] However, asymmetry of topography is not uncommon.

The dipoles of centrotemporal spikes and their clinical significance

Centrotemporal spikes have been studied with EEG single or multiple dipole modelling computerized techniques mainly by Grecory, Wong *et al.* from Canada,[359,360,799,816–820] van der Meij *et al.*[781–784] from the Netherlands, Baumgartner, Graf, Lischka and colleagues[71,72,491] from Austria, and Yoshinaga

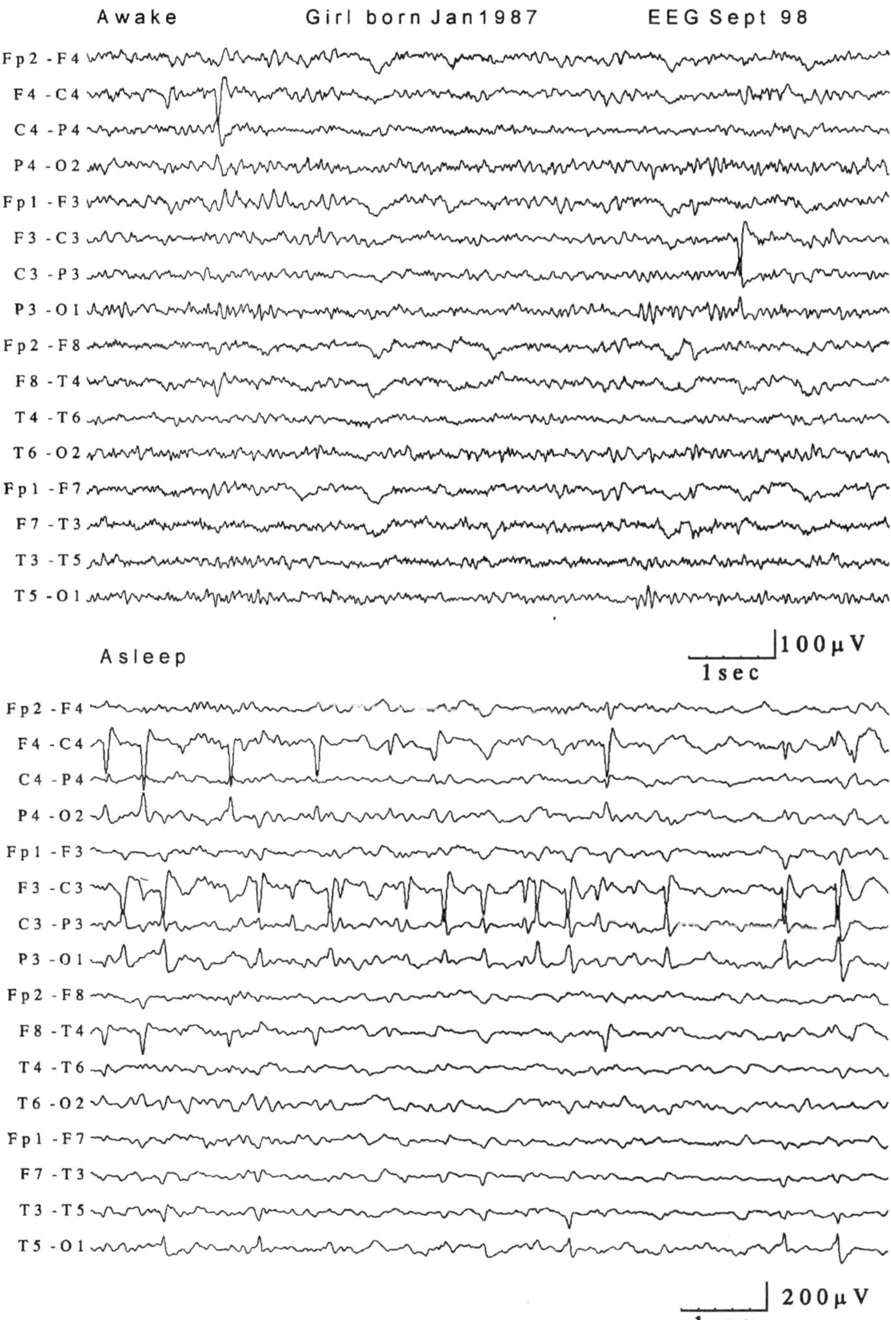

Fig. 5.3a. Right and left centrotemporal (central) spikes of a child with Rolandic seizures in remission for 3 years (case 4.25).
Note that centrotemporal spikes are highly activated by sleep. They are also activated by tapping her fingertips (Fig. 5.3b).

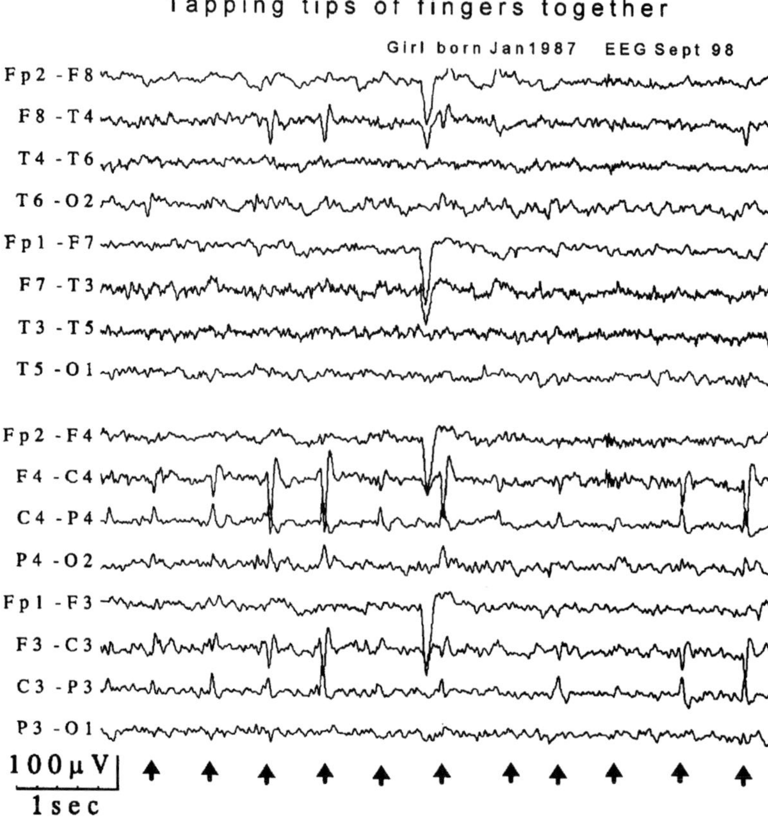

Fig. 5.3b. Same child, same EEG as in Fig. 5.3a. Bilateral evoked central spikes by self-tapping the tips of her fingers together. Arrows indicate tapping of tips of fingers together.

with associates[832–834] from Japan. The consensus is[359,491,781,817,832–834] that the main negative spike component of CTS can be usually modelled by a single and stable tangential dipole source along the Rolandic region with the negative pole maximum at the centrotemporal and the positive pole maximum at the frontal regions. It was hypothesized that centrotemporal spikes arise from a single generator which is oriented tangential to the surface.[359] The generator is most likely situated in the inferior bank of the Sylvian fissure, [817] the anterior wall of the central sulcus[72] or at the bottom of the sensory cortex.[834] It is also agreed that frequently the major centrotemporal negativity is preceded by a small spike with the positive pole in the centrotemporal and the negative in the frontal regions.[359,781] This CTS tangential dipole and its location has been confirmed with magnetoencephalography by Baumgartner *et al.*, 1995[71] and more recently in a detailed study by Minami *et al.* 1996[536] from Japan (Fig. 5.4).

This dominant and stable horizontal dipolar topography centred near the lower region of the Rolandic sulcus was found nearly exclusively in children with typical Rolandic seizures while atypical cases or CTS in symptomatic patients appear to have a more complex distribution of more than one dipoles.[799,832] Grecory and Wong[360] found that CTS with a frontotemporal dipole (group A) were associated with a lower incidence of clinical abnormality than nondipole CTS (group B). Thus, in 99 children of group A frequent seizures (10 per cent), developmental delay (18 per cent), school difficulties (34 per cent) and abnormal neurological examination (22 per cent) were less significant

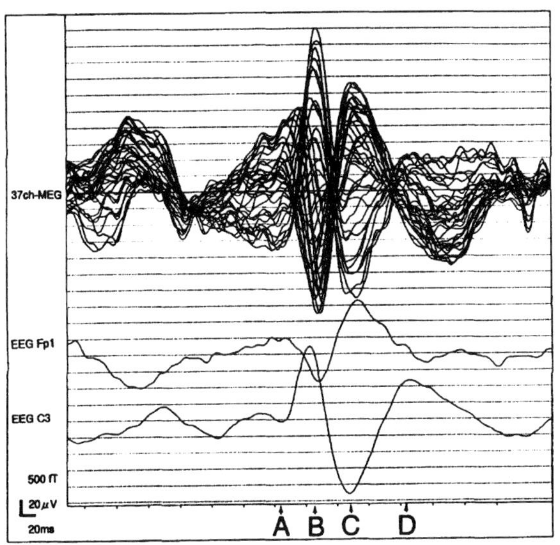

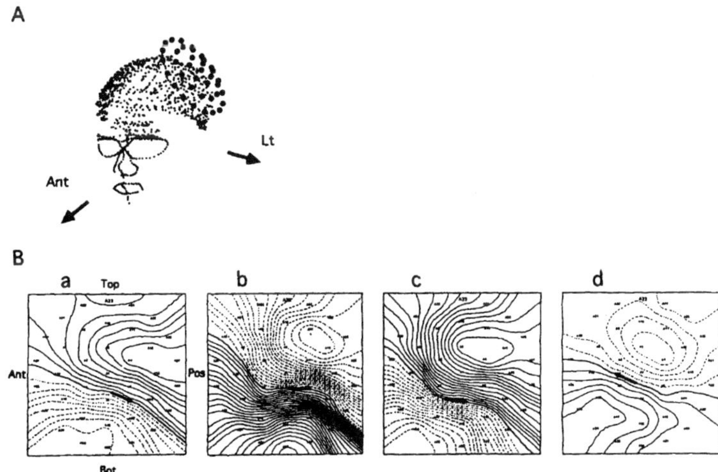

Fig. 5.4. Upper. Actual 37-channel magnetoencephalographic (MEG) recordings, and electroencephalogram (EEG) recorded at Fp1 and C3.
(A), (B), (C), and (D) indicate the four portions of polarity reversal.
Lower: (A) The 37-channel sensor locations of magnetoencephalography (MEG) in the left centrotemporal region of a patient's head. Ant = anterior; Lt = left. (B) MEG isocontour maps at four portion. (a), (b), (c) and (d) correspond to phase reversal portions (A), (B), (C) and (D) in upper figure. Magnetic flux exits from the continuous-line area and enters the dotted-line area. The contour step is 200 femto-Tesla. The arrows denote the estimated equivalent current dipole (ECD), with the positive pole at the arrowhead. Ant = anterior; Pos = posterior; Top = top of head; Bot = bottom of head. (a) Preceding small positive wave. (b)Prominent negative sharp wave. (c) Following positive wave. (d) Negative slow wave.
[From Minami et al., Ann Neurol 1996: 39:326–334 with the permission of the authors and the editor.]

than in group B of 267 children with frequent seizures (55 per cent), developmental delay (55 per cent), school difficulties (60 per cent), and an abnormal neurological examination (63 per cent). Similar were the results of Yoshinaga *et al.*[832] who studied three groups; Rolandic seizures ($n = 14$), other types of epilepsy with centrotemporal spikes ($n = 15$) and epilepsy with focal spikes in other areas ($n = 13$). The spike dipole in each group was analysed using the dipole tracing method. Only the spikes of Rolandic seizures were characterized by constantly stable dipoles which were strictly localized in the Rolandic area. However, van der Meir *et al.*[781–784] found that the quantitative properties of centrotemporal spikes were similar in various groups of children to normal or abnormal neurological state, without seizures or seizures manifesting either with oropharyngolaryngeal or hemifacial symptoms. Also, Legarda and Jayakar[476] correlated two specific spike features: (a) dipole fields, and (b) exact location of maximum negativity, with the presence or absence of clinical seizures in 42 neurodevelopmentally normal children with 'Rolandic (central)' spikes. Thirty-three (79 per cent) presented with seizures. Seventeen of 21 children revealing dipoles (81 per cent) and 16 of 21 patients without dipoles (74 per cent) had seizures. Children with high central (C3/C4) foci were just as likely to present with seizures (10 of 15, 67 per cent) as were those with low central (C5/C6) foci (23 of 27, 85 per cent) ($P < 0.10$). The majority of their study subjects (27 of 42, 64 per cent) revealed maximum negativity in the low central region (C5/C6), and the dipole feature was as likely to be associated with high central foci (seven of 15, 47 per cent) as with low central foci (14 of 27, 52 per cent). They concluded that 'although Rolandic spikes are a reliable indicator of potential epileptogenicity, neither their exact location nor dipolar distribution help to further define the population with clinical seizures.' Furthermore, Baumgartner *et al.*, 1996[72] studied the functional organization of the interictal spike complex in Rolandic seizures and compared it with somatosensory evoked potentials after median nerve stimulation that provided a biologic marker for the location of the central sulcus in 12 patients with Rolandic seizures. They used multiple dipole modelling to assess the number, the three-dimensional intracerebral location, and the time activity of the underlying neuronal sources. Although the interictal spike complex could be modelled by a single tangential dipolar source in seven patients, in the remaining five patients, two sources – a radial and a tangential dipole – were necessary adequately to explain the interictal spikes. The tangential source was located deeper than the radial source and was characterized by a frontal positivity and a centroparietal negativity with a phase reversal across the central sulcus, suggesting that the interictal spikes originated in the anterior wall of the central sulcus. The radial source showed a single electronegativity over the ipsilateral central region, which would be compatible with involvement of the top of either the pre- or postcentral gyrus. Both sources showed biphasic time patterns with an average latency difference of 30 ms. They concluded that in some patients with typical Rolandic seizures, the interictal epileptiform spike complex is generated by multiple, simultaneously active neuronal populations within the central region and that epileptiform activity is propagated between these two adjacent cortical areas.

Varma *et al.*, 1997[787] have recently proposed that the characteristics of the slow wave may be more important than the sharp wave of the CTS complex. They compared the morphological features of interictal spikes in three patients with Rolandic seizures and three patients with symptomatic localization related epilepsies. Two-second epochs centred at the peak negativity of the sharp waves were analysed from a referential montage during stage I sleep. The epochs from the two groups were compared using parametric and information theory analysis. Information analysis determined the likelihood of correctly identifying the clinical group based on their interictal spikes. Standard parametric, morphological and spectral analyses were also performed. There was no significant difference in the morphology of the sharp wave between the two groups. However, the two groups could be separated by information contained in the after-going slow wave which also showed significant morphological and spectral differences.

Dipoles in routine EEG

The dipoles of the CTS can be studied in routine EEG with the referential and Laplacian montage that

I personally prefer (Fig. 5.2). Gibbs and Gibbs[327] had already observed in routine EEG recordings that 'negative spikes in the midtemporal region usually spread as positive spikes to both frontal areas, and as lower amplitude positive spikes to both parietal regions' (plates 196, 215; (page 214).[327]

Frequency and pattern of occurrence of the centrotemporal spikes

Centrotemporal spikes are usually abundant on awake and mainly sleep EEGs.[61,99,125,128,145,153–155,170,171,193,194,260,267,326,327,355,438,483,484,508,512,562,586,620,687,767] They may be singular but more frequently they occur at irregular repetitive rates as long clusters of usually around 5–10 spikes in 3–15 s. Their average frequency in awake EEGs is 4–20 per minute[99,170,260,767] and this is two to five times higher in slow sleep (Table 5.1). However, these are only indicative numbers as the frequency of centrotemporal spikes fluctuates significantly in the same or subsequent EEG and sometimes appears nearly continuous in one part of the record to disappear in another part, probably depending on arousal levels. Also, it should be emphasized that there is unanimous agreement that frequency of CTS is by no means related to the clinical state. This fact is well known and well established from the very first reports of Rolandic seizures[125,128,267,483,508,562] and it is consistent with the finding that more than 90 per cent of children with CTS, often bilateral and abundant, may not have seizures.[153–155,260,327,438,512,586] It is not unusual to have a normal awake EEG or an EEG with a few scattered CTS after a typical Rolandic seizure while subsequent EEGs show 'marked deterioration' both in frequency and amplitude of CTS which may also occur in other locations. It is this 'deteriorating EEG' that often leads to inappropriate introduction, increase or change of anti-epileptic drugs in children who are seizure-free (see illustrative case 4.1). Centrotemporal spikes may persist for years, usually 3–5, after remission of seizures and they nearly always disappear after the age of 16 years.

Activation and facilitation of the centrotemporal spikes by sleep

Centrotemporal spikes of Rolandic seizures or in normal children with CTS but without seizures increase during sleep by a factor of 2–5[53,54,61,78,99,126,145,170,171,188,190,193,194,234,260,317,326,355,439,512,687,767] (Table 5.1) without disturbing the sleep organization.[61,99,145,170,171,193,194,355,687,767] Furthermore, CTS may also occur only during sleep in 3–35 per cent[512] of the cases with Rolandic seizures which necessitates sleep EEG in children suspected of Rolandic seizures who have normal routine awake EEG. It is interesting that Lombroso[508] who had the highest rate, 35 per cent, of CTS occurring only during sleep concluded[508] that 'the effect of drowsiness and sleep in activating an otherwise absent or inconspicuous midtemporal spike focus is considerably less evident than for anterior spike foci typically found in psychomotor epilepsy. In only 35 per cent was a midtemporal focus evidenced in sleep only, though sleep often activated such foci already present in the waking state'.

Table 5.1. Spikes per minute in awake and all sleep stages[99,170,767]

	Ten children with CT spikes and seizures	Ten children with CT spikes only[99]
	Spikes/min	Spikes/min
Awake	10.6, (4)*	13.1
Stage I [(and II)]	40.6, (16) [12.8]**	31.7
Stage II	44.6	34.5
Stage III and IV	55.6, (22)[21.3]	57.7
REM	40.9, (11)[7.2]	14

Open numbers are from the study of Bernardina and Beghini, 1976[99]; *numbers in parentheses are from Clemens and Majoros, 1987[170] and **numbers in brackets from Terzano *et al.*, 1991[767].
Eeg-Olofsson *et al.*[260] found that normal children with CTS but without seizures had 8.4 CTS/min when awake, which increased to 15.6/min in sleep.

Gibbs and Gibbs,[326,327] long ago emphasized the need for 'EEG recordings to be made in the waking and sleeping states. This statement may sound dogmatic, but it is supported by comparison of recordings awake and asleep in many thousands of cases and it is basic to the present discussion. To put the matter figuratively, sleep takes the blanket off the brain and reveals seizure discharges and underlying disorder that rarely appear in the waking state'[326]

Bernardina and Beghini (1976)[99] studied polygraphically the nocturnal sleep of 20 neurologically normal children with typical centrotemporal spikes. There were two groups. Group A had 10 children with centrotemporal spikes and Rolandic seizures, while group B had 10 children with centrotemporal spikes only, without seizures. The cyclic organization of sleep and the percentages of the different stages were normal in all 20 subjects. However, CTS were facilitated during all stages of NREM sleep by a factor of three to five times. Sleep facilitated only CTS, unilateral or bilateral, that pre-existed in the awake states. Sleep did not induce new CTS foci at other localizations or at the other side. The only differences between the two groups were: (1) REM sleep facilitated the CTS only in those with Rolandic seizures (Table 5.1), and (2) spontaneous generalized discharges were induced by sleep in three children with Rolandic seizures.[99] None of the 20 children of the two groups had spontaneous generalized discharges in alert stages.

Clemens and Olah (1987)[171] compared polygraphic all-night sleep records of 11 children with Rolandic seizures and eight normal controls. Basic properties of sleep organization and electromorphology were preserved in both groups. The only detectable difference of 17 quantitative sleep parameters measured was that children with Rolandic seizures had more waking in the first half of the night.

Clemens and Majoros (1987)[170] in another report of the 11 children with Rolandic seizures, confirmed the results of Bernardina and Beghini, 1976[99] regarding the facilitation of CTS in all stages of sleep (Table 5.1). Furthermore, they showed that peak activation for every stage of sleep was in the first cycle of sleep. This was followed by marked decrease in the second cycle and another moderate increase in the third cycle. Thus, maximum spike/min ratios mainly occurred in the first cycle of stages III and IV of sleep. Stages 1–2 on the descending slopes of consecutive cycles showed a decrease in spike density during the night, as opposed to the increasing rate of activation of the same stages on the ascending slopes. The periods of maximum activation were in the first 2 h of sleep with another near the end of the night sleep. This is consistent with the clinical observations that most of the Rolandic seizures occur mainly in the first hour of sleep followed by the period before awakening. The authors concluded that 'the actual drive of spiking as well as seizures in Rolandic seizures is the functional overweight of sleep-inducing mechanisms'.[170]

Also, Baldy-Moulinier (1992)[61] found no significant changes of sleep organization in 19 children studied. 'The only particularity is a longer REM latency during the first cycle (mean latency = 136.11 min)' attributed to the 'tremendous increase of epileptic discharges immediately after sleep onset and during the different stages of NREM sleep in the first cycle'. In the presented histogram of a child with Rolandic seizures the number of CTS are at least twice as frequent in the first cycle of sleep as opposed to the following NREM and REM cycles.[61]

Terzano *et al.* (1991)[767] studied from all night polygraphic EEGs the 'discriminatory' effect of a cyclic alternating pattern of sleep on interictal spikes in 10 patients with focal symptomatic seizures and 10 children with Rolandic seizures. Interictal EEG paroxysms were analysed with respect to the two arousal states of non-rapid-eye-movement sleep: (a) the cyclic alternating pattern (CAP), expressed by biphasic EEG periodic activities and related to long-lasting fluctuations between greater (phase A) and lesser (phase B) arousal levels; and (b) the non-CAP (NCAP), manifested by an unchanging EEG pattern reflecting a relative stable state of arousal. Interictal symptomatic spikes were mainly enhanced during CAP, particularly in phase A. Conversely, there were no significant differences in spike activation between CAP and NCAP for Rolandic seizures. The authors concluded that 'the intense activity of the Rolandic foci induced by sleep as such could be explained on the basis of the greater dependence of these functional cortical EEG abnormalities on the degree of synchronization during sleep'.

Activation and inhibition of CTS by external stimuli, hyperventilation and photic stimulation

The consensus is that CTS are not influenced by eyes opening and closing, hyperventilation or photic stimulation. However, according to Y. Gastaut[314] the CTS 'block to fist clenching' is 'facilitated by release of the fist after a sustained contraction' and 'they frequently accompany the other Rolandic activities that react similarly, notably beta rhythm and its sub-harmonic variety, the mu rhythm' (see details in Appendix 1, page 100). The 'blocking of CTS by hand and finger movements' has also been studied by Niedermeyer and Naidu (1989).[571,572] They reported that 'clenching fist or repeatedly performing alternating closure and opening of the contralateral hand' may block central spikes 'in some but not all cases of Rolandic seizures' and never occurred 'in children with CTS caused by structural lesions (especially in cerebral palsy)', though this could occur in passive hand movements of four girls with severe Rett's syndrome.

Fonseca *et al.* (1996)[292] examined the influence of tongue and hand movement, tactile stimulation and cognitive tasks on the discharge rate of CTS in 35 children. Eighteen had non-febrile convulsions and 12 had Rolandic seizures. Tongue movement had a marked, more than 50 per cent, inhibitory effect on CTS and this was more significant for patients with Rolandic seizures. The other significant reduction occurred in left sided CTS during right hand movements and looking at coloured spots. A similar inhibitory effect on EEG centrotemporal spikes by mouth and tongue movements was described by Colamaria *et al.*, 1991[173] in a child with CTS and status epilepticus manifesting as anterior operculum syndrome.

Extreme somatosensory evoked potentials/spikes

The most common, after sleep, form of activation of the centrotemporal spikes is by somatosensory stimulation mainly of the fingers of the hands or toes and heels of the feet. These extreme somatosensory evoked potentials (ESEP) which in EEG appear as giant evoked spikes are usually elicited at the same side of the spontaneous unilateral CTS with contralateral stimulation. Like the normal somatosensory evoked potentials, their location depends on the site and side of stimulation (Figs. 5.3b, 5.5 and 5.6) but their size and morphology is identical to that of the CTS.

These evoked spikes, corresponding to mid or long latency somatosensory evoked potential, usually have a latency of 35–80 ms depending on the height of the individual and the site of the stimulation.[659] They persist during sleep.[208]

ESEP may occur in EEG with or without spontaneous functional spikes. ESEP, like CTS, occur in children with or without seizures, with idiopathic or symptomatic seizures and disappear with age.

De Marco alone[201–205] and with associates[206–208,563,759,760] was the first to describe giant spikes evoked by somatosensory stimuli in the feet or hands of children with or without seizures, even at a stage when the EEG was otherwise normal. They showed that these were exaggerated mid- or long-latency somatosensory evoked potential[563,760] and call them extreme somatosensory evoked potentials (ESEP). De Marco and Tassinari, 1981[208] detailed the results of the evaluation of 15,000 children referred for an EEG mainly because of behavioural, speech and educational problems who were tested for ESEP customarily by tapping the heel. One hundred and fifty five children (1 per cent) had ESEP. Age of the first EEG recording of ESEP varied from 1 to 13 years with a peak at 4–8 years (91 per cent of the cases). ESEP could be the only EEG abnormality, and spontaneous spikes appeared at a later age stage, usually between 1 and 4 years after the first EEG with ESEP, initially during sleep and subsequently also while awake. The morphology and topography of the spontaneous focal spikes and the ESEP were strikingly similar.[208] Of those without seizures that were followed up, 15 per cent developed fits that were mainly versive and diurnal. Spontaneous spikes and ESEP later disappeared at around the age of 10–14 years, usually 1–3 years after the remission of seizures.[208] De Marco proposed that this combination of ESEP and seizures and their evolution constitute another syndrome of benign partial childhood epilepsy which he called 'benign partial epilepsy with extreme somatosensory evoked potentials', as detailed in Chapter 16. What is relevant in this section is that amongst the reasons that De Marco and Tassinari, 1981[208] considered in their differentiation of this proposed

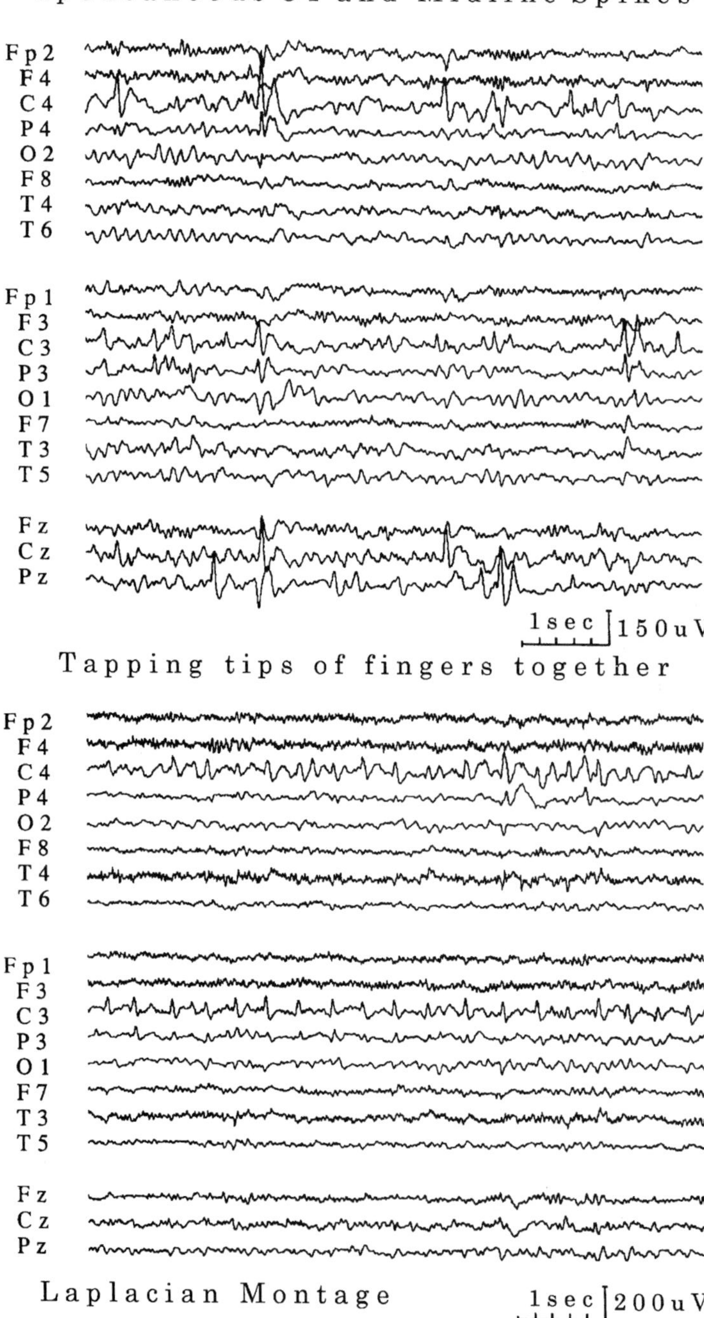

Fig. 5.5. From video-EEG of illustrative case 4.3 (Chapter 4).
Upper: Spontaneous central and midline spikes (C4, C3, C2, P2).
Lower: Synchronous central spikes (ESEP) are elicited at C3 and C4 when she taps the tips of her fingers together.

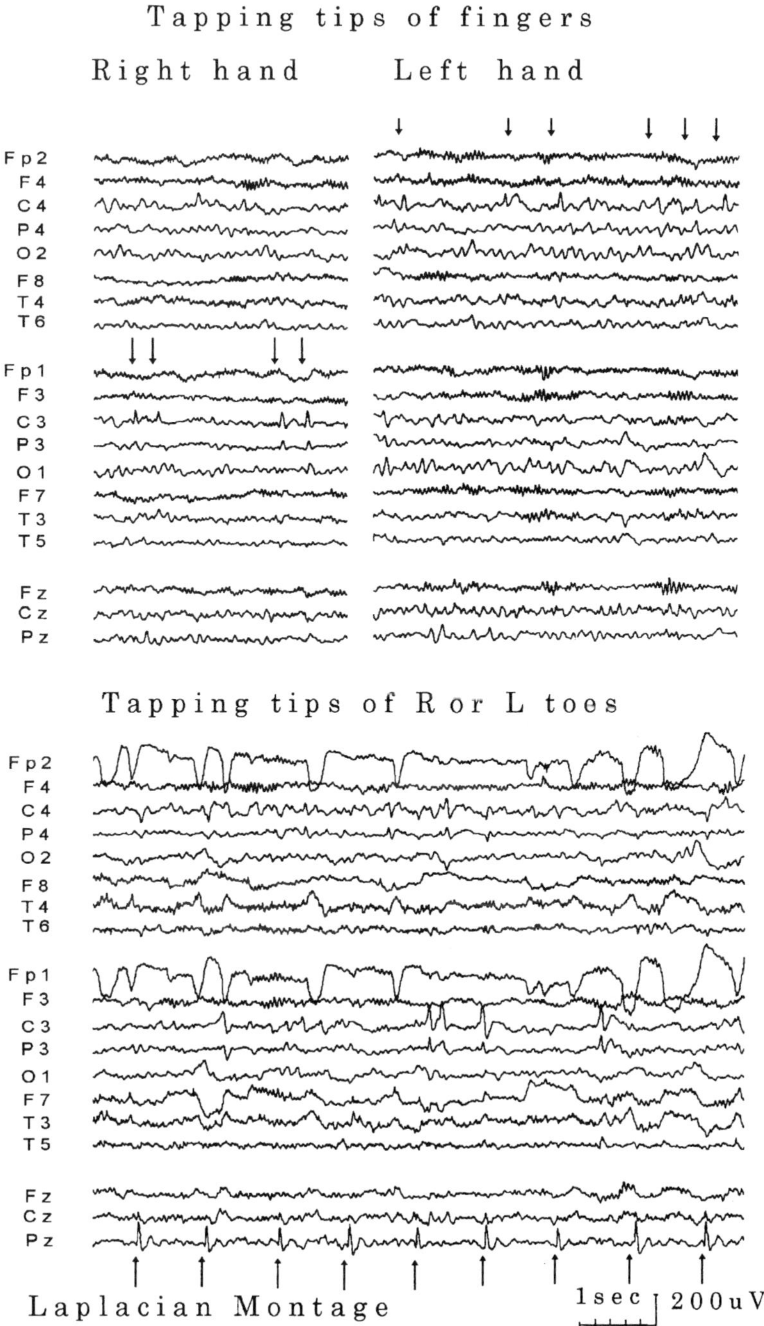

Fig. 5.6. Same patient, from the same video-EEG of Fig. 5.5.
Upper: Central spikes (ESEP) are elicited from contralateral stimulation (tapping the fingers) of each hand (arrows).
Lower: Tapping of the toes of the right or left foot elicits giant ESEP in the Pz midline electrode (arrows).

new syndrome from Rolandic seizures was that: 'Finally, and most important, ESEP have been observed in only one case of benign epilepsy with Rolandic foci out of more than 100 such cases examined by one of us' (De Marco,1980).[202] This is at variance with my experience. Our results indicate that tapping the fingers evokes time-locked giant somatosensory sharp and slow waves (ESEP) in the corresponding brain locations in approximately 15 per cent of children with CTS with or without Rolandic seizures (Figs. 5.5 and 5.6). These different results are most likely due to different techniques of stimulation applied by De Marco and ourselves. We mainly stimulate the fingertips of the hands which is more likely to produce ESEP in children with CTS because the lateral central gyrus is the main location of the cortical hyperexcitability in these children (recall the homunculus of Penfield). Conversely, De Marco *et al.*[201–208,563,759,760] mainly stimulate the heels of the feet which should be less sensitive in children with Rolandic seizures for the above reasons but probably more sensitive in children with midline and parietal spontaneous spikes. This also explains their findings that ESEP are mainly recorded from the posterior midline (Pz) electrode.[208]

According to De Marco *et al.*[201–208,563,759,760] 'the ESEP are of high amplitude spikes sometimes reaching 400 μV, involving the parietal and parasagittal regions with maximum amplitude in the hemisphere opposite to the stimulated site'. However, regarding the location of ESEP an explanation is needed here. ESEP elicited from stimulation of the feet, as preferred by De Marco,[208] are mainly located in the posterior midline electrode (Pz) as expected from the cortical representation of the foot, and lateralization is not obvious in EEG recordings with a 10/20 system electrode placement (see Figs. 5.5 and 5.6). Conversely, ESEP elicited by stimulation of the fingers are in EEG recordings of the 10/20 system always contralateral to the stimulation site with a maximum amplitude in the C3/C4 electrode, as again expected from the cortical representation of the hand (see Figs. 5.5 and 5.6).

Fonseca, Tedrus *et al.*[290–292] from Brazil also extensively studied the reactivity of centrotemporal spikes and ESEP. In a recent report (1994)[290] they tested 6500 children aged 2–15 years by consecutive taps applied to both hands and feet using a tendon reflex hammer. The locations of the hands and feet when the stimulus was delivered, signified above, are not stated. Of these 6500 children, 186 (2.9 per cent) had ESEP but only 75 of them also had seizures. The remaining 111 patients without seizures had the EEG because of minor behavioural and scholastic problems. Of the 75 patients with seizures, 31 (16.7 per cent) had febrile convulsions only. Of the other 44 children (23.7 per cent), 21 were boys, who had non-febrile seizures and seven also had a previous history of febrile convulsions. In these 44 patients with non-febrile seizures, ESEP were evoked from stimulation of the feet in 42 and of the hand in 11. In 39 of these 44 cases the EEG also showed spontaneous focal spikes, which occurred predominantly in the parietal regions in 24. Spontaneous epileptiform activity was recorded in 39.6 per cent of the patients without epileptic seizures and 85.3 per cent with seizures. The clinical characteristics of these patients are described in the Chapter 16.

More recently, Manganotti and colleagues, 1998[522] detailed neurophysiological findings of these 'extreme somatosensory evoked potentials' in six patients with clinical features of Rolandic seizures. Both tapping and electrical stimulation in the fingers produced scalp evoked potentials in all subjects, characterized by a spike followed by a slow wave, similar in morphology and scalp distribution to the spontaneously occurring spikes. This paroxysmal activity was sensitive to stimulus rate; the number of evoked spikes was inversely related to the frequency of stimulation, being maximal at 1 Hz and disappearing at high frequencies of 10 Hz. Spontaneous spikes disappeared during high-frequency stimulation but were present during low-frequency stimulation. Averaged somatosensory evoked potentials at 3 Hz stimulation showed a late high-amplitude component, identical in morphology and distribution to the single evoked spike. The authors concluded that evoked and spontaneous spikes share common cortical sensorimotor generators.

Musumeci *et al.*[555]and Ferri *et al.*[276] reported a 7-year-old boy with fragile-X syndrome and seizures who had 'Rolandic epileptiform potentials during sleep and hand tapping as well as ESEP'.

Robertson *et al.*, 1988[681] described EEG findings for seven girls with Rett's syndrome. Central spikes occurred in five of the seven girls. They appeared to be age related and could be evoked by tactile stimulation in two patients.

Yamagata *et al.*, 1997[827] reported a 10-year-old girl with Rolandic seizures who had spontaneous centrotemporal spikes which could also be induced by blinking irrespective of surrounding light conditions. This indicated that centrotemporal spikes were probably elicited by the somatosensory stimuli produced by tapping between the eyelids.

Techniques to elicit extreme somatosensory evoked potentials/spikes

It should be emphasized that any type of mechanical or electrical stimulus can elicit ESEP in susceptible children provided that it is properly applied. It must be abrupt and strong enough (without being uncomfortable) and delivered in the appropriate sensitive body region. Percussing distal parts of legs (toes and heel) or arms (palms and mainly tips of fingers) with a reflex hammer or with the plantar tips of the examiner's fingers is very effective in eliciting ESEP. A hammer can also be connected to a channel of the EEG so as to mark the exact timing of the stimulus and measure the latency of the evoked spike. Electrical stimulation with digital electrodes, similar to orthodromic sensory nerve testing, and of the nerve, similar to antidromic sensory nerve testing, are equally effective for ESEP, but this is only for research purposes and should not be needed in routine EEG as it is not more efficient than the mechanical stimulation described above which is a more child friendly method.

The way that I test for ESEP in children was influenced by an observant technician, Ms Ioannidou in Aghia Sophia hospital for Children in Athens, 1981. She observed that a child had EEG spikes every time when he was tapped, out of boredom, the EEG bed with the tips of one or the other hand. These were consistently reproduced by the examiner by abruptly and firmly striking with the palmar tips of his fingers the palmar tips of the child's fingers. It is important that the produced stimulus is brief, firm and abrupt, and the method is similar to eliciting a Hofmann reflex in the upper limbs or a Rossolimo reflex in the lower limbs. Though we also use the same method by tapping the plantar surface of the tips of the toes, this was not systematically investigated. I have found that an easy way to test this activation in routine EEG for ESEP is to ask the child to tap together the palmar surface of the tips of the fingers of both hands together. The child should be instructed to strike them with sufficient strength and at random intervals of varying frequency. This may elicit either bilateral or unilateral giant spikes (Fig. 5.6). Tapping with an electrical hammer is another way we use to obtain and study children who may dislike electrical stimulation for ESEP.

Ours was not a new discovery. De Marco, long before us as detailed above and in Chapter 16, had already published significant papers on his experience[201–204,206–208,563] which in 1981 included 15,000 children tested with his method of activation which again came from an observant technician: 'a discharge of bilaterally synchronous and symmetrical spikes and waves' was induced in a non-epileptic child with a normal resting EEG 'when the technician inadvertently brushed the external border of the foot' (De Marco and Negrin, 1973).[207] Since then, they use a reflex hammer, striking with the same strength as that for obtaining tendon reflexes the lateral and medial aspect of the heel of one and then the other foot. 'Tapping of the fingertips was performed in half of the subjects'.[208]

EEG functional spike-sharp wave foci in other than the centrotemporal regions in children with Rolandic seizures or with centrotemporal spikes

An age-related cortical epileptogenicity and not a 'migration of spikes'

It is well established[87,102,129,249,277,286,308,326,327,386,438,512,603,605,608,793] that centrotemporal spikes may co-exist in the same EEG with independent functional spikes in other locations such as occipital (O2, O1), midline (Fz,Cz,Pz), frontal (Fp2, Fp1, F3, F4) or parietal (P3,P4). The sharp waves in these other locations may be unilateral or bilateral, independent or synchronous with the CTS and have the same morphology and other characteristics of the CTS (Figs. 5.7 and 5.8). They are also exaggerated by sleep and they are age-related.

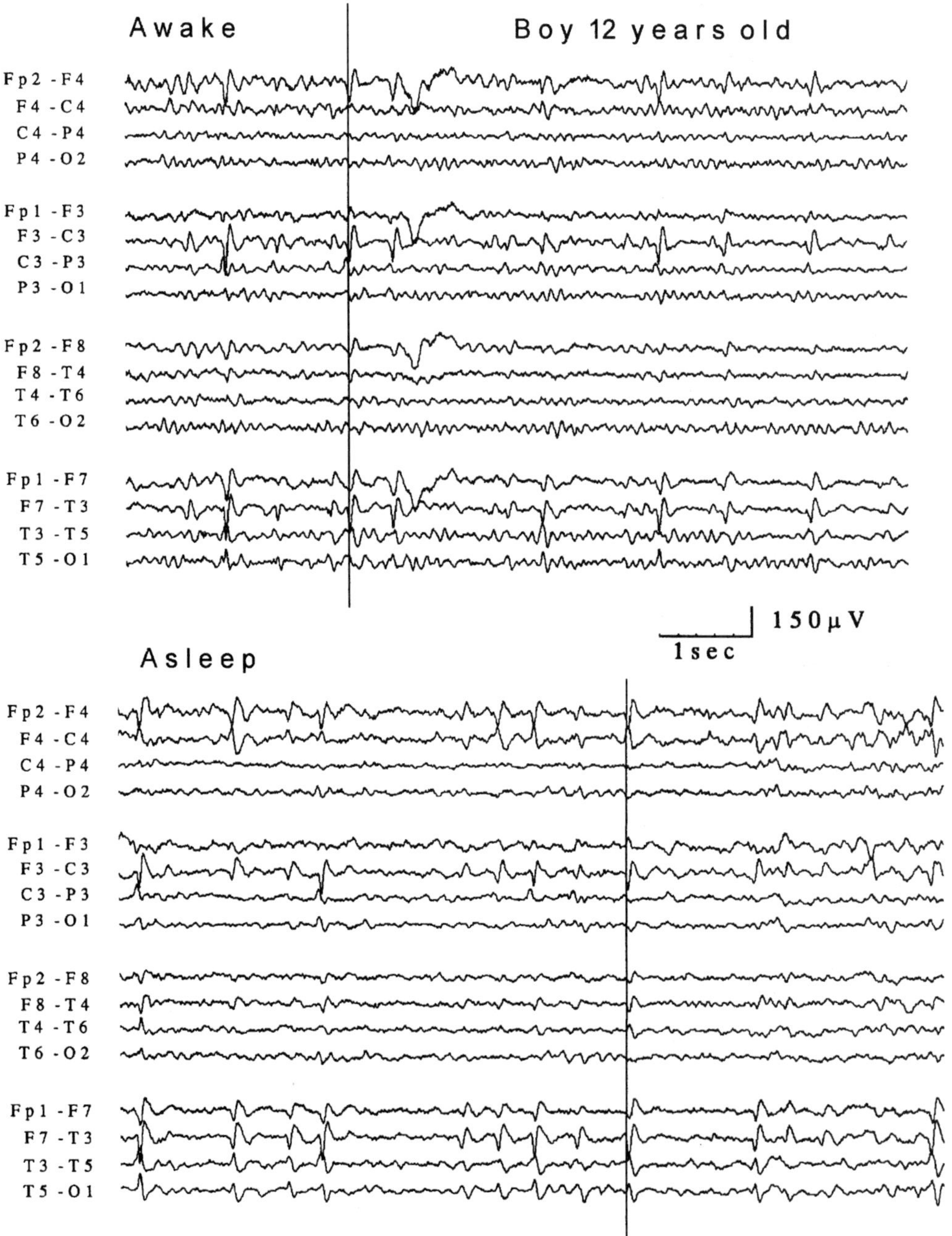

Fig. 5.7. Left centrotemporal spikes with a synchronous right frontal spike during awake and sleep EEG of a 12-year-old boy with a recent single nocturnal hemifacial seizure progressing to secondary GTCS. He also had some brief diurnal attacks of speech arrest at age 10 years.

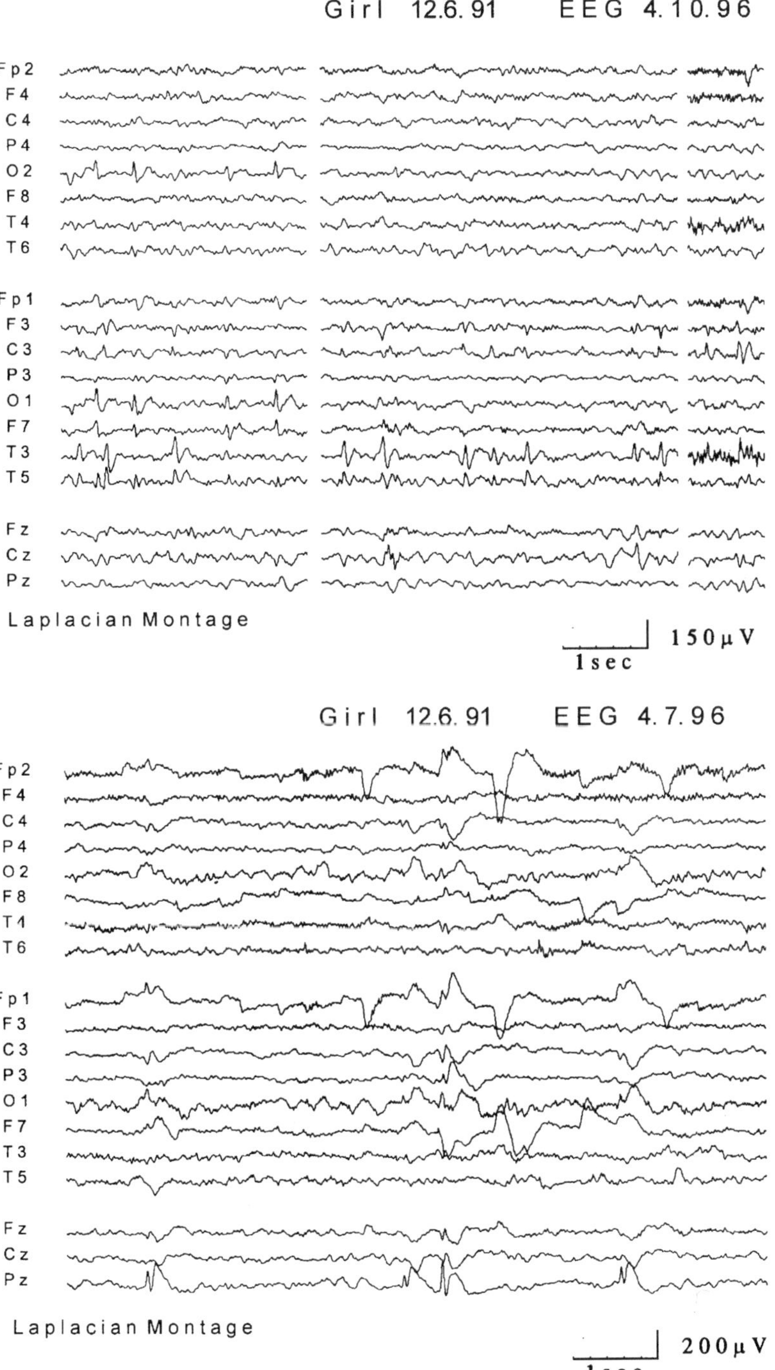

Fig. 5.8. Centrotemporal, posterior temporal, midline and occipital spikes in EEG of a 6-year-old girl with infrequent, nocturnal Rolandic seizures and probably early onset benign childhood occipital seizures.

The commonest situation is where these different spike foci occur in longitudinal EEG either preceding or less frequently following the appearance of centrotemporal spikes. That occipital spikes often precede the appearance of centrotemporal spikes is detailed in Chapter 10. This is a natural evolution which is expected, as peak age at onset is 5 years for occipital and 8–9 for centrotemporal spikes.

This age-dependent disappearance of functional spikes from one location and their appearance in another location is called by some experts 'migration of spikes', a term first used by Gibbs *et al.* 1954[326]. Blume[130] has argued against, Andermann and Oguni[41] in favour of migration of spikes. My opinion is that 'migration of spikes' is an unfortunate term and we should cease to use it. The spikes do not migrate. They are born and die in the same location of cortical hyperexcitability which results from an age-dependent derangement of the maturational process. This is mainly occipital in early childhood and centrotemporal in middle childhood. It does disappear with age when maturation is completed. Exceptionally there may be a low generalized seizure cortical threshold at a later age to explain the generalized discharges and infrequent GTCS that may occur in 2 per cent of the patients later in life. A similar view has been previously expressed by Luders *et al.*, 1987[512] as follows: 'It seems that the main pathogenetic factor is a genetically determined diffusely increased cortical epileptogenicity whose EEG or clinical expression is governed by maturational factors. Sharp waves and/or seizures occur exclusively in childhood, and it is likely that its focal expression is due to selective rates of maturation of the different cortical areas.'[512]

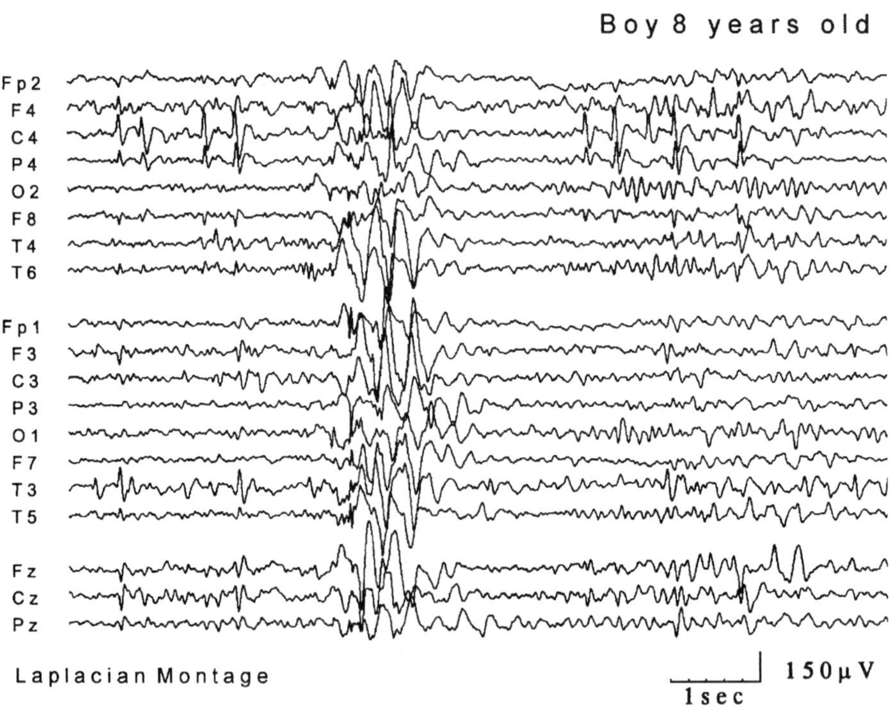

Fig.5.9. Centrotemporal spikes and a brief generalized discharge of microspikes and slow waves without ictal clinical manifestations. Also note that the right sided spike is mainly central (C4) while the left one is mainly midtemporal (T3).

Generalized discharges in children with Rolandic seizures, centrotemporal spikes or both

There is great disagreement between authors[78,99,102,512] regarding the occurrence of generalized discharges in Rolandic seizures with a reported prevalence varying from as low as 0 per cent[512] to as high as 54 per cent.[78] Because of these contradictory results I reviewed my reports of 250 routine awake EEGs of 72 children with Rolandic seizures (see Chapter 4). Only five EEGs of three patients (4.2 per cent) had brief generalized bursts of 3–5 Hz slow waves intermixed with small spikes (Fig. 5.9). These lasted for 1–3 s, were not associated with clinical manifestations and occurred at a later stage when children did not have seizures. These findings are compatible with the above expressed view that age-related 'focal seizure sensitivity' diffuses at a later stage. Additionally, I could not find any EEG of any child with Rolandic seizures that had the typical 3–4 Hz spike and slow wave of absence epilepsy. Conversely, only three of more than 100 children with typical absence epilepsy that I investigated with video-EEG had CTS in their EEG, but none had clinical features of Rolandic seizures. However, one of the 72 children with Rolandic seizures developed later in life brief absences and infrequent GTCS (Fig. 5.10; see also illustrative case 4.26) and we have also reported a woman with eyelid myoclonia with absences that had Rolandic seizures as a child.[362] These cases are probably no more than what we would expect from coincidence or from an exceptional development of diffuse cortical excitability. We have also reported the co-existence of aggressive functional spike foci, centrotemporal spikes and generalized spike-wave discharges in children without seizures complaining of episodic dizziness and headache (see Chapter 16).[7]

Irrespective of my experience, brief generalized discharges of spike and slow wave, particularly in sleep recordings, of children with Rolandic seizures are well reported.[99,102] They are usually of no clinical significance as they are not associated with ictal clinical manifestations. Generalized discharges can also occur in normal children with CTS but no seizures.[154] In particular, Cavazzuti *et al.*[154] reported that school children with CTS could later develop generalized discharges and vice versa.

The highest percentage of generalized discharges often associated with clinical manifestations in Rolandic seizures was reported by Annette Beaumanoir *et al.*, 1974.[78] This is a well performed longitudinal study of 26 children with Rolandic seizures which were exhaustively investigated with all types of EEG while awake and during sleep. A routine EEG was performed every 8 months; 15 children had 4–36 h tele-EEG supplemented with audio and video recordings and 10 had overnight EEG.

In routine EEG all 26 children showed centrotemporal spikes although these occurred less often when the child was engaged in some kind of activity. In addition 14 children had brief, less than 3 s, generalized discharges of 3–4 Hz spike and slow wave that were synchronous or asynchronous and often more apparent on the right. 'In two patients a generalized 3 Hz spike and slow wave discharge triggered by hyperventilation lasted 8–9 s without any apparent clinical concomitant.' 'In another patient an EEG performed shortly after a generalized nocturnal seizure revealed petit mal status that was arrested with IV diazepam.' In tele-EEG, 11 of 15 Rolandic seizure patients had brief 3–4 Hz synchronous and generalized spike and slow wave discharges that occurred without any detectable cause and 'were occasionally accompanied by clinical manifestations: halting speech could sometimes be identified in the tape recorded voices, or an involuntary twitch, usually facial, could be seen. These clinical disturbances were always brief and would not have been noticed without the aid of audio and video. Indeed, even with such aids, most paroxysms had no clinical expression at all. However, within a few seconds after the discharge, there was some kind of speech or motor impairment.'[78] Moreover, six patients had 3 Hz generalized discharges of spike-wave lasting for more than 6 s and accompanied clinically by typical absences. 'These were rare in the waking and active state, never occurring more than twice every 5 h.'[78] In four patients, two of whom had tele-EEG captured absences, 'activation procedures triggered absences with typical clinical and EEG manifestations.'[78] All 10 patients that had overnight sleep EEG showed bilaterally synchronous and symmetrical discharges of spike and

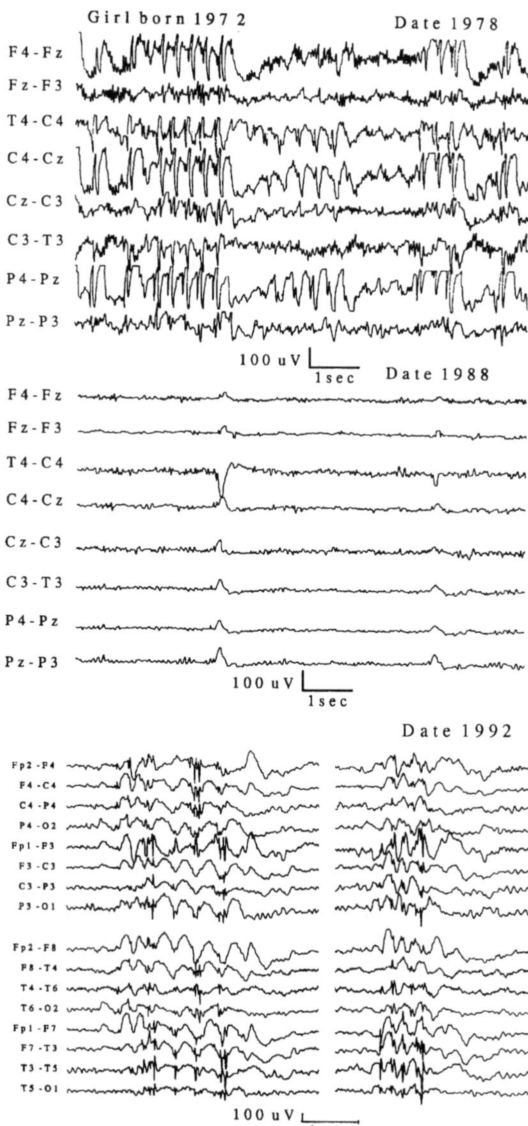

Fig. 5.10. Longitudinal EEG of a girl with nocturnal Rolandic seizures as a child (illustrative case 4.26 in Chapter 4). At age 19 years, after the remission of Rolandic seizures and centrotemporal spikes, she developed two GTCS on awakening.

Upper: EEG at age 6 years. Note the marked and nearly continuous abnormality of spike and slow waves, mainly in the right centrotemporal region.

Middle: EEG at age 16 years. Centrotemporal spikes disappeared and the illustrated sample shows the only abnormality recorded.

Lower: Video-EEG at age 20 years showed frequent brief generalized spike/polyspike and slow wave discharges. These were not associated with cognitive impairment, tested with breath counting. However, occasionally there was a concomitant eyelid fluttering with the generalized discharge.

In addition, there were brief runs of single sharp and slow waves, independently in the left but more frequently the right midtemporal electrodes.

slow wave or polyspikes and slow waves during stages II and III of sleep. These were not observed in REM sleep.

In the same report of Beaumanoir *et al.*, 1974[78] 11 of 26 patients, adults and children with typical absence seizures alone (12 patients) or associated with GTCS (12 patients) and atypical absence epilepsy (two patients) had unilateral or bilateral CTS. Furthermore, four of 26 adult patients with 'occasional focal (one case), focal and generalized (three cases), generalized (22 cases) idiopathic convulsions' had Rolandic spikes.

Beydoun *et al.* 1992[102] retrospectively reviewed 3 years of EEG records and found 50 EEGs of 41 patients who had centrotemporal spikes. Nineteen of them had Rolandic seizures. Six (14.6 per cent) of the 41 children, including two (10.5 per cent) of the 19 with Rolandic seizures, had generalized discharges. These were brief 4–6 spike or polyspike waves (four children) or 3 Hz generalized spike-wave (two children). The authors do not clarify whether these generalized discharges occurred while awake or during sleep. In an illustrative example of a discharge, this is of 1 s duration, consists of mainly slow waves with interspersed small spikes and occurred during drowsiness. The authors concluded that 'the presence or absence of these EEG features was not predictive of the clinical course. The high incidence of generalized spike-wave discharges in children with Rolandic seizures suggests a possible relation in the expression of these two EEG traits.'

Background abnormalities

By definition of an idiopathic seizure-syndrome, background EEG should be normal and this is true for the majority of the children with Rolandic seizures. The rule is that centrotemporal spikes appear in a relatively well organized EEG, with well formed alpha rhythm and no excess or focal slow activity. However, exception is the rule in medicine. Frequent, focal slow activity may be seen in regions with highly firing CTS.[129] In my experience with idiopathic Rolandic seizures, excess of mainly posterior slow waves that may also have some lateralization is often seen in EEGs of children before the appearance or after the disappearance of CTS. Beaumanoir *et al.*, 1974[78] found that EEGs of 19 out of 26 children with Rolandic seizures had 'rhythmical 4 Hz activity of low voltage that was often bilateral in the parieto-occipital areas'. I have also seen children with localized slow waves in the anterior regions which caused me worry regarding an underlying structural lesion. A normal high resolution MRI, subsequent normal background EEG with CTS and more importantly an excellent evolution proved that my initial worries were wrong. These children with focal EEG slow wave abnormalities, focal spike waves or both also had an equally good prognosis with those where the EEG background was normal (see illustrative cases in Chapter 4). Also the case reported on page 95 with ictal video-EEG clearly demonstrates background abnormalities in routine EEG prior to the discovery of CTS.

Centrotemporal spikes in normal children

Table 5.2 shows the prevalence of centrotemporal, occipital and other functional focal spikes in 6392 normal children from four main studies.[154,260,331,586] I have divided them into two groups. Those of school age of 5–6 to 12–14 years and those that are younger, 1–2 to 4–5 years. The following general conclusions can be drawn:

(a) Functional focal spikes occur in 2–4 per cent of normal children and this prevalence may be higher if central spikes were included by Gibbs and Gibbs and if sleep EEGs were performed in the studies of Cavazzti *et al.*[154] and Okubo *et al.*[586]

(b) Centrotemporal and occipital are the main spike locations. In the whole age group of children from 1 to 14 years, centrotemporal are 9.7 times more frequent than occipital spikes. Frontal spikes are rare.

(c) Spike location, at least for the two most common of them, is age related. Thus, in school-age children centrotemporal spikes (median = 2.3 per cent) are probably 10 times or more frequent than occipital spikes (median = 0.2 per cent). Conversely, occipital spikes prevail in younger children below the age of 6 with a median prevalence of 0.9 per cent which is three times as frequent at that of the centrotemporal spikes (median 0.3 per cent). This age-dependent prevalence is very important and explains well the peak age at onset of Rolandic seizures (the clinical representative of the centrotemporal spikes) and the Panayiotopoulos syndrome (the main clinical representative of the occipital spikes).

Table 5.2. EEG spike foci in normal children

Authors	Year	Age range	Number	CTS %	OS %	FS %	GD %
EEG spike foci in normal children from age 5 and 6 years to 12 and 14 years							
Gibbs and Gibbs[331]	1967	5–14	1076	0.7*	0.3	0	0.1
Eeg-Oloffson *et al.*[260]	1971	6–15	533**	2.1***	0	0.6****	
Cavazzuti *et al.*[154]	1981	6–13	3726	2.4	0.1		1.1
Okubo *et al.*[586]	1994	6–12	1057	3.5	0.2	0.1	1.0
Sum/median			6392	2.2	0.1	0.1	1.0
EEG spike foci in normal children from age 1 and 2 years to 4 and 5 years							
Gibbs and Gibbs[331]	1967	2–4	726	0.3*	0.8	0.1	0.1
Eeg-Oloffson *et al.*[260]	1971	1–5	210	0.5	1.0	0.0	0.3
Sum/median			936	0.3	0.9	0.1	0.3

*This prevalence by Gibbs and Gibbs[331] refers to mid-temporal rather than to centrotemporal spikes.
**Of these 533 children 110 who were older than 13 years did not have occipital or centrotemporal spikes. This means that for the 423 children between ages 5 and 13 years the prevalence of centrotemporal spikes was 2.6 per cent.
***This prevalence of 2.1 per cent is derived from eight children with centrotemporal spikes only. There were an additional three children in this age group who had centrotemporal and frontal spikes which means that the prevalence of CTS in this study is 2.6 per cent.
****These were three children who had frontal spike foci together with central, mid-temporal and centrotemporal spikes. There were no children with frontal spike foci only.
CTS = Centrotemporal spikes; FS = Frontal spikes; OS = Occipital spikes; GD = Generalized discharges.

Gibbs and Gibbs (1967)[331] found that amongst the EEGs of 1802 normal children aged 2–14 years the prevalence of midtemporal spikes was 0.53 per cent as compared to 0.4 per cent for occipital and 0.03 per cent for frontal spikes. The prevalence was higher (0.7 per cent) for children aged 5–14 years as compared with 0.3 per cent for those aged 2–4. These numbers do not include central spikes.

Eeg-Olofsson *et al.* (1971)[260] performed awake and sleep EEGs in 743 well defined normal children aged 1 to 15 years. Fourteen children (1.9 per cent) had definite focal spikes. Centrotemporal spikes alone (nine children) or with frontal spikes (three children) occurred in 1.6 per cent. More precisely, centrotemporal spikes were found in only one (0.5 per cent) of the 210 children aged 1–5 years and in 11 (2.6 per cent) of the 6–15 year age group. Three of these children with centrotemporal spikes also had frontal spikes in their EEG. The mean age of children with centrotemporal spikes was 8.6 ± 2.8 (median 8) years. Two (0.3 per cent) children aged 2 and 5 years had right sided occipital spikes. It is also interesting that two of the children with centrotemporal spikes developed paroxysmal activity during IPS which was localized in the posterior regions.

Cavazzuti *et al.* (1980)[154] did a large scale EEG study in 3726 out of approximately 20,000 school children aged 6–13 years in Modena, Italy. Eight channel EEG was recorded during 'wakefulness, at rest and hyperventilation'. All children were neurologically normal and had no history of epileptic seizures. Epileptiform EEG patterns were found in 131 cases (3.54 per cent). The prevalence of CTS was 2.4 per cent. There were 50 children with midtemporal, 27 with Rolandic or parietal and 11 with bilateral midtemporal and/or Rolandic/parietal spikes. Additionally, two children had occipital spikes. Another 41 children had generalized discharges of the 3 Hz spike and slow waves discharges (four cases) or multiple spike and slow wave complexes (37 cases). Half of the subjects with EEG abnormalities had behaviour problems and/or slight psychomotor ability disturbances. Follow-up studies over an 8–9 year period demonstrated the spontaneous disappearance of the EEG abnormalities, usually within school age or, at the latest, during adolescence. Only four of the 88 children with centrotemporal spikes had abnormal EEG by the age of 15–16 and none after the age of 17–18 years. In a few subjects a change of the location of spikes or their evolution into generalized discharges or vice versa was observed. Only two of the 87 normal children with centrotemporal spikes developed 'grand mal' seizures. There is no information of whether these seizures were nocturnal or diurnal but the authors comment that 'In these last two subjects we observed diffusion of the previously unilateral EEG abnormalities and the appearance of generalized discharges of multiple spike and slow wave complexes in connection with the beginning of the clinical epileptic syndrome.' Also that 'we have not observed the development of partial epilepsy in our subjects'.[78] Five of the 41 children with generalized discharges developed absences (one), myoclonic jerks (one) or GTCS (three)

Okubo *et al.* (1994)[586] performed a similar study in Japan also recording with eight channel EEG during waking, at rest and hyperventilation in 1057 healthy children aged 6–12 years of an elementary school. Epileptiform discharges, detected in 53 children (5.0 per cent), consisted of centrotemporal spikes (37 cases, 3.5 per cent), generalized spike and slow wave complexes (10 cases, 1 per cent), occipital spikes (two cases, 0.2 per cent), frontal spikes (one case, 0.1 per cent), and a combination of multiple spike and slow wave complexes and focal spikes (two cases). The occurrence of a positive past history of febrile convulsions was higher (18.9 per cent) in children with compared to those without epileptiform discharges (9.4 per cent). Also, using the Rutter scales for teachers and parents, there were no statistically significant differences regarding emotional and behavioural problems between these two groups. Only two (5.3 per cent) of 38 siblings of children with CTS had centrotemporal spikes in their EEG which is by far less than needed to support 'an autosomal-dominant genetic factor for centrotemporal spikes in waking EEGs of healthy children' (see genetics of Rolandic seizures in Chapter 4). Conversely, the occurrence of generalized discharges in siblings of probands with generalized discharges was very high (four of nine, 44.4 per cent), implicating genetic factors.

Centrotemporal spikes in other conditions of children with or without seizures

Centrotemporal spikes and functional spikes in other locations is a frequent EEG finding in children with or without seizures, in the normal or abnormal neurological state. For example, Kellaway, 1980[438] reported that in a cohort of 35,458 children aged 1 to 16 years who were referred for EEG studies, 2724 (7.7 per cent) showed unilateral or independent bilateral foci of spikes or sharp wave and another 802 (2.3 per cent) had multiple foci in the same or heterogeneous regions of both hemispheres. Amongst 2724 with unilateral or independent bilateral foci, 40 per cent were temporal (91 per cent had seizures), 23 per cent central (38 per cent had seizures), 29 per cent occipital (54 per cent had seizures) and 8 per cent frontal (75.4 per cent had seizures). Thus, centrotemporal spikes may occur in a number of diverse conditions from normal children to those with one or a few Rolandic seizures and to a more severe variety of organic brain diseases.

Centrotemporal spikes of the same morphology and other characteristics described in children with Rolandic seizures are often found in a variety of unrelated brain disorders where they also occur in the same age groups and frequently are facilitated by sleep. In this respect it should be reminded that the first recognition of their functional character by Y. Gastaut, 1952[314]was made in children with organic brain diseases such as 'certain infantile athetoses' and 'spastic diplegias'. There was no reference in this report to neurologically normal children and the two illustrated cases suffered from 'Little syndrome' and 'chronic epilepsy with left hemiplegia who underwent hemisphrectomy'. Furthermore, Y. Gastaut[314] concluded about their functional character was mainly influenced by the possibility that these 'prerolandic spikes', as she called them, were the result of an excessive reaction of the prerolandic cortex to the projecting proprioceptive impulses from the intense spasticity or dystonia that these children had (see Appendix 1, page 100).

Also, in the initial reports of Gibbs and Gibbs[326,327,330,331] and Smith and Kellaway[732] (see the excellent review by Kellaway, 1980)[438] children with central or mid-temporal spikes frequently had mental retardation and cerebral palsy with or without epileptic seizures. Thus, Gibbs and Gibbs, 1967[331] in a later review of their findings emphasized that 'mental retardation and cerebral palsy are amongst the most outstanding non-epileptic symptoms of patients with mid-temporal spiking. Birth injury is slightly more common.' They estimated that 13 per cent of children with mid-temporal spikes had cerebral palsy and 16 per cent had mental retardation.[331] Headache was found in 11 per cent of children with mid-temporal spikes and 13 per cent of children with normal EEG.[331] Kellaway,1980[438] found that 'from 203 children with Rolandic (central) spikes 25.4 per cent had Rolandic seizures, 32 per cent had abnormal neurological findings or mental retardation and 42.6 per cent had no seizures with no intellectual or neurological deficit'.[438]

Amongst 136 children older than 3 years of age who had febrile convulsions Kajitani *et al.*, 1981[430] found that 21 (4.2 per cent) of them had CTS, a prevalence which is just above that of normal school-age children (upper limit of reported prevalence 3.5 per cent, see Table 5.2).

Centrotemporal spikes also occur in a number of diverse and unrelated conditions such as fragile X syndrome,[276,444,554–556,674] Rett syndrome[299,376,572,573,679,681,790,830] and Fukuyama type congenital muscular dystrophy.[823]

In all these conditions the centrotemporal spikes appear in the same age group as for Rolandic seizures, are often exaggerated by sleep and usually disappear after late teens. The EEG frequently shows marked background or focal abnormalities of slow waves and other forms of epileptiform activity such as polyspikes, in the same or subsequent EEG. These children may or may not have seizures.

Age-dependence and evolution of the centrotemporal spikes

Centrotemporal spikes, as all other functional spikes, are age-dependent, that is they appear at a certain age of maturation and have a short life span with normalization of the EEG after a few years.

The age at onset of centrotemporal spikes is mainly from 3 to 13 years with a peak at 8–9 years. This is shown in Fig. 5.11 where the cumulative results of Gibbs and Gibbs[327,329,331] (388 children with centrotemporal spikes and 318 with occipital spikes) and Kellaway[438] (1736 subjects with centrotemporal and 790 with occipital) are put together by approximation. It should be realized that this histogram reflects the tendency of the spikes to disappear with time and the addition of new cases which are two opposing factors. The prevalence of centrotemporal spikes gradually increases from the first year of age to peak at age 8–9 years and gradually decline afterwards.

The 'life span' of centrotemporal and other functional spike foci is limited. The consensus is best summarized by Kellaway[438] as follows: 'Longitudinal studies of children with spike foci show that all such foci, regardless of locus, tend to disappear with increasing age or the passage of time. The rate and degree of attrition vary somewhat depending on location, but for all foci there is an initial period of 1–2 years of a high attrition rate with 50–60 per cent of the children losing their focus within 12 months of its first demonstration. Within 5 years only about 15–22 per cent of the foci are still present.' Though Kellaway[438] refers to centrotemporal and other 'functional' foci in other locations indiscriminately of neurological status which could be normal or abnormal, the same results are obtained from other longitudinal studies from normal school-age children[154] or children with Rolandic seizures.[127,128,328,483,498,504,562] Thus, Cavazzuti *et al.*, 1980[154] in a longitudinal study of school-age children over 8–9 years found that midtemporal (50 cases), Rolandic or parietal (27 cases) and occipital spikes (two cases) 'spontaneously disappeared, usually within school age or, at the latest, during adolescence.' Similarly, Lerman and Kivity-Ephraim , 1981[485] studied focal epileptic EEG discharges, mainly centrotemporal and occipital spikes, in 100 children not suffering from seizures and confirmed that these are age-dependent, tending to disappear during the teenage years.

A similar rate of attrition of centrotemporal spikes and normalization of EEG with age in children suffering from Rolandic seizures is well documented in all relevant reports.[127,128,328,483,498,504,562]

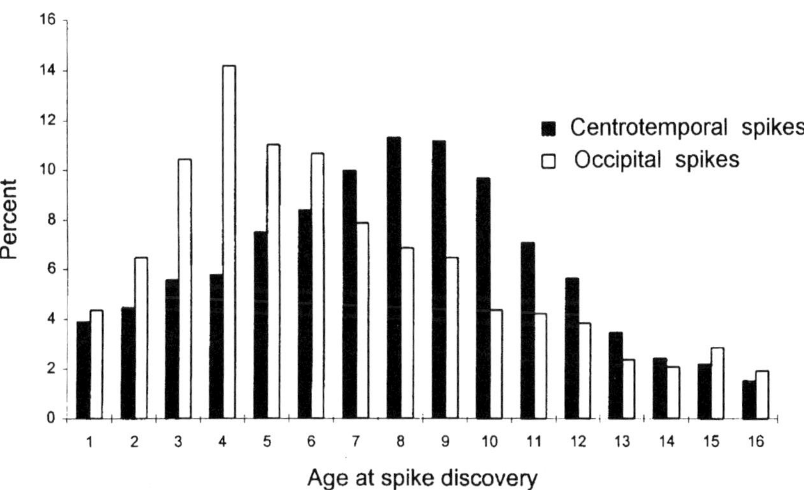

Fig. 5.11. Age-related prevalence of occipital spikes and centrotemporal spikes in EEG of subjects with or without seizures. This was estimated by approximation from the combined data of Gibbs et al.[326] *and Kellaway*[438] *(see text).*

Note that the peak age of first discovery of the occipital spikes is much earlier (3–5 years) than that of the centrotemporal spikes (7–10 years). These correspond to the peak age at onset of the Panayiotopoulos syndrome (peak at 5 years) and Rolandic seizures (7–10 years).

Ictal EEG of Rolandic seizures

There are only a few seizures recorded with EEG.[23,25,135,178,195,196,372,401,481,538,682,797,801,812]

Figures 5.12a, 5.12b and 5.12c show EEG samples from an ictal video-EEG of a Rolandic seizure that was recorded at St. Thomas' Hospital by technician Mr S. Rowlinson who has the rewarding task to video-EEG nearly all patients referred for possible or definite seizures. This was a routine video-EEG after partial sleep deprivation of a nine and a half-year-old girl. The following are extracts of her clinical history detailed by Dr C D Ferrie, consultant paediatric neurologist:

> Case 5.1. This is a nine and a half-year-old normal girl, top of her class. She had 5–10 seizures that started at age 8 years mainly in successive nights. All occurred approximately half an hour after she has gone to sleep; on one occasion the attack occurred just as she got up from bed to go to the toilet after waking up half an hour into her sleep. She is totally unaware of the attacks apart from the one on her way to the toilet when she felt slightly light-headed prior to losing consciousness.
>
> Her parents feel that they can predict when she is about to have an attack because she feels nauseated for a day or so prior to this and also does not seem quite herself. She looks rather pale and gets tired easily.
>
> The very beginning of the seizures was never witnessed. Her parents are aware of them because they have a baby alarm in her room and they hear a strange gurgling noise. They find her unresponsive, drooling saliva, her face twisted or deviated to one side followed by unilateral clonic convulsions. Her first seizure was prolonged for 40 min and was slightly unusual in that she had definite repeated ictal vomiting during it.
>
> She had two routine awake EEG. The first was normal and the second was reported as showing runs of occipital intermittent rhythmic delta waves interpreted elsewhere as suggestive of localized or systemic pathology.
>
> I am fairly strongly of the opinion that these are benign childhood partial seizures ... I will first try to confirm this with a sleep EEG.

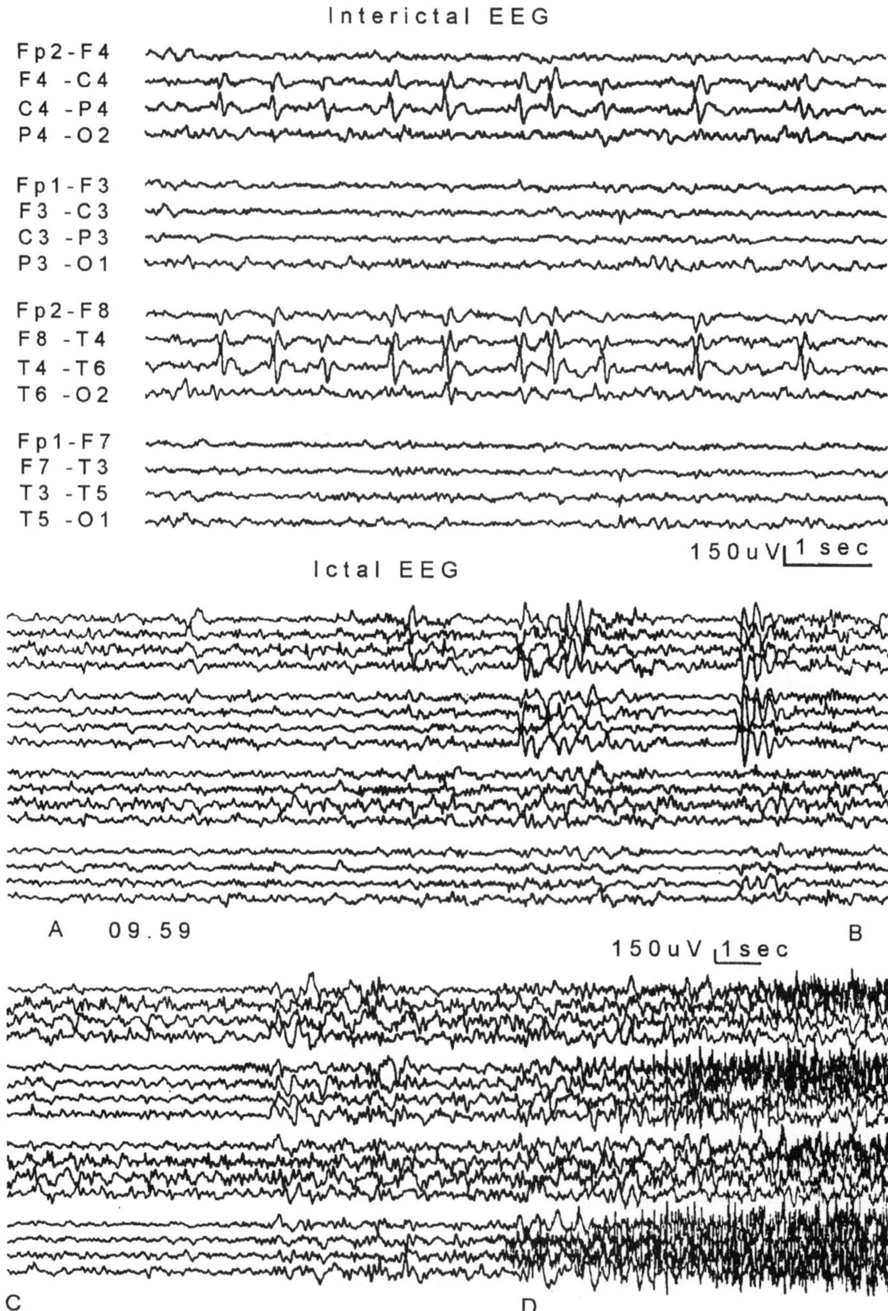

Fig. 5.12a. Upper: Interictal video EEG with frequent right centrotemporal spikes. Also note small left sided centrotemporal spikes.
Middle and lower: Ictal video-EEG. Prior to the seizure the centrotemporal spikes remitted (A) with the appearance of small spikes and slow waves in the same regions (B and C) before the onset of the clinical manifestations of the seizure (D) (see details in Fig. 5.12b). Numbers denote actual time (minutes and seconds). See details of clinical events in text.

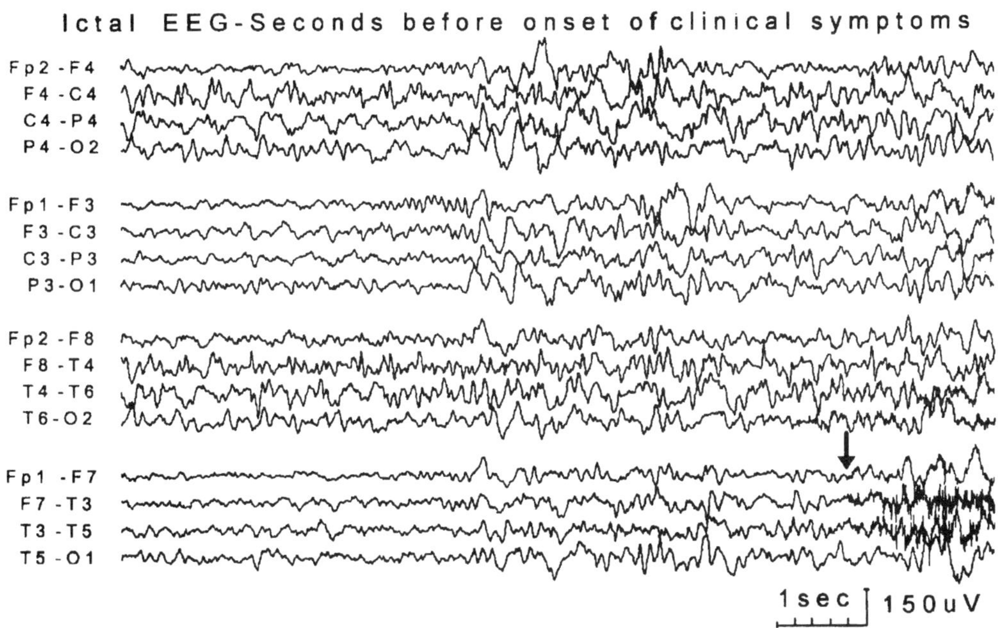

Fig. 5.12b. From Fig. 5.12 a. Details of the onset of the discharge prior to the ictal events. Arrow indicates onset of clinical manifestations (note muscle artefacts on the left)

The interictal awake EEG had normal background with frequent right sided CTS that became abundant during sleep. Infrequent small spikes also occurred independently in the left posterior temporal electrode (Fig. 5.12a). Brief 2–4 s generalized discharges of sharp slow waves intermixed with small spikes were recorded only during sleep. These were not associated with clinical manifestations.

The seizure occurred 5 min after onset of sleep. Before the seizure the girl was in stage II of sleep, lying on her stomach with the right side of the face in the pillow. Clinically the first manifestation was a tonic contraction of the left facial muscles (see onset of muscle artefact over the left temporal channels at D in Fig. 5.12a and 5.12b) with head moving left and upwards. Simultaneous with the tonic contraction, there was fast clonic jerking only of the left eyelid while both eyes were semi-opened. Within seconds and while the face was in tonic contraction to the left, the left eyelid showed fast clonic contractions, and there was a tonic backwards arching of the trunk with flexion of the legs at the knees. This was followed by a prolonged generalized clonic phase that lasted for 4 min and 39 s. During this phase, the child was stiff with fast, low range flexion clonic spasms of the proximal muscles of all limbs and jaw. The eyes were opened in the middle position and did not demonstrate any movements. Gradually, the clonic convulsions became less intense and slower, more apparent in the upper limbs and jaw.

The electrical event lasted for 6.5 min. It started in the right central and midtemporal regions with 2–3 Hz slow waves and irregular, random and monophasic medium voltage fast rhythms and spikes intermixed and superimposed on the slow waves (A to D, Figs. 5.12a and 5.12b). This activity tended to spread and the amplitude of the fast rhythms and spikes rapidly increased before the first clinical manifestation which occurred 30 s from the onset of the EEG ictal changes (D in Fig. 5.12a and arrow in Fig. 5.12b). The clonic phase was characterized by generalized polyspikes interrupted by slow waves at 5–7 Hz, gradually slowing to 4–5 Hz and finally to 1–2 Hz (Fig. 5.12c). The polyspike discharges were maximal posteriorly with some right sided emphasis. The electrical event of

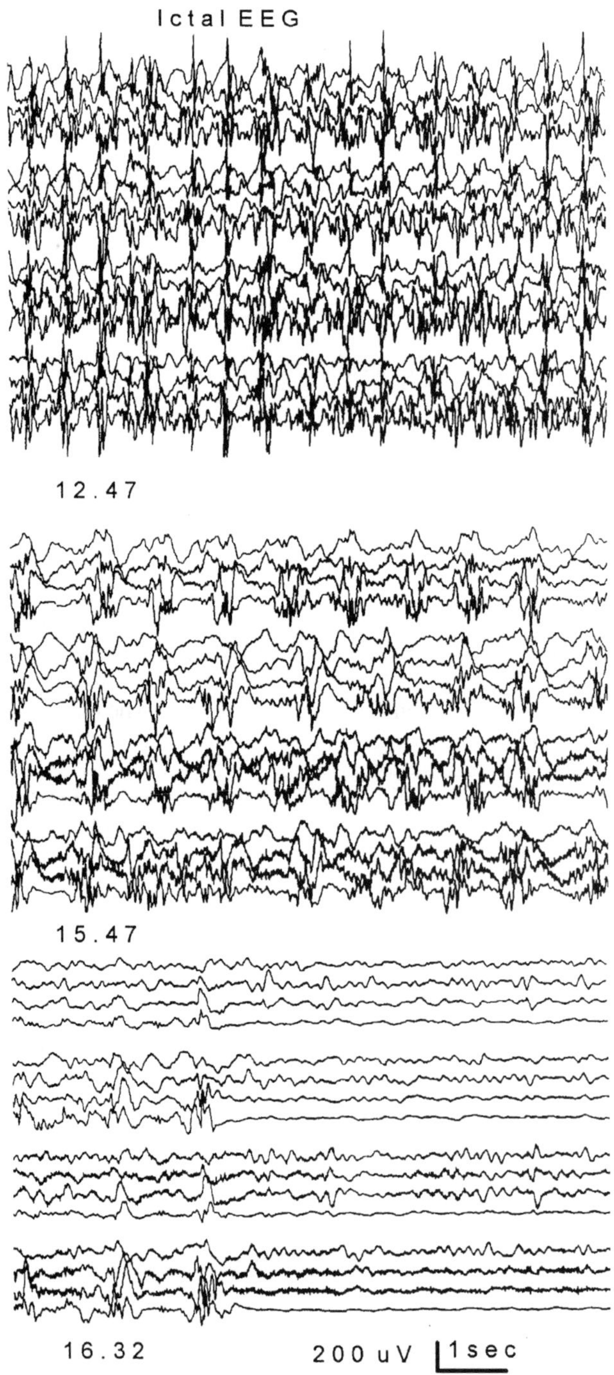

Fig. 5.12c. The end of the seizure of patient in Fig. 5.12a and 5.12b. Numbers denote actual time (minutes and seconds). See text.

polyspikes and slow wave at 1–1.5 Hz continued for 60 s after the cessation of the clinical events. During the last 10 s these were localized mainly over the left posterior regions.

post-ictally the record was dominated by generalized 1–2.5 Hz slow activity. post-ictal CTS appeared after 5 s and were of longer duration and of rather higher amplitude. The first run of sleep spindles was recorded 28 min post-ictally.

Dalla Bernardina and Tassinari (1975)[196] reported the ictal EEG of a child with Rolandic seizures during a partial motor hemifacial seizure in phase II of natural sleep.

Ambrosseto and Gobbi (1975)[25] recorded a seizure of a 10-year-old boy during the drowsy state of awakening. This consisted of turning of the eyes and head to the opposite side of the EEG ictal activity with tonic extension of the limbs followed by unilateral clonic jerking; 30 s later, his eyes and head turned to the other side and he had ipsilateral clonic jerks. The child became cyanosed and there was post-ictal deep sleep.

Roger *et al.* (1990)[682] reported the ictal EEG of an 8.5-year-old boy with a 40 s seizure at stage II of sleep. This consisted of rhythmic spikes involving 'secondarily the vertex and the left temporal regions'. Clinically there was tonic contraction followed by clonic jerks of the right facial muscles.

Lerman (1992)[481] refers to a diurnal seizure recorded in one of his patients: 'it began with local decremental activity followed by dense spikes in the centrotemporal area during the tonic phase and 'spike-waves' in the clonic phase, with no spread and no post-ictal slowing. The whole episode lasted less than 1 min'.

Watanabe (1996)[797] described two cases: The first is of a 9-year-old girl who had a seizure during stage II of sleep. 'Low voltage semi-rhythmic alpha activity appeared from the left midtemporal region which propagated to other areas with increasing amplitude and decreasing frequency. Seven s later, the right corner of her mouth was drawn downward to the right. Ten s later, she opened her eyes. Fifteen s later, her head rotated to the right, followed by GTCS.' The other case of Watanabe[797] is a diurnal simple partial seizure of a 9-year-old girl. The attack consisted of speech arrest and salivation. EEG showed ' a burst of repetitive spikes in the right and left midtemporal and central regions' with the 'dipole showing negativity in the midtemporal and positivity in the frontal regions' for less than 30 s.

Westmoreland, 1998[801] illustrated the ictal EEG of a 10-year-old boy with a diurnal seizure that started with numbness of the right side of the mouth progressing after approximately 10 s to 'lips quivering, head and eyes to the right' followed by clonic movements of the right side of the face. The ictal discharge of rhythmic fast activity started from the left mid-temporal regions after a cluster of left interictal mid-temporal spikes.

Wirrell (1998)[812] also reported a diurnal ictal seizure of an 8-year-old girl with focal spikes in the left centrotemporal-parietal region during the tonic phase evolving to spike and wave during the clonic phase.

Horita and Maekawa (1993)[401] reported a 9-year-old boy with Rolandic seizures and 'right centro-parietal spikes'. During polysomnography, he had 'a partial seizure of the left face with impaired consciousness'. On the ictal EEG, a low-voltage fast discharge was initiated in the right frontal area followed by a diffuse rhythmic high voltage discharge at 5–6 Hz.

Boulloche *et al.* (1990)[135] reported a 5-year 4-month-old patient with clusters of oropharyngolaryngeal seizures consisting of sialorrhea and speech arrest. 'EEG showed repeated bilateral centrotemporal spikes-waves discharges which sometimes were associated with bilateral facial clonic contractions synchronous with anarthria and sialorrhea. Consciousness was preserved.' Transient pseudo-bulbar palsy (anterior opercular syndrome) resulted from seizures: loss of identifiable speech, drooling with difficulties in swallowing, absence of palatal movements and of the gag reflex. Intellectual functions remained normal. Seizures resolved within a few weeks after treatment with sodium valproate and carbamazepine.

Gutierrez *et al.* (1990)[372] reported a subclinical ictal event in Rolandic seizures with multiple spike and wave discharges appearing as a reverse dipole that was electropositive in T3–C3 and negative in F3. They postulated that the seizure discharge originated in the depths of the sylvian fissure involving folded cortical areas. Similarly, Silva *et al.*, 1995[728] describe a 15-year-old boy with Rolandic seizures. A 45 s subclinical ictal electrographic discharge was electropositive in T4 while interictal right sided mid-temporal spikes were electronegative in the same locations.

Appendix 1

A misleading element of the electroencehalographic semiology: the prerolandic spikes without focal significance. [314]

By Mme Y. Gastaut

I am grateful for this translation from the French to Dr M. Koutroumanidis, Neurologist and Clinical Neurophysiologist.

This report concerns very brief variations of biphasic potential difference, occurring over the prerolandic regions where they take the form of a spike. They are unilateral or bilateral and, in the latter case, asynchronous or synchronous, asymmetric or symmetric (asymmetry of amplitude and not of topography). They are sporadic but can be grouped in brief volleys assuming a pseudo-rhythmic appearance. They do not react to eye opening but they block to fist clenching and, on the contrary, they are facilitated by release of the fist after a sustained contraction. They frequently accompany the other Rolandic activities that react similarly, notably beta rhythm and its sub-harmonic variety, the mu rhythm (rythme en arceau). These prerolandic spikes can often be presented as an isolated arched wave.

These (prerolandic spikes) reflect, without any doubt, an excessive mode of reaction of the prerolandic cortex to the projecting proprioceptive afferents, following the observations of Gay and Gellhorn (1949) in the cat and the ape, and of Dowson (1951) and Gastaut (1952) in humans.

They (prerolandic spikes) are observed in (the context of) direct prerolandic hyperexcitabilities, provoked by a local irritation, but also in indirect (hyperexcitabilities), provoked by a sustained bombardment of proprioceptive afferents; this is why they can be observed in subjects bearing an irritative lesion in the Rolandic areas as well as in those who present a dystonic muscular disorder characterized by an intense but discontinuous spasticity, or by paroxysmal variations of tone. Thus, they constitute the characteristic element of the dystonic disorders of subcortical origin: a) of certain infantile athetoses, where they are manifested in between the abnormal movements; b) mainly of the spastic diplegias where they are evidently bilateral, less when a hemiparesis is superimposed, which by cancelling out the tonic spasms of the one side of the body, suppresses the spikes of the opposite hemisphere, resulting in the apparently contradictory situation of spikes ipsilateral to hemiplegia.

The error not to be committed is to confuse these 'functional' prerolandic spikes with those which accompany certain focal cortical lesions, and make of this, a sign of 'latent' epilepsy, or of cortical scar with 'epileptogenic potential'. Taking again the example of hemiplegia developed on the ground of bilateral spasticity, which is the case in a number of infantile encephalopathies, the error which should not be committed is to consider the 'functional' spikes over the sound hemisphere as a manifestation of a focal lesion; a point of view which would lead to suppose a lesion ipsilateral to the hemiplegia or, for example, to deny because of bilateral (EEG) alterations an otherwise indicated by important contralateral EEG abnormalities hemispherectomy.

(Work from the Laboratory of Neurobiology of the Faculty of Medicine, Marseilles. Pr agrege: H. Gastaut.)

Fig.1 was an example of prerolandic spikes in two cases of Little syndrome with right and left hemiparesis respectively. In both cases the spikes were on the same side as the hemiparesis.

Fig. 2 was an EEG of 'a chronic epileptic with left hemiplegia, to whom hemispherectomy was offered. There are important diffuse abnormalities in the right hemisphere while the left presents only prerolandic spikes that disappear during clenching of the fist. These spikes, considered as functional, did not contraindicate the operation which has been entirely successful.'

Part III
Occipital seizures and related epileptic syndromes

Chapter 6. Occipital seizures: The symptoms

Chapter 7. Occipital epilepsies: The syndromes

Chapter 8. Early onset benign childhood occipital seizures: Panayiotopoulos syndrome

Chapter 9. Late onset benign childhood occipital seizures or late onset idiopathic childhood occipital epilepsy

Chapter 10. Occipital spikes, occipital paroxysms and other electroencephalographic findings in children with benign childhood occipital seizures. Occipital spikes in normal children and those without seizures

Chapter 11. Benign childhood occipital seizures and related epileptic syndromes: Historical aspects and literature review

Chapter 12A. Epilepsies characterized by seizures with specific modes of precipitation (reflex epilepsies): General aspects

Chapter 12B. Idiopathic photosensitive occipital seizures

Chapter 13. Benign childhood occipital seizures and related epileptic syndromes: Personal studies

Benign Childhood Partial Seizures and Related Epileptic Syndromes. C P Panayiotopoulos
©1999 John Libbey & Company Ltd., pp. 103–117.

Chapter 6

Occipital seizures: The symptoms

Definition

Occipital seizures originate from an epileptic occipital focus that is triggered spontaneously or by external visual stimuli. Elementary visual hallucinations are the commonest and most characteristic ictal symptom, most likely the first and often the only seizure clinical manifestation. Ictal elementary visual hallucinations mainly consist of small multi-coloured circular patterns that often appear in the periphery of a temporal visual hemi-field, becoming larger and multiplying in the course of the seizure, frequently moving horizontally towards the other side and lasting for seconds to 1–3 min, rarely longer. Elementary visual hallucinations may progress and co-exist with other occipital seizure symptoms such as illusions of ocular movements and ocular pain, pursuit-like tonic deviation of the eyes, eyelid fluttering or repetitive eye closures and oculoclonic-epileptic nystagmus. Complex visual hallucinations, visual illusions, and other symptoms from more anterior ictal spreading occur in the seizure progress which may terminate with hemiconvulsions or generalized convulsions. Ictal blindness, appearing *ab initio* or less commonly after other occipital seizure manifestations, usually lasts for 3–5 min though status amauroticus may occasionally occur. Complex visual hallucinations, without the emotional and complicated character of temporal lobe seizures, originate from the junction of the occipital with the parietal and temporal lobes. They may be the first ictal symptom, often follow elementary visual hallucinations and progress to other ictal clinical manifestations as above. Consciousness in not impaired during the elementary and complex visual hallucinations, blindness and other occipital seizure symptoms (simple partial seizures) but may be disturbed or lost in the course of the seizure usually prior to convulsions. Ictal vomiting, occurring at onset or the course of an occipital seizure, may originate from extra-occipital spreading. post-ictal headache, often with other migraine-like symptoms such as vomiting and photophobia, is probably more frequently associated with occipital than any other partial seizures and may occur even after brief visual seizures. Frequency of occipital seizures varies from daily to once per life. Visual seizures, particularly if they are associated with post-ictal headache, imitate migraine with aura, basilar and acephalgic migraine for which they are commonly mistaken though their true epileptic identity cannot easily escape clinical scrutiny.

Introduction

The cardinal symptoms of occipital seizures are mainly visual and occulo-motor. Visual symptoms include elementary and complex visual hallucinations, blindness, visual illusions and pallinopsia. There may also be sensory hallucinations of ocular movements and ocular pain. Ictal oculo-motor symptoms include tonic deviation of the eyes (more pursuit-like than oculotonic), oculoclonic or nystagmus and repetitive eyelid closures or eyelid fluttering. Some of these ictal manifestations are primarily generated in the occipital cortex or in the neighbourhood of the occipital-parietal and temporal lobes. Seizures may spread from the occipital to other more anterior regions of the brain generating symptoms from the temporal, parietal and frontal lobes and secondary hemi or generalized convulsions. Ictal vomiting and ictal or post-ictal headache are frequently associated with occipital seizures. Occipital seizures manifesting with elementary visual hallucinations, blindness, vomiting and headache alone or in combination may imitate migraine, which is the reason that they are often mistaken for migraine with aura, acephalgic or basilar migraine.[370,611,618,625,795]

Avanzini[55] has comprehensively reviewed the anatomical and functional properties of the occipital lobes in relation to occipital seizures. Plant[658] has detailed the anatomy and physiology of eyelids.

Abbreviations

GTCS = Generalized tonic–clonic seizures
MRI = Magnetic resonance imaging
CT Scan = Computed tomography scan
SPECT = Single photon emission tomography
EBOS = Early onset benign childhood occipital seizures
LBOS = Late onset benign childhood occipital seizures

Historical aspects of occipital seizures, visual hallucinations and blindness

Gowers (1885)[352] found that 119 of 1000 patients with epileptic seizures had a 'special sensory aura' which in 81 patients was referred to as 'the organ or sense of sight'. He divided the patients with ocular and visual warnings into those with

(a) a sensation in the eyeball itself, (b) diplopia, (c) apparent increase or diminution of the size of objects, (d) loss of sight and (e) distinct visual sensations.

Loss of sight preceded loss of consciousness in 26 patients, and one patient was blind for 1 h. Lights, colours, a ball of light, a flash or a glare was perceived by 46 patients. In one patient, the seizures began with dazzling red and white stars and progressed to a vision of an old woman. Another patient first saw bright coloured lights followed by the image of a girl.

It is also interesting that the first scientific evidence of photosensitive epilepsy by Gowers (1881)[351] refers to occipital seizures induced by bright light. This patient was a man, with 'bright blue lights, like stars–always the same' preceded GTCS that were elicited 'at any time by looking at a bright light, even a bright fire. The relation is intelligible since the discharges apparently commenced in the visual centre'.

Terminology

Visual hallucinations are subjectively experienced images in the absence of an actual external stimulus
Elementary visual hallucinations consist of single, usually geometric forms, spots or lines
Complex visual hallucinations consist of objects, faces or scenes
Percept is the mental image or product of perception of any object in space
Phosphenes are subjective sensations of light due to non-luminous stimulation of the retina. Phosphenes are also used to denote visual percepts from stimulation of the visual cortex with electrical stimulation, in which case they are usually coloured spots or circles[709]
Visual illusions are misinterpreted false percepts of real external images
Palinopsia is the persistence or recurrence of visual images after the exciting stimulus has been removed
Stereoscopic vision is the normal accurate depth perception achieved with binocular vision
Teleoscopic vision refers to visual illusions that the objects appear far away and small

Visual hallucinations and other visual seizure symptoms

Elementary visual hallucinations

The elementary visual hallucinations of idiopathic occipital seizures[611,618,625] are detailed in Chapters 9 and 13 and in my experience they are not different from those of symptomatic occipital seizures. Ictal elementary visual hallucinations are usually stereotyped for each patient, often lasting for seconds and rarely to more than 1–2 min. They consist of mainly bright multi-coloured, rarely dichromatic or monochromatic, predominantly circular patterns of spots, circles or balls. Bright red, yellow, blue and green appear to predominate. Coloured square, triangular and rectangular or star-like shapes, alone or in combination with circular patterns, are infrequent. Individual elements of the visual hallucinations are usually multiple (tens or hundreds) but 1–4 may also occur. Their size varies from 'spots' to occasionally the size of a coin or a small ball. They may multiply and increase in size in the course of the seizure and may progress to other non-visual occipital seizure symptoms and more rarely to extra-occipital manifestations and convulsions.

Similar descriptions, 'colours, a ball of light',[352] several small spheres, white in the centre with an intermediate zone of blue and outside this a ring of red',[396] 'balls of fire but redder than any fire',[396] 'round bright coloured object rotating in front of his left eye', [651] dominate all relevant reports[51,57,74,220,304,313,352,396,404,513,602,608,611,625,651 ,700,797,804,811] from the time of Gowers[352] and Holmes.[396] These coloured and circular elementary visual hallucinations are more likely to originate from the primary visual cortex as demonstrated by electrical stimulation studies of patients with occipital epilepsies[486,651] and in intracortical microstimulation of the visual cortex of blind people for purposes of visual prosthesis.[709]

Other seizure descriptions have included stars, triangular or polygonal and more rarely streaks or lines, again generally coloured.[513,648,650,694] Flickering, flashing, pulsating or twinkling lights are also occasionally described and are more likely to originate from the lateral convexity of the occipital cortex.[647,648,694]

Penfield and Rasmussen[651] gave the following descriptions from stimulation in or near the calcarine fissure on the pole of the occipital lobe: 'Red, green and yellow lights', 'Red and blue light moving slowly', 'Coloured stars', 'Stars', 'Star before each eye', 'Diamonds', 'Star, Two stars', 'Wheels', 'Colours, like an attack', 'Fawn and blue light', 'Lights like an attack', 'Blue, green, and coloured discs', 'Colours advancing', 'Coloured balls. When repeated he reported light', 'White mark on contralateral side and red spot ipsilateral side', Red and blue wheels', 'Flashing in eyes and red mark'. The same authors[651] remarked: 'In general, it would appear that the calcarine image was more often coloured while images produced from the secondary visual zone more often consisted of colourles light','The colour images seen may be summarized as red, green, yellow, pink, blue, fiery, gray and fawn', 'The visual contours were simple and unreal ...The descriptions run as follows: a brilliant ball, a star, a streak, a wheel, a spot or a flash, a shadow, a light' and they further clarify:

> The sufferer from ophthalmic migraine may have experienced something similar and yet the detailed zigzag outlines of migraine images have not been described to us.[651]

Elementary visual hallucinations are usually unilateral, contralateral to the side of the epileptic focus, appearing in a normal, blind or damaged hemifield[694] and often increasing in numbers and size as the seizure progresses. However, they may also be seen in the centre and obscure the visual field. Unilateral visual hallucinations may be moving horizontally towards the other side in which case their appearance may be ipsilateral to the epileptogenic focus.[57,513] Less frequently, the movement is rotatory, peripheral, random, approaching or moving away from the patient.[513,648,694]

According to the stimulation studies of Penfield and Rasmussen:[651] 'Visual movement was more frequently present than absent. The image might remain still but more often it moved slowly in a certain direction or it danced, flickered, or whirled'.[651]

Elementary visual hallucinations are brief, lasting seconds to less than 2 min, though rarely they may last much longer.[370,396,795]

Elementary visual hallucinations may be the only seizure manifestation but they often progress to other ictal symptoms such as complex visual hallucinations, oculoclonic seizures, tonic deviation of the eyes, eyelid fluttering or repetitive eye closure, impairment of consciousness, experiential phenomena, hemi-anaesthesia and unilateral or generalized convulsions.

They may be infrequent or occur several times per day.

Ludwig and Marsan (1975)[513] found that 47 per cent of patients with an occipital EEG focus of mainly symptomatic occipital epilepsy had visual hallucinations. 'The more common visual aberration, the simple visual aura, included reports of elementary sensations of light and colour in simple or gross form. These descriptions were quite variable amongst patients with respect to colour, morphology, position in space, and type of movement; however, in any one particular patient only one or at the most two visual patterns predominated, remaining constant through the years as a prelude to a seizure with no change in their own inherent qualities. A panoply of colours was reported; green, red-orange, white, yellow, purple-black, silver, red, and polychromatic. Morphologies or contours perceived included; a line or streak, a square, flashing light, zigzag lines of light, a spot, stars, a circle, ball of lights, dust-like particles, spark, non-specific design or pattern, and a disk with star-like projection. Movement of the image was present rather often and was described either as rotatory horizontal, peripheral, random or in a direction away from or toward the patient. Simple visual phenomena had lateralizing features at their onset in 2/3 of patients. In the remaining 1/3 images were diffuse or described as directly in front of the patient. Stationary auras were contralateral to the epileptogenic focus. In horizontally moving auras the cerebral focus is ipsilateral to the side of origin and contralateral to its terminus'.

Repeated elementary visual seizures in the form of status epilepticus have been described but are exceptional.[308,795] Walker *et al.* 1995[795]described a 31-year-old man with occipital simple partial status epilepticus also misdiagnosed as migraine: From age 13 years, he had episodes of simple partial status epilepticus occurring twice a month. These typically consisted of elementary visual hallucinations of flashing lights obscuring his left visual field for a period of 2 days, associated with a severe frontal headache that progressed to complex partial seizure symptomatology or secondarily generalized convulsions. EEG showed that a single sharp/slow wave discharge over the right occipital lobe was associated with the perception of a flash of light in the left visual field. High-resolution MRI revealed that the right hemisphere and right caudate nucleus were smaller than the left and there was an abnormal gyral pattern in the right parietal region. Despite these remarkable clinico-EEG-MRI features this patient was diagnosed for many years as having migraine.

Complex visual hallucinations

Complex visual hallucinations as the first, opening symptom of occipital seizures are less common than elementary visual hallucinations, maybe less than 10 per cent. They probably originate from the occipito-parietal-temporal junction and they are likely to be more frequent in symptomatic than idiopathic occipital epilepsy.

Complex visual hallucinations may take the form of persons, animals, objects, figures or scenes. They may be a face or a limb, a number or a letter, static or moving, normal in size, smaller or larger than normal, vividly real, outlined or distorted or of changing shape and dimension and progressing to more complex visual hallucinatory experiences. They may be familiar, friendly or frightening, unfamiliar and grotesque. They may or not be related to past visual experience and connected with past events. They may appear in a small or large area of a hemifield or in the centre and the whole of the visual field. They may be static, moving horizontally, expanding or shrinking, approaching or moving away. In patients with visual field defects due to structural brain lesions, complex visual hallucinations appear in the defective visual field.[63,131,312,313,447,448,465,466,486,513,700,738,746,749,796,811]

An influential report on the subject is by Lance, 1976[465] and the subject has been recently effectively reviewed by Kolmel, 1993.[448] Lesser *et al.*, 1998[486] found that 'formed visual illusions were elicited upon stimulation of electrodes located at the lateral occipital-posterior temporal junction implying higher order processing in this region. Visual responses were described as a white question mark or the outline of a person's head in the hemifield contralateral to the stimulated eye'. Colour may be normal or the figures or pictures may be colourless, and they may appear distorted to take the form of grotesque images. More often, they are weak in colour and stereotypical in appearance, which allows differentiation from visual hallucinations of other causes.[447]

An interesting but extremely rare ictal complex visual hallucination is autoscopia (or heautoscopy) which means viewing one's own image, viewing oneself.[177,746] This mirror self image looks 'real', usually undistorted, silent and brief or recurrent, from the present time or from the past, framed or performing complex tasks.

Complex visual hallucinations including ictal autoscopia probably originate from occipito-parietal and occipito-temporal junction areas.[64,131,448,459,474,746] In two patients reported by Penfield *et al.*[650,651] habitual complex visual hallucinations could be elicited by stimulation of the right posterior temporal regions.

Visual illusions

Ictal visual illusions are most likely generated from the non-dominant parietal regions.[459] However, they are encountered in patients with occipital epilepsy probably from spreading to the parietal neighbouring regions.

Visual illusions are misinterpretations, false percepts, of real external images.[164,448] These distorted images (metamorphopsia)[164,166] involve changes in size, dimension, shape, proportions, position, colour, illumination and movement, alone or in combination. Changes in perception of object size (dysmegalopsia) are common, the percepts being smaller (micropsia) or larger (macropsia) than the real image. Objects may be distorted in shape, pulled, compressed or rotated in lateral or vertical directions (dysmorphopsia). They may appear in black and white (achromatopsia), in one colour (monochromopsia), and be hazy and dark or highly illuminated and bright. Motion and speed may be affected with or without distortion of direction (horizontal, vertical or rotated, approaching or moving away). Movement is faster or slower. Moving objects may appear stationary and vice versa.

Visual illusions also entail changes in spatial interpretation affecting stereoscopic vision. 'Far objects appear near, near ones far, and convex ones concave, or vice versa (pseudoscopic vision)'.[166]

Ictal visual illusions may occupy part or the whole visual field and are probably more likely to be associated with symptomatic than idiopathic occipital seizures.

It should be emphasized that visual illusions may be an entirely normal phenomenon. Abe *et al.*[4] examined the prevalence of episodic macropsia, micropsia, and distortions of time perception in 3,224 high-school students aged 13 to 18 years. About 9 per cent of the students reported having experienced one or more types of episodic illusion within the past 6 months. The prevalence of probable migraine was more than three times higher in students with episodic illusions than in those with no episodic illusions. Experiencing more than one type of illusion was found to be associated with probable migraine. Illusions appeared only during fever or while falling asleep in 25 per cent of a subsample of 1315 students.

Palinopsia (visual perseveration)

Palinopsia, that is persistence or recurrence of visual images after the exciting stimulus has been removed, is an interesting form of visual illusion associated with non-dominant posterior parieto-temporal lesions that interfere with mechanisms of visual synthesis.[165,475,513,550,746] Ictal palinopsia of an object or scene occurs in a defective left hemifield or field quadrant and is persistently or recurrently perceived despite actual disappearance of that image from either visual fields.

That palinopsia may be the first seizure symptom has been unequivocally demonstrated with ictal EEG recordings by Lefebre and Kolmel[475] in a case with post-traumatic seizures. Lateralized long-latency visual perseveration was associated with synchronous temporo-parietal epileptic discharges. Similarly, Muller *et al.*1995[550] reported three patients with right sided posterior cortical lesions and ictal palinopsia documented with simultaneous EEG. In this respect their case 1[550] is of interest. This was a woman with a right posterior cerebral artery infarct. She had several attacks of palinopsia consisting of faces or scenes persisting or reappearing within minutes into her hemianopic left visual field. Illustrative ictal EEG shows paroxysmal rhythmic fast activity starting from the posterior temporo-parietal regions.[550]

Palinopsia may also be a manifestation of migraine.[680]

It is interesting that palinopsia is also referred to as an ictal symptom in late onset benign childhood occipital seizures (LBOS) by Gastaut and Zifkin.[313] Fourteen per cent of their 63 patients had visual illusions 'including micropsia, metamorphopsia and palinopsia'. Whether these patients had normal or abnormal neurological state and brain scan cannot be deduced. It is also not clarified whether these patients had a good or bad prognosis.

Palinopsia was described by one of my patients who had one single secondary GTCS.

This was an 18-year-old normal, intelligent student who had no family or personal history of seizures or migraine. He rushed to catch the train back home after a hard day's work. He was hungry and thirsty. He looked at a small video display unit of travel information and, after he looked away, the image of the screen persisted in the right upper corner of his vision and nearly simultaneously, started flashing at a rate of 3–5 Hz for 2 s. This was followed by visual illusions of the walls of the station and the passengers closing in on him, ending within 5 s with a generalized tonic–clonic seizure. Routine EEG, sleep deprivation EEG and MRI were all normal. No medication was prescribed. Two years later he remained well with no further visual or other seizures.

Blindness (amaurosis)

Blindness (amaurosis) is a common ictal or post-ictal symptom of idiopathic and symptomatic occipital seizures.[21,56,67,70,313,335,396,404,418,423,450,459,513,605,609,647,649,651,694,698,700,716,811,837] Ictal blindness and less frequently ictal hemianopia occurred in 34.6 per cent of patients with symptomatic occipital epilepsy. It has been reported in 22 of 60 patients with post-traumatic visual fits,[694] 10 of 25[811] and 12 of 42[700] patients with intractable occipital epilepsy. In neurosurgical series, it appears that ictal blindness is due to contralateral seizure spread to involve both occipital lobes[67,700,811] which was also reported by Penfield and Erickson.[647] Salanova *et al.*[700] stated that 'whether or not ictal blindness is due to inhibition of the visual cortex by the seizure discharge is unknown'. In idiopathic occipital seizures ictal blindness may be found in approximately two thirds of the patients.[313,418,605,609] Ictal EEGs during blindness demonstrate seizure activity[77,313,370,519] or relative flattening.[215]

Blindness may follow the visual hallucinations and progress to other ictal epileptic symptoms but often it occurs as an initial or the only ictal seizure manifestation with abrupt onset. The duration of ictal blindness is usually longer, 3–5 min, than that of ictal visual hallucinations but it may last for hours or days (status epilepticus amauroticus). Hemianopia may be an ictal and is certainly a frequent post-ictal manifestation of occipital seizures as vividly described by Holmes.[396]

Ayala (1929)[56] is the first to report 'status epilepticus amauroticus', as he named it, in a 34-year-old man with a history of alcoholism, left sided motor partial seizures and secondarily GTCS. Sixteen years after neurosurgery, which had good effect on his seizures, he began having attacks of complete blindness, lasting 1–2 min, without loss of consciousness or any other symptoms. These attacks, alternating with GTCS, became more frequent, culminating in continuous blindness lasting 15 days and punctuated by motor partial and secondary GTCS. Light perception and then sight returned 4 days later. Ayala considered this 'status epilepticus amauroticus' to be either a seizure equivalent or the result of ischaemia secondary to interference with occipital lobe circulation.

Barry *et al.* (1985)[67] reported five patients, aged 13 to 74 years, four having brain structural lesions, for whom ictal blindness (three patients) or homonymous hemianopia (two) lasting from hours to days was documented with ictal simultaneous EEG monitoring. Ictal blindness occurred when seizure propagation involved the contralateral occipital lobe.

Kuzniecky,[459] emphasizing that ictal and post-ictal amaurosis cannot always be clearly separated, mentions 'a patient with post-ictal amaurosis lasting hours following brief ictal occipital seizures. In other cases, patients with fixed hemianopsia may report amaurosis suggesting post-ictal involvement of the unaffected occipital lobe.'[459]

Rarely, frequent seizures of amaurosis may lead to permanent visual deficits.[21] Onset of ictal blindness in adulthood nearly always indicates structural lesions.[67,423,459,694,698,700,811] In children with late onset benign occipital seizures, ictal blindness is commoner after visual hallucinations symptom[313] but it has also been reported in symptomatic cases.[335] Gilliam and Wyllie (1995)[335] reported that six of seven consecutive patients 'who experienced amaurosis as a prominent feature of their seizures' had MRI abnormalities including ischaemic, traumatic and space-occupying lesions, with five limited to the parietal-occipital region. The mean age of seizure onset was 4 years and four patients experienced severe post-ictal headache and nausea. Six patients had unilateral, posterior interictal spike and slow wave complexes. They rightly concluded that the 'constellation of ictal amaurosis, occipital paroxysms, and post-ictal migrainous symptoms does not necessarily signify a benign, non-lesional epilepsy'.

In one of 12 neurosurgical cases with ictal blindness reported by Salanova *et al.*[700] ictal blindness lasting several minutes started at age 11 years and it was the 'sole manifestation of her seizures for several years before she developed complex partial seizures'. She had a left occipital oligodendroglioma removed at age 35 years after which she remained seizure free.

In patients with post-traumatic epilepsy, ictal amaurosis has been mainly associated with damage to the visual association cortex than to the calcarine area itself (Russell and Whitty, 1955[694]). Of 10 patients reported by Kuzniecky *et al.*, 1997[457] with occipital lobe developmental malformations and onset of seizures before the age of 15 years, six had visual hallucinations and one with occipital cortical dysplasia had ictal and post-ictal blindness.

Bauer *et al.*[70] reported two patients, in one of whom blindness manifested as an aura prior to tonic–clonic seizures; the interictal EEG exhibited a spike-wave focus bi-occipitally. In the second patient blindness occurred post-ictally. An ictal SPECT, carried out at the onset of the seizure, demonstrated marked hyperperfusion in both occipital regions.

The view that post-ictal blindness, after mainly convulsive seizures, is 'chiefly' seen in children[450] is contradicted by many reported cases in adults.[457]

An interesting rare variation of ictal blindness is 'white ictal blindness'. The patient cannot see because everything is white 'like a white sheet in front of your eyes' said one of my patients with severe symptomatic occipital epilepsy who also had independently elementary visual hallucinations of flashes and coin-like shapes of yellow, red and blue for 30 s to 1 min. They would appear in the left visual field, spread to occupy the whole visual field and move around him from left to right. These were often followed by complex visual hallucinations of 'dark, distorted faces' that he does not recognize or more complex scenes that he cannot define. LOC often follows without convulsions but often with incontinence of urine. CT brain scan showed marked hypodensity around the right parieto-occipital regions.

Another of my patients with idiopathic photosensitive and spontaneous occipital seizures would wake up from sleep either with elementary visual hallucinations or white blindness (all white) before generalized convulsions (see illustrative cases, Chapter 12B).

Non-visual manifestations of occipital seizures

Deviation of the eyes, oculoclonic seizures, epileptic nystagmus

Deviation of the eyes often but not necessarily followed by ipsilateral turning of the head is the commonest, 40–50 per cent, non-visual symptom in occipital seizures.[63,131,551,552,604,648,694,700,701,746,751,808,810,811] However, ictal deviation of the eyes, smooth (pursuit-like) or violent, tonic (oculotonic), clonic (oculoclonic) or both, may originate from any cortical epileptogenic focus either directly or through secondary propagation.

Contraversive tonic deviation of the head and eyes due to occipital seizures, spontaneously or electrically induced, was first documented by Foerster and Penfield (1929),[285] and Penfield and Jasper,[648] and has been studied with surface and depth EEG by Takeda *et al.*[751] and with stereo-EEG by Munari *et al.*[551] In all 16 patients of Munari *et al.*[551] ocular deviation occurred within 10 s of seizure onset. It was mainly tonic associated with rapid ictal EEG discharge (14 patients) and less often clonic associated with slow pseudorhythmic spikes. The ictal discharge originated in the medial occipital cortex, above or below the calcarine sulcus, and was always contralateral to the direction of eye movement. Ictal eye and head deviation is a consistent finding in all neurosurgical series of occipital epilepsy.[131,552,700,701,808,810,811]

Rosenbaum *et al.* (1986)[688] comprehensively reviewed the relevant literature and concluded that in occipital epilepsy the focus is contralateral to the direction of head turning. They also reported adult with seizures consisting of stereotyped deviation of the head to the left, with conjugate leftward deviation of the eyes after a delay of 1 to 5 s followed by complex visual hallucinations. Ictal EEG started with rhythmic 4–5 Hz activity in the right occipital electrode. They suggested that 'motor phenomena can result from a discharge in the visual cortex without implicating visual pursuit or extra-occipital spread'.

The consistent lateralization of occipital seizures with deviation of eyes and head is contrary to similar ictal symptoms of frontal or temporal lobe seizures where the direction of head movement is equally likely to be ipsilateral or contralateral to the EEG focus[584] though the views are conflicting.[531] The epileptogenic focus is more likely to be contralateral to the movement of the head and the eyes if consciousness is not impaired[531] or if it is the initial ictal symptom[825] even in seizures of frontal or temporal lobe origin. Ipsilateral head or eye deviation occurred in three of 26 patients with symptomatic occipital epilepsy reported by Williamson *et al.*[811] and one of 42 of Salanova *et al.*[700] According to Munari *et al.*[551] this may be due to early spread to the ipsilateral occipital lobe.

I am not aware of any study comparing ictal deviation of eyes, head or both of occipital versus extra-occipital origin. The following conclusions are derived from my personal experience supplemented by relevant reports in the literature. This would need verification with well designed comparative studies.

In occipital epilepsy the deviation of the eyes is usually pursuit-like or tonic, rarely clonic, and different from the oculoclonic ictal symptoms that are often seen in partial motor seizures of extra-occipital, mainly frontal origin. Occipital oculotonic seizures are similar to a voluntary, pursuit-like turning of the eyes to one side that by itself could not be considered as an abnormal movement by witnesses. This is opposed to ictal ocular symptoms of extra-occipital origin, which mainly look unnatural. In extra-occipital seizures the eye movement is more violent, and there is usually an upwards deviation associated with ipsilateral eyelid tonic or clonic convulsions often spreading to other facial, neck and shoulder muscles of the same side. The movement of the eyes is simultaneous or follows the movement of the head with neck and shoulder muscles often involved. Tonic–clonic deviation of the eyes occurs simultaneously with tonic or clonic convulsions of the ipsilateral facial muscles (as is for example the case in hemifacial Rolandic seizures).

Ictal pursuit-like or oculotonic symptoms in occipital epilepsy usually follow visual symptoms and mainly elementary visual hallucinations but may also occur *ab initio*. In this stage, consciousness is often but not invariably impaired. This phase may progress to unilateral clonic seizures of the face and the extremities with or without progression to generalized tonic–clonic seizures. Ictal oculotonic symptoms in benign childhood occipital seizures are described in Chapters 8, 9 and 13.

Forced eyes and head turning has also been described in eyelid myoclonia with absences (EMA),[628] an idiopathic generalized epileptic syndrome characterized by the triad of eyelid myoclonia associated with brief absences, generalized discharges of 3–6 Hz polyspikes and slow waves which are brief (usually 3–4 s) precipitated mainly by eye-closure and photosensitivity. 'I will be looking over there and the sunshine will be coming through on that side. And my head, without me even knowing, it automatically turns, you can not stop it and it goes like this and your head has an automatic reaction to go back to the sunlight and start flickering the eyes and you try to pull yourself away...', one of our patients with EMA explained. This description may be arbitrarily taken as indirect evidence of self-induction although this is strongly denied by the patients. To us, this is similar to the well known phenomenon of the 'attraction movement when light is presented and other manifestations of the optic fixation reflexes when volitional movements of the eyes are unattainable or weak'[628]

Ictal nystagmus (epileptic nystagmus) has been the subject of many reports.[101,295,301,378,432,433,638,675,770,777] It is mainly a horizontal[295,301,378,433,770] and rarely a vertical[432] nystagmus. The rapid phase of the nystagmus is opposite to the epileptic focus, and in the same direction as the eye and head deviation, which may co-exist, precede or follow. Most of the reported cases are adults with severe symptomatic seizures originating from the posterior cerebral regions[295,432,433,770] though children have also been reported.[378,433] Harris *et al.*, 1997[378] reported an infantile case in which epileptic nystagmus was first noted at 10 days of age. Electronystagmography showed a right-beating nystagmus with predominantly linear slow phases that traversed the midline. Neuroimaging revealed dysplasia of the left middle temporal gyrus extending posteriorly into the parieto-occipital cortex. The right hemisphere and subcortical structures appeared normal. Perfusion studies demonstrated interictal hypoperfusion with ictal hyperperfusion in the left temporal lobe. Electrocorticography demonstrated spiking over the left temporal-parieto-occipital region. Following extensive surgical resection of this area and weaning of anti-convulsants, the child has remained seizure-free without nystagmus. The authors concluded that their case demonstrates the cortical origin of epileptic nystagmus, and shows that the infant cortex has functioning efferent connections to brainstem oculo-motor centres from 10 days of age.

However, epileptic nystagmus may also be an ictal symptom of typical or atypical absences[623,798] as we have demonstrated with video-EEG recordings in our department.[623]

Rosenberg *et al.*, 1991[689] reported a rare case with bilateral papillary constriction and internal ophthalmoplegia as the only physical manifestation of a partial sensory seizure. The onset and offset of each attack corresponded distinctly with an electroencephalographic discharge of the left temporo-occipital region.

Forced eyelid closure and eyelid blinking

Forced eyelid closure and eyelid blinking is an interesting ictal clinical symptom described in all neurosurgical series.[63,459,551,648,700,751,811] According to Willamson,[808] based on his experience from intractable occipital epilepsies, eyelid closure and eyelid blinking is an early ictal sign and has a forced quality that may be distinguished from the more casual blinking associated with many other seizure types.

In my experience from idiopathic occipital seizures, ictal eyelid blinking is not rare. It occurs after the phase of visual hallucinations, at a stage when consciousness is impaired and heralds the impending secondary generalized convulsions (see illustrative cases in Chapter 19). However, it may also occur alone, be inconspicuous in appearance and not suspected as a seizure event, documented only with video-EEG recordings in occipital photosensitive patients (see Chapter 12B).

Eyelid opening, 'eyes widely opened', is also another well described symptom in patients with nocturnal seizures of occipital origin,[74] but this may also be a symptom from other cerebral locations such as mesial temporal structures. Widened palpebral fissures with fixed staring and dilated pupils is amongst the typical symptoms of mesial temporal lobe seizures.[809]

It should be emphasized that eyelid opening, eyelid closure and eyelid fluttering or blinking (or eyelid myoclonia) are more common ictal symptoms in idiopathic generalized epilepsies with absences that are easily diagnosed on clinical and EEG evidence.[623,628]

Sensory hallucinations of ocular movements and pain

A sensation of ocular movement in the absence of detectable motion is considered rare.[399,700,746,811]. Holtzman and Goldensohn, 1977[399] reported two patients with hallucinating of eye movement as the earliest manifestation of their seizures. The characteristic feature is a unilateral sensation of eye movement in the absence of eye movement, oscillopsia or nystagmus. The first patient, a physician with an arteriovenous malformation in the medial portion of the right occipito-parietal fissure, had frequent seizures starting stereotypically with a flickering sensation in his left eye either alone or followed by left sided hemiconvulsions. There were no eye movements or changes of the pupil. 'Sometimes it slows down and stops and there is no further seizure. Sometimes it goes very fast and is followed by a sensation of heaviness in the left half of my body. During this flickering sensation I do not see any flashes, there are no changes in light. I could perform my normal duties. I have been reading, writing, and concentrating on my scholastic work. I have been driving and I have performed my normal work'. The second patient had a large left tentorial meningioma compressing the occipital lobe. He had attacks of a strange feeling of vibrating pulsations in his left eye without eye movements. Duration varied from a few to as long as 45 s and were associated or followed by inability to concentrate or think and visual blurring from the left eye. The flickering sensation 'started out very slowly and then gradually built up in amplitude'. He also had 'paroxysmal alexia that later became continuous' and incomplete right superior quadrantanopia.

These hallucinating of ocular movement and ocular sensations may not be rare. They occurred in two of my 13 patients with idiopathic occipital epilepsy (Chapter 9). One, a boy of 10 years, had visual hallucinations in the right eye, associated with a feeling that 'draws my right eye and my head to the right'. In the other, elementary visual hallucinations are associated with 'tension in eyes. Feels similar to when you look up into your eyebrows as hard as you can. The aura continually tries to move to the left and at a slight tilt upwards. This involuntary movement of the eyes causes the pain described above. The motion to the left seems out of your control. It can be resisted but this adds to nausea and general pain'. Neither himself nor the witnesses could confirm any such movement of the eyes.

Ictal vomiting (ictus emeticus)

Considered exceptionally rare[229,282,371,414,417,453,537,559]or dismissed as a non-seizure or migrainous event, ictal vomiting eluded physicians until its frequent association with early onset benign childhood occipital seizures (EBOS) was unequivocally documented by Panayiotopoulos.[603,605] Ictal vomiting was previously considered an extremely rare occurrence in epilepsies, with only 16 cases found in a recent report of two additional patients.[229] The consensus reached from ictal recordings of mainly symptomatic epilepsies is that ictal vomiting is activated from the non-dominant temporal lobe and insular.[229,282,371,414,417,453,537,559] Though this may be partly true in symptomatic epilepsies, it does not explain its scarcity in adults who commonly have right sided temporal lobe seizures, or why most of the reported cases show bilateral epileptogenic foci and why ictal recordings with mainly left sided abnormalities exist.[793] These indicate that ictal vomiting may require more than one contributing factor. Furthermore, it does not explain why ictal vomiting is a main seizure manifestation of idiopathic childhood occipital seizures[150,192,270,277,367,370,443,517,793,826] and why although some right sided preponderance is apparent this is not always the case.[615] We offered three possible explanations: (a) vomiting is triggered by focal cortical epileptic discharges, (b) it is the result of a vomiting-inducing substance released by the cortical electrical discharge and (c) both epileptic cortical manifestations and vomiting are the result of a neurotransmitter mediated process which is excitatory both for the vomiting centre (or the chemoreceptor trigger zone) and the cortex.[603] We favoured the third possibility but this is only an assumption.

Irrespective of pathogenetic mechanisms, it is important to recognize that ictal vomiting is unequivocally associated with early onset benign childhood occipital seizures[150,192,270,277,367,370,443,517,615,793,826] but it may also occur in other benign childhood partial seizures with extra-occipital EEG foci.[603,622] In our studies ictal vomiting occurred in 24 out of 900 patients with epileptic seizures (2.7 per cent).[603,622] Only three had evidence of symptomatic partial seizures (one with mental retardation, one with hemiplegia and one with hydrocephalus). From the other 21 children with idiopathic partial seizures, 12 had EBOS. The remaining nine children had unilateral central spikes that were also elicited with somatosensory stimuli (two), midline spikes (two), frontal spikes (one), ill sustained photoparoxysmal response (one) or consistently normal EEGs (three). These nine patients have been followed up for many years and are detailed in a recent a report[622] and in Chapter 16. All but one child had nocturnal seizures. All seizures in all patients manifested with ictal vomiting, eye deviation and unilateral clonic convulsions with or without impairment of consciousness. The median onset of seizures was 5 years and seizure life span was brief with three children having a single fit, three having 2–3 and only one child having many seizures prior to the initiation of medication. Prognosis was excellent with no seizures and good development in the long follow-up period.[622] Ictal vomiting did not occur in any of 67 children with centrotemporal spikes only.[603]

Ictal vomiting in EBOS may occur at any stage of the ictus, usually at the beginning but it may also occur later before the convulsive phase of the seizure.[192,277,603,605,608,615] These findings have been confirmed world-wide.[192,270,277,367,443,517,793] In more recent reports ictal vomiting occurred in 70 per cent of 113 children with EBOS reported by Ferrie *et al.*[277] and in all 56 children with EBOS reported by Caraballo *et al.*[150] Furthermore, ictal vomiting has also been recently well documented in reflex occipital photosensitive seizures, some of which may also be benign.[370] There is no reference to ictal vomiting in the neurosurgical series of occipital seizures.[131,700,701,808,811]

Recently, Viani *et al.* 1995[792] studied seizures and polygraphic patterns of 18 patients with Angelman's syndrome. Seven patients had partial seizures with eye deviation and vomiting, similar to those of the EBOS. They suggested that Angelman's syndrome occurs in most of the patients as a non-progressive, age-dependent myoclonic encephalopathy with a prominent occipital involvement.

Headache

The association of headache with epileptic seizures is often neglected despite well documented evidence of ictal but more commonly of post-ictal headache.[69,132,186,232,408,471,699,710,835] Ictal and mainly post-ictal headache appears to be more often associated with occipital than any other type of partial seizures.[602,618,710]

Ictal headache, 'a sensation of bifrontal pressure, vague ache in the head, sharp stabbing retro-orbital pains or a sensation of electricity passing through their head',[710] is unlikely to be confused with migraine headache. However, post-ictal headache, which occurs in 10–40 per cent of patients with partial or generalized seizures, may be indistinguishable from migraine particularly if associated with vomiting and photophobia. [186,618,710]

Ictal headache

The following case by Gowers in1879[350] is an example of ictal headache which is masterly diagnosed:

> Gowers presented a 30-year-old man who 'was well until two months before he was first seen (April, 1878), when one morning something seemed very brilliant before him, "as if he had a polished plate on his breast." He felt giddy, but did not fall; he sat down, bathed his head, and was better, but afterwards felt extreme pain in his eyes, "as if they were bursting." Subsequently he had slight attacks, almost daily, of the following character. "A pain commences in the neck, goes across the head, comes down between the eyes, and is felt on each side of the bridge of the nose. If walking, the road or path seems to get narrower

> and narrower, so that he hardly knows where he is going, and simultaneously his sight fails; he feels with a stick to see if he is not getting off the path. The pain at the top of the head and in the eyes is something awful, and the eyes seem to throb. The loss of sight is not complete; he can only see just before him; nothing on either side; but he can generally see better to the right than the left." During the three days before he was first seen, at the commencement of the attacks, as the sight was going, he had a flickering of light, "like a gold serpent", in the eye, moving in all directions very fast; seen with both eyes he thought, but more before the left eye than the right. The pupils were equal. Acuity of vision normal. I thought that there was a very slight defect in the left field on the temporal side, but I could not, even on very careful examination, be sure of it. He was treated with bromide and belladonna, and the attacks ceased, except that once or twice he had a slight flickering before the eyes. He had, however, several attacks of pain on the top of his head, coming on suddenly, and he often had pain at the back of the neck. He was seen repeatedly during the next three months, and continued free from attacks. Five months after he was first seen (as I subsequently learned) he had a fall, and afterwards most severe pain in the right side of the head just above the right eyebrow, darting through the head. His manner became altered, and his speech confluent, words being run together. He also had delusions, fancying that persons were in the room who were not. He then became comatose for a day or two, and died'. A post-mortem examination revealed a right occipital and posterior parietal lobe tumour, probably a sarcoma.

Gowers[350] concluded that the 'Headache was such as sometimes comes in epileptic seizures – paroxysmal... The tumour was in the sensory region of the brain and the paroxysmal symptoms were acute pain and a transient disturbance of vision...'

Documentation of ictal headache can be found in the reports by Blume and Young[132], Isler *et al.*[408] and Saint-Hilaire *et al.*[699] The best review with historical aspects is by Isler *et al.*[408] Young and Blume[132,835] found that 24 (2.8 per cent) of 858 of their patients with seizures had ictal pain confirmed, in some of them, with ictal recordings. Like Gowers (1901)[351] they divided their patients into those with unilateral pain (10 patients), cephalic pain (11 patients) and abdominal pain (three patients). Only two of the 11 patients with cephalic pain described the pain as throbbing. Others described it as sharp or steady, but many were unable to ascribe a quality to it. Cephalic pain initiated the seizure in eight patients and accompanied other ictal symptoms in three. It was unilateral in seven but there was no relation between side of the headache and the seizure origin. All patients had partial seizures. The nature and location of the EEG abnormalities varied considerably from patient to patient but four patients had occipital EEG foci interictally. In two of these, the right occipital and the right posterior temporal regions were the origins of the recorded seizures with cephalic pain. They reported three illustrated cases. The first was a 21-year-old woman who had onset of seizures at age 12 years. Seizures began 'with a throbbing, left parietal headache immediately followed by hearing a beeping noise'. Her arms trembled and she saw flashing coloured lights in the left visual field. After this she lost consciousness and had a GTCS. EEGs showed independent bi-occipital and posterior temporal spikes, maximal on the right side. The second was a 46-year-old man who had late onset seizures due to a lesion in the right temporo-occipital region. 'A sharp, severe headache in the right supra-orbital area' was followed by loss of consciousness with deviation of the head and eyes to the left and then a GTCS. The third was a 20-year-old woman who had GTCS from early childhood until the age of 16 when she had seizures that 'began with a sharp, pain in the left temple that then spread to both temporal regions'. She then experienced a sensation of 'needles picking the scalp' especially in the vertex. She would then lose consciousness, stare blankly and have automatisms. EEGs showed occasional sharp waves in the right temporal region. The authors suggested that the headache may be due to free fatty acid release.

Seven of 100 adult patients with seizures studied by Schon and Blau[710] had headaches preceding seizures. One described a sensation of bifrontal pressure associated with mood depression for 2 days prior to a seizure and another one had right frontal headache, tiredness and urinary frequency for 3 days prior to a fit. The other five patients complained of a vague ache in the head, sharp stabbing retro-orbital pains or a sensation of electricity passing through their head for seconds to 5 min before their seizures.

Diaz and Diaz, 1976[232] studied 'paroxysmal epileptic headache' which they defined as 'an episode of pain that starts suddenly, in a varying area that is usually the same for the same patient, of medium to high intensity, lasting from a few seconds to minutes and, rarely, hours; the episode subsides spontaneously and tends to recur'. This was found in 32 of 125 patients with epileptic seizures. Headache lasted from 30 s to 4 h but in the majority (62 per cent) this was 15 min or less. Pain was severe in 24 patients and moderate in eight. Average age of onset was 11 years, with 80 per cent of cases presenting it in the first or second decade of life. Paroxysmal headache persisted for a maximum of 41 years and a minimum of one month, with an average of six years. The authors concluded that epileptic paroxysmal headache can be the only epileptic symptom (31 per cent) or be associated with other ictal manifestations, independently (56.2 per cent) or simultaneously (12.5 per cent). EEG studies showed main localization in the temporal lobes (56 per cent). 'Treatment with hydantoine, primidone and methylsuccimide gave excellent results.[232]

Ictal headache, mainly orbital, is described in early and mainly late onset benign childhood seizures (see Chapters 8 and 9). Kivity and Lermann[443] reported that in five of nine children with diurnal prolonged seizures of EBOS type these were heralded by headache which in some cases was very severe.[443] Ictal headache was found in 13 per cent and post-ictal headache in 16 per cent of 113 children with EBOS.[277]

Post-ictal headache

Post-ictal headache occurs in half of patients after GTCS of any cause.[710] Of 100 patients with seizures studied by Schon and Blau[710] post-ictal headaches occurred in 51 and it was invariably associated with the seizures in 32 of them. It was mainly bilateral (36 patients), throbbing (16), usually lasting for 6–72 h. Major seizures (17 patients had major seizures only and another 12 both minor and major seizures) were more often associated with post-ictal headache than minor attacks (13 patients had minor seizures only). Nine of the 100 patients also had migraine and in eight 'a typical, albeit a mild, migraine attack was provoked by fits'. The post-ictal headache in those without migraine (40 patients) was accompanied by vomiting (11 cases), photophobia (14) and vomiting with photophobia (four). Furthermore, post-ictal headache was accentuated by coughing, bending and sudden head movements and relieved by sleep. The authors concluded that 'it was, therefore, clear that seizures provoke a syndrome similar to the headache phase of migraine in 50 per cent of epileptics' and proposed that 'post-ictal headache arises intra-cranially and is related to the vasodilatation known to follow seizures'. It is also interesting that nine of 51 patients with post-ictal headache had visual symptoms in association with their seizures. In seven of them ' it took the form of a visual aura, flashes of light (six) and blurring of vision (one) lasting 3–10 min. The other two patients had post-ictal blurring of vision.

D'Alessandro *et al.*[186] studied headaches amongst 174 patients, older than 16 years, who had complex partial seizures (94 patients), simple partial seizures (49), simple and complex partial seizures (nine), absences (19) and myoclonic jerks (three). post-ictal headache was found in 23 patients who all had complex partial seizures. post-ictal headache was mostly bilateral (15 patients), and usually prolonged for more than 1–6 h (14) with symptoms such as nausea, vomiting, pallor, dizziness, drowsiness and photophobia occurring in 10 patients. post-ictal headache always occurred after seizures in 13 and occasionally in 10 of the 23 patients. There was no statistical difference regarding interictal headache between the above seizure groups of patients which suggests that post-ictal headache does not have a genetic basis.

post-ictal headache after partial seizures without GTCS appears to be a common occurrence in symptomatic occipital and other forms of partial fits[602,620,694,710] but it is mainly emphasized and probably more common in idiopathic occipital seizures.[304,313,618]

Russell and Whity[694]in their study of 60 patients with visual seizures due to brain wounds commented:

> 'It is interesting that in four cases in this series unformed hallucinations were followed by severe headache, sometimes throbbing and unilateral, the whole sequence resembling what might be

called a traumatic migraine. However, we were not able to recognize any special physiological or anatomical features in these unusual cases.'

post-ictal headache after visual seizures is a consistent symptom in one third of patients with late onset benign childhood occipital seizures (LBOS) without preceding convulsions. This post-ictal headache occurs immediately or after 5–10 min from the end of the visual hallucinations. The duration and severity of the headache appears to be proportional to the duration and severity of the preceding visual seizures. The headache may be diffuse, of mild to moderate intensity, but in most patients it is strong, pulsating and may be associated with nausea, vomiting, photophobia and phonophobia. Thus, the post-ictal headache of some patients with LBOS may be indistinguishable from migraine.[213,215,313,620] (see also Chapter13).

post-ictal headache, after simple partial visual seizures, occurred frequently in my patients with LBOS (see Chapter 13).[618] This was moderate but more often severe headache, mainly bilateral, rarely unilateral, pounding or throbbing. Even simple, elementary visual hallucinations of less than 1 min duration could be followed by severe headache, often indistinguishable from migraine headache associated with nausea, vomiting, photophobia and phonophobia. It was longer and more severe with visual seizures of longer duration. Other similarities with migraine headache is that in some patients this started 3–15 min after the end of visual hallucinations, a phenomenon known in migraine as the free interval.[123] post-ictal headache was equally common in those with or without a family history of migraine, probably indicating that post-ictal symptoms do not depend on a predisposition to migraine.

Ictal clinical symptoms from occipital seizure propagation

Seizure discharges originating from an occipital focus may remain localized, or spread to the other occipital lobe and often to more anterior ipsilateral cerebral regions through infra-sylvian and supra-sylvian propagation. It is reported that infra-calcarine occipital foci will propagate to the temporal lobe causing complex partial seizures whilst supra-calcarine foci will induce seizures that tend to propagate to the parietal and frontal areas giving origin to predominantly motor seizures.[751]

Infra-sylvian spread to the ipsilateral medial temporal lobe appears to be the most common, around 50 per cent in neurosurgical series, documented with intracranial EEG recordings.[63,131,700,751,811] Ictal clinical manifestations consist of various combinations of symptoms such as epigastric-visceral sensations, nausea, belching and autonomic signs, olfactory-gustatory hallucinations, experiential phenomena, fear and panic, impairment of consciousness, eyes widely open with a fixed stare, oral-alimentary automatisms (lip smacking, chewing, swallowing, tooth grinding), reactive, stereotyped automatisms or both, deviation of head and eyes, and tonic and dystonic postures.

Infra-sylvian spread to the ipsilateral lateral temporal lobe is associated mainly with auditory and complex visual hallucinations and language impairment if in the dominant hemisphere.

Supra-sylvian spread is less common, 12–38 per cent in neurosurgical series, resulting in lateral or medial frontal lobe seizure symptoms. Sensory and motor symptoms are the commonest from the lateral supra-sylvian and complex posturing from the medial supra-sylvian spread.

Some patients may have more than one type of ictal propagation involving ipsilateral and sometimes contralateral infra-sylvian and supra-sylvian structures.[808]

Seizure propagation to other regions representing association cortex or parietal lobe may occur and the semiology may represent activation or inhibition of related functional structures.[459] Contralateral spread to the other occipital lobe is associated with ictal blindness.[700,808,811]

It is this complex seizure propagation that causes the 'clinical pleomorphism' of occipital epilepsy described by Ludwig and Marsan.[513] 'Clinical pleomorphism was more apparent than is commonly conceived; thus, although the incidence of visual auras was relatively high (47 per cent), epigastric, psychic, somatic, and other sensory phenomena were not infrequently encountered. Ictal motor patterns were most commonly (53 per cent) non-focal or absent, but partial or focal motor attacks and psychomotor seizures were amply represented'.

These results and conclusions are based on thorough studies of patients who have intractable occipital seizures that are mainly due to structural lesions of the occipital lobes. Therefore, the pattern and direction of the seizure propagation may be influenced not only by the epileptic focus but also by the anatomical and functional integrity of the surrounding cerebral tissue. It may be different in pure forms of idiopathic occipital epilepsy where for example complex partial seizures with temporal lobe symptomatology were conspicuous by their absence in the 16 patients with late onset idiopathic occipital epilepsy that I studied (see Chapter 13).

Occipital seizures from recent reports of occipital epilepsy in neurosurgical series

Williamson *et al.*[811] studied clinical characteristics, seizure spread patterns, and results of surgery in 25 patients with occipital lobe seizure origin. Symptoms and signs served to identify occipital lobe origin in 22 (88 per cent) patients included elementary visual hallucinations, ictal amaurosis, eye movement sensations, early forced blinking or eyelid flutter, and visual field deficits. Eye or head deviation, or both, was observed frequently and was contralateral to the side of seizure origin in 13, but three patients exhibited ipsilateral deviation in some or all their seizures. After these initial signs and symptoms, clinical seizure characteristics resembled those of seizures originating elsewhere. Seizures typical of temporal lobe origin with loss of contact and various types of automatic, semi-purposeful activity occurred in 11 patients. Seizures in three patients exhibited asymmetrical tonic or focal clonic motor patterns characteristic of frontal lobe seizures. Eleven of the 25 patients had, on two occasions, two or more distinctly different seizure types. Scalp EEGs were seldom helpful for occipital localization and were frequently misleading. Intracranial EEGs correctly identified occipital seizure origin in most, but not all, patients and also confirmed that the variability in clinical seizure characteristics was related to different seizure spread patterns, medially or laterally above and below the Sylvian fissure, both ipsilateral and contralateral to the occipital lobe of seizure origin. Eighteen patients had occipital lobe lesions detected with computed tomographic or magnetic resonance imaging scans or both.

Blume *et al.*[131] reported the results of epilepsy surgery in the posterior cortex of 19 patients. Visual phenomena were the most common initial ictal symptoms, occurring in 13 (68 per cent) patients. Twelve patients had complex partial seizures that were always without warning in two, always following an aura, usually visual in seven and with or without warning in three. Scalp EEG identified the origin of most recorded seizures in 12 (63 per cent) of the 19 patients. An interictal spike focus appeared in 15 patients (79 per cent), and always correlated with the epileptogenic lobe as defined by scalp and/or subdural-recorded seizures (14 patients) or by clinical analysis and CT brain scan (one patient).

Salanova *et al.*[700] reported the electroclinical manifestations, electrocorticography, cortical stimulation and outcome in 42 patients with surgery of occipital lobe epilepsy. In more than two-thirds of the patients the clinical manifestations indicated the occipital onset of the seizures. Seventy-three per cent experienced visual seizures. Elementary hallucinations were the most common and 12 also had ictal blindness. Other occipital manifestations included: contralateral eye deviation, blinking, a sensation of eye movement and nystagmoid eye movements. Intra-operative cortical stimulation elicited a habitual visual seizure in 37 per cent of 29 patients. Lateralizing clinical features were seen in almost two-thirds of patients: contralateral head deviation occurred in half, 59 per cent had visual field defects contralateral to the epileptogenic area and 64 per cent had abnormal imaging studies ipsilateral to the side of surgery. More than one-third of patients exhibited more than one seizure type, suggesting ictal spread to temporal or frontal lobe: 50 per cent had typical temporal lobe automatisms, and 38 per cent exhibited focal motor seizure activity. Surface EEG recordings showed posterior temporal-occipital epileptiform discharges in 46 per cent of patients. Only 18 per cent had electronegative spiking limited to occipital electrodes. Large epileptogenic areas were often found on intracranial recording with depth electrodes and on electrocorticography. Pre-excision electrocorticography spiking was restricted to the occipital lobe in only 13 out of 34 patients. More often spiking also involved the posterior temporal and posterior parietal regions.

Benign Childhood Partial Seizures and Related Epileptic Syndromes. C P Panayiotopoulos
©1999 John Libbey & Company Ltd., pp. 119–132.

Chapter 7

Occipital epilepsies: The syndromes

Definition

Occipital epilepsies are a heterogeneous group of syndromes characterized by seizures originating in one or both occipital lobes (Table 7.1). Aetiology may be idiopathic, structural or metabolic. Syndromes of idiopathic occipital epilepsy are genetically determined, often age-related and manifest with occipital seizures that may be spontaneous only, precipitated by external visual stimuli only or both. There may be also an idiopathic low threshold sensitivity manifested with situation-related occipital seizures. In idiopathic occipital epilepsy, neurological, mental and neuroimaging state is normal. In idiopathic occipital epilepsy, seizures may manifest with visual or non-visual symptoms. Elementary visual hallucinations, deviation of the eyes and ictal vomiting, alone or in combination, are the most frequent ictal manifestations. Progressing to temporal lobe seizure symptomatology is rather exceptional though the pathogenesis of ictal vomiting is not certain. Frequency of seizures is syndrome related. They are age-related and well controlled with appropriate anti-epileptic drugs if necessary. Background inter-ictal EEG is normal. Occipital spikes and occipital paroxysms spontaneous, evoked or both are often abundant but disappear with age frequently long after cessation of occipital seizures. Idiopathic occipital seizures, because of visual hallucinations, vomiting and headache, imitate migraine with aura, basilar and acephalgic migraine for which they are often misdiagnosed. Metabolic or other derangement such as eclampsia may have a particular predilection for the occipital lobes and cause either situation-related occipital seizures or permanent occipital lesions leading to symptomatic occipital epilepsy. Syndromes of symptomatic occipital epilepsy include any condition where occipital seizures are caused by structural lesions situated in the occipital lobes. Structural occipital lobe lesions may be congenital, residual, or progressive resulting from vascular, neoplastic, metabolic, hereditary, congenital, inflammatory, parasitic, systemic diseases and infections. Patients with symptomatic occipital epilepsies often but not invariably have neurological deficits that may be static or progressive depending on the underlying cause. Brain imaging usually demonstrates occipital structural lesions, but on many occasions this would require high resolution new generation MRI techniques, and results may also be normal for some patients suspected to have symptomatic occipital epilepsy (cryptogenic occipital epilepsy). The discovery of the underlying cause of symptomatic occipital epilepsies may need haematology, biochemistry, screening for metabolic disorders, molecular DNA analysis or even skin or other tissue biopsy. Background EEG is usually abnormal with posterior lateralized slow waves. Unilateral occipital spikes and occasionally occipital paroxysms occur and there may be photosensitivity, but there are also fast multiple spikes either posterior or generalized and these are often facilitated by sleep. Symptomatic occipital seizures may start at any age and at any stage after or during the course of the primary disorder. They may be the first symptom manifestation of a devastating course such as in Lafora disease. Frequency, severity and response to treatment varies considerably from good to intractable and progressive, mainly depending on the underlying cause and extents of the lesions. Symptomatic occipital seizures may imitate the idiopathic ones particularly at onset. However, they are more aggressive, more complex and they often progress to temporal lobe semiology. They may also imitate migraine but because of other co-existent symptoms and signs, they are less likely to be misdiagnosed as migraine.

The definition proposed by the Commission refers to occipital seizures rather than to occipital epileptic syndromes[177]

Occipital lobe epilepsies are classified by the Commission[177] amongst the localization-related (focal, local, partial) epilepsies and epileptic syndromes and are defined as follows.

'Occipital lobe epilepsy syndromes are usually characterized by simple partial and secondarily generalized seizures. Complex partial seizures may occur with spread beyond the occipital lobe. The frequent association of occipital lobe seizures and migraine is complicated and controversial. The clinical seizure manifestations usually, but not always, include visual manifestations. Elementary visual seizures are characterized by fleeting visual manifestations which may be either negative (scotoma, hemianopsia, amaurosis) or, more commonly, positive (sparks or flashes, phosphenes). Such sensations appear in the visual field contralateral to the discharge in the specific visual cortex, but can spread to the entire visual field. Perceptive illusions, in which the objects appear to be distorted, may occur. The following varieties can he distinguished: a change in size (macropsia or micropsia), or a change in distance, an inclination of objects in a given plane of space and distortion of objects or a sudden change of shape (metamorphopsia). Visual hallucinatory seizures are occasionally characterized by complex visual perceptions (e.g. colourful scenes of varying complexity). In some cases, the scene is distorted or made smaller, and in rarer instances, the subject sees his own image (heautoscopy). Such illusional and hallucinatory visual seizures involve epileptic discharge in the temporo parieto occipital junction. The initial signs may also include tonic and/or clonic contraversion of eyes and head or eyes only (oculoclonic oroculogyric deviation), palpebral jerks, and forced closure of eyelids. Sensation of ocular oscillation or of the whole body may occur. The discharge may spread to the temporal lobe, producing seizure manifestations of either lateral posterior temporal or hippocampoamygdala seizures. When the primary focus is located in the supracalcarine area, the discharge can spread forward to the suprasylvian convexity or the mesial surface, mimicking those of parietal or frontal lobe seizures. Spread to contralateral occipital lobe may be rapid. Occasionally the seizure tends to become secondarily generalized.[177]

Classification of occipital epilepsies

Occipital epilepsies are classified in Table 7.1 where I follow the same principles and when possible the same nomenclature as that of the Commission on Classification and Terminology of the International League Against Epilepsy.[176,177] It would be wrong to propose a new classification system. All we need is to improve the existing scheme and this is attempted in Table 7.1.

Occipital seizures are partial (focal, local) and therefore all occipital epilepsies are by definition localization-related. They are divided in idiopathic and cryptogenic/symptomatic. Cryptogenic are suspected symptomatic epilepsies where the underlying cause cannot be revealed by the available means of investigations. Because of high resolution brain imaging and progress in other fields of medicine the number of cryptogenic epilepsies decreased dramatically in favour of the symptomatic ones.

Table 7.1. Occipital epilepsy syndromes

Occipital seizures are partial (focal, local) and therefore all occipital epilepsies are by definition localization-related.

Idiopathic occipital epilepsies

Localization-related (focal, local, partial) occipital syndromes

Early onset benign childhood occipital seizures or Panayiotopoulos syndrome

Late onset benign childhood occipital seizures or Late onset idiopathic childhood occipital epilepsy

Occipital epilepsy or occipital seizures precipitated by specific modes of activation

Idiopathic photosensitive occipital epilepsy or Idiopathic photosensitive occipital seizures.

Idiopathic fixation-off sensitive (scotosensitive) epilepsy or Idiopathic fixation-off sensitive (scotosensitive) seizures

Symptomatic occipital epilepsy secondary to structural lesions, hereditary diseases

Residual occipital structural lesions of any cause

Pre- peri- or post-natal lesions

Post-traumatic, infectious, inflammatory, vascular insults, of any cause

Progressive or static space occupying lesions

Arteriovenous malformations, cavernous angioma and other vascular malformations

Malformations of cortical development

Intra- or extra-occipital lobe tumous, benign or malignant

Sturge-Weber disease

Metabolic

Some metabolic diseases have a particular predilection to cause occipital lobe damage that may generate occipital seizures

Mitochondrial encephalomyopathy, lactic acidosis and stroke-like episodes (MELAS)

Coeliac disease

Situation-related occipital seizures

(a) Isolated occipital seizures occurring only when there is an accumulation of precipitating factors that alone could not be sufficient to induce an occipital seizure. An example of this is patients, mainly children and adolescents, having isolated occipital seizures due to prolonged video-game exposure (mental excitation, concentration and fatigue together with photic and pattern stimulation), hunger, sleep deprivation and other precipitating factors. These patients are not photo or pattern sensitive.

(b) Occasional occipital seizures following migraine aura (migraine with aura, acephalgic or basilar migraine).

Normal persons and or patients with migraine may have an occipital seizure by a rather aggressive photic stimulation in EEG departments. These are detailed in the relevant chapters and they are also examples of situation-related epilepsies.

(c) Occipital seizures occurring only when there is an acute metabolic or toxic event such as eclampsia, non-ketotic hyperglycaemia, alcohol or drugs.

Epidemiological aspects of occipital epilepsy syndromes

The precise incidence and prevalence of occipital epilepsies is not known. They are more common in children than in adults because of the benign childhood occipital seizures that mostly remit. In neurosurgical series prevalence is around 5 per cent of operated patients.[459] This is comparable with demographic studies.[521] Manford *et al.*, 1992[521] in a prospective community-based study of newly diagnosed epileptic seizures found that of 594 patients with definite epileptic seizures, 160 (26.9 per cent) had seizures with a clinically localisable onset: 36 (22.5 per cent) frontal, 52 (32.5 per cent) central sensorimotor, 43 (27 per cent) temporal, nine (5.6 per cent) frontotemporal, and 10 each (6.3 per cent) parietal and other posterior cortex. This may be an underestimation as partial seizures in this population are much less (22.5 per cent) than generalized seizures.

The prevalence of idiopathic occipital seizures in children with onset of seizures before the age of 13 years is approximately 4.3 per cent.[605] Capizzi *et al.*[147] found that of 168 children with symptomatic partial seizures 19 (11.3 per cent) had occipital symptomatic epilepsy.

In my studies, (Chapter 13), excluding three patients with IGE and visual hallucinations, the prevalence of occipital epilepsy of any cause amongst 1360 patients with epileptic disorders was 4.6 per cent (63 patients). Amongst these 63 patients with occipital epilepsy 25.4 per cent had definite (nine patients) or possible (seven patients) non-photosensitive idiopathic occipital epilepsy with visual hallucinations, 38.1 per cent (24 patients) had early onset benign childhood occipital seizures, 27 per cent had symptomatic occipital epilepsy (17 patients) and 9.5 per cent (six patients) had idiopathic photosensitive occipital epilepsy. However, there should be some bias in my studies as severe forms such as Lafora or more common forms such as post-traumatic or tumorous symptomatic occipital epilepsy are conspicuously absent.

Cryptogenic/symptomatic occipital epilepsies

The syndromes of idiopathic occipital epilepsy are detailed in the subsequent chapters on benign childhood partial seizures.

Cryptogenic and symptomatic occipital epilepsies are beyond the scope of this book but I felt that I should present a brief description of some of them, particularly:

(a) Those that may be significant in differential diagnosis such as symptomatic occipital epilepsy of malformations of cortical development or coeliac disease.

(b) Others that have been over-emphasized particularly regarding the relation of occipital epilepsy and migraine such as MELAS.

(c) Others because they are offered for comparison and discussion such as eclampsia-related occipital seizures.

In chronic symptomatic occipital epilepsies structural abnormalities are more commonly low-grade glial tumours, gliosis and porencephaly.

There are four major publications on 98 patients with intractable occipital lobe epilepsy of neurosurgical series[110,131,700,811] and occipital epilepsies have been reviewed recently by Sveinbjornsdottir and Duncan,[746] Williamson,[808] Williamson *et al.*,[810] Salanova *et al.*,[701] Munari *et al.*,[552] Andermann *et al.*[42] and Kuzniecky.[459] Aicardi's[15] book on 'Epilepsy in children' is a unique source of knowledge for all.

An historical reminder of symptomatic occipital epilepsy

I cannot resist the temptation of reproducing in this book one of the most remarkable descriptions of symptomatic occipital epilepsies, of a type that we often lack in our technological days with the tight formats of the published reports, which often miss important clinical details that are the key points in diagnosis and management. This comes from Gordon Holmes 1927[396] on 'visual epilepsy':

VISUAL EPILEPSY. Attacks to which this term may be applied have been frequently observed. They have been well described by Gowers, who in his last paper on the subject recorded two cases in which I was able to observe the patients during several attacks. Since the war there have been more opportunities of investigating such attacks. The cortical visual centres lie around the calcarine fissures, that in each hemisphere corresponding to the homonymous halves of the two retinae and receiving therefore impressions from the opposite halves of the visual fields. It is definitely determined, too, that there is a detailed localization in each cortical visual area, its posterior part corresponding to macular or central and its anterior part to peripheral vision, while the upper part of the area receives impressions from the lower part of the field and the lower from the upper. Perceptions due to the irritation of any part of the visual cortex are projected to the corresponding point in the field of vision. and consequently if the discharge spreads over the cortex the phenomena perceived appear to the patient, to move through the opposite half of the binocular field of vision. This can be illustrated by one of Gowers' cases in which I was able to observe the patient during many attacks, some of which lasted 10 min or longer. They commenced with the appearance of several small spheres, white in the centre with an intermediate zone of blue and outside this a ring of red, immediately to the left of the point at which the patient gazed; from here they moved either at a uniform rate or in jerks to the left and downwards. As the patient remained conscious during the attacks he was able to indicate the position to which he referred them. When the spectra passed further from the fixation-point the colours disappeared from them. Almost immediately after their appearance vision in the left halves of the fields became dim and the loss quickly amounted to a left complete hemianopia which persisted for several minutes after the attacks ceased, then disappearing gradually from the centre towards the periphery. In all attacks the eyes deviated towards the left and the head turned in the same direction as soon as the visual spectra appeared. This deviation of the eyes and head was at first tonic but later became clonic; it could be controlled to some extent by the patient. In some of the attacks at least it was probably secondary to the visual spectra, the gaze being directed reflexly towards the point in space to which the spectra were projected. This man had in all probability cerebral tumour, but its position in the brain was not determined. Gowers assumed that the symptoms were due to a lesion in the neighbourhood of the angular gyrus. Gowers records in the same lecture another case, that of a girl, aged 9, who was under my observation for some years. She had been, since receiving an injury to her head at the age of 31 years, subject to right-sided epileptiform attacks. Most of which began with the appearance of a bright light in the right halves of her visual fields, which she spoke of as 'twinkles', probably because it scintillated. Frequently there were colours in it. As soon as it appeared she invariably brought her hand to the outer side of her right eye 'to rub it away'. Her head and eyes turned slowly to the right, she lost consciousness and developed tonic and clonic spasms in her right limbs. On regaining consciousness there was a defect of vision in each eye to the right of the fixation-point, occasionally a complete hemianopia which cleared up quickly. Mr. Sargent discovered a cyst, probably the result of a traumatic haemorrhage, in the left angular gyrus, but it is possible that there were other lesions nearer the calcarine area. Similar attacks of visual epilepsy have been frequently observed in men who had received gunshot wounds of the occipital region. Several such cases informed me that some time after the infliction of the wound, or on regaining consciousness after it, they saw light or stars though they were often temporarily blind. A study of phenomena associated with the later stages of such wounds is more instructive. One of my patients was wounded over the pole of the right occipital lobe in 1916, as a result of which he has still a small left-sided paracentral scotoma, chiefly in the upper quadrants. Since being wounded he has been subject to fits, all of which begin with flashes of light to the left of his fixation-point, apparently just outside the scotoma. He describes the flashes as shell bursts or 'balls of fire but redder than any fire', which dance about to his left; then vision to his left becomes hazy, everything seems to be receding into the distance, his left arm and later his left leg become numb and he loses consciousness. On one occasion on which I was able to examine him immediately after a seizure there was for a time a left-sided hemianopia. In another man with a similar wound near the right occipital pole, the fits began with the appearance of very 'bright lights of all colours' in the left of the point on which the eyes were directed. They grew brighter and brighter until he lost consciousness. He exteriorized these visual sensations so vividly that on a few occasions he assaulted nurses who came to his assistance, as he thought they were 'flashing those lights in front of my eyes'. In a third man, who had a piece of metal embedded near the anterior end of the left calcarine fissure, the epileptiform attacks commenced with the appearance of a dull black patch which he referred to the lower part of the outer canthus of his right eye. Next flashes of lightning appeared in the same place and often persisted for 10–15 min. Simultaneously, or somewhat, later in the severer attacks, his right limb became numb and powerless and he lost consciousness. I have observed a large number of similar cases, in all of which the traumatic lesion lay near and frequently injured the calcarine visual area. There seems,

> therefore, little doubt that these relatively simple and crude visual phenomena must be attributed to a discharge spreading over the receptive visual cortex. I have never seen them occur as primary phenomena in epileptiform seizures due to injury or disease of other portions of the brain. They may obviously result from discharges spreading back to the occipital cortex from the parietal or temporal lobes, but then they are preceded by motor or sensory aurae. It is probable that purely negative phenomena may occur in patients subject to visual epilepsy ; one man with a gunshot wound of the right occipital region informed me that while reading he sometimes lost his sight to his left side, and another, also with a right occipital injury, that while in a cinema he suddenly became unable to see to his left, but I have not had an opportunity of examining a patient during temporary primary hemianopia.

Following this, Holmes differentiates the visual occipital seizures from the 'complex or highly organized subjective visual sensations that do not result directly from lesions of the occipital cortex' such as of the blind and of those originated from the temporal lobe:

> 'More complicated subjective visual phenomena are frequently associated, as Hughlings Jackson originally pointed out, with local lesions in the neighbourhood of the uncus of the temporal lobe, but they are different in origin and nature to those we are studying. I refer to them here only for purpose of contrast.
>
> These uncinate epileptic seizures frequently begin with subjective smells and tastes, which are almost invariably of an unpleasant, usually of an extremely disagreeable, character; often there is, too, an epigastric sensation which may account to actual nausea. Then comes that peculiar mental state which Jackson called the 'dreamy state' or 'intellectual aura' characterized by a feeling of unreality of the present or familiarity with the events of the moment as though they had been experienced before. Often visions which the patient associates with the past come up. A patient whom I had under observation always saw, in this stage a woman with a red cloak approaching nearer and nearer until, as the spectre reached her, she lost consciousness. In other cases, the vision may be of a scene tinted with a tone of familiarity, a building or a similar object. In such cases the visual hallucinations, for to these the term hallucination can be applied, is only part of the intellectual aura of Jackson and is obviously the result of more complicated cerebral and psychological processes than the perception and projection of lights and colours.'

Malformations of cortical development[460]

Previously often escaping available brain imaging, disorders of malformations of cortical development are now recognized as a common cause of symptomatic partial seizures (localization-related symptomatic epilepsies) including occipital seizures thanks to high resolution MRI. Salanova *et al.*[700] found that one fifth of their neurosurgical series of occipital epilepsy patients had developmental pathology on neuroimaging studies, histology or both. It was occasionally missed by MRI and proven only by histology.[700] More recently, Kuzniecky *et al.*[457] described the clinical spectrum, treatment, and outcome of 10 patients with occipital lobe developmental malformations and seizures. Mean age of seizure onset was 8 years and there was a strong correlation between the presence of visual auras, the scalp EEG pattern, and the subtype of underlying pathology. Magnetic resonance imaging showed cortical developmental malformations in all patients, with heterotopia, polymicrogyria and focal cortical dysplasia being the most frequent malformations. Despite the presence of occipital lobe structural malformations in all patients, visual field deficits were present in only two. The clinical manifestations were similar to patients with other structural lesions involving the occipital lobe. Interictal EEG often showed low-voltage, fast-spiking activity over the occipital lobe resembling ictal like activity. Conversely, patients with developmental cystic lesions had a paucity of interictal discharges over the occipital regions. MRI showed evidence of focal lesions involving the occipital lobe, with or without concurrent occipital horn dilatation. Those patients who underwent cortical resections were seizure-free or showed major improvement at a mean follow-up of 3.5 years. The authors concluded that 'intracranial stimulation studies and the low frequency of pre- and postoperative deficits suggest that some degree of cortical visual reorganization may occur in patients with occipital lobe malformations.' Also, 'occipital lobe cortical developmental malformations should be sought as a cause of symptomatic occipital lobe epilepsy even though they may become symptomatic after childhood.'

Symptomatic occipital epilepsy and coeliac disease, with or without occipital calcifications

Symptomatic occipital epilepsy in coeliac disease (CD) is probably the most likely of all to imitate clinically and EEG late onset benign childhood and idiopathic photosensitive occipital seizures. This interesting association between occipital seizures and CD with or without bilateral occipital calcifications has been well documented mainly by Italian authors who have also formed the Italian Group on coeliac disease and epilepsy.[341–345,409,788] This brief account is based on their newly published book on 'epilepsy and other neurological disorders in coeliac disease'[341] which is highly recommended for further reading.

Coeliac disease is a common permanent gluten-sensitive enteropathy that is genetically determined, modified and provoked by dietary habits with gluten-containing food such as cereals, bread, pasta and biscuits. It may manifest with classical or single malabsorption symptoms or single nutrient deficiencies or is asymptomatic. Though onset is more common in childhood, CD may present in adult life as anaemia, metabolic bone disease, diarrhoea or weight loss. Tests for IgA anti-gliadin antibodies with a 75 per cent detection sensitivity and the more sensitive IgA anti-endomysium antibodies (95 per cent sensitivity) are used for screening. Small-bowel biopsy demonstrating crypt hyperplasia and flat mucose is still essential for confirmation. Management consists of life-long complete eradication of gluten from the diet. For those few with confirmed coeliac disease who may not benefit from a scrupulous gluten-free diet, prednisolone 5–20 mg daily is often beneficial.

Diverse epileptic conditions with onset in childhood and early adolescence have been reported in patients with symptomatic or asymptomatic coeliac disease. These include severe epilepsies such as Lennox–Gastaut syndrome, myoclonic epilepsies with ataxia[104,510] but more frequent symptomatic occipital epilepsy.[22,184,288,341–345,409,516,788].

In an epidemiological study on the 'frequency of epilepsy in coeliac disease and vice versa' Vascotto and Fois[788] found that of 2627 patients with typical CD 21 (0.79 per cent) had seizures and 12 also had cerebral calcifications. Mean age at diagnosis of CD = 5.9 years. Of 993 with atypical CD 18 (1.8 per cent) had seizures and 11 also had cerebral calcifications. Mean age at diagnosis of CD = 9.7 years. Of 169 subjects with silent CD, six (3.5 per cent) had seizures and three also had cerebral calcifications. Mean age at diagnosis of CD = 10 years. Conversely, of 1210 with various types of seizures, CD was found in 10 patients and three of them had cerebral calcifications. Thus, the overall prevalence of epilepsy in CD was 1.15 per cent (the authors quote a 0.5–1 per cent prevalence of epilepsy in a paediatric population) and half of them showed cerebral calcifications. Vascotto and Fois[788] concluded that the length of time that these children were exposed to gluten is significant for the development of seizures and cerebral calcifications.

Gobbi, Bertani and the Italian Working Group (IWG) on Coeliac Disease and Epilepsy[342] have reported 63 patients and reviewed another 192 patients from the literature. These 255 patients were divided into four groups. Group 1 consisted of 143 cases with coeliac disease, epilepsy and cerebral calcifications, group 2 (69 cases) had CD and epilepsy without cerebral calcifications, group 3 (33 cases) had epilepsy and cerebral calcifications without CD and group 4 (10 cases) had CD and cerebral calcifications without epilepsy. In general, age at onset of epilepsy ranged between 1 and 28 years with a mean at around 6 years with most of the patients starting seizures between 4 and 13 years. Seizures are mainly partial and the occipital are by far the most common. However, generalized tonic–clonic seizures and absences may occur from onset of epilepsy. In most of the patients, seizures started before the detection of CD and the institution of the gluten-free diet (GFD). However, there were also cases where seizures started after GFD and these were more likely to be symptomatic, drug-resistant occipital epilepsy. Initial ictal seizure symptoms were mainly elementary visual hallucinations and the evolution was benign in around 1/3 to 1/4 of the patients also with EEG normalization. However, the majority progress to other seizure types and an epileptic encephalopathy with delayed mental development after an initial relatively good response to treatment. Severity of epileptic seizures is not proportional to the severity of cerebral calcifications.

EEG abnormalities initially consisted mainly of occipital paroxysms, occipital spikes or generalized discharges. IPS activation of occipital spikes was not uncommon. Multi-spike discharges in sleep EEG often betrays their symptomatic character.

The authors concluded that 'Although clinically heterogeneous, epilepsy in CD is usually localization-related, originating from the occipital lobe, and the course is usually drug-resistant. It is frequently characterized by an early and apparently benign initial phase followed by an epileptic encephalopathy after a seizure-free interval. GFD seems to control the seizures if started near the onset of epilepsy and early in childhood, confirming the hypothesis of a relation between CD and epilepsy in these patients.'[342] They also emphasized that in a few patients occipital seizures may have a benign course and speculated that in these benign cases the evolution of the seizures is CD-independent, and that the epilepsy and CD association is casual or genetically linked.[342]

Triulzi[775] reviewed the neuroradiological findings in coeliac disease, epilepsy and cerebral calcifications. These are cortical-subcortical serpiginous calcifications mainly bilateral and located in the parieto-occipital regions. They may extend to more anterior regions and may increase during the evolution before starting GFD. There is no leptomeningeal enhancement and there is no associated brain atrophy. There is no enlarged subependymal-periventricular vessels or enlarged ipsilateral choroid plexus. They are well illustrated with CT brain scan but MRI usually fails to reveal them though they may be detected as hypointense lesions with T2-weighted MRI. The author concluded that neuroradiological features of these patients are markedly different from those of the Sturge–Weber syndrome which show enhancement of the pial angioma detected with CT and MRI, calcium deposits beginning in the subcortical white matter and limited to the site of the enhancing angioma showing on T2-weighted MRI as linear hypointense signals within the cortex and associated progressive localized cerebral atrophy.

A history of gastro-intestinal symptoms, nutritional problems, a positive family history of CD and an atypical Sturge–Weber syndrome without a cutaneous nevus should raise the possibility of this syndrome. Occipital seizures in Sturge–Weber syndrome are rare.[49]

Lafora disease[96,684]

Lafora disease is an autosomal recessive disorder amongst the progressive myoclonic epilepsies, characterized by the presence of Lafora bodies (PAS-positive diastase resistant polyglucosan inclusions) found in brain, skin, liver and other body tissues. It has recently been mapped to chromosome 6q24. Onset of the disease is around the age of 14 years (common range 8–18 years) mainly with occipital, myoclonic and generalized tonic–clonic seizures.[5,6,316,685,758,771,773] Occipital seizures occur in 30–50 per cent of the patients; they may be spontaneous or photically induced and consist of complex and elementary visual hallucination. At the initial stages Lafora disease may imitate idiopathic generalized epilepsies, with myoclonic jerks, GTCS and generalized discharges of polyspikes and slow waves, spontaneous or photically induced, and a relatively normal EEG background. Occipital involvement is indicated by occipital polyspikes and visual seizures, but these rarely occur without co-existing myoclonic seizures, GTCS and EEG generalized discharges which are also often induced by IPS. Background EEG may be abnormal before onset of seizures[5,6] but may also be normal at the initial stages of the disease.[758] Cognitive decline is relentless either before or soon, within months, after the onset of seizures, and death is unavoidable within 1–10 years.

Lafora disease should be suspected when onset of occipital seizures is combined or followed by myoclonus and progressive mental decline.[316,684] Confirmation of the diagnosis is often made by the detection of Lafora bodies in the eccrine ducts of the sweat glands in axillary skin biopsy.

Symptomatic occipital epilepsy due to mitochondrial disease (MELAS)[388]

Mitochondrial encephalomyopathy, lactic acidosis and stroke-like episodes (MELAS) is a maternally inherited mitochondrial cytopathy due to a point mutation in the mitochondrial leucine (UUR) transfer

RNA gene at position 3243. Point mutations in myoclonic epilepsy with ragged red fibres (MERRF) usually occur within the tRNA-Lys gene at position 8344. MELAS and MERRF mutations are heteroplasmic and although there is considerable overlap in the clinical presentation of the A3243G and A8344G mutations, they do seem to be distinct syndromes.[163]

MELAS is characterized by recurrent brain stroke-like episodes mainly in the posterior cerebral regions which are often precipitated by metabolic stress, exertion and fatigue. There are multiple and heterogeneous lesions, preferentially in the occipital lobes, that not do not correspond to the vascular territories of main cerebral arteries.

According to Hirano and Di Mauro[388] cardinal 'clinical features of MELAS include: (a) stroke-like episodes at a young age (typically before 40 years of age); (b) encephalopathy manifested as seizures, dementia, or both; and (c) mitochondrial dysfunction with lactic acidosis, ragged-red fibres, or both. In addition, to secure the diagnosis, at least two of the following clinical features should be present: normal early development, recurrent headaches, or recurrent vomiting. Other commonly encountered manifestations include myopathic weakness, exercise intolerance, myoclonus, ataxia, short stature, and hearing loss. It is uncommon for more than one family member to have the full MELAS; in most pedigrees, there is only one patient with MELAS with oligo-symptomatic or asymptomatic relatives in the maternal lineage.

The pathophysiology of stroke-like episodes in MELAS is uncertain. It may be due to one or a combination of factors such as local metabolic alterations, abnormal cerebrovascular reserve, increased lactate in both the occipital and temporal lobes, impaired auto-regulation secondary to the impaired metabolic activity of mitochondria in the endothelial and smooth muscle cells of blood vessels,[168] cerebral hyperaemia and fluctuating CO_2 reactivity which is possibly a consequence of local lactic acid production.[361]

Patients with MELAS frequently manifest seizures, myoclonus and ataxia; therefore, they may closely resemble individuals with MERRF. In a review[389] of 110 reported patients with MELAS, myoclonus was noted in 38 per cent, seizures in 96 per cent and ataxia in 33 per cent.[389] However, stroke is the distinguishing clinical feature of MELAS. In patients with MELAS seizures are not infrequently the initial clinical manifestation (28 per cent). The seizures are sometimes associated with stroke-like episodes and it is suggested[389] 'that the increased metabolic demands imposed by the seizures provoke some MELAS strokes, and that it is likely that the cerebral lesions cause the seizures, thus establishing a vicious cycle. Sometimes febrile episodes accompany the seizures, raising the hypothetical possibility that the added metabolic stress of the febrile illness can precipitate seizures.'[389]

Hirano and Pavlakis[389] found that information about seizures was available in 42 of the 110 reported patients with MELAS.[389] Only six had visual seizures, 26 had both generalized and partial seizures, 10 had generalized seizures only (including one patient with absence seizures). Partial seizures were predominantly motor (21 patients) and, less commonly, visual (six patients), temporal (three patients), auditory (one patient), or sensory (one patient). At least six individuals developed status epilepticus. Myoclonus is generally less common and less severe in patients with MELAS than in patients with MERRF.[389]

Considerable interest in the association of migraine and occipital seizures in this syndrome come from Andermann and collaborators.[35,40,257] Andermann in a more recent review maintains that there is a 'syndrome of malignant migraine, epilepsia partialis continua and predominantly occipital lesions' that 'has been shown to be characteristic of MELAS'. However, it is not even certain that these patients of Andermann *et al.*[35,40,257] suffered from MELAS. None of the four illustrative cases[35,257] had conclusive confirmation of MELAS, 'the diagnosis was based on a strong clinical suspicion of mitochondrial encephalopathy'[35]and no new cases have been reported since the initial report of 1986[40] despite the authors continuing interest.[35] Also, these patients cannot be considered as characteristic of MELAS where occipital seizures are relatively rare (14 per cent as opposed to 50 per cent for motor partial seizures) despite the predominant occipital involvement of the pathological process. Headaches are common in MELAS but this does not mean that they are migraine. MELAS causes significant brain changes which may lead to stroke-like episodes and these are unlikely to be painless. A comparison with eclampsia also manifesting with severe headaches and occipital seizures, which in this case are mainly reversible, may be convincing.

Pre-eclampsia and eclampsia

Pre-eclampsia is a multi-system disorder associated mainly with hypertension, proteinuria, oedema, haemoconcentration, hypoalbuminemia, abnormalities of hepatic function or coagulation, and increased urate levels. Approximately 4 per cent of women with untreated pre-eclampsia develop eclampsia which is a potentially fatal disease. Symptoms and signs arise because of vasospasm caused by exaggerated vascular responsiveness to circulating angiotensin and catecholamines. There is a selective vulnerability of the occipital lobes during eclamptic hypertensive encephalopathy. This is demonstrated in pathological specimens with multiple petechial haemorrhages in cortical patches or subcortical haematomas mainly in occipital lobes. Also, recent MRI and functional brain imaging studies demonstrated extensive but reversible bilateral abnormalities of the cortex but mainly of the white matter in the posterior cerebral regions indicative of subcortical oedema without infarct.[20,162,546,711] These are similar to those of hypertensive encephalopathy

Neurological symptoms of eclampsia include seizures, headache, blindness and impairment of consciousness. Headache often associated with vomiting may be the first symptom. Seizures may be generalized or visual partial with secondary GTCS. Cortical blindness may also be ictal.[347,381,520,660] Plazzi *et al.*[660] reported two women with eclampsia who continued having visual seizures long after their recovery from the acute stages of eclampsia. Ictal elementary visual hallucinations lasting for seconds were multi-coloured circles or squares.

Differential diagnosis and investigations of patients with occipital lobe epilepsy

The diagnosis of occipital seizures should not be difficult and these should be first differentiated from migraine, normal phenomena and psychogenic or other causes unrelated to seizures. A thorough neurological evaluation also including visual field testing may reveal relevant deficits in symptomatic occipital epilepsy. Occipital seizures in an otherwise normal child are most likely to be idiopathic while in an adult these are mainly symptomatic and their cause should be thoroughly investigated. For all partial seizures, in adults or children, I always ask for an EEG and MRI. The EEG is essential as it may show occipital spikes, occipital paroxysms or photosensitivity in favour of an idiopathic syndrome. Conversely, it may raise suspicions of a symptomatic cause with unequivocal focal slow waves, accelerating fast rhythms or generalized polyspikes and slow waves. Worsening of the background EEG is also significant for diagnosis. When routine EEG is normal, an EEG after partial sleep deprivation recording during sleep and awakening is essential. The MRI is also mandatory as symptomatic occipital seizures may initially or for years deceive us into thinking they are truly idiopathic (see the following two illustrative cases). Unsuspected residual or progressive lesions, tumours, vascular malformations and malformations of cortical development are all shown with MRI. CT is much inferior to MRI and insensitive to focal cortical dysplasia. Conversely, calcifications of coeliac disease may be missed with MRI but this is rare.

Illustrative cases of symptomatic occipital epilepsy imitating idiopathic occipital epilepsy

The following two cases illustrate the difficulties that we have sometimes to differentiate symptomatic from idiopathic occipital epilepsy even when CT brain scan and MRI are available. For both cases, it was only after a high resolution 3D MRI that the correct diagnosis was made.

Case 7.1. This normal woman, born in 1969, was referred to me in 1992 with a diagnosis of migraine associated with epilepsy. At 9 years of age she started to have frequent episodes of visual hallucinations and headache on awakening between 5.30 and 6.30 a.m. every one to two months. The visual hallucinations consisted of vivid, flashing multi-coloured lights and circular patterns which occupied her visual fields and obscured her vision (Fig. 9.2). Severe unilateral headache followed 1–2 min later, described as like pressure behind one eye, often associated with vomiting. On many occasions and within 1–2 min from the onset of the visual hallucinations there was loss of consciousness associated with 'the right arm rising up above her head and jerking about', 'a strange feeling as if she was going to die', and 'convulsions with tongue biting'.

She was seen by five consultant neurologists who attributed the episodes of visual hallucinations and headache to migraine, whereas the associated episodes of loss of consciousness were diagnosed as basilar migraine, genuine epileptic seizures triggered by the migraine, or a coincidence of migraine and epilepsy. Neurological examination was normal. A sleep EEG, at age 23 years, showed, only on awakening, long runs of right sided occipital spikes with some partial attenuation with eyes open. Four previous routine EEGs were reported as showing mild non-specific abnormalities. Computed tomography of the brain and MRI in 1992 were reported as normal.

She never received any anti-epileptic treatment as a result of the above diagnostic considerations of migraine and because of family and personal fears regarding side effects. She only had small doses of carbamazepine 200–400 mg daily at age 19 years which she shortly abandoned.

At age 26 years, she had approximately two visual seizures per month on awakening that 'now take the form of blurring of vision and nausea' which progress to secondary generalization five to six times yearly. A new EEG reported that in addition to the 'very active right occipital spike focus there were some infrequent spikes in the left anterior temporal regions'. A new high resolution 3D MRI showed some minor and residual brain lesions in the right occipital lobe.

There is no family history of epilepsy. Her father has severe migraine.

One intelligent young man with occipital seizures and mild EEG abnormalities in the occipital regions had initially an MRI that was reported as normal but one year later, a new high resolution MRI performed for research purposes showed 'white matter lesions and mild atrophy of ventricular system and subarachnoid space wider than normal' of yet unknown cause. Neuroophthalmological evaluation and visual evoked response are entirely normal. Two EEGs, one during sleep and the other on awakening, showed some non-specific bilateral posterior slow waves with right sided emphasis. This highly intelligent man gives the most remarkable description of his visual seizures and of their progression.

Case 7.2. This 22-year-old intelligent student had at age 15 years a television-related visual seizure and from age 17 years infrequent visual simple partial seizures and on two occasions secondary GTCS. His description of the events is superb:

'The first episode that I recall, occurred when I was fifteen years old. I was sitting in a chair watching television when I literally saw a very bright yellow object (looking very much like an image of the sun) move across my left visual field. It started from the temporal side and moved repeatedly across to the nasal side at a fast oscillatory rate (several times per second) and then disappeared after about 3 min. I initially exclaimed out loudly 'What is that?' before lapsing into an episode of about 5 min of impaired consciousness. I recall almost nothing during these 5 min apart from the movements of the visual image starting and then disappearing until I was suddenly aware of family members asking me if I was all right. Once I regained full consciousness, I was a little disorientated and unbalanced because I could not see properly out of my left eye for another 20 min or so. When I regained full vision, I had no residual symptoms apart from a slight headache.

In the subsequent years, I have suffered on six to seven occasions with a similar type of partial seizure that I have described in detail below as the '20/07/97' seizure. All of these episodes except one has been at night and several months have always elapsed between them. On two occasions, May 1992 and August 1995, I have completely lost consciousness and suffered a full tonic–clonic convulsion immediately after suffering the same type of seizure symptoms as 20/07/97. The additional notable symptom that I suffer from, which seems to happen every time I have had the six to seven epileptic episodes, is clusters of momentary left visual field disturbances that always occur in the first few hours after waking up. The disturbance is like a momentary flickering or blurring of vision (always in the left temporal field only) with a simultaneous brief feeling of slight unsteadiness. Several of these moments can occur within, for example, a 10 min period and then several again over a similar period one or more hours later. There is no fixed pattern or any other related symptoms such as headache or nausea etc. These clusters also occur independently of the seizures and are thus more frequent than them, I would estimate that every 2–3 months I suffer from them. One unexplained feature is that the vast majority of times this occurs on Sunday mornings. The only thing I can think of is that I often watch television till very late on the night before as it is a Saturday and then I sleep in an irregular pattern for the rest of the week because I wake up late usually between 11 a.m. to noon on the Sunday. Thus, there may be a combination of irregular sleeping and excess television that produces these, although if this is true I would expect them to possibly occur more frequently than they do.

Apart from this I am perfectly healthy and do not suffer from any major (frequent, long lasting or very severe) headaches or any other symptoms/illnesses.

20/07/97 Seizure – Diary of events

19/07/97 – Saturday

Slept at 02:20 in the morning, mainly due to watching television till late.

20/07/97 – Sunday

8 a.m. Woke up spontaneously, went back to sleep.

12.30p.m. Woke up and got up, had bath, got dressed. During getting dressed, several episodes of visual flickering.

2.15p.m. Another cluster of visual flickering while using computer.

10p.m Prepared to go to sleep by getting undressed, and getting into bed.

10.33p.m. Not having got to sleep, sudden awareness of rapidly oscillating vague dark disproportionate face like figures moving forward and back in the temporal field of the left eye. Simultaneous feeling that the left jaw and shoulder are moving inwards towards the eye. Adjusted body position to lie flat on my back with head looking upwards and forwards, noticed time and also a chink of light at the door out of my right eye. Concentrating on the visual hallucination of the left eye becomes very frightening, therefore I begin to try and concentrate on the door seen by right eye. Inwards movement of shoulder/jaw ceases after less than 1 min but constant oscillation of intensely frightening face like image continues. Become aware after 1–2 min of occasional involuntary twitching eversion/dorsiflexion movements of left foot and left index finger and wrist.

10.37p.m. Suddenly the visual hallucination ceases completely. I noted time out of my right eye. Got up and switched on the light. Noticed that I had almost no vision in the left eye, only blackness. Right eye is normal as is physical motion of the body. I drew a visual fields estimate by self-assessment (left homonymous hemianopsia).

10.45p.m. Vision gradually completely returns to left eye over 1–2 min. Switch off light and try to get to sleep. There is no immediate headache.

11.15p.m. Unable to sleep because of development of a severe headache which makes head feel very heavy and tight, focus of pain is on the right occipital area. Generalized exacerbation of pain on shaking head from side to side. Sharper throbbing pain also noticed simultaneously over the whole forehead and in both eyeballs especially when pressed. Overall it feels like the head is full of too much pressure which is causing pain. Decide to get up and write down detailed version of all events.

12.00a.m. Get into bed to sleep. Right occipital headache and heaviness of head still persist although sharper throbbing pain frontally has subsided. Eyeballs are still sore and painful if pressed.

21/7/97 – Monday 8.30 a.m. Got up and went into St.Thomas's for an EEG.

Summary

3–4 min of visual hallucinations followed by 8–10 min of left visual loss followed by 30 min of sharp frontal and posterior headache followed by 1 h or more of a dull generalized headache and pain in eyeballs on pressure.

Treatment with carbamazepine (retard) 400 mg bd started after the last seizure. He had no further visual seizures of any type in the following 6 months.

Illustrative cases of symptomatic epilepsy with ictal vomiting

The following are the only three symptomatic cases that had ictal vomiting amongst the 418 patients

I reported.[603] They illustrate that diagnosis is easy based on clinical symptoms. All had abnormal neurological signs, CT brain scan and in two EEGs showed significant localized slow activity.

> Case 7.3. This 4-year-old boy was born prematurely with difficult delivery. There is moderate delay of psychomotor development and he is hyperkinetic. From age one and a half years he developed infrequent nocturnal seizures of waking up with eyes deviated to one side followed by generalized convulsions. At age 4 years he had another nocturnal seizure with prolonged for 15 min deviation of the eyes, choking-like movements, vomiting and inability to speak without convulsions. A sleep EEG next morning showed no consistent abnormalities. CT brain scan was abnormal with mild and diffuse cortical atrophy.

> Case 7.4. This boy born with Caesarean section has hydrocephalus, mental retardation and left hemiplegia. At age 8 years he started having infrequent diurnal seizures and once during sleep 'stomach upset' and vomiting followed within 1 min by loss of consciousness. CT brain scan was grossly abnormal. EEG showed high amplitude bursts of slow waves on the right.

> Case 7.5. This girl has right sided hemiparesis and had right sided convulsions in the first days of her life. At 11 months old she had a nocturnal seizure with vomiting and cyanosis followed by right sided convulsions. CT brain scan was abnormal and EEG showed high amplitude delta waves on the left.

Treatment of patients with symptomatic occipital epilepsy

Drug treatment is similar to that for other partial epilepsies such as temporal lobe epilepsy.

The drug of choice is carbamazepine, phenytoin, phenobarbitone and clobazam in that order. Topiramate is probably the best of the new drugs. Vigabatrin is also effective but its use in occipital seizures may be restricted by the side effect of irreversible visual field defects. In my experience neither sodium valproate nor lamotrigine was helpful.

Regarding neurosurgical treatments, the published experience is rather limited in comparison with temporal lobe epilepsy. Williamson *et al.*[811] reported that resection of the lesions in 16 patients produced excellent results in 14 (88 per cent). Five patients had temporal lobectomies, with good results in three, but poor results in two. Two patients with unlocalized seizures had complete section of the corpus callosum, one with a good result and the other with poor results. Blume *et al.*[131] reported the results of epilepsy surgery in the posterior cortex of 19 patients. Fourteen (74 per cent) obtained a significant reduction in seizures after posterior corticectomy, six (32 per cent) were seizure-free over a median follow-up of 3.7 years (range, 1 to 14 years). Salanova *et al.*[700] reported that 23 patients underwent only occipital resections; five had only temporal resections, so as to preserve the visual fields, and the remaining 14 patients had extensive resections, which included the posterior temporal or posterior parietal regions. A follow-up period of 1 to 46 years (mean 17 years) was available for 37 patients. Forty-six per cent became seizure free and 21 per cent had a significant reduction in seizure frequency. A better outcome was observed in those patients in whom there was no post-resection electrocorticographic or surface EEG epileptiform discharge, or who exhibited an occipital lobe lesion.

Idiopathic occipital epileptic syndromes

Benign childhood occipital seizures and related epileptic syndromes

The syndromes of idiopathic occipital epilepsy are classified in Table 7.1. Benign childhood occipital seizures and related epileptic syndromes have been largely neglected despite their remarkably sound and fascinating clinical and EEG features and the fact that some of them may be as benign as the benign Rolandic seizures if appropriately differentiated from migraine with aura, acephalgic and basilar migraine as well as cryptogenic and symptomatic epilepsies.

Based on an extensive review of the literature and my personal experience, benign childhood occipital seizures (BCOS) have two distinctly different clinical phenotypes:

(a) The early onset benign childhood occipital seizures (EBOS) or Panayiotopoulos syndrome;

(b) The late onset benign childhood occipital seizures (LBOS) or late onset idiopathic childhood occipital epilepsy.

Idiopathic benign photosensitive occipital seizures (IPOS) are another interesting manifestation of an age-related seizure susceptibility with some patients having photically induced occipital seizures alone or combined with spontaneous fits.

The following chapters present the clinical and EEG features of these variants of benign childhood occipital seizures and attempt their differentiation from other diseases that they may imitate or be mistaken for, such as:

(a) Migraine with aura, basilar and acephalgic migraine;

(b) Symptomatic and cryptogenic occipital epilepsies also including coeliac disease.

Historical aspects, literature reviews and my personal experience are also detailed.

Benign Childhood Partial Seizures and Related Epileptic Syndromes. C P Panayiotopoulos
©1999 John Libbey & Company Ltd., pp. 133–147.

Chapter 8

Early onset benign childhood occipital seizures: Panayiotopoulos syndrome

Definition

Early onset benign childhood occipital seizures (EBOS) or Panayiotopoulos syndrome is the second in frequency after the Rolandic seizures manifestation of a childhood seizure susceptibility syndrome that is age related and may be genetically determined. The cardinal features of Panayiotopoulos syndrome are infrequent, often single, partial seizures manifested with deviation of the eyes, vomiting or both which frequently progress to hemi- or generalized convulsions. Ictal behavioural changes, irritability, pallor and eyes widely open are common. Retching, coughing, speech arrest, cyanosis, oropharyngolaryngeal movements, and incontinence of urine may occur less often. Consciousness is usually impaired or lost either from the onset or during the course of the seizure but in a few children it may be preserved throughout the fit. The seizures may last for a few minutes to hours (partial status epilepticus) and they are usually nocturnal. The clinical ictal symptoms are the same irrespective of whether the seizures are nocturnal or diurnal. Onset is between 1 and 12 years of age with a peak at 5 years and remission usually occurs within one year from onset. The mean total number of seizures is three with a maximum of 15. Prognosis is excellent. The early onset BOS is the most benign of all seizure syndromes despite the highest frequency of status. The likelihood to continue having seizures after the age of 12 is less than that for febrile convulsions. The EEG shows occipital paroxysms (Figs. 8.1a, 8.1b, 8.1c) which in routine recordings occur when the eyes are closed because of fixation-off sensitivity (FOS). Other patients with EBOS may have only random occipital spikes and some may have occipital spikes or paroxysms in sleep EEGs alone and a few may consistently have normal EEGs. Centrotemporal and giant somatosensory evoked spikes may occur simultaneously with occipital paroxysms in the same EEG with morphologically similar sharp and slow waves in other locations such as midline, parietal and frontal (Fig. 8.2). These multi-focal sharp waves are more frequently seen in serial EEGs where occipital spikes are usually first to appear. Frequency, location and persistence of occipital spikes and paroxysms do not determine clinical manifestations, severity and frequency of seizures or prognosis. Occipital spikes may occur in 0.5–1.2 per cent of normal mainly pre-school age children. They are age dependent with a peak at 4–6 years of age. They often persist despite clinical remission and usually disappear before the age of 13. Age-dependent occipital spikes frequently occur in a variety of organic brain diseases with or without seizures and children with congenital or early onset visual and ocular deficits.

A typical case of nocturnal EBOS is a 5-year-old child who wakes at night vomiting. There is deviation of the eyes to one side and consciousness is impaired. This lasts half an hour terminating with hemiconvulsions. The next morning the child is back to normal. The EEG is grossly abnormal with occipital paroxysms lasting as long as the eyes are closed and demonstrating FOS (Figs. 8.1a, 8.1b, 8.1c). Two similar nocturnal seizures occurred in the same year. Progression to convulsions was prevented with rectal application of diazepam. No more seizures of this or any other type occurred but the EEG remained abnormal until the age of 9 years.

A typical case of diurnal EBOS is a 5-year-old child who while at school, suddenly feels unwell, becomes agitated and is pale. Within 10 min he starts vomiting and gradually becomes less responsive with eyes deviating to one side. This state lasts for 1 h and ends with hemiconvulsions in the accident and emergency department of the nearest hospital. Though a more serious neurological condition was feared by the paediatricians, the child gradually recovers and within hours he is entirely normal. An EEG two days later showed occipital paroxysms. Despite the fact that no treatment was initiated the child developed well with no seizures although EEGs continued to be abnormal for years after cessation of fits.

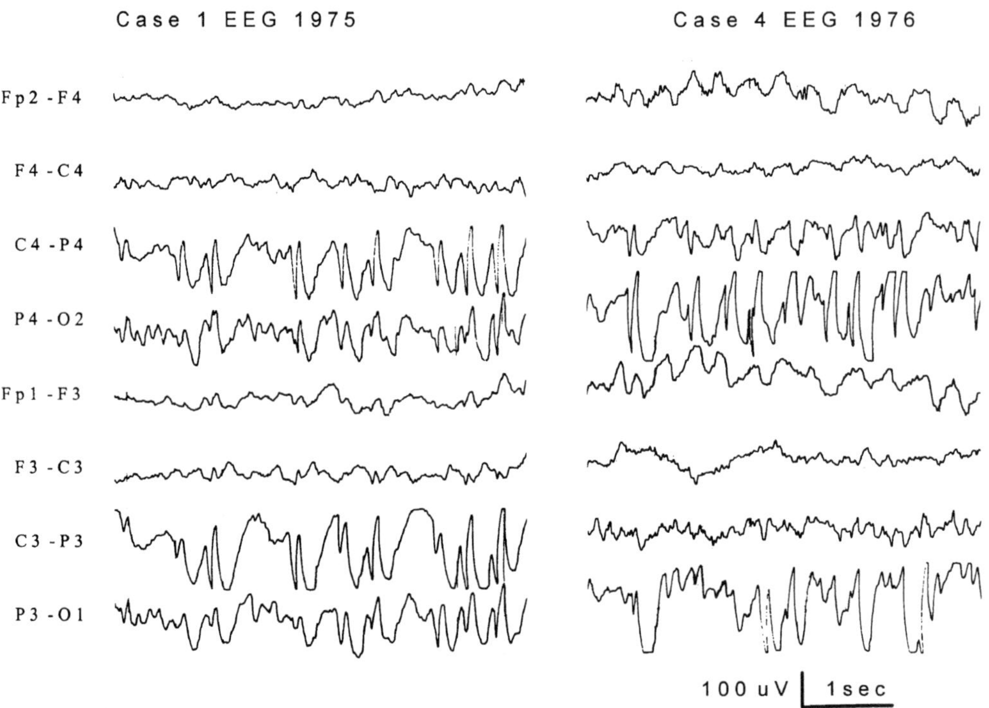

Fig. 8.1a. Occipital paroxysms in the first two children with Panayiotopoulos type early onset benign occipital seizures that I published in Neurology, 1981[600] as cases 1 and 4. Note the similar morphology and distribution of the occipital paroxysms.

There was also ample demonstration of FOS as also shown in the next two figures, Figs. 8.1b and 8.1c. Occipital paroxysms occurred immediately after closing of the eyes, lasting as long as the eyes were closed. The EEG normalized immediately after opening of the eyes and as long as the eyes were open. The occipital paroxysms became continuous in darkness even when the eyes were open.

All these EEG were recorded in a chip eight channel, ink pen EEG machine.

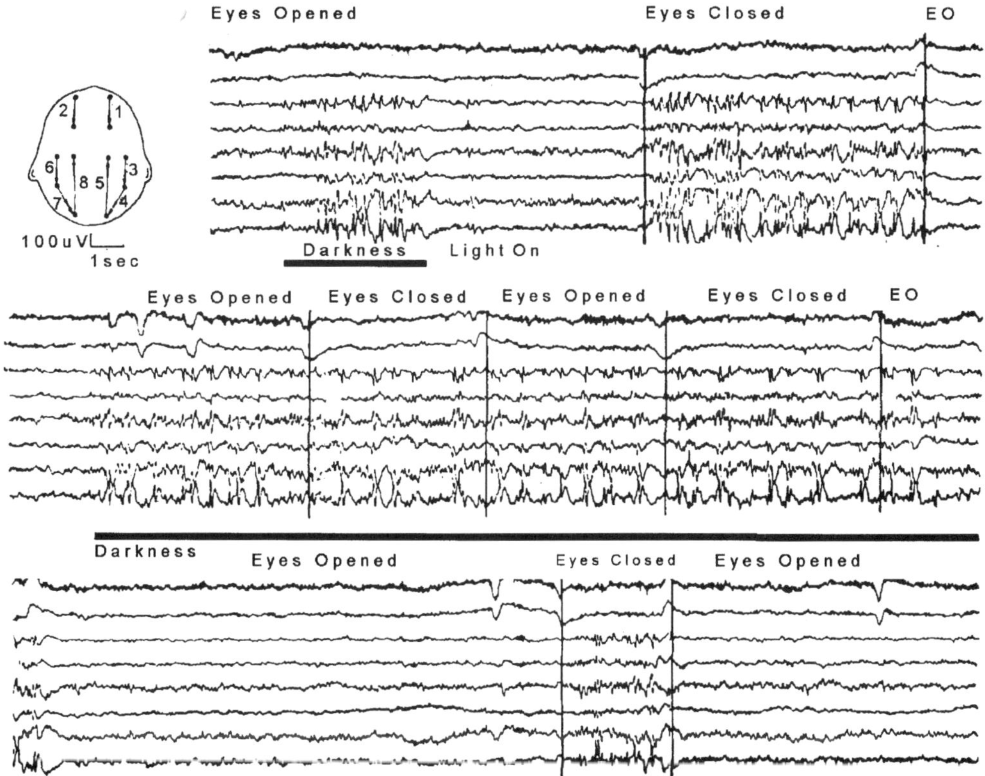

Fig. 8.1b. EEG of case 1 in 8.1a. The occipital paroxysms consistently occur when the eyes are closed and disappear when the eyes are opened, provided that the lights in the recording room are on. Darkness (remember that this should be total darkness) has the same activating effect on occipital paroxysms which appear again when eyes are open and the lights are switched off. Opening and closing of the eyes in darkness does not interfere with the occipital paroxysms which are continuous thus excluding the participation of other than visual stimuli. EEG recording in total darkness is annotated with the horizontal black thick line.
Modified from Panayiotopoulos, 1981[600] with the permission of the editor of Neurology.

Introduction

The early onset benign childhood occipital seizure susceptibility syndrome (EBOS)[86,150,192,270,367,443,517,600,602,603,605,606,608,630,636,793,797] is not yet recognized by the Commission[177] although it is more common, more benign and easier to diagnose than the LBOS. Though the identification[600,602] of the EBOS was due to the associated severe EEG occipital spikes, the syndrome is more often revealed by characteristic clustering of clinical manifestations which are rarely seen in other epileptic syndromes and may also occur without EEG occipital spikes.[608]

Synonyms and abbreviations

EBOS = Early onset benign childhood occipital seizures

Synonyms

Early onset benign childhood epilepsy with occipital paroxysms[605]
Benign nocturnal childhood occipital epilepsy[606]
Panayiotopoulos type of benign childhood occipital epilepsy[150,270,271]
Panayiotopoulos syndrome[12]

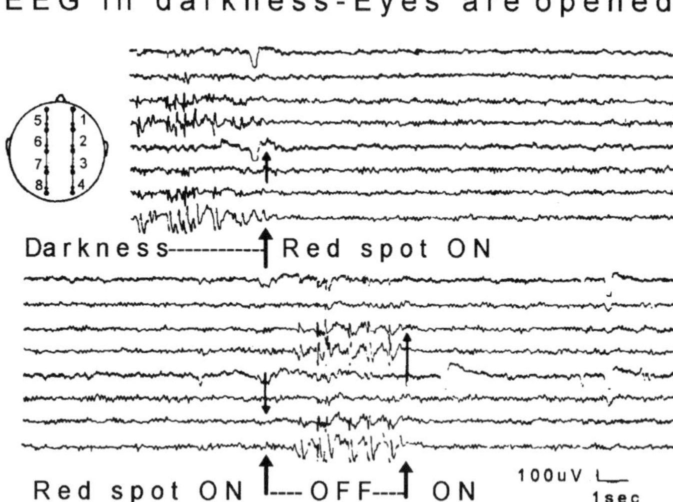

Fig. 8.1c. EEG of the same child as in 8.1a and 8.1b. Recording in darkness with eyes remaining continuously open. The occipital paroxysms are inhibited by fixating on a spot of red light (created by the light of an opthalmoscope showing through the finger from a distance of approximately 2–3 m).
Modified from Panayiotopoulos,1981[600] with the permission of the editor of Neurology.

The early onset benign childhood occipital seizures, so vigorously denied even today by some of experts,[36] is a syndrome that should be logically expected. We already know that centrotemporal spikes occur in 2–3 per cent of normal children at a peak age of 8–9 years and they are associated with Rolandic seizures,which are their clinical model. Similarly, we already know that occipital spikes occur in 0.5–1 per cent of normal children at a peak age around 4–5 years (Fig. 8.4). It would be logical to predict that occipital spikes, second in frequency after the centrotemporal ones, would also have a clinical prototype. This is what I have described and detail in this chapter.

Prevalence

It appears that Panayiotopoulos syndrome is the second most common syndrome of benign childhood partial seizures after Rolandic seizures. EBOS are 2–4 times less frequent than RS.

Panayiotopoulos[605] found 16 children with EBOS (3.8 per cent) amongst 418 patients with onset of seizures before the age of 13 years. Ninety four (22.5 per cent) had benign childhood partial seizures with 72 having Rolandic seizures and two LBOS. Thus, EBOS had an estimated prevalence of 17 per cent amongst the benign childhood partial seizures; it was 4.5 times less frequent than Rolandic seizures and eight times more frequent than LBOS.[605]

With improving awareness, prevalence of EBOS is expected to increase. No such case of EBOS was recognized in retrospective studies of children with occipital paroxysms[180,287] although children also had 'neurovegetative symptoms' which were significantly more common than the visual hallucinations.[287] Recently, Fejerman[270] in a large scale study found 130 (60.2 per cent) children with Rolandic seizures, 56 (26.3 per cent) with Panayiotopoulos type EBOS and 18 (8.4 per cent) with Gastaut type LBOS. Nine additional patients (4.2 per cent) had combining features of Rolandic seizures and EBOS. Similarly, Guerrini *et al.*[368] found that 11 of their patients with benign occipital seizures had EBOS and only four had LBOS. Maher *et al.*[517] also found a higher incidence of EBOS (14 patients) in relation to LBOS (one patient) with another five patients having symptoms of both EBOS and LBOS.

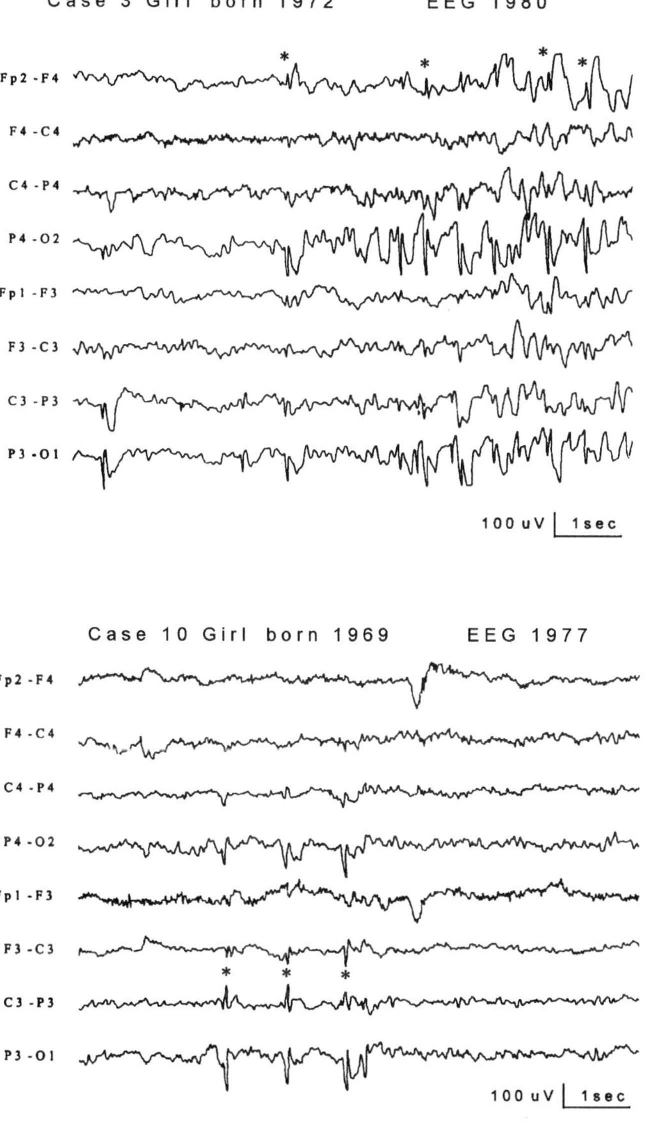

Fig. 8.2. These are also EEGs from my studies in Athens of case 3[605,606] *and 10,*[606] *see Table 13.1 (Chapter 13). Upper: Occipital spikes of case 3 occur synchronously with right frontal spikes (asterisks). Lower: Occipital spikes of case 10 occur synchronously with left central spikes (asterisks).*

I would expect that the prevalence of EBOS is around 25 per cent of all benign childhood partial epilepsies and 2.5 times less frequent than Rolandic seizures. I base this assumption on the prevalence of occipital spikes in children (29 per cent) as opposed to 63 per cent for centrotemporal spikes and 8 per cent for frontal spikes according to the findings of Kellaway.[438] However, the prevalence of occipital spikes in normal children (0.2 per cent) is 9.7 times less frequent then that of centrotemporal spikes (2 per cent) (see page 193).

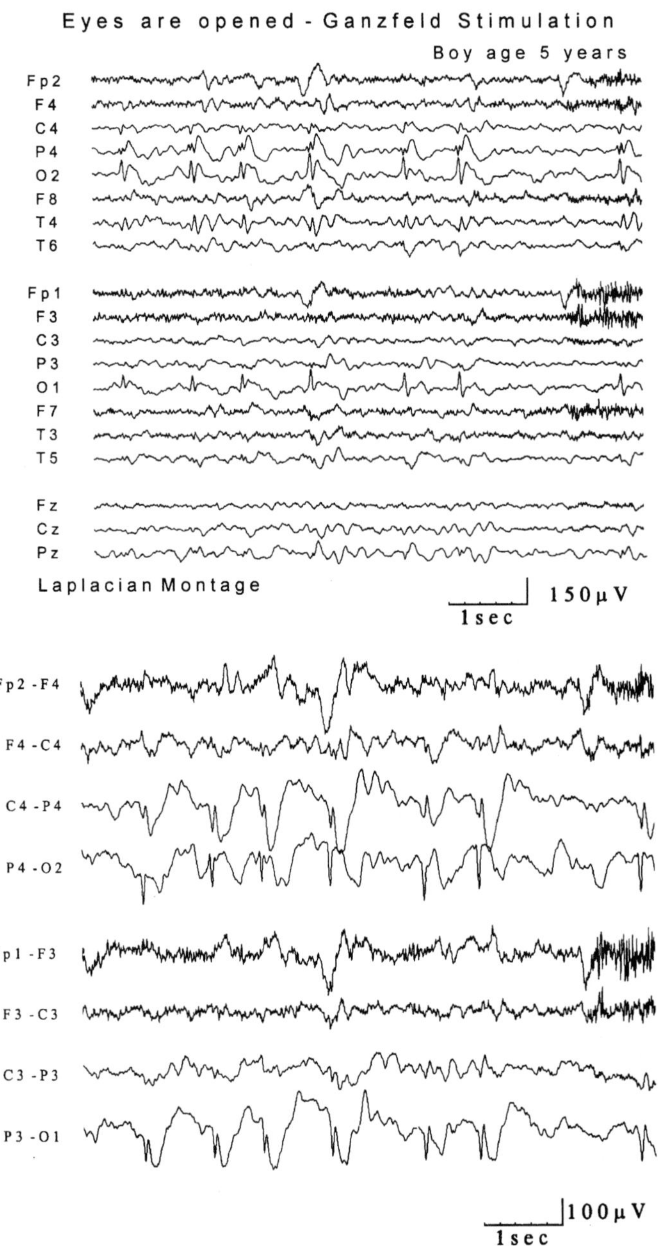

Fig. 8.3. This EEG of illustrative case 18 (page 145) would not exist under the present recommendations to paediatricians in the UK – not to ask for an EEG after the first seizure.
There are frequent clusters of occipital spikes during eyes closed that demonstrate FOS with Ganzfeld stimulation (achieved by asking the child to look at a white paper in front of him).
The same EEG sample is shown in Laplacian montage (upper) and bipolar montage (lower) for comparison. Note the dipoles of the right occipital spikes. Also the right occipital spike negativity spreads to the right midtemporal T4 electrode (upper).

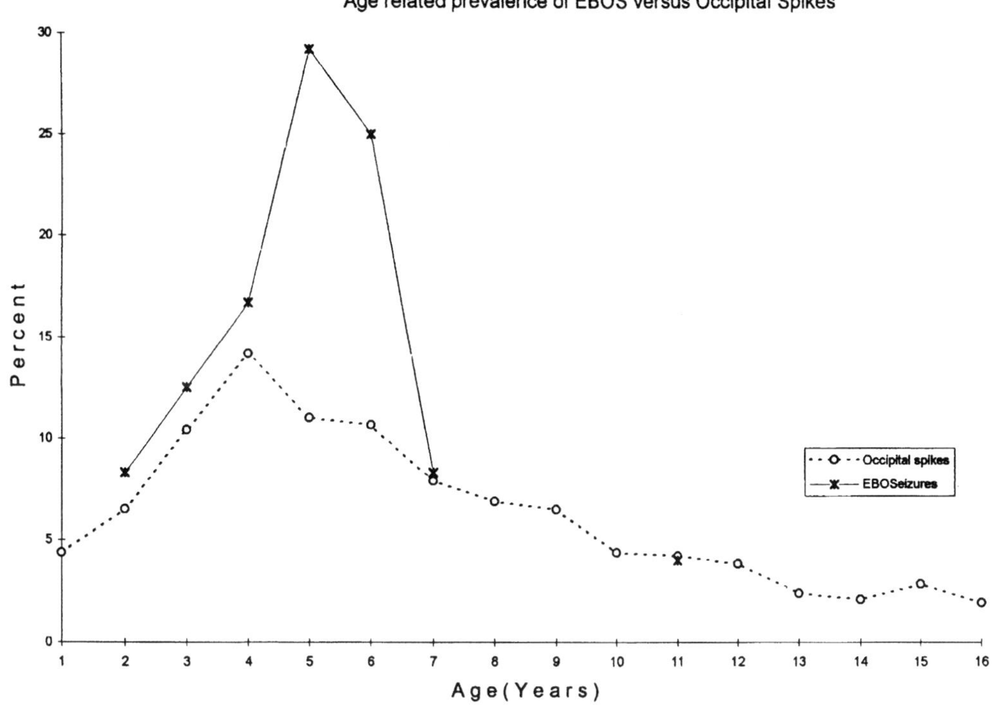

Fig. 8.4. Age at first discovery of occipital spikes in children as calculated from the studies of Gibbs et al.[326] *and Kellaway*[438] *compared with the age at onset of seizures in 24 children with Panayiotopoulos syndrome of early onset benign childhood occipital seizures.*
Note the remarkable similarities between the two curves.

Clinical features of EBOS

Ictal vomiting (ictus emeticus)

Considered exceptionally rare[229,282,371,414,417,453,537,559,772] or dismissed as a non-seizure or migrainous event, ictal vomiting eluded physicians until its frequent association with EBOS was unequivocally documented by Panayiotopoulos.[603,605,606] Ictal vomiting in EBOS may occur at any stage of the ictus, usually at the beginning but may also occur later before the convulsive phase of the seizure[603,605,606,608,615] as confirmed in all subsequent reports.[150,192,270,277,367,443,517,793]

In recent studies, ictal vomiting occurred in 70 per cent of 113 children with EBOS reported by Ferrie and colleagues[277] and in all 56 children with EBOS reported by Caraballo *et al.*[150]

Headache

Though headache was not initially described in EBOS,[605] it appears that it may occur either in the ictal or post-ictal phase[277,443] though this is much less common than in LBOS. Kivity and Lermann[443] reported that in five of nine children with diurnal prolonged seizures of EBOS type these were heralded by headache which in some cases was very severe.[443] Ictal headache was found in 13 per cent and post-ictal headache in 16 per cent of 113 children with EBOS.[277]

Deviation of the eyes and other convulsive features

Unilateral deviation of the eyes is, with ictal vomiting, amongst the most common ictal manifestation described in 13 of 16 patients (81.3 per cent) by Panayiotopoulos[605] and confirmed in all other reports.[12,86,150,192,270,272,277,367,443,517,793]

The deviation of the eyes is usually slow, more of a shifting of the eyes to one side (pursuit-like) which often horizontally move to their extreme, and can hardly be seen in the corner through the opened eyelids. This is not associated with any other convulsive features of the eyes or eyelids though the head may also turn axially towards the same side. This pursuit-like deviation of the eyes may be brief for minutes or prolonged for hours, continuous or less often intermittent with eyes returning into midline and tonically deviated again towards the same side. The eyelids remain open, but may be semi- or widely open without any clonic movements or jerks.[74] There are no hemifacial spasms or dystonic movements of any type at this stage where consciousness is often but not invariably impaired.

Thus, these occipital oculotonic ictal symptoms are differentiated from extra-occipital ictal ocular symptoms, where the tonic deviation of the eyes often occurs simultaneously with tonic or clonic convulsions of the ipsilateral facial muscles (as is for example the case in the hemifacial seizures of Rolandic seizures). In extra-occipital ictal ocular symptoms the eye movement is usually more violent, there is usually an upwards deviation, the ipsilateral eyelid goes into tonic or clonic convulsions and these also often involve other facial muscles ipsilaterally. The movement of the eyes is simultaneous or follows the movement of the head. Neck and shoulder muscles may be simultaneously involved.

Deviation of the eyes may occur without vomiting in 10–20 per cent of the patients.[74,195,277,600,605,636]

This phase of eye deviation, vomiting or both may progress to unilateral hemi-clonic convulsions of the face and the extremities in 25 per cent[277]–37 per cent.[605] The whole seizure ends with a GTCS in nearly half of the patients.[605]

Occasionally, in some children eyes may be widely open and remain in the midline before other convulsions occur, as is the case with the patients described by Beaumanoir.[74]

Impairment of consciousness

Consciousness is impaired in 80–90 per cent of seizures either from the onset or more commonly during the course of the fits.[277,605] This may be mild or moderate with the child retaining some ability to respond to verbal commands but often unable to speak. Severe disturbance of consciousness with complete unresponsiveness is less common at the beginning of the seizure, usually occurring with convulsions. In 10–20 per cent of the seizures consciousness is preserved throughout the ictus.[277,605]

Visual hallucinations and blindness

There is undue emphasis on whether visual hallucinations occur or not in EBOS.[36,43] What difference would this make to the diagnosis? Even if we assume that all children with EBOS, in all their seizures have ictal elementary visual hallucinations, there are many more dramatic differences between EBOS and LBOS. In Panayiotopoulos syndrome seizures are prolonged, usually over 10–30 min, often nocturnal, infrequent, mainly 1–3 in duration with a short active life span, usually less than one year and of excellent long-term prognosis. Conversely, in LBOS seizures are short, usually seconds to less than 1–3 min, mainly diurnal, frequent, often daily, with a protracted active life span of a 5 year median and of uncertain prognosis (see Chapter 13). The argument that visual hallucinations in EBOS are not reported because children are too young or seizures are nocturnal may be partly true. However, this does not explain the fact that older children with EBOS even in diurnal seizures do not describe visual hallucinations while these are well reported by younger children with LBOS even when they precede nocturnal secondary generalized convulsions. The following are reports of children with EBOS who have visual hallucinations but this does not signify anything other than their occipital origin.

Amongst the illustrative cases of 63 patients of Gastaut and Zifkin[313] there was a 10-year-old boy who had a single nocturnal seizure with nausea and vomiting followed by generalized convulsion. 'Several minutes after it ended, nausea and vomiting recurred and were followed by a loss of vision lasting several minutes. An EEG performed the next day and another 1 month later were both normal.'[313]

Five of 18 patients of Beaumanoir[74] had diurnal seizures characterized by visual symptoms and nocturnal seizures mainly manifested with unilateral oculoclonic convulsions.

Iwasaki *et al.* (1992)[410] reported the case of an 8-year-old boy who had attacks of vomiting followed by loss of consciousness and elementary visual hallucinations consisting of red and blue colours. He sometimes complained of constriction of visual field for 10 to 20 s, as if a curtain had fallen following the visual hallucination of a bright light spot. The EEG showed occipital paroxysms suppressed by eyes opening in an illuminated room, but not in a dark room.

Ferrie *et al.*[277] described 12 children who had 'ictal tonic deviation (eight children) or vomiting (11 children) and ictal visual symptoms (12 children)' as an overlap group of EBOS and LBOS. The age of onset was later (mean = 6.9 years), remission occurred later (mean age = 10.3 years) and seizures were more than in the pure form of 113 children with EBOS. Some of these 12 children with typical attacks of EBOS later developed LBOS. Similarly, Yalcin *et al.*[826] reported that some of their patients with EBOS had visual hallucinations prior to ictal vomiting and eye deviation.

None of the 16 children I reported[605] and another eight children I examined more recently with EBOS had visual hallucinations of the type seen in the LBOS. One of my first patients[600] with two nocturnal seizures typical of the EBOS at age 5, had 2 years later eight diurnal, less than a minute, episodes of 'dizziness' in which the environment seemed to move away from her and return to her with increasing speed. Two of them progressed to automatisms and loss of consciousness without convulsions (see illustrative case 1, page 146).[600] Two other patients revealed on questioning that they saw a diffuse coloured light when concentrating with closed eyes.[636]

Other ictal clinical manifestations

What are probably more common than appreciated are other autonomic symptoms such as pallor which I was able to detect in all patients with diurnal attacks when I specifically enquired. Autonomic are usually the first symptoms, together with behavioural changes such as the child becoming very quiet, vacant or restless, agitated or feeling sick.

Automatisms, aphemia, retching, coughing and oropharyngolaryngeal symptoms are uncommon, less than 10 per cent, and occur together or follow the more characteristic ictal manifestations of vomiting, deviation of the eyes and impairment of consciousness.[277,605]

Duration of seizures and partial status epilepticus

The most interesting feature of EBOS is the frequent occurrence of partial status epilepticus which occurs in more than one third of the patients and may be singular, the only clinical event in a child's life.

That seizures may be prolonged for more than half an hour (partial status epilepticus) was already known from our initial reports in 1980–1981[600,636], documented in all of our subsequent publications[602,603,605,606,630] and confirmed world-wide.[192,270,271,277,367,443,517,793]

The exact duration of the nocturnal seizures cannot be estimated as their onset may be long before the first apparent clinical manifestations. Approximately two thirds of the seizures last for 6–10 min but in the other one third the duration is prolonged for more than half an hour to 3–12 hours.[192,270,271,277,367,443,517,602,603,605,606,630,793] The initial stage of diurnal partial status epilepticus is inconspicuous, with the children just feeling and looking unwell. They are pale, quiet or agitated or complain that they are sick and vomit. Occasionally they may also have headache. This is followed by impairment of consciousness, deviation of the eyes or both, often ending with hemiconvulsions or GTCS. post-ictally, children may complain of headache but usually they return to normal after a few hours of sleep. I am not aware of any child with EBOS having more than one GTCS at the end of this state.

Partial status epilepticus in EBOS was found in eight of 16 children,[605] three of 19,[517] nine of 56[270] and 50 of 113 with EBOS.[277] In the study by Ferrie *et al.*[277] partial status epilepticus was exclusively during sleep (64 per cent), in the awake state (28 per cent) or both (8 per cent). The mean duration was 2.3 h (with a standard deviation of 2.8 h). In 10 per cent of the cases there was no impairment of consciousness. Partial status epilepticus terminated with hemiconvulsions (34 per cent) or GTCS (16 per cent). One third ended without generalized convulsions probably because of the appropriate use of diazepam in more than half of all cases. Partial status epilepticus was the only clinical event in the child's life in two of eight children in our report[605] and in five of nine children reported by Kivity and Lerman.[443]

Partial status epilepticus in EBOS has been vividly described as 'cerebral insult-like'[630] and 'stormy onset'[443] EBOS because they may imitate more serious neurological conditions.

Circadian distribution

Seizures are mainly nocturnal. All 16 children reported by Panayiotopoulos[605,606] had nocturnal seizures, with five of them also having diurnal seizures. In another report of ours, a child had diurnal seizures only.[630] Maher *et al.*[517] had 16 children with nocturnal seizures, one with nocturnal and diurnal and two with diurnal only. Nine children reported by Kivity and Lerman[443] had prolonged episodes of impairment of consciousness, vomiting, headache, deviation of the eyes and other convulsive seizures. Two of them were nocturnal and seven diurnal seizures. In the multicentre study of Ferrie *et al.*[277] two thirds of seizures were nocturnal.

Age at onset and sex

Age at onset varies from 1 to 12 years with a consistent median in all studies at around the age of 5 years (Fig. 8.4).[150,277,605] There is a single case with onset at 14 years[368] but this must be entirely exceptional.

My initial impression that girls[605] were more frequently affected than boys was probably due to small numbers as both sexes are equally affected in the study of 113 children with EBOS.[277]

Frequency of seizures and evolution

The number of seizures suffered by these children with EBOS is remarkably small and the prognosis appears excellent, as shown in long prospective studies with some children having more than 15 years follow-up.[277,605] Also, frequency of seizures and prognosis are not influenced by partial status epilepticus with which EBOS is more frequently associated than probably any other epileptic syndrome.[150,192,277,367,443,517,605,608,793]

In the initial prospective study[605] five (31.3 per cent) of 16 children had only one seizure. The median number of seizures was three, mean 3.6 (SD = 3.5) and range 1–12. These have been confirmed in all other reports.[150,192,277,367,443,517,793] Ferrie *et al.*[277] found a range of 1–15 seizures, a median of 2 and a mean of 3 (SD = 2.4) with thirty four (30.1 per cent) of 113 having a single seizure only.

For those children with more than one fit, the last occipital seizure usually occurs within 1 year and rarely 2 years from onset.[277,605] I know of only one child who had his first diurnal occipital partial status epilepticus at the age of 6 years, developed two brief nocturnal seizures of the Rolandic type at the ages of 7 and 8 and had another typical diurnal occipital partial status epilepticus at the age of 12 years, 3 months after stopping treatment with phenobarbitone.

Four (3.5 per cent) of 113 children developed typical Rolandic seizures after remission of the occipital seizures and only one (0.9 per cent) of 113 patients (case 11 of Panayiotopoulos[605]) had infrequent GTCS after the age of 19 years.[277]

Mental and neurological state and neuroimaging

By definition of an idiopathic syndrome, all children with EBOS have normal neurological and mental state. Brain imaging (CT brain scan or MRI) when performed is normal.[277,368,605]

Genetics

Usually, there is no family history of similar seizures but Kuzniecky and Rosenblatt[458] reported a family with three out of four children probably having early onset BOS.[458] EEG occipital spikes were also detected in the fourth youngest child and 26 per cent of mainly younger members of this family. In the study of Ferrie *et al.*[277] there was a 7 per cent history of epilepsy in first degree relatives; in two this was identified as Rolandic seizures and in another as BOS. A high incidence of febrile convulsions may exist with reported incidence of 30 per cent[793] and 16 per cent.[277]

Differential diagnosis

Children with Panayiotopoulos syndrome merit, like those with the Rolandic seizures, a precise diagnosis which can easily be achieved from characteristic clustering of clinical and EEG findings. There is a combination of autonomic disturbances, vomiting and deviation of the eyes which may last for hours, occur mainly during sleep and often progress to convulsions. A more severe neurological condition may be suspected during the ictus, particularly if this is prolonged, but the post-ictal entirely normal state of the child should be reassuring. These clinical features rarely occur with this sequence in other forms of epilepsies[370,603]and when combined with EEG occipital paroxysms are probably pathognomonic for this entirely benign childhood seizure susceptibility syndrome of the EBOS.

Similar seizures may rarely occur in symptomatic occipital epilepsy which are diagnosed on abnormal neurological and mental symptoms, abnormal brain imaging and EEG background abnormalities (see illustrative cases in Chapter 7). Angelman's syndrome[792] or any other symptomatic epilepsy that may manifest with similar seizures of eye deviation and vomiting, should not be difficult to diagnose based on other symptoms and signs. In our studies only three of 900 patients with seizures had evidence of symptomatic partial seizures (one with mental retardation, one with hemiplegia and one with hydrocephalus).[603,622] These are described as illustrative cases in Chapter 7.

However, similar ictal symptoms to those of EBOS have also been described[622] in other children with extra-occipital 'benign' spikes which have an equally good prognosis as EBOS. Nine of such patients that I have studied had unilateral central spikes which were also elicited with somatosensory stimuli (two), midline spikes (two), frontal spikes (one), ill sustained photoparoxysmal response (one) or consistently normal EEG (three).[622] Furthermore, ictal vomiting has also been recently well documented in idiopathic occipital photosensitive seizures, some of which may also be benign.[370]

Treatment

Treatment cannot be effectively evaluated in a syndrome such as early onset BOS where the natural course may be of only one seizure. In the collaborative study of Ferrie *et al.*,[277] there was no evidence of superiority amongst monotherapy with phenobarbitone, carbamazepine, sodium valproate or no treatment. Therefore, although there is no consensus on treatment, children with Panayiotopoulos syndrome should not need medication. The parents of those with partial status epilepticus may be advised to use rectal diazepam in case of recurrence.[621] A year course of treatment, mainly with carbamazepine, may be recommended but most likely it is not needed.

I am often concerned that I treated some of these children with EBOS with anti-epileptic drugs, barbiturates or carbamazepine for years. However, this was in the 1970's when we knew nothing about EBOS. We saw only the dramatic clinical features of partial status epilepticus lasting for hours and an occipital electrical status epilepticus on EEG when the eyes were closed. There is no justification now, close to 2000, for such an aggressive treatment. We now know a good deal, though not all about the Panayiotopoulos syndrome.

Relation of EBOS to LBOS, Rolandic and other benign childhood partial seizures: a unified concept

The unified concept of all benign childhood partial seizures as an age-related seizure susceptibility syndrome is overemphasized in this book and detailed in Chapter 3 and 18.

That children with occipital paroxysms may also have in the same or subsequent EEG centrotemporal spikes has been emphasized in many reports.[277,308,326,386,603,605,608,793] This was also signified by Herranz Tanarro *et al.* (1984)[386] who concluded that 'benign occipital epilepsy is related to childhood epilepsy with Rolandic paroxysms' on the basis that 13 (41.9 per cent) of 31 children with occipital paroxysms also had 'functional spike-wave focus of temporo-Rolandic localization'. Clinically, 10 children were seizure-free with minimal brain dysfunction in eight of them and two were diagnosed as having basilar migraine. Only four patients suffered from febrile convulsions while the 17 other patients had visual, motor or vegetative partial seizures, and even generalized fits. This association of EBOS and Rolandic seizures has also been reported by Gastaut[308] in a 7-year-old child who at the age of 4 years had 'an adversive seizure to the right, followed by nausea, vomiting and diarrhoea, before losing consciousness for over an hour. Since then numerous other nocturnal attacks of right hemifacial twitching, salivation and anarthria had occurred. EEGs showed occipital paroxysms and left centro-temporal spikes.' One of the 18 patients of Beaumanoir[74] also had 'Rolandic seizures prior to the onset of the occipital ones' and two patients had one brother each with Rolandic seizures.

Regarding EBOS, four of the 16 children with EBOS that we reported[603,605] also had 'centrotemporal spikes either in the same or subsequent EEG and one showed additional frontal spikes'.[603] Additionally, three children had Rolandic seizures with occipital and centrotemporal spikes.[605] It was also apparent that some children initially had seizures typical of EBOS and later developed Rolandic seizures (see illustrative case 14, and Fig. 8.5).[605,608]

These findings have been confirmed by Vigevano and Ricci[793] who reported 14 children with EBOS, six of whom had centrotemporal spikes together or independently of the occipital spikes. Ferrie *et al.*[277] found that from 113 children with EBOS 29 (25 per cent) had centrotemporal spikes, eight (7 per cent) had frontal spikes, three giant somatosensory evoked spikes and 14 (12 per cent) diffuse discharges. Four children developed Rolandic seizures after remission of EBOS.[277] Similar associations have also been confirmed more recently by Guerrini *et al.*,[368] Ferraro *et al.*[274] and Fejerman *et al.*[272]

A unified concept for all benign childhood partial epilepsies has been proposed,[609] as detailed in Chapters 3 and 18.

Illustrative cases of Panayiotopoulos syndrome

The nocturnal early onset benign childhood occipital seizures (EBOS) and the risk of misdiagnosing more serious forms of epilepsies later in life are best illustrated with the following case.

> Case 2 of Table 13.1 (case 4 of reference[600]). This 27-year-old intelligent woman had only two seizures in her life at age 6 years. Both occurred during sleep. In the first one she was found by her parents vomiting vigorously, eyes turned to one side, pale and unresponsive. She was taken to hospital and her condition remained unchanged for 3 h from onset before developing a generalized tonic–clonic seizure. She gradually improved and was normal next morning. The second seizure occurred 4 months later. She woke up and told her mother that she wanted to vomit and then vomited. She was able to speak and reply. Within minutes her eyes turned to the right but she was still responsive. In particular, her mother who was on her left asked 'where am I?', 'there, there' the child replied indicating to the right. Ten minutes later she closed her eyes and became unresponsive. Generalized convulsions occurred 1 h from the onset. She recovered quickly. Her EEGs showed occipital paroxysms (Fig. 8.1a) but normalized by the age of 8 years.
>
> She and her sister had infrequent classical vasovagal syncopal episodes. After one such syncopal episode at age 16 years, this was misdiagnosed as temporal lobe epilepsy in a major paediatric neurological hospital in the USA.
>
> At age 27, she is well, has successfully studied and works in business administration.

The following case is presented because the epileptic seizure was reliably witnessed by his parents from onset with behaviour and autonomic disturbances which would be difficult to attribute to seizure activity before the motor partial events. The EEG had occipital paroxysms but the report was rather alarming and unhelpful.

Case 18 of Table 13.1. This 6-year-old normal boy had a benign occipital childhood seizure at age 4 years while in the train on his way from England to France for holidays with his parents who vividly describe the events: 'he was happily playing and asking questions when he started complaining that he was feeling sick, and became very pale and quiet. He did not want to drink or eat. Gradually he was getting more and more pale, kept complaining that he felt sick and became restless and frightened. 10 min from the onset his head and eyes slowly turned to the left. The eyes were opened but fixed to the left upper corner. We called his name but he was unresponsive. He had completely gone. We tried to move his head but this was fixed to the left. There were no convulsions. This lasted for another 15 min when his head and eyes returned to normal and he looked better although he was droopy and really not there. At this stage he vomited once... In the ambulance, approximately 35 min from the onset, still he was not aware of what was going on although he was able to answer simple questions with yes or no. In the hospital he slept for three quarters of an hour and gradually came around but it took him another half to an hour before he became normal again'.

Two MRIs were normal. Despite occipital paroxysms (Fig. 8.3) which should suggest EBOS, the reporting physician was not helpful: 'Very active spike and slow wave discharges over both post-central regions. The appearances are those of focal epilepsy but the focus is difficult to lateralize. Possibly left more than right.' A similar prolonged episode, preceded by behavioural changes, occurred 8 months later at school. He received no medication. Since then he has been well.

Prolonged episodes, simple and complex partial motor status epilepticus, imitating cerebral insults, are common. They are usually nocturnal (see case 2), rarely diurnal or combined. They may be solitary, i.e. the only clinically detected epileptic event in the life of a child. Single diurnal partial status epilepticus is best illustrated with the following case.

Case 17 of Table 13.1[630]. This normal British girl of Chinese origin, born 8.5.84 had on 21.2.90 one single, prolonged (7–8 h) episode of vomiting, impairment and loss of consciousness, deviation of the eyes and generalized convulsions. The events are described as follows:

13.30 She became suddenly unwell after running a race at school. She had just finished running. Vomited. Complained that she wanted to be sick again. All of a sudden she stood still, urinated and lost control of herself. She was helped to walk to the school bus. Unable to climb the steps but on arrival at the school she was able to walk up the stairs. Laid on the floor.

14.30 Unconscious. Eyes widely open and deviated to one side. Limp and pale. Not responding to commands. In the ambulance: Bubbles in her mouth and dribbling of saliva.

16.15 Taken to St.Thomas' Hospital, London. Twitching (all four limbs) and unresponsive. Diazepam 2 mg intravenously. Admitted. Unconscious over the next 4–5 h. Gradually the level of consciousness improved.

22.00 Conscious and well. No medication was prescribed.

In the last communication with her two years later she is well. There is no family history of migraine or epilepsy.

The epileptic nature and the length of the seizure may not be apparent in some children with EBOS, manifesting with mainly vomiting and autonomic ictal symptoms as illustrated with the next case.

Case 19 of Table 13.1. This normal boy, born 19.2.88, had in December 1993 'a vomiting episode and could not get up, went to the bathroom, was said to be conscious, but then turned his head to the left and for a few seconds became vacant; although the episode was said to have lasted for a few seconds it was not until half an hour later that he was back to normal'. EEG showed abundant occipital and frontal spikes that were also triggered together imitating generalized discharges.

In February 1995, he had a similar episode where 'he had a lot of coughing, felt sick and vomited. He went to the toilet and back to his bed and had another episode where he was looking to the right. He looked pale and returned back to his normal self within 3–4 h.' A new EEG was similar to the previous one but spike foci were less active.

No medication was prescribed and the child was well for the next year of follow-up.

Visual symptoms or other partial in addition to the motor seizures are extremely rare in children with EBOS. This is illustrated in the following case which has the longest follow-up, from 1973 to 1997, and is the first case where the activating role of the elimination of central vision and fixation (FOS) was demonstrated in her EEG (case 1 of Panayiotopoulos, 1981).[600]

Case 1 of Table 13.1. This normal woman, born in 1967, had at age 5 years a nocturnal seizure of vomiting and tonic deviation of the eyes. She was limp, unable to speak and recovered within 15 min without convulsions. A similar nocturnal episode occurred 9 months and one year later. The last one was not associated with vomiting. The child was awaken by a strong feeling of 'dizziness', eyes deviated to the left, followed by a similar deviation of the head. No convulsions occurred and she was well within 15 min. At age 7 and 8 years she had brief diurnal episodes during which she felt dizzy, the environment appeared to move slowly away from her and then come back towards her with increasing speed. Occasionally this was followed by impairment of consciousness and automatisms. On a few other occasions she complained of rotatory vertigo. On questioning, she thought that these episodes were precipitated by darkness or when her eyes were closed. I was unable to reproduce them. She had never experienced generalized convulsions or headache. There is no family history of migraine and epilepsy. EEG occipital paroxysms and FOS were demonstrated in all her EEGs up to the age of 16 years when she had her first normal EEG (Figs. 8.1a, 8.1b and 8.1c). Last communication with her was in 1997: She is well and has obtained two University degrees in Mathematics.

The next case is to demonstrate that some children may have the clinical manifestations of EBOS without EEG documentation of occipital paroxysms or occipital spikes.[608]

Case 23 of Table 13.1. This normal boy, born 10.5.88, had his first seizure at age two and a half years. 'He vomited in the back of the car and on being taken out was very pale and had his eyes open but not obviously looking at anything and was unable to stand or sit. He continued to retch. His mother took him to a friend's house, over 30 to 45 min away, where he held his head and cried, rolling on the floor and lost control of his bladder. He returned to his normal self after about 4 h having had a sleep in the interim. A second episode occurred 4 months later when he woke after an hour's sleep in the evening with his eyes wide open but not obviously taking anything in visually for a period of half an hour, vomited and went off to sleep. Three similar nocturnal episodes occurred in the following 4 months. No more attacks after initiation of treatment with carbamazepine.' His awake and sleep EEGs were entirely normal.

One of the best arguments I used in favour of the benign character of EBOS is the frequent occurrence of EBOS with Rolandic seizures. This is well illustrated in the following case with multiple benign occipital paroxysms, centrotemporal spikes, frontal spikes and somatosensory evoked spikes.[605,608] Her first seizure at age 7 years was typical of EBOS while the second fit, one year later, was a typical Rolandic seizure:

Case 14 of Table 13.1. This normal girl was born in 1975. Two febrile convulsions occurred at ages 2 and 3 years old. At 7 years she had a prolonged nocturnal seizure which started with vomiting and impairment of consciousness during sleep. She was taken to hospital with vomiting and unresponsiveness; subsequently her eyes deviated to the right followed by right sided convulsions. The whole episode lasted for more than 3–4 h. She was well in the next morning and was discharged 4 days later with phenobarbitone 3 mg/kg. An EEG 6 days later showed some diffuse slow waves 3–5 Hz. Significant EEG abnormalities appeared 3 months later with long runs of high amplitude spike and slow wave paroxysms in the right occipital electrode which attenuated on opening the eyes. Two additional, less active foci of smaller amplitude spikes were recorded from the left occipital and right frontal electrode simultaneously with the right occipital spikes. Treatment changed to carbamazepine 15 mg/kg. Another episode occurred one year later, at age 8, during a mild febrile illness; she woke up in the morning with oropharyngolaryneal movements, eyes turned to the right, tried but was unable to speak. This lasted for approximately 10 min. No further seizures occurred in the long follow-up. Her last EEGs in 1988–1991 were normal but previous EEGs had shown multiple spike foci in the left frontal, left and right central electrodes with no further occipital paroxysms. In one but not other EEGs (Fig. 8.5) tactile stimuli consistently elicited contralateral somatosensory evoked spikes with a delay of the negative peak of 50 ms. The last abnormal EEG in 1986 showed independent high amplitude spikes mainly in the left and less often in the right central electrode. Evoked spikes were not elicited. In addition, high amplitude atypical spike and slow wave generalized discharges were recorded with a higher amplitude anteriorly and left. In the last follow-up in 1991, age 16 years old, she was well with normal EEG, successfully attending high school.

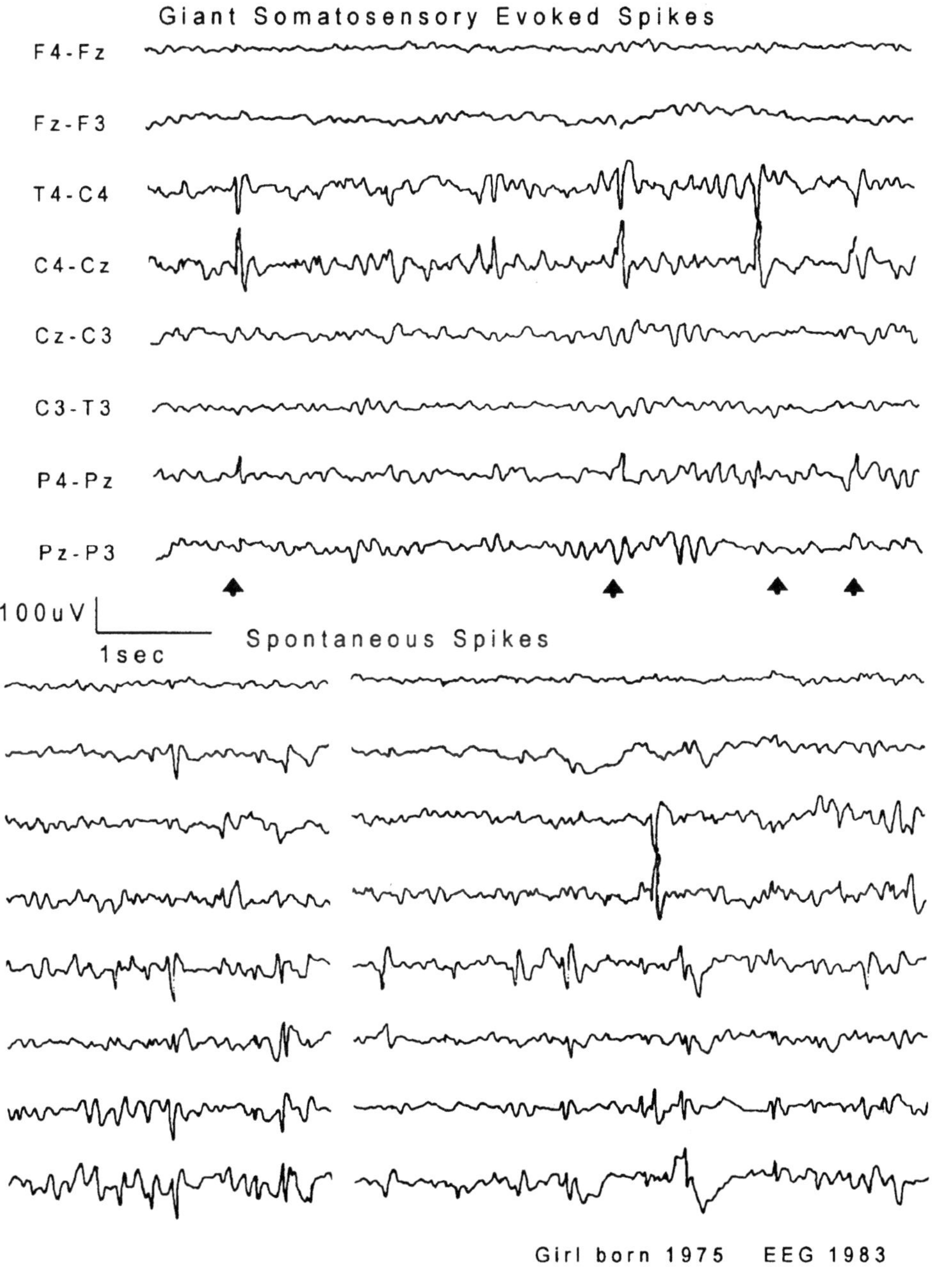

Fig. 8.5. EEG of illustrative case 14 at 8 years of age. Note spontaneous spike foci and giant somatosensory spikes evoked by tapping the fingers of the left hand (arrows). There were no spikes evoked by tapping the fingers of the right hand, the sole of the foot or the toes. Earlier EEG had occipital spikes alone or simultaneously with frontal spikes.

Benign Childhood Partial Seizures and Related Epileptic Syndromes. C P Panayiotopoulos
©1999 John Libbey & Company Ltd., pp. 149–172.

Chapter 9

Late onset benign childhood occipital seizures or Late onset idiopathic childhood occipital epilepsy

Definition

Late onset benign childhood occipital seizures (LBOS) or late onset idiopathic childhood occipital epilepsy is a rare manifestation of a childhood seizure susceptibility syndrome with an age-related onset, often age-limited and may be genetically determined. Seizures mainly manifest with elementary visual hallucinations, blindness or both. They are usually frequent, diurnal and mainly lasting for seconds to less than 3 min. Elementary visual hallucinations are the commonest and most characteristic ictal symptom, most likely the first and often the only seizure clinical manifestation. Ictal elementary visual hallucinations mainly consist of small multi-coloured circular patterns which often appear at the periphery of a visual field, becoming larger and multiplying in the course of the seizure, frequently moving horizontally towards the other side and lasting for seconds to 1–3 min, rarely longer. Elementary visual hallucinations may progress and co-exist with other occipital symptoms such as sensory illusions of ocular movements and ocular pain, tonic deviation of the eyes, eyelid fluttering or repetitive eye closures. Complex visual hallucinations, without the emotional and complicated character of temporal lobe seizures, visual illusions, and other symptoms from more anterio-laterar ictal involvement, may rarely occur *ab initio* or from seizure progress which may terminate with hemiconvulsions or generalized convulsions. Ictal blindness, appearing *ab initio* or less commonly after other occipital seizure manifestations, usually lasts for 3–5 min. Consciousness is not impaired during the elementary and complex visual hallucinations, blindness and other occipital seizure symptoms (simple partial seizures) but may be disturbed or lost in the course of the seizure usually prior to convulsions. Occipital seizures of LBOS may infrequently progress to other extra-occipital manifestations such as hemiconvulsions and hemiparaesthesia. Spreading to produce symptoms of temporal lobe involvement is exceptional and may indicate a symptomatic cause. Episodes of loss of consciousness and falls may rarely occur without convulsions. post-ictal headache, mainly diffuse but also severe, unilateral and pulsating or indistinguishable from migraine headache, often occurs in one third of the patients and in 10 per cent of them it may be associated with nausea and vomiting. Headache, mainly orbital, may also be ictal, often preceding the visual or other seizure symptoms in a small number of patients.

Age at onset is from 3 to 16 years with a mean age of around 8 years. Girls and boys are equally

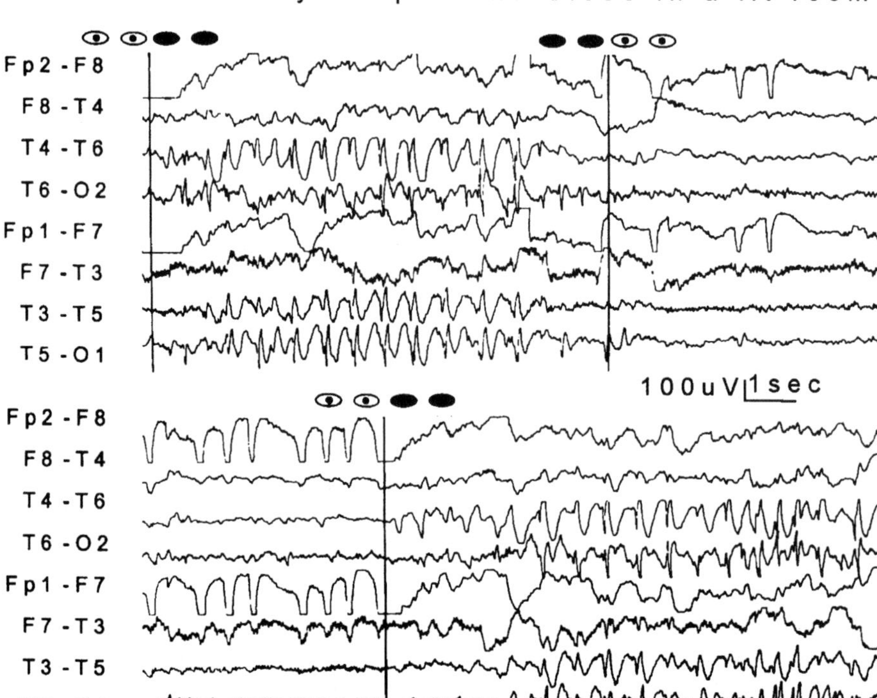

Fig. 9.1a. This patient (case 24 of Table 13.3) was the subject of my report in 1980[599] to question the concept of basilar migraine causing ischaemic lesions and secondary epileptogenesis proposed by Camfield et al.[146] This was also the first case report documenting FOS of the occipital paroxysms. His clinical history is detailed on page 164 as case 24, and he is one of only three patients with LBOS and occipital paroxysms that I saw in the last 25 years.
Occipital paroxysms occur only when the eyes are closed in routine EEG with the lights of the room on. Also, compare the reactivity of occipital paroxysms to darkness and fixation-off in Figs. 9.1b and 9.1c of the same patient.
From Panayiotopoulos, 1980[599] with the permission of the editor of Neurology.

affected. Prognosis is relatively good with remission often occurring within 2–4 years from onset for approximately 50–60 per cent and a dramatically good response to treatment mainly with carbamazepine in more than 90 per cent. However, 30–40 per cent of patients may continue having visual seizures and infrequent secondary generalized tonic–clonic convulsions particularly if not appropriately treated with carbamazepine. The late onset BOS, because of a combination of visual hallucinations, blindness and headache, may be misinterpreted as migraine particularly if the ictus is long.

The EEG shows occipital paroxysms demonstrating fixation-off sensitivity (FOS) (Figs. 9.1a, 9.1b and 9.1c) but others may have only random occipital spikes, some may have occipital spikes in sleep EEGs alone and a few may consistently have normal EEGs. Centrotemporal, frontal and giant somatosensory spikes may occur but less often than in Panayiotopoulos syndrome. Ictal EEG is characterized by regression of occipital paroxysms and the sudden appearance of an occipital discharge which consists of fast rhythms, fast spikes or both. This is of much lower amplitude than that for the occipital paroxysms.

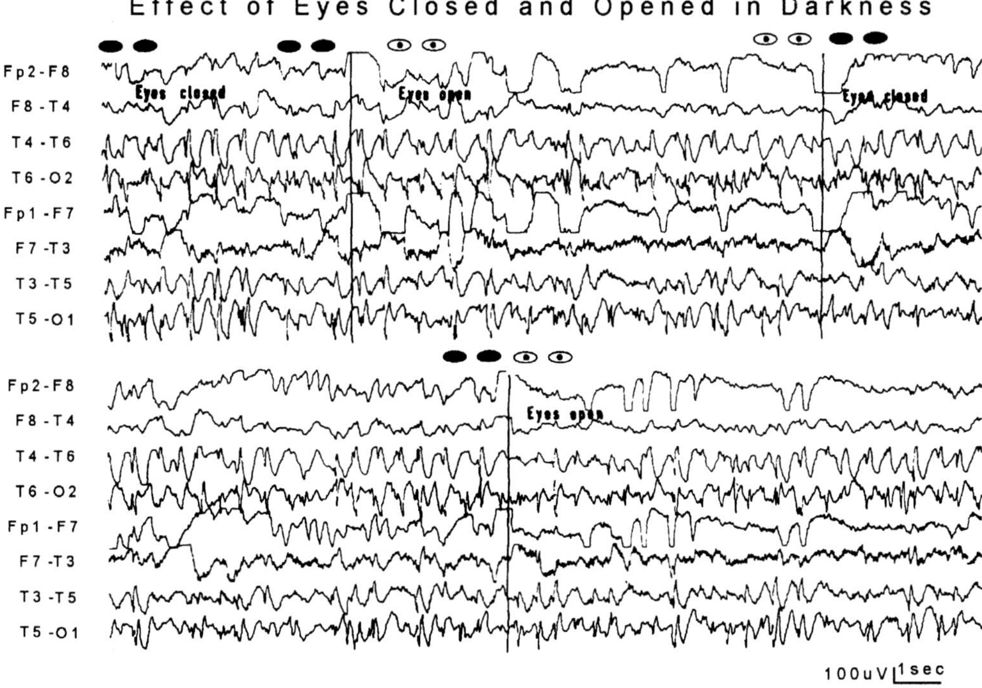

Fig. 9.1b. Same patient as in Fig. 9.1a. In total darkness, the occipital paroxysms are continuous irrespective of whether the eyes are closed or opened, thus excluding the participation of proprioceptive impulses in their generation.
From Panayiotopoulos, 1980[599] with the permission of the editor of Neurology.

Exclusion criteria for late onset benign childhood occipital seizures

The following exclusion criteria should apply:

a. Cryptogenic or symptomatic epilepsies of any aetiology. Their detection often requires a high resolution MRI.
b. Generalized epilepsies.
c. Photosensitive patients with syndromes of idiopathic generalized epilepsy (IGE). Patients with regional occipital photosensitive seizures (idiopathic photosensitive occipital seizures) may be different from LBOS although they are most likely related within the framework of a benign childhood partial seizure susceptibility syndrome (see Chapter 12B).

Abbreviations

EBOS =	Early onset benign childhood occipital seizures (Panayiotopoulos syndrome)
LBOS =	Late onset benign childhood occipital seizures
RS =	Rolandic seizures
IGE =	Idiopathic generalized epilepsies
GTCS =	Generalized tonic–clonic seizures
FOS =	Fixation-off sensitivity

A typical case of the late-onset BOS is an 8-year-old child who starts complaining of elementary visual hallucinations that consist of unilateral multi-coloured small circles lasting for a few seconds. Their

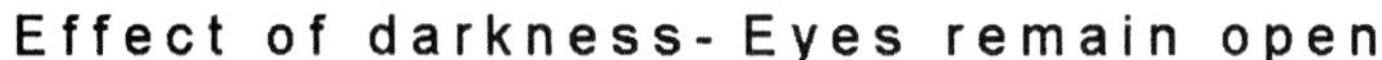

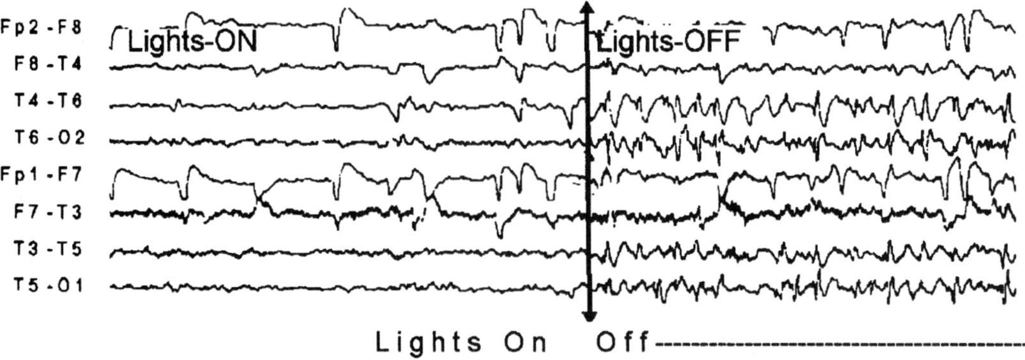

Effect of fixation in darkness-- Eyes open

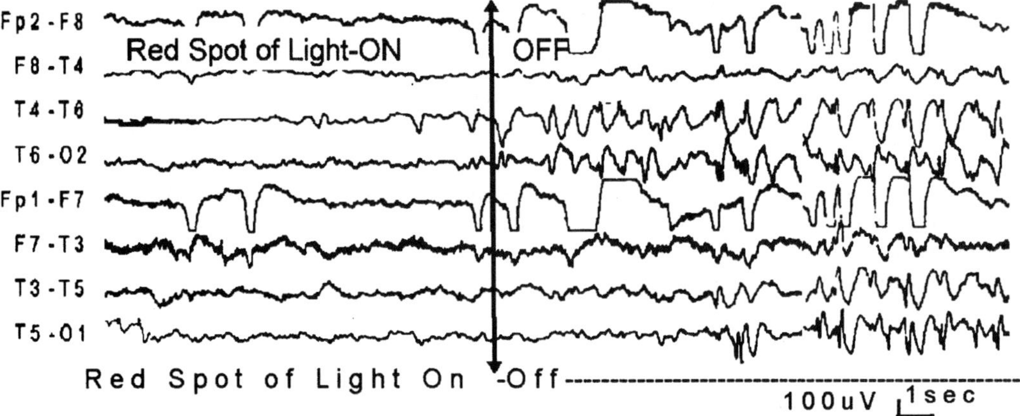

Fig. 9.1c. Same patient as in Fig. 9.1a. Recording with eyes continuously open. The occipital paroxysms are induced by darkness (upper) and inhibited by fixation on a red spot of light (bottom). Modified from Panayiotopoulos (1980)[599] with the permission of the editor of Neurology.

frequency and duration increased over the next few months and these symptoms were also followed by diffuse headache. The diagnosis of migraine with aura was made and relevant treatment was initiated without success. On the contrary, the child had two episodes where the same visual hallucinations became so intense as to obscure his vision followed by deviation of the eyes and head. An EEG showed bilateral occipital paroxysms when the eyes were closed. MRI was normal. The child had two episodes of complete blindness without convulsions. The diagnosis of basilar migraine was suspected but visual seizures continued, one of them ending with GTCS. No more seizures of any other type occurred after treatment which carbamazepine which continued for 3 years. At age 20 years, the patient attends university, is well, and free of seizures with no treatment and normal EEG.

Synonyms

LBOS = Late onset benign childhood occipital seizures or Late onset idiopathic childhood occipital epilepsy

Synonyms

Childhood epilepsy with occipital paroxysms[177]
Benign partial epilepsy of childhood with occipital spike-waves[304]
Benign epilepsy of childhood with occipital paroxysms[310]
Basilar migraine, seizures and severe epileptiform EEG abnormalities[146]
Childhood epilepsy with migrainous phenomena and occipital paroxysms[602]
Migraine and epilepsy with infantile onset and EEG findings of occipital spike-wave complexes[213]
Infantile epilepsy with occipital focus and good prognosis[74]
Late onset benign childhood epilepsy with occipital paroxysms[605]
Gastaut type of benign childhood occipital epilepsy[270,271]

Introduction

Late onset benign childhood occipital seizures,[74,192,287,296,302–306,308,313,319,344,367,386,560,605,608,620,621,625,753,763,797] though less common, of uncertain prognosis and most unlikely to be the main natural representative of childhood occipital spikes, is the only syndrome of 'childhood epilepsy with occipital paroxysms' recognized by the Commission on Classification and Terminology of the International League Against Epilepsy.[177] The Commission[177] defined this as follows:

> 'The syndrome of childhood epilepsy with occipital paroxysms is, in general respects, similar to that of benign childhood epilepsy with centrotemporal spikes. The seizures start with visual symptoms (amaurosis, phosphenes, illusions, or hallucinations) and are often followed by a hemiclonic seizure or automatisms. In 25 per cent of the cases, the seizures are immediately followed by migrainous headache. The EEG has paroxysms of high amplitude spike waves or sharp waves recurring rhythmically on the occipital and posterior temporal areas of one or both hemispheres, but only when eyes are closed. During seizures, the occipital discharge may spread to the central or temporal region. At present no definite statement on prognosis is possible.'

This definition, which needs extensive revisions, is based entirely on a well performed retrospective study of Gastaut (1981,1982,1985,1987)[302–306,308,310] and an update by Gastaut and Zifkin (1987).[313] It should be emphasized that an accurate description of LBOS may not be possible at this stage of our knowledge. In Gastaut's series[310,313] not all patients were idiopathic, cases with photosensitive seizures alone were included and some had syndromes of mainly generalized epilepsies. This is because by the inclusion criteria of these authors, patients could have (a) occipital paroxysms and seizures, (b) occipital seizures with or without occipital spikes, with or without photosensitivity, with or without neurological or brain scan abnormalities, with or without other forms of generalized or partial seizures.[310,313] These are detailed in Chapter 11. Studies that preceded[146,220,326,327,599,735] and followed[18,52,74,167,180,192,214,223,225,287,296,340,367,386,458,514,560,568,574,753,763,766] the reports of Gastaut [302–306, 308,310,313] are also mainly retrospective, refer to small numbers of individual patients, data are grouped together with EBOS and the main emphasis is either on the non-specificity of EEG occipital paroxysms regarding the diagnosis of LBOS or the relations with migraine. Therefore, the following presentation of LBOS is based on significant but not yet conclusive evidence, as is also indicated by the final words of Gastaut,[310] one of the greatest epileptologists of the last half of this century:

> 'It does exist, even though it is a rare condition and though an accurate prognosis is difficult to determine.'[310]

My own prospective studies alone and with colleagues[596,599–602,604,605,607,608,611,618,620,621,625,629,635,636] over the last 25 years have substantially influenced this presentation of LBOS (see personal studies, Chapter 13).

Prevalence

Late onset benign childhood occipital seizures appear to be rare with a probable prevalence of 0.2–0.9 per cent of all epilepsies, 2–7 per cent of benign childhood partial seizures and 10–20 per cent of all benign childhood occipital seizures. Despite my interest in this condition, I have seen only *3 cases with visual seizures and occipital paroxysms* that would meet the criteria of the idiopathic 'childhood epilepsy with occipital paroxysms' as proposed by the Commission on Classification and Terminology of the International League Against Epilepsy.[177]

Gastaut[302–306,308,313] initially reported that LBOS are one quarter as frequent as Rolandic seizures but later in 1992,[310] having seen only seven cases in 4 years, accepted that it is rare.[310] Only five of 18 cases with occipital seizures and occipital paroxysms reported by Beaumanoir[74] had seizures characterized by visual symptoms. Panayiotopoulos[605] found only two cases of LBOS (0.5 per cent) amongst 418 patients with onset of seizures before the age of 13 years. Ninety four (22.5 per cent) had benign childhood partial seizures with 72 having Rolandic seizures and 16 EBOS. Thus, LBOS had an estimated prevalence of 2.1 per cent amongst the benign childhood partial seizures and was 36 times less frequent than Rolandic seizures and eight times less frequent than EBOS.[605] This low prevalence of LBOS is also apparent from the small numbers of patients reported in the literature with this condition.[287,386,560,568,763,797] Amongst 107 neurologically normal children with partial seizures, Deonna *et al.* 1986[225] found only one (0.9 per cent) child with LBOS compared to 38 (35.5 per cent) Rolandic seizure cases. Maher *et al.*[517] found that from 20 patients with benign occipital seizures, 14 had EBOS, one had LBOS and five had symptoms of both EBOS and LBOS. In two recent studies[270,368] of 311 children with benign childhood partial seizures, 200 (64.3 per cent) had Rolandic seizures, 80 (25.7 per cent) EBOS and 22 (7.1 per cent) LBOS. Nine additional patients (2.9 per cent) had combined EBOS and Rolandic seizures. Thus, in four studies[270,368,517,605] EBOS was found in 119 (82.6 per cent) patients as opposed to 25 of LBOS (17.4 per cent). Only, Dalla Bernardina *et al.* (1993)[192] found that LBOS was slightly less frequent than EBOS. Amongst 33 children with idiopathic occipital lobe epilepsy 14 (42.2 per cent) probably had LBOS, eight (24.2 per cent) had prolonged nocturnal seizures of EBOS type and another 11 (33.3 per cent) had 'partial occipital seizures often spreading to motor areas and frequently associated with Rolandic or hemiconvulsive seizures'.

In my studies, excluding three patients with IGE and visual hallucinations, the prevalence of occipital epilepsy of any cause in a population of 1360 patients was 4.6 per cent (63 patients). Amongst these 63 patients with occipital epilepsy, only three (4.7 per cent) had the combination of idiopathic visual seizures with occipital paroxysms. Conversely, 24 patients (38.1 per cent) had Panayiotopoulos syndrome (see Chapter 13 on personal studies).

Clinical features of late onset benign childhood occipital seizures

Visual seizures

Visual seizures are the most typical and usually the first ictal symptom of LBOS.[74,192,287,296,302–306,308,313,319,344,367,560,599,605,608,618,620,621,625,753,763,797] They were well described by Gastaut[302–306,308] and Gastaut and Zifkin,[313] who found visual seizures in 75 per cent of their patients and also concluded that 'They did not have similarities to the migraine visual aura'. Based on their observations, reports by other authors and the descriptions of my patients[618] (see pages 164–172), the following may accurately represent the visual seizures of LBOS.

Elementary visual hallucinations

Elementary visual hallucinations, occurring as an initial seizure symptom in probably more than two-thirds of the patients, are characterised by their morphology, colour, location and spread, movement and duration, and progress to other seizure manifestations. They are usually multi-coloured and circular, appearing in the periphery of a hemifield or centrally, multiplying in numbers, enlarging or both, moving horizontally to the other side, flashing or static.[618] They may be the only ictal

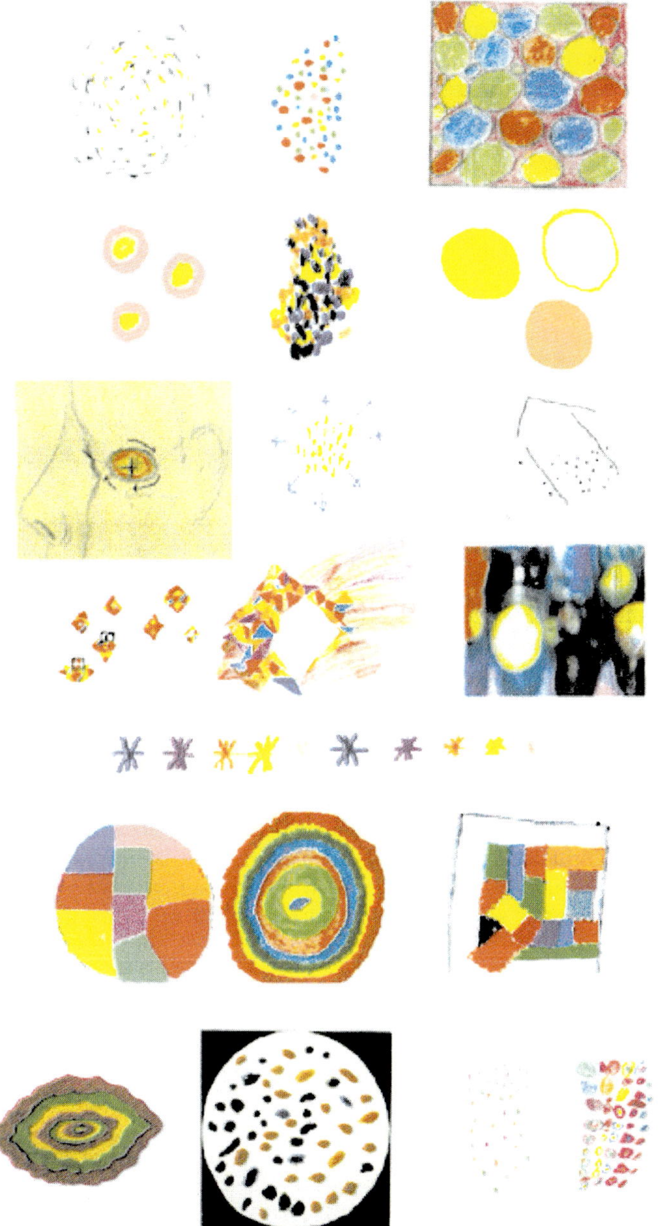

Fig. 9.2. Elementary visual hallucinations as illustrated by my patients.
Two upper rows from left to right are those of cases 24–29 consecutively. Third row from left to right: cases 33,30,32 (pages 164–172). Fourth row: left and middle are the visual hallucinations of case 31 without (left) and just prior to secondary GTCS (page 169). On the right, these are the visual hallucinations of a case with symptomatic visual seizures that could well be mistaken for idiopathic prior to a high resolution MRI (case 7.1, page 129). Fifth row from left to right: the visual hallucinations of a recently seen young patient with probably idiopathic occipital epilepsy (case 34, page 171). Sixth row from left to right: the visual hallucinations in photosensitive visual seizures of patients 36, 39 and 35 (Chapter 12B). Seventh row: the visual hallucinations of four cases with symptomatic visual seizures (Chapter 7).

manifestations or progress to other seizure symptoms. Figure 9.2 illustrates the visual hallucinations as perceived by patients with idiopathic and symptomatic occipital seizures with or without occipital paroxysms, spontaneous or provoked. This visual symptomatology, considering all its components together, is markedly different from migraine visual aura.[618]

Morphology: They are mainly circular, simple spots, circles or spheres. Squares, rectangles or star-like shapes are rare. They are small and usually numerous. They may be large and singular.

Colour: As a rule they are brightly multi-coloured, all colours. Red, yellow and blue are probably more common. Only one of my patients had visual hallucinations consisting of dark spots, some also show squares or linear patterns, others have monochromatic patterns but this is the exception.[618]

Background: The background is usually of the surrounding environment but some patients describe it as shiny and whitish. A child described his multi-coloured visual hallucinations as appearing against a black background.

Location: They are usually unilateral appearing in a temporal visual hemifield but they also frequently start from the centre of the vision.[618]

Movement: They may be static multiplying in numbers, size or both. Moving horizontally towards the opposite side is often described and this movement may be slow or fast, occurring once or repetitively. Moving towards or more rarely away from the eyes may be described by those with central visual hallucinations. The individual elements also appear often to move, changing positions and intensity between them.

Vision: The elementary visual hallucinations may obscure the vision in the space that they occupy although the visual perception of the surroundings usually remains intact. However, as they progress, vision may also be distorted as though being viewed through broken magnified lenses or getting out of focus.

Duration: The elementary visual hallucinations are mainly brief, for 5–15 s, rarely exceeding 1–2 min, if they occur alone without other occipital or extra-occipital spreading. However, there are rare reports that the visual seizures may last much longer, as is the case with one of my patients who for years had brief visual seizures lasting for seconds to 1–2 min; however his last ever fit manifested exclusively with his habitual elementary visual hallucinations lasting for 20 min (case 24). It is interesting that another patient of mine (case 27) who also had onset of brief visual seizures, later experienced infrequent similar seizures prolonged for 20–30 min (see illustrative cases on page 164–172).

Seizure stereotype: For any one patient, in every seizure, the elementary visual hallucinations have a fingerprint with a stereotypic appearance regarding morphology, colours, location, movement and the other characteristics detailed above. Most of the patients also know at what stage of their visual hallucinations secondary generalization is probably unavoidable. What is different in seizures of the same patient is the duration. This may be extremely brief, these are the commonest, or prolonged with or without secondary generalization.

Complex visual hallucinations and visual illusions

Complex visual hallucinations appearing from seizure onset are much rarer, probably occurring in less than 10 per cent of the patients. They may emerge from elementary visual hallucinations although a distortion of the visual image as described above may occur as they progress. Complex visual hallucinations usually take the form of a face or figures which again may have the same location and sequence as those of the elementary visual hallucinations. They do not have the emotional and other characters of those associated with temporal lobe semeiology. Gastaut and Zifkin[312,313] emphasized 'an unusual hallucination of a 1- or 2-digit number' noted by three of their 63 patients.

Ictal visual illusions such, as micropsia, metamorphopsia and palinopsia, most likely generated from the non-dominant parietal regions,[459] though described by Gastaut and Zifkin[313] may not be part of

LBOS or else are extremely rare. They are probably more likely to be associated with symptomatic than idiopathic occipital seizures.

Blindness or partial visual loss

Blindness[313,418,605,618] is probably as common an ictal symptom as elementary visual hallucinations. It may occur alone and be the only ictal event in patients who may, at other times, have visual hallucinations without blindness. Blindness is sudden, total and usually lasts on average longer than the visual hallucinations, usually 2–5 min if alone. The case quoted by Panayiotopoulos, 1980[599] is characteristic with a combination of brief, for seconds, visual seizures of elementary visual hallucinations or infrequent episodes of blindness lasting for minutes (case 24, page 164). In one patient of Gastaut (case 3)[308] blindness 'lasted for 45 min followed by a 2 min dysphasia and a major convulsion'. Some patients may describe an impairment of visual awareness before the appearance of visual hallucinations (see illustrative case 30, page 168). Post-ictal blindness, hemianopia and other partial visual loss is well established after visual seizures with or without secondary generalization.

Non-visual ictal symptoms

Deviation of the eyes and oculoclonic seizures

Deviation of the eyes, usually following elementary visual hallucinations and often but not necessarily associated with ipsilateral turning of the head, is the commonest, around 70 per cent, non-visual symptom in LBOS. This motor partial seizure, a well known ictal symptom of occipital origin, usually starts after but may also occur while visual hallucinations persist. It may be mild but more often it is severe and progresses to hemiconvulsions and GTCS. That children with benign occipital seizures may have motor partial seizures *ab initio* is well established. Five of 18 patients of Beaumanoir[74] had diurnal seizures characterized by visual symptoms and nocturnal seizures mainly manifested with unilateral oculoclonic convulsions. Also Dalla Bernardina *et al.* (1993)[192] had 11 (33.3 per cent) of 33 patients with 'partial occipital seizures often spreading to motor areas and frequently associated with Rolandic or hemiconvulsive seizures'. Whether these cases have a better prognosis and shorter seizure life span than those of LBOS with elementary visual hallucinations, has not been examined. This is another grey area or an overlapping between LBOS and EBOS. Ferrie *et al.*[277] in their study of 113 patients with EBOS had an additional 12 patients who manifested with ictal visual symptoms and tonic eye deviation or vomiting. These showed important differences in comparison to the 113 cases of EBOS. Age at onset (6.9 ± 2.5 as opposed to 4.6 ± 1.7 years for EBOS) and age of last seizure (10.3 ± 3.8 as opposed to 5.6 ± 2 years for EBOS) were later, number of seizures was higher for (6 ± 3 as opposed to 3 ± 2 for EBOS) and more patients had ictal (67 per cent as opposed to 13 per cent for EBOS) and post-ictal (42 per cent as opposed to 16 per cent for EBOS) headache.

Forced eyelid closure and eyelid blinking

Forced eyelid closure and eyelid blinking, an interesting ictal clinical symptom of occipital seizures, occurred in six of 63 patients reported by Gastaut and Zifkin.[313] It occurred in two of 11 patients with LBOS in my series (cases 30 and 31, pages 168 and 169). This was after the phase of visual hallucinations, at a stage where consciousness was impaired and heralded the impending secondary generalized convulsions. Case 30 (page 168) is a characteristic example. He had numerous brief visual seizures and on seven occasions these progressed to GTCS in a stereotypical manner. They start with elementary visual hallucinations which instead of stopping, spread gradually in all directions, become bigger and bigger, vision gets obscured and 5 min later he loses consciousness. At this stage eyelid flickers occur for a few seconds followed by generalized convulsions.

Eyelid opening, 'eyes widely opened', is also another well described symptom in patients with nocturnal seizures of occipital origin,[74] but this may also be a symptom of Rolandic seizures. Widened palpebral fissures with fixed staring and dilated pupils are amongst typical symptoms of mesial temporal lobe seizures.[809]

Sensory hallucinations of ocular movements and pain

A sensation of ocular movement in the absence of detectable motion is a rare occurrence in LBOS and mainly occur in the progress of elementary visual hallucinations. They occurred in two of my patients with LBOS. In a boy of 10 years, elementary visual hallucinations in the right eye were associated with a feeling that 'draws my right eye and my head to the right' (case 26, page 166). In another case, elementary visual hallucinations were associated with 'tension in eyes. Feels similar to when you look up into your eyebrows as hard as you can. The aura continually tries to move to the left and at a slight tilt upwards. This involuntary movement of the eyes causes the pain described above. The motion to the left seems out of your control. It can be resisted but this adds to nausea and general pain.' (case 31, page 169)

Ictal clinical symptoms from occipital seizure propagation

Elementary visual hallucinations or other ictal symptoms at the opening seizure phase may progress to hemi or generalized convulsions without other noticeable partial seizure manifestations in between. According to Gastaut and Zifkin[313] visual seizures are often followed by other, non-visual seizure symptoms such as hemiconvulsions (43 per cent), complex partial seizures (14 per cent), dysphasia, dysaesthesia, adversive convulsions (25 per cent) and generalized tonic–clonic seizures (13 per cent). In my studies, I have not seen cases of LBOS with typical complex partial seizures of temporal lobe symptomatology either from onset or secondary, which may suggest that such a situation is extremely rare and may indicate a symptomatic cause.

Ictal vomiting (ictus emeticus)

Ictal vomiting, which is one of the most prominent symptoms in EBOS, appears to be extremely rare in LBOS. Ictal vomiting is not mentioned amongst detailed descriptions of ictal symptoms in LBOS by Gastaut[302–306,308,310] and Gastaut and Zifkin.[313] Ferrie *et al.*[277] described 12 children who had 'ictal tonic deviation (eight children) or vomiting (11 children) and ictal visual symptoms (12 children)' as an overlap group of EBOS and LBOS. Zung and Margalith,1993[837] reported a seven-year-old boy who 'experienced several episodes of complete visual loss, accompanied by gastro-intestinal symptoms and a sensation of fright, but with preservation of consciousness'. These episodes ended abruptly with visual recovery and no post-ictal phenomena. CT brain scan was normal and interictal EEG showed occipital paroxysms.

Headache

Ictal headache, mainly orbital, is a rare occurrence. However, post-ictal headache is a consistent symptom in one third of LBOS even without preceding convulsions. This post-ictal headache occurs immediately or after 5–10 min from the end of the visual hallucinations. The duration and severity of the headache appear to be proportional to the duration and severity of the preceding seizures. The headache may be diffuse, of mild to moderate intensity, but in most patients it is strong, pulsating and may be associated with nausea, vomiting, photophobia and phonophobia. Thus, the post-ictal headache of some patients with LBOS may be indistinguishable from migraine[213,215,618] as it is also not that uncommon in other cryptogenic/symptomatic occipital seizures (see Chapters 7 and 14).

Impairment of consciousness

Visual seizures, even the prolonged ones, are simple and are clearly described by the patients. Impairment of consciousness usually occurs at the onset of other ictal manifestations following the visual hallucinations or blindness. In some cases loss of consciousness associated with falls may occur independently and without convulsions (see illustrative case 26, page 166).

Circadian distribution

Visual seizures are predominantly diurnal and occur at any time of the day. Longer seizures with or without secondary hemi- or generalized convulsions tend to occur after awakening or often during sleep. Thus, some children may have numerous diurnal visual seizures and only a few exclusively nocturnal or on awakening secondary GTCS.

Precipitating factors

By excluding patients with idiopathic photosensitive occipital seizures from LBOS, there are no apparent precipitating factors for most of them. These patients according to the EEG reactivity of the occipital paroxysms suffer from fixation-off sensitivity. However, only a few may report that clinical seizures are precipitated in going from bright light to darkness or darkness itself (see fixation-off sensitivity and scotosensitive seizures in Chapter 10).[81,313]

Age at onset and sex

Boys and girls appear to be equally affected. The mean age at onset is around 8 years of age with a range from 3 to 16 years. Though reported age at onset varies from 15 months to 19 years, it would be difficult to accept such an early onset of visual hallucinations as 15 months or a late onset after the age of 16 years, which are beyond the age boundaries of other syndromes with benign partial seizures.

Frequency of seizures

In untreated patients, brief visual seizures are frequent, often several per day or weekly. However, propagation to other seizure manifestations such as focal or more generalized convulsions is much less frequent, monthly, or exceptionally yearly. Seizures cease or dramatically reduce after appropriate medication which, in my experience, is carbamazepine.

Prognosis

Prognosis of LBOS is not as clear and predictive as with EBOS or Rolandic seizures, though the response to treatment with carbamazepine as a rule is usually excellent with either cessation or dramatic reduction of visual and other seizures.[618]

That some children with LBOS can do well, with an age-limited susceptibility to seizures, has been unequivocally demonstrated by many authors from the times of Gibbs and Gibbs,[326,327] but more specifically by Gastaut,[302–306,308,313] and subsequent authors with long follow-up.[18,52,74,167,180,192,213,223,225,287,296,340,367,386,458,514,560,568,574,753,763,766] Also, it is well documented in the above reports that other children may do badly despite clinico-EEG features indistinguishable from those with good prognosis.

Available data may indicate that more than 60 per cent of children will go into remission in their late teens. For another 30–40 per cent infrequent visual seizures and occasional secondary generalization may occur later in life after treatment withdrawal. For the remaining few, seizures may continue in adulthood and become difficult to control. The problem is that we do not know exactly the extent of the good or bad prognosis and the possible differentiating factors between them. My suggestion is that some of these patients with bad prognosis may have minor occipital structural lesions, escaping CT brain scan and old generation MRI detection. Therefore, they suffer from symptomatic occipital seizures, not idiopathic LBOS. This is another good reason why a high resolution MRI should be obtained for these patients. In this respect, I refer to one of my patients who did badly[611] though she could easily fulfil the criteria of LBOS applied by Gastaut and Zifkin.[313] She had three CT brain scans in her life and an MRI in 1993 that were normal. It was only a year ago that a 3D MRI showed some minor residual lesions in the right occipital lobe, confirming that she has symptomatic occipital epilepsy imitating LBOS (see case 7.1 of symptomatic occipital epilepsy, page 129).

Gastaut in 1982[302–306] reported 'full remission of seizures in 92 per cent before the age of 19 years' and concluded that it is 'a benign form of epilepsy, although less so compared to Rolandic seizures where full cure occurs before the age of 15 years in all cases'. This relatively good prognosis was also confirmed in a later report by Gastaut and Zifkin.[313] I quote: 'Prognosis was usually good but not as good as for Rolandic seizures. Complete seizure control was achieved in 60 per cent of the patients with any type of antiepileptic medication. In none of our cases have the seizures persisted into middle adulthood, and other types of recurring seizures in adulthood were seen in only three patients. The prognosis, as expected, is poorer in patients with other evidence of cerebral disturbance such as mental retardation or abnormal CT scans, or whose EEGs show an additional secondary epileptiform disturbance. Complete seizure control with anticonvulsant drugs was achieved in 38 patients (60 per cent), and seizures persisted in three patients followed beyond age 19. Seizure control may be achieved, although the epileptiform EEG may persist for several months or years after the seizures have ceased.' Subsequent reports by other authors, some in long prospective studies, confirmed this relative, but not invariably, good prognosis of LBOS.[18,52,74,167,180,192,213,223,225,287,296,340,367,386,458,514,560,568,574,753,763,766]

The main opposition to a good prognosis of LBOS came from studies of patients with EEG occipital paroxysms who did not necessarily suffer from LBOS. Newton and Aicardi[18,568] studied 16 patients with 'the EEG abnormality of occipital sharp and slow waves significantly or completely suppressed by eye-opening. All had seizures consisting of transient loss of consciousness. Most experienced additional grand mal, partial (simple or complex), or clonic fits. Response to treatment was poor initially in nine and subsequently in 11. Learning difficulties were present in 10 children'. Newton and Aicardi[18,568] rightly concluded that these *'cases illustrate the wide range of clinical disorders that may accompany the EEG abnormality and indicate that the prognosis associated with this EEG pattern is not necessarily benign'*. This was confirmed by Cooper and Lee[180] in another retrospective study who also concluded that: 'This study suggests that reactive occipital epileptiform activity is not uniformly associated with a benign course and that other factors are involved in determining prognosis of the epilepsy'. Similar also were the results of Talwar *et al.*[753] on a retrospective study of patients who were selected only because of EEG occipital paroxysms irrespective of underlying cause. Therefore, these studies[18,180,568,753] showed that occipital paroxysms are not specific for LBOS and that they can occur in many other conditions associated or not with epileptic seizures, such as patients with cryptogenic and symptomatic seizures or syndromes of generalized epilepsy. Prognosis for such a heterogeneous group of patients, selected because of EEG occipital spikes only, varied widely from excellent to extremely bad (as expected). The non-specificity of occipital spikes, also occurring in normal children, is well known from the times of Gibbses's (see Chapter 10).

It is of concern that even, in 1997,[36] these reports[18,180,568,753] were misinterpreted as indicating that 'the benign course of EBOS and LBOS is by no means always found'.[36] Let me re-emphasize the point. Aicardi and Newton[18,568] did not investigate prognosis of idiopathic clinical forms and certainly not of the EBOS. More explicitly, they showed that EEG occipital paroxysms are not specific as they occurred both in idiopathic and symptomatic epilepsies. Accordingly, prognosis was variable.

Another warning came from reports of children with clinico-EEG features similar to those of LBOS which are due to demonstrable brain structural lesions,[335,457] the closest example being those with coeliac disease and occipital calcifications.[338,340,343–345] These children, despite clinical similarities to idiopathic LBOS, suffer from symptomatic occipital epilepsy that is usually but not invariably associated with a bad prognosis (see Chapter 7).

Another concern is from three reported cases of LBOS that later developed continuous spike-waves during slow-wave sleep (CSWS) with or without clinical and mental deterioration.[52,762] Aso *et al.* (1987)[52] reported a normal boy who at the age of seven had occipital seizures with visual hallucinations of flickering lights and non-visual symptoms of tachypnea, pallor, generalized motor symptoms and unresponsiveness and an EEG with occipital paroxysms. This later evolved to CSWS without psychomotor change or atonic seizures. More recently, Tenenbaum *et al.* (1977)[762] reported an atypical and rather aggressive seizure and behaviour evolution in two boys with clinical and EEG features of LBOS. Both boys experienced severe cognitive deterioration associated with CSWS. One child showed global improvement in behaviour and partial restoration of cognitive functions after control of seizures and normalization of the EEG.

In my experience, in three cases with clinical features of LBOS and occipital paroxysms (cases 24–26, on pages 164–167) that I followed from onset to as many as 22 years, remission was achieved by all, response to treatment was excellent in all, but the duration of seizure life span varied significantly from 1 to 12 years.[605,608] A similar pattern of long duration of active seizures, well suppressed by treatment, appeared to be the case in five other children with clinical manifestations of LBOS but with either normal or untypical EEG occipital abnormalities (cases 27–31, pages 167–169). Also, on page 171 I report adult patients who had onset of visual seizures in late childhood or early adolescence which were indistinguishable from the clinical features of LBOS but continued having seizures despite showing a normal brain scan. It is possible that these patients have subtle occipital lesions that may be detected with new generation MRI.

Therefore, my conclusions are:

(a) Patients with LBOS have frequent visual seizures and infrequent GTCS which may well be controlled with carbamazepine but the seizure life span is usually long and

(b) Patients with features of LBOS who do not do well may suffer from symptomatic occipital epilepsy that may be revealed only with high resolution, new generation MRI.

Mental and neurological state and neuroimaging

By definition of an idiopathic syndrome, all children with LBOS should have normal neurological and mental state. Brain imaging should include high resolution, last generation MRI which should also be normal.

Genetics

These are not known for LBOS. Usually, there is no family history of similar seizures in LBOS. There is equivocal evidence that there may be an increased incidence of epilepsies or migraine. This is by no means certain.

Kuzniecky and Rosenblatt (1987)[458] reported a family with three out of four children having symptoms more like early than late onset BOS. All had EEG occipital spikes that were also detected in the fourth youngest child and 26 per cent of mainly younger members of this family.

Nagendran *et al.* (1990)[557] reported a family with LBOS. The youngest boy had at age 7 years visual hallucinations of 'seeing coloured spots' lasting 5–10 min and followed by several hours' drowsiness. They occurred twice per day but ceased with administration of sodium valproate. His youngest sister had at age 6 years two GTCS in one night. 'She admitted seeing brightly coloured spots. Her attacks have been difficult to control. Lately her attacks comprise visual loss for some 30 s'. Both had EEGs with occipital paroxysms. Their middle brother had centrotemporal spikes in the EEG but was asymptomatic. The oldest brother had occipital slow waves at age 11 years. The mother said that she had 10 attacks of visual disturbances between the ages 10–20 years. The father had some major convulsions at age 31 years which did not recur. Both parents had normal EEG.

A family history of epilepsy was found in 36.6 per cent, migraine in 15.9 per cent and 14 per cent of the patients had febrile convulsions in Gastaut and Zifkin's report.[313]

Pathophysiology

The following brief references to pathophysiology of benign occipital seizures, elementary visual hallucinations and post-ictal headache are addressed as thoughts and indications derived from clinical observations rather than claiming any firm scientific evidence.

Though expert opinions[36] assume that in EBOS and LBOS 'the pathophysiology is the same', this is not known for either of them and I could not find any incontrovertible evidence for this in the literature.

Gastaut and Zifkin[313] speculating on the pathophysiology of LBOS wrote that: 'Any discussion of the pathophysiology of benign epilepsy with occipital paroxysms must consider both the genesis of the interictal and ictal neuronal discharge in the absence of any evident lesion and also the pattern of ictal spreading of this discharge that is responsible for the clinical symptoms'. My opinion is that the pathophysiology of the benign childhood occipital seizures is similar to that of Rolandic seizures and other childhood benign partial epilepsies. I explain this on the basis of an age-dependent cortical excitability due to a mild and reversible derangement of the brain maturation process. The difference between the various forms of benign childhood partial seizures is due to a different age and maturation dependent location, but the pathophysiology is the same. This hypothesis also explains why occipital paroxysms and spikes often co-exist with similar spike foci in other cortical areas such as centrotemporal or frontal as well as giant evoked somatosensory potentials in the same or subsequent EEG. That occipital paroxysms may be bilateral and synchronous is not against this cortical hyperexcitability which is driven simultaneously by 'fixation-off sensitivity'. This is not a new view. Luders *et al.*, 1987[512] suggested that 'It seems that the main pathogenetic factor is a genetically determined diffusely increased cortical epileptogenicity whose EEG or clinical expression is governed by maturational factors' and further stated that 'the focal nature of the EEG is most probably due to different cortical areas reaching the stage of active epileptogenicity at different times (in general the occipital areas do so before the centrotemporal regions)'.[512] Also, long before us Sorel and Rucquoy-Ponsar (1969)[735] reached the same conclusion in a report on 'functional epilepsies of maturation'.

Occipital paroxysms according to the above thesis are due to a cortical hyperexcitability, which is age and maturation dependent. However, Gastaut and Zifkin[313] expressed different views in favour of a subcortical excitability. They hypothesized that the occipital paroxysms are due to a subcortical, thalamocortical, mechanism. I quote: 'In order to explain the rhythmic spike and wave complexes seen with eye closure or IPS over an intact occipital lobe, Gastaut (1950)[300] proposed a thalamocortical mechanism, driven by a thalamic pacemaker. Ludwig and Ajmone-Marsan (1975)[513] suggested that bilateral, rhythmic, synchronous occipital spike and wave complexes in epileptic patients could be the result of an atypical 'centrencephalic' disturbance, similar to that responsible for generalized 3 Hz spike and wave complexes, which we have seen in 19 of our patients. A subcortical mechanism in the electrogenesis of these occipital spike and wave complexes is also suggested, for two reasons. First, there is the absence of discernible occipital lesions. Second, there is a resemblance between the interictal occipital spike and wave complexes and (a) the normal posterior slow waves of youth, and (b) the posterior delta rhythm often found in association with typical spike and wave complexes in classic absence. The response to IPS at 3 Hz in some photosensitive patients, in whom occipital and posterior temporal bilateral spikes are seen prior to generalization (Gastaut,1950),[300] also suggests a similar subcortical mechanism.'

I cannot agree with this view. The patients described by Ludwig and Ajmone-Marsan (1975)[513] with bilateral, rhythmic, synchronous occipital spike and wave complexes were entirely different from those of children with benign occipital seizures. These were mainly adults, possessed the lowest incidence of visual or other auras, the highest percentage of nonfocal seizures (mainly GTCS) and 'the highest incidence of metabolic abnormalities acting as probable causative epileptogenic agents'.[513] Furthermore, the absence of 'a discernible lesion' is compatible with the functional nature of these cortical spikes and not in favour of a subcortical mechanism. Additionally, regional occipital photosensitivity is well established as a cortical phenomenon.[616] More significantly, the occipital paroxysms are bilateral because they are activated by fixation-off sensitivity[599,600] which is unlikely to act through a subcortical, thalamocortical, mechanism.

What is the pathophysiology of elementary visual hallucinations? That the location and seizure generation of elementary visual hallucinations is in the visual cortex is unanimously accepted and documented through ictal surface or deep EEG recordings.[313,513,648,694,700,746,811] This is also in accordance with their remarkable similarities with the 'phosphenes' elicited on intracortical microstimulation of the visual cortex in blind people for the purposes of visual prosthesis.[709] In these experiments, the size of phosphenes ranges from a 'pin-point' to a 'nickel', at levels of stimulation near threshold, and phosphenes have distinct colours such as yellow, blue or red but not green, becoming white, greyish or yellowish at increasing level of stimulation. Phosphenes do not flicker. Visual phenomena caused by after discharge become more diffuse, gradually expanding and becoming multi-coloured.

In migraine with aura, Russell and Olosen[693] suggested that 'cortical spreading depression remains the most likely explanation' of the gradual and contiguous spread of symptoms. This cannot be the explanation for rapidly developing epileptic, ictal elementary visual hallucinations which have the same pathophysiology as any other partial seizures.

Another aspect refers to the spread of occipital seizure discharges to the other side or more anterior regions. This has been well studied and detailed elsewhere for symptomatic occipital epilepsy (Chapters 6 and 7) and may be similar for EBOS and LBOS. However, we have to accept that the occipital discharge may be facilitated, obstructed or modified by structural lesions of the brain as opposed to the LBOS that are generated in a normal brain substrate. This may explain the relatively low incidence in LBOS of secondary seizures with temporal lobe symptomatology which are common in symptomatic occipital epilepsy. Also that approximately 90 per cent of children with EBOS manifest with ictal symptoms such as vomiting which are rarely seen in symptomatic occipital epilepsies.

What is the pathophysiology of post-ictal headache? This is even more difficult to explain but essential to understand and investigate. The observation is that post-ictal headache is very common even after minor visual seizures and it is often indistinguishable from migraine headache.[313,618,694,710] In my studies, post-ictal headache was not more common in those with family predisposition to migraine.[618] It may be that the seizure discharge in the occipital lobes triggers a genuine migraine headache through trigeminovascular or brain stem mechanisms.[313,618,800]

According to Gastaut and Zifkin,[313] 'the post-ictal migrainous symptoms of some attacks may be explained by a persistence in the territory of the posterior cerebral and basilar arteries of the initial vasodilation accompanying the occipital ictal activity in children with impaired or labile cerebrovascular autoregulation who are predisposed to migraines'. This hypothesis is the converse of the theory of Camfield *et al.* (1978),[146] since we suggest that occipital seizure is responsible for the migraine and not vice versa.'

Treatment

Starting medication

Unlike other benign childhood partial seizures that may not need treatment, late onset childhood occipital seizures should be treated because seizures are frequent irrespective of whether they are as brief and mild as the visual ones. Secondary generalization is probably unavoidable without medication. There is no tendency of the visual seizures to reduce or stop without medication. Carbamazepine may be the drug of choice. In my experience, all seizures stopped or dramatically reduced within days after appropriate treatment with carbamazepine.[618] However, Gastaut and Zifkin[313] concluded that 'Almost all available anticonvulsants have been tried without any one being the obvious drug of choice. The rapid response to clobazam is noteworthy. In seven of nine patients in whom it was used, both seizures and interictal spikes ceased after only several days of treatment.'

It is known that carbamazepine may exceptionally induce in children with Rolandic seizures new type of fits such as absences, absence status, atonic and myoclonic jerks with an exaggeration of EEG abnormalities that tend to become generalized.[149,230,406,752] These carbamazepine-induced clinico-EEG features imitate atypical benign childhood epilepsy.[149] I have seen a similar case and this is described in Chapter 17. However, I have never seen and I am not aware of any reported cases where this side effect of carbamazepine occurred in benign childhood occipital seizures but the numbers of patients may be small and the possibility remote. Non-epileptic myoclonic jerks and tic-like movements (sniffing, coughing, or sighing) may also be induced by carbamazepine[11,754] but this again may be very rare. Rectal diazepam may prevent secondary GTCS in patients with prolonged visual seizures as in case 30 (page 168).

Patients with LBOS may seek medical attention only after their first secondary hemi or generalized convulsion. Despite many visual seizures, these patients are usually not treated because the minor seizures are ignored or dismissed as migraine. This is well documented in the illustrated case reports below.

Stopping medication

The problem is not when to start and what medication to give in LBOS, which is clarified above. The difficulty is when to stop medication as the EEG is an unreliable indicator of possible relapse. Certainly, drug withdrawal is not considered if the patient continues having even brief and mild visual seizures which should be sought for thoroughly by the physician. My practice is to attempt slow reduction, usually 2–3 years after the last visual or other minor or major seizure. Withdrawal is at a rate of 10 per cent of the existing dosage every month but if visual seizures reappear the drug is restored to its original dose. I exhaustively inform the patient that if visual seizures recur upon withdrawal of medication, this means that their liability to seizures is still active and continuation of drug treatment is mandatory.

Differential diagnosis

The differential diagnosis of children with LBOS is mainly from cryptogenic/symptomatic occipital epilepsy including those associated with coeliac disease and migraine with aura, basilar or acephalgic migraine. In view of the significance of such a differentiation and the frequent misdiagnosis with these conditions, I have reviewed them in detail in various chapters of this book. I have also emphasized that symptomatic occipital epilepsy need not manifest with neurological or visual deficits and often imitates LBOS. High resolution MRI studied by experienced neuroradiologists often gives the answer. A normal CT brain scan is unreliable.

The differential diagnosis of LBOS from metabolic diseases such as hyperglycaemia, mitochondrial disorders such as MELAS and MERFF or Lafora disease should not be difficult and these are discussed in Chapter 7.

The most frequent misdiagnosis of LBOS is for migraine with aura, basilar and acephalgic migraine. This is the reason why two chapters (15 and 16) of this book are devoted to these disorders and their differentiation from LBOS. Occipital seizures may imitate migraine with aura, basilar and acephalgic migraine but their epileptic nature cannot escape clinical scrutiny.

Electroencephalography

Interictal and ictal EEG findings are detailed in the following Chapter 10.

Illustrative cases of late onset benign childhood occipital seizures

The following patient is probably the first published case of late onset BOS in which FOS was demonstrated (Panayiotopoulos, 1980).[599] He is presented because of characteristic features (which are strikingly different from those of the early onset BOS), the relatively resistant and frequent visual seizures, the less favourable outcome when compared with early onset BOS, the long follow-up (22 years) and finally because the case should have been seen as a link (Panayiotopoulos, 1980)[599] between the reports of Camfield *et al.* (1978)[146] and Gastaut (1982).[304]

> Case 24 of Table 13.3. This intelligent man, born in 1965, has had a 22 year regular follow-up from 1976. His clinical and EEG manifestations (Figs. 9.1a, 9.1b, 9.1c, 9.2) have been reported extensively.[599–601,605,608]
>
> I first saw him in June 1976 aged 11 years. He had excellent performance at school and did not have a

family history of epilepsy but his mother had two episodes of migraine with visual aura in her late 30s. From January to June 1976, he complained of brief episodes of visual hallucinations consisting of 'millions of small, very bright, coloured mainly blue and green, circular spots of light which appear on the left side and sometimes move to the right (Fig. 9.2).' These episodes occurred about once a week, lasted no more than 1 min, and were not accompanied by altered consciousness, headache, or vomiting. His father, a physician friend, was concerned about two other episodes in March 1975 and May 1976, during which 'his eyes were turned to the right, his right arm appeared rigid and there was loss of consciousness for a few seconds.' These were not related to any visual disturbances. In May 1976, while asleep, he was found on the floor without explanation. He was given phenobarbital, 30 mg three times daily.

For the next 6 months he continued to have the visual hallucinations, now followed by post-ictal right-sided headaches and vomiting for 1 or 2 h. In two of these episodes, he was dysphasic and may have been slightly confused but could understand conversation. These two brief episodes were not followed by headache or vomiting. Three other episodes of complete blindness occurred immediately after he dived into the sea: 'Everything went suddenly black, I could not see and I had to ask other swimmers to show me the direction to the beach.' The blindness cleared in 1 or 2 min and was followed by right-sided headache and vomiting. Only once was an episode of blindness preceded by visual hallucinations. He was treated with cyclohexyl-2-methylamino-propranol-phenylethyl barbiturate, 50 mg three times daily, and attacks ceased.

Since age 14, he experienced short-lived simple visual hallucinations on three occasions only. In addition, at the age of 16 he once awoke from sleep with his habitual elementary visual hallucinations in the left visual field, fell asleep again, and later he had a witnessed left motor partial seizure with secondary generalization followed by post-ictal confusion, vomiting, and prolonged headache. At the age of 23, on one occasion he awoke from sleep with his habitual elementary visual hallucinations in the left visual field which lasted for 20 min. The next morning he had unilateral headache and nausea.

By April 1992 he had become a solicitor, suffered a manic-depressive illness in 1993 but when I last saw him (July 1996) he was well with no seizures, migraine or psychosis.

Neurologic examination remained entirely normal, but EEG showed gross abnormalities of occipital paroxysms in two EEGs performed within the first 6 months after I first saw him (Figs. 9.1a, 9.1b, 9.1c). All subsequent EEGs over the years were normal. Skull radiograms, a CT brain scan and later in 1994 an MRI were normal.

The next case is the only other patient with LBOS and occipital paroxysms that I saw in Athens amongst 418 patients with seizure onset before 13 years of age.[605]

Case 25 of Table 13.3. This intelligent girl, born in 1970, started having frequent, often daily episodes of elementary visual hallucinations at age 9 years. These consisted of brilliant coloured spots in front of her left visual field. Their duration was seconds to as long as 1 min. The longest ones were followed by diffuse headaches of moderate intensity for a quarter to half an hour. This was initially diagnosed as migraine with aura but one year later and within a month she had a similar episode of elementary visual hallucinations lasting longer, the coloured spots becoming larger and more dense followed after 2–3 min by deviation of the eyes to the left which progressed to left sided hemiconvulsions. An EEG showed clusters of high amplitude occipital spikes mainly on the right and mainly when the eyes were closed. Her parents refused treatment despite another four nocturnal hemiconvulsions. Therapy with carbamazepine started at age 14 years after another diurnal seizure at school with the same sequence of events as the first one.

All seizures stopped and she remained free of seizures until the last follow-up at age 22 years. An MRI at age 20 years was normal. The EEG normalized at age 14 years and treatment was withdrawn at age 20 years.

All subsequent cases are from my prospective studies in St. Thomas' Hospital from 1989, which continue.

In these 10 years I saw only one patient fulfilling the clinical and EEG criteria of LBOS. In this case occipital paroxysms occurred only once in his EEG (Fig. 9.3). Three of the video-EEG recordings showed bilateral, high amplitude sharp-slow wave occipital paroxysms when eyes were closed or open provided that central vision was eliminated binocularly (patient 'looking through' +10 spherical lenses, underwater goggles fixed with semi-transparent tape, darkness) (Fig. 9.3). However, all his subsequent alert and sleep EEGs, one 7 days later with no medication and the others annually from

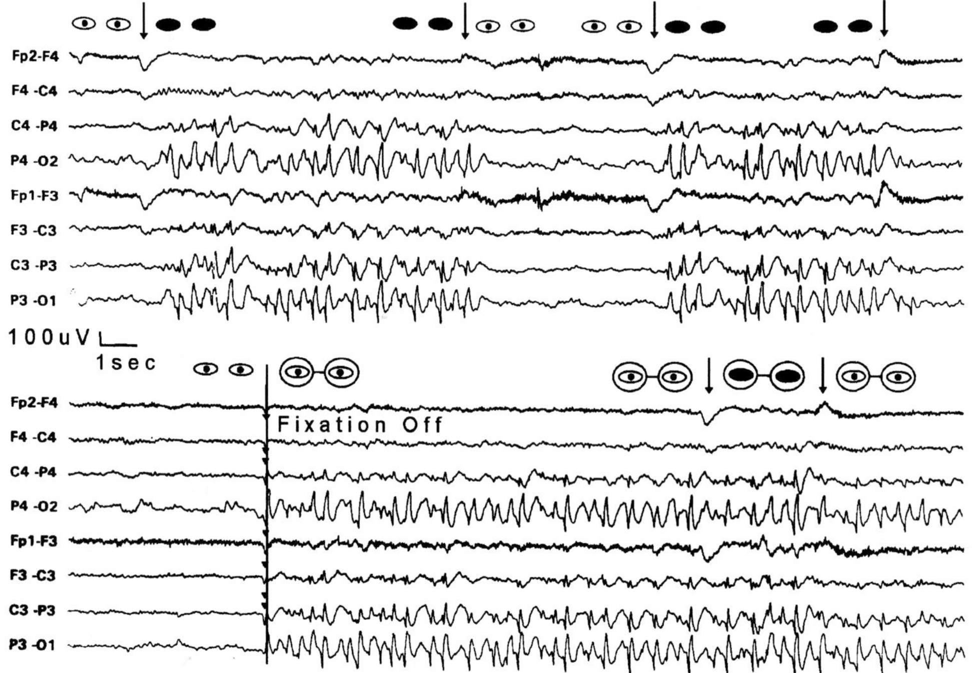

Fig. 9.3. From video-EEG of patient 26. Occipital paroxysms occur as long as fixation and central vision are eliminated by any means (eyes closed, darkness, + 10 spherical lenses, Ganzfeld stimulation). Under these conditions, even in the presence of light, eyes opening is not capable for inhibition. Conversely, occipital paroxysms are totally inhibited by fixation and central vision.
Symbols of eyes open and close without glasses is when fixation is possible (routine EEG recordings in a lit room).
Symbols of eyes open and closed with glasses is when fixation and central vision are eliminated by any of the above means.

1990 to 1998, were normal. This indicates that LBOS may occur without documented occipital paroxysms. This case is also interesting because of brief episodes of falls with loss of consciousness without convulsions.

Case 26 of Table 13.3. This normal boy, born 24.1.80, had from age 10:

(a) Brief, infrequent episodes of complete blindness without warning or impairment of consciousness.

(b) Frequent (1–3 per week), transient visual disturbances lasting for 10–30 s. He is unable to define his visual experiences which he calls 'visions'. 'It looked like a rectangle filled with coloured small circles. This time I saw the colours. They were blue, green, red and yellow (Fig. 9.2). While I was reading I started seeing the words stuck all together. I blink a lot to see more clearly. It is a familiar vision, sometimes bright or dark. It replaces, obscures the real images. They are large objects, probably people, which I cannot identify.' 'They are always in my right eye and draw my right eye and my head to the right'.

(c) Four brief (1–2 min) episodes of loss of consciousness without convulsions whilst sitting or standing. He falls down and becomes unresponsive, but there are no post-ictal symptoms. One episode was witnessed in hospital as 'clumsiness, vacant, unresponsive for a minute or so'. No convulsions. Another one was witnessed by his parents: 'He was next to us in a shop. We heard a bang and saw him on the ground. Colour white not blue. He was out for a few seconds.'

No further episodes occurred after initiation of treatment with carbamazepine which was stopped 3 years later. He is a good student. Last follow-up at age 18 years. He is well, no treatment, normal EEG and normal MRI.

Four patients had the clinical features of LBOS with visual seizures but never demonstrated occipital spikes or occipital paroxysms in numerous alert and sleep EEGs. The following two cases are presented because of the difficulty in differentiating them from acephalgic or basilar migraine and consistently normal EEG (Panayiotopoulos *et al.*, 1997).[625]

Case 27 of Table 13.3: This normal boy, born in 1981, had onset of weakly episodes of visual hallucinations at age 8 years. The hallucinations were brief for 5–15 s and consisted of 3–4 concentric spherical rings of red and yellow moving from the left to the right visual field and repeating the same course again after their disappearance on the right. On other occasions there was only one coloured ball moving continuously from left to right (Fig. 9.2). The colours were faint at onset becoming more intense and brilliant as the seizure progressed. There was no impairment of consciousness, convulsions or headache.

The diagnosis of acephalgic migraine was made elsewhere.

Since age 10 years, on four occasions, the same concentric rings were bigger (double in size) followed the same course from left to right but the duration of the seizure was longer for 1 min probably associated with left hemianopia. On three more occasions these were more prolonged for 2–3 min followed by left sided tonic deviation of the head with clonic movements of the left face and arm. This was followed by loss of consciousness with cyanosis. The patient does not think that he was losing consciousness, only that he was unable to speak when people were talking to him. This lasted for 10 min. Post-ictally he was exhausted, wanted to sleep and had severe headache for 4–5 h. One such episode occurred within minutes after looking at the lights of a car from close distance. At this stage the diagnosis of occipital lobe seizures was suspected.

No further seizures of any type occurred when carbamazepine 600 mg daily was initiated at age 11 years up to the age 14 years. However, in his follow-up at age 16 years he admits to infrequent, brief simple visual hallucinations as above that are more likely to occur after watching television or playing video games for long periods. The longer of them are occasionally followed by diffuse headache of moderate intensity for 10–15 min and once he felt sick. In the last follow-up (July, 1998) he tells me of an interesting change in his seizures. He had three of them in the last year and they were stereotyped lasting for nearly an hour each (50–55 min he told me). They started with left sided blurring of vision, 'whitish like a fog', together with 'small clouds of colours, mainly red' and mixed with small coloured circles. There was no progression to other symptoms but when the blurring of vision and the visual hallucinations cleared, he had left sided throbbing headache which started 5–7 min after the cessation of the seizures and lasted for half an hour. What does this development signify? Does this herald the end of the story, as I would suggest based on my experience from case 24, or is this now turning to migraine with visual aura, as others would prefer? Let us wait and see the progress. Meanwhile I have asked for a 3D MRI, a new EEG and I increased carbamazepine to therapeutic range.

Three EEGs, alert and sleep, at the active stage of his seizures were normal. A high resolution MRI was also normal.

Case 28 of Table 13.3: This boy, born 8.5.1983, started having brief seizures of visual hallucinations 2–3 daily at the age of 7 years which occurred every day. They consisted of brilliant, multi-coloured spots and circles lasting for a few seconds (Fig. 9.2). There was no loss of consciousness or convulsions.

On 2–3 occasions, his vision went black, he felt himself spinning around and that big coloured balls were covering his body. He felt he was on the ground because 'my legs gave way' and this lasted for 1–2 min. Post-ictally he was pale, tired and had a headache.

Routine and sleep EEG, MRI and CT brain scan were normal.

A diagnosis of basilar migraine was made elsewhere and treatment with Pizotifen was initiated with no effect. The visual hallucinations remitted after starting carbamazepine 200 mg bd and reappeared again when carbamazepine was stopped for 3 months at age 12 years. Presently (April 1998) he is free of seizures on the same medication.

A paternal sister has epilepsy from the age of 16 years of age but we do not know its type. His mother has migraine with visual aura which she describes very well. This is a classical visual aura with the zigzag lines and shimmering lights. This lasts for approximately 20 min before she has the headache.

He has learning difficulties which are mainly or exclusively expressed in writing. Otherwise he is normal.

The third case of possible LBOS without occipital paroxysms from St. Thomas' Hospital is presented because of onset of seizures in middle teens, misdiagnosis of various forms of migraine and migralepsy, and his intelligent description of the visual fits and their progression to GTCS, from visual hallucinations, to eyelid flickering and impairment of consciousness. This slow progression from visual fits to GTCS may be interrupted by rectal application of diazepam.

Case 30 of Table 13.3. This intelligent boy, born July 1980, started having from age 14 years elementary visual hallucinations with or without secondary generalized convulsions. He divides these events and their sequence into three periods:

The 'period of vulnerability', as he calls it, is the first to occur. This lasts for approximately 5–10 s and is described as 'sight deteriorates very slightly as it does before the aura, but flashing does not start. It is a reduction of visual awareness around ten per cent'. This happens about twice a day but only lasts for seconds. It started occurring 2 years after onset of his seizures.

This may be followed by elementary visual hallucinations. Suddenly and in the centre of his vision, there is a rounded small area filled with a maximum of ten yellow rounded spots (Fig. 9.2). The diameter of this central area is approximately 2–3 cm and the background is probably shiny, like steam on the road on a hot day. The yellow spots are small. The colour is a strange yellow unlike the normal one. The yellow spots change in intensity between them. These visual hallucinations remain the same throughout the whole period. They may last for a few seconds to usually up 3 min. They occur approximately once per month and 95 per cent on awakening and rarely in the afternoon hours. They are followed by headache approximately 15 min after the disappearance of visual hallucinations. The longer their duration, the more severe is the headache. It may last for half an hour but usually up to 3 h. It is bilateral and pulsating. Only once was this associated with vomiting which was probably due to drug administration. There is photophobia and phonophobia during the headache phase.

He had seven secondary generalized convulsions that were all preceded by visual hallucinations. The first occurred at age 14 years and the last three at age 17 years with the recent one being prevented by diazepam rectally. There are stereotypes. They start with the vulnerability phase which is followed by his visual hallucinations which instead of stopping, start spreading gradually to all directions in his visual field. They become bigger and bigger, retain the same unnatural yellow colour, become even bigger, are bizarre and obscure his vision. Finally, his vision is obscured and the images are distorted as through magnifying lenses and he describes it himself as 'tunnel vision'. They last longer, up to 5–10 min. At this stage he tells his mother to call the ambulance, he loses consciousness and eyelids flicker for a few seconds before progressing to generalized convulsions. This is followed by severe post-ictal confusion and severe headache. He is back to his normal self probably after 3–4 h of sleep.

Only once, after his first seizure, did he describe experiential phenomena (saw book of his life pages turning backward with pictures getting younger and younger but this has not happened since).

Another interesting symptom is that when in complete darkness in his room, he has some visual changes which, understandably, he cannot describe well. He says that the darkness is not the same, it is getting greyish, and this immediately stops when he looks at the LED of a watch or some light coming through doors that he leaves purposely semi-open.

Possible precipitating factors are hunger 'when I miss my meals' and lack of sleep.

Two high resolution MRI of the brain were normal.

An EEG at age 16 years was reported as normal. However, a subsequent EEG at age 17 showed on awake, an excess of diffuse 2–4 Hz slow activity and brief generalized bursts of sharp theta with occasional larval spikes. This was mainly seen on eyes closed and during elimination of central vision and fixation. A sleep EEG showed some brief, half a second, generalized discharges of spike and slow wave of higher amplitude in the anterior regions which occurred during stage I–II of sleep.

He has two older paternal and two maternal half-brothers. One of the paternal half-brothers had a history of 'flashing lights' in his late teens and the other had severe headaches and he had passed out on a few occasions in his late teens. I have no more information about them. The other problem is that both his father and his two paternal half-brothers are highly sensitive when they miss their meals. His mother tells me that they start shaking and they may become aggressive.

He was treated with Propranolol 40 mg daily from age 15 to 17 years without any benefit to seizures or headache. There is not the slightest hint of any visual seizures or any type of visual symptoms, headaches or any other related events since starting medication with carbamazepine 400 mg bd in October 1997 up to the time I last saw him in January 1998.

The next, fourth case, of visual seizures in normal persons starting at late childhood or early/middle teens, without occipital spikes and with normal MRI, is also of interest as seizures continue in adult life and also because of the characteristic occipital progression from visual to other seizure manifestations and GTCS.

Case 31 of Table 13.3. This musician, born 29.6.1976, started having visual seizures at age 12 years. These are well described by him:'Bright colours in centre (red, yellow, orange triangles with a shade of green merging to a star or rectangle-like shape). The whole area is rotating rapidly in each of its separate components and as a whole. Tension in eyes. Feels similar to when you look up into your eyebrows as hard as you can. The aura continually tries to move to the left and at a slight tilt upwards. This involuntary movement of the eyes causes the pain described above. The motion to the left seems out of your control. It can be resisted but this adds to nausea and general pain. After 20–30 s colours become less bright and less concentrated resulting in flashes of light in a more general field of vision. These flashes of light last for a shorter time (10 s approximately). After this the area in which this has been seen is blind. You can hardly see. This lasts from between 1 and 5 min,' 'strong pulsating headache, mainly like being stabbed in the eye, follows for 10–12 h'.

These visual seizures were initially very frequent every day or week but they gradually reduced to 1–2 per year probably as a result of treatment which started at age 16 years with sodium valproate 500 mg bd. An interesting feature is that these visual seizures usually come at night after he switches out the light.

In addition he had 12 nocturnal secondary generalized convulsions. The first occurred at age 16 years, the last at 21. He wakes up with a sense of fear and violently spinning around for approximately 2–3 s, followed by his habitual visual hallucination which ends up with 'an explosion of colours that flicker in the centre of my eyes like a flash camera' for another 10 s (Fig. 9.2). Then, he becomes unresponsive, eyes stare and dilate followed by slow repetitive eye closures for 1 min before progressing to secondary GTCS.

CT brain scan, MRI, sleep and three awake EEGs were normal. He was initially diagnosed as having 'atypical migraine' and an expert epileptologist stated that 'his first GTCS began rather like migraine with visual phenomena'. He also suffers from bipolar affective disorder. There is no family history of migraine or epilepsy.

The following patient has a particular and 'unusual form of idiopathic regional occipital epilepsy which may be misdiagnosed as migraine with aura' which we recently reported.[10] Her visual seizures were identical to those of LBOS but the EEG occipital paroxysmal abnormalities were different from any other published case and unique in our experience.

Case 29 of Table 13.3. This normal woman, born 7.10.1973, started having at age 12 brief, monthly, nocturnal seizures of visual hallucinations. The seizures would wake her up with bright, flashing, multi-coloured, circular lights at a frequency of 6–10 Hz (Fig. 9.2). The colours were mainly orange, red, white and lasted for approximately 3–5 s, then any object in front of her became slightly blurry and moved slowly from right to left for another 3–5 s. Severe post-ictal, non throbbing headache and vomiting followed for several hours. These seizures were initially misdiagnosed as migraine with aura. Occipital lobe epilepsy was suspected when one year later the visual hallucinations were followed by generalized convulsions. She had one to two occipital simple partial seizures with secondary generalization every year despite treatment with sodium valproate 700 mg nocte. Carbamazepine 400 mg nocte was added at age 18 with complete control of all seizures with the exception of two secondary generalized convulsions at age 20 when she stopped medication for 3 months.

Neurological examination and high resolution MRI were normal.

She has a maternal half-brother with generalized tonic–clonic seizures on awakening. His father had absences as a child and late onset generalized tonic–clonic seizures. Another brother suffers from common migraine. Her mother had 'migraine' as a teenager. There is no relevant medical history in her remaining two brothers and four maternal half-brothers.

All her EEGs from age 12 years show identical abnormalities which are always induced by eye-closure and consist of brief paroxysms of alpha-like fast rhythms intermixed with low voltage bi-occipital spikes (Fig. 9.4). They occur immediately after closing of the eyes (eye closure state) and their duration does not exceed 5 s. Occasionally, squeak alpha rhythm without occipital spikes occurs on eye-closure.

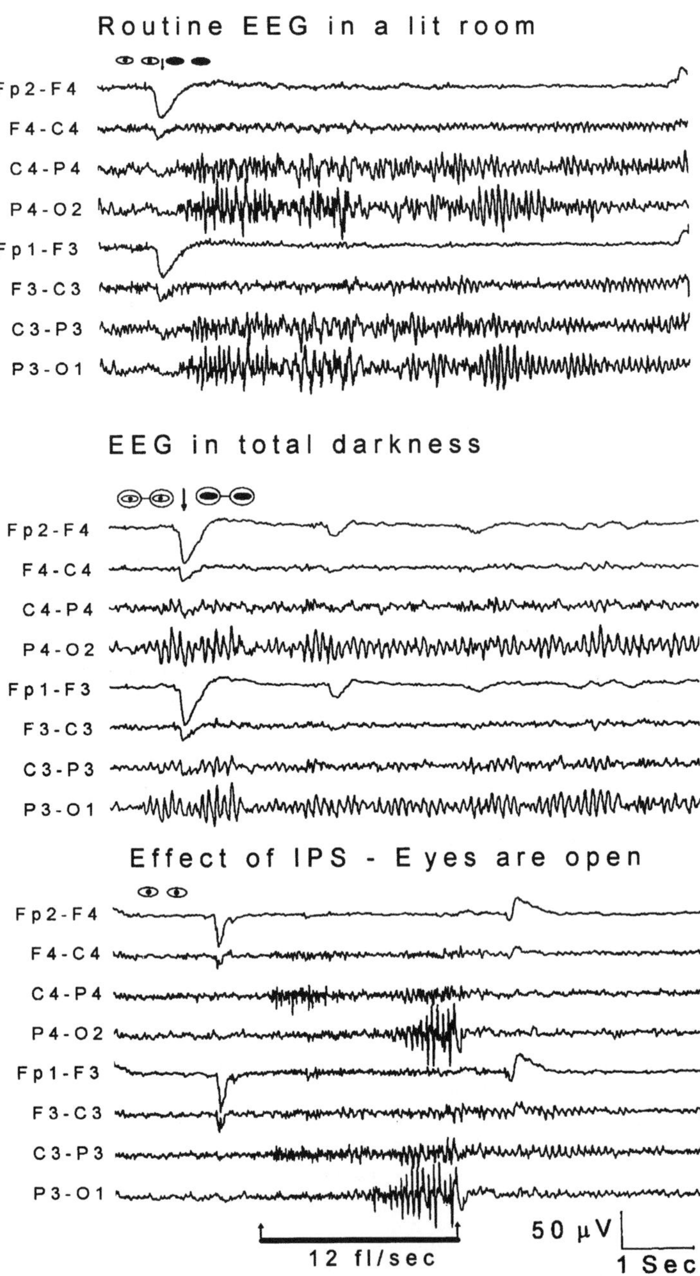

Fig. 9.4. Video-EEG of patient 29 with idiopathic regional occipital sensitivity. Note fast occipital spiking immediately after eye-closure which does not persist for more than a few seconds (top). This is inhibited in darkness (middle). These are eye-closure, not eyes-closed, related abnormalities. Photic stimulation evokes time-locked spikes (bottom).

Modified from Agathonikou et al., 1997[10] *with the permission of the authors and the editor of the Journal of Epilepsy.*

The EEG paroxysms never occurred when closing of the eyes was performed in conditions of complete darkness (underwater goggles covered with opaque tape), and elimination of central vision and fixation in the presence of light (underwater goggles covered with semi-transparent tape) (Fig. 9.4). Also, they never persisted in the eyes-closed state. Intermittent photic stimulation evokes time-locked occipital spikes with eyes closed or open (Fig. 9.4).

Sleep EEG was normal except for some brief runs of posterior fast rhythms intermixed with occipital spikes during stage I of sleep.

Her last EEG in 1998 showed timed-locked occipital spikes during IPS. The resting EEG was normal.

Finally, there were another two normal cases that should be classified according to the criteria of Gastaut and Zifkin[313] in LBOS because of visual seizures in late childhood. They did not have occipital spikes and CT scan was normal. They are both of interest though they have an entirely different course than expected for a benign condition with seizures continuing in adult life.

Case 32 of Table 13.3. This normal lady, born 6.8.72, had four GTCS in 2 years from age 11. All occurred within 15 min from awakening and were preceded by visual hallucinations which she describes at age 25 years as follows: 'Fuzzy vision starts in the bottom right hand corner of my *right* eye. (At 12 years old this used to look like the head of a person in my *left* eye.) This distorts my focus and vision, almost like being very drunk with no balance. The black dots travel across my *right* eye, they do not get bigger but get more dense interrupting my vision (Fig. 13.2). Images in front of me seem to become more 3D and more "real". This lasts for 10 s by which time I know that I am going to have a seizure so I lie down and black out.' Attacks of 'fuzzy vision which is less severe than my aura can happen at any time of the day and continue infrequently'. There are no obvious precipitating factors.

She was free of GTCS from 13 to 25 years and medication with carbamazepine stopped at age 15 years despite her continuing to have infrequent visual seizures. She had two GTCS within 3 weeks at age 25 years without apparent precipitating factors. She had the same sequence of visual seizures preceding GTCS which happened again after awakening. She had post-ictal headache only after GTCS.

Great grand mother had 'epilepsy' and mother 'severe migraine'.

An EEG at age 25 years was of excellent organization but showed infrequent and brief bursts of medium amplitude sharp and slow wave exclusively in the anterior regions and time-locked occipital spikes to IPS. MRI was not possible because she could not tolerate the tube.

Case 33 of Table 13.3. This intelligent man born 7.9.36 started having visual seizures with or without secondary GTCS at the age of 13 years. The onset is with a rotating concentric circle of bright yellow in the centre, red in the middle and black outside. This is the size of the eye, appears in the left temporal hemifield and rotates clockwise (Fig. 13.2). He tries to fight against it unsuccessfully, his eyes and head turn to the left and this may last for a minute or be longer, for 3 min, and progress to secondary GTCS. He used to have approximately four secondary GTCS every year until the age of 31 years when control was achieved mainly with primidone and phenytoin. Despite having 4–5 visual seizures per year, he was advised to stop medication at age 53 years. His visual seizures became more frequent, lasted longer and finally he had a secondary GTCS at work 10 months later. With phenytoin 300 mg daily he remained free of any seizures until his last follow-up one year later (Sept. 1991). An EEG in 1973 was normal. An EEG in 1990 showed excess of theta. CT brain scan in 1990 is normal.

At the time of completion of this book I saw another patient with visual seizures starting in early teens which I could not include with the other 63 patients because of its late arrival. I quote from my notes:

Case 34. She was born in 1981 and developed well. There is no family history of seizures or migraine.

She has a very interesting history of elementary visual hallucinations that twice progressed to secondary generalization.

Elementary visual hallucinations: They started sometime in the summer of 1997, that is when she was 16 years old. She describes them very well. They appear in the temporal field of her left eye. They consist of small star-shapes or balloons that are brilliantly multi-coloured. The predominant colours are red, blue and yellow (Fig. 13.2). Initially, there are a few of them in line, the one after the other with interchanging-flashing brilliance amongst them. They slowly move to the right side, the one after the other, with increasing speed as they progress. While the first ones disappear to the right new ones appear, probably bigger and probably with increasing brilliance, on the left moving with increasing speed to the right. These seizures lasts for seconds to a maximum of 2 min, and they may be associated with mild bitemporal headache which last as long as these are present. There are no post-ictal events. There is no impairment of consciousness. These episodes occurred once every week or month. They do not have any particular cicardian distribution. There are no particular precipitating factors. She did not ask advice about them.

Secondary generalization: This occurred twice. The first was on 25.11.97 and the other one on 12.2.98. On the first occasion, she was eating with her mother. Suddenly, she said 'here they are again, I am dizzy' and within 2 min the same visual hallucinations as described above became more brilliant and probably of bigger size. This was followed by buzzing in the ears and she then lost consciousness. Her mother told me that her eyes turned to the *left* (she insists that this was the side), she became unresponsive and probably there was some left sided tonic contraction of the face. She gradually fell over to the right side. Her mother finally laid her down. There were no convulsions. She was unresponsive for another 2 or 3 min and it took her approximately 10–15 min before completely recovering from the post-ictal state. She was subsequently tired and had a moderate headache, which was bitemporal and lasted for another 2–3 h. She was taken to the hospital. She was prescribed no medication.

She continued having these monthly or weekly elementary visual hallucinations as described above until February 1998 when she had the second secondary generalization. She was in the family car with her father driving. She told her mother that she was again in that previous state and within 2 min the same events happened as before. The only difference is that her eyes turned to the *right* she had bitten her mother's fingers although there were no obvious convulsions, and the post-ictal confusion was much shorter.

After these episodes, she rightly started treatment with carbamazepine, which she now receives 200 mg tds. No further episodes minor or major occurred after this.

She is a good student. Her neurological examination is normal.

EEGs were within normal limits. She also has a CT brain scan, which is reported as normal. She could not tolerate the tube for MRI.

Chapter 10

Occipital spikes, occipital paroxysms and other electroencephalographic findings in children with benign childhood occipital seizures. Occipital spikes in normal children and those without seizures

Brief description, definitions and clarifications

The interictal EEG manifestations of the early[277,600,605,606] and late onset benign childhood occipital seizures (BOS)[304,313,599,600] are identical and as fascinating as their clinical features (Figs. 10.1a and 10.1b). The EEG marker of benign occipital seizures (BOS) is occipital paroxysms defined as 'long runs of repetitive high amplitude sharp and slow wave complexes in the occipital regions which are morphologically similar to the centrotemporal spikes'.[608] The word 'paroxysm' in EEG terminology is a 'Group of waves which appears and disappears abruptly and which is clearly distinguished from background activity by different frequency, morphology or amplitude'. The individual complexes of the occipital paroxysms show a diphasic spike component with a main surface negative peak in the occipital electrodes and of an amplitude often exceeding 200 µV. This is followed by a smaller positive peak and a high amplitude negative slow wave. Occipital paroxysms are bilateral and synchronous but unilateral and predominantly right sided or random occipital spikes often occur. Occipital paroxysms appear and persist only when the eyes are closed and may not be recorded in children who keep their eyes open during the EEG. This is because the occipital spikes are activated by the elimination of fixation and central vision (fixation-off sensitivity).[599,600,602,604] These children are not photosensitive clinically or during intermittent photic stimulation (IPS). However, occasionally at a later stage of their disease, when occipital paroxysms decline, IPS may provoke some time-locked occipital spikes.

Occipital paroxysms may persist long after remission of clinical seizures[304,605] but also they may not be detected interictally during the active seizure phase.[304,367,368,605,608,793] Also, some children may have random occipital spikes that do not have the repetitive character of occipital paroxysms. Centrotemporal, frontal or somato-sensory evoked spikes in the same or mainly in subsequent EEGs may be recorded particularly in the Panayiotopoulos syndrome.[277,308,386,603,605,608,793] Brief general-

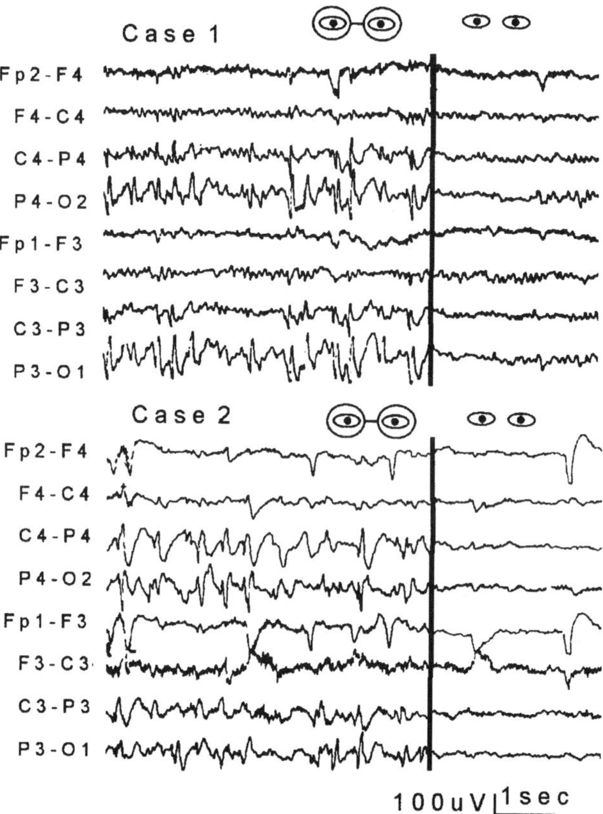

Fig. 10.1a. Occipital paroxysms of a child with EBOS (upper) and a child with LBOS (bottom) that I reported in 1981 in Neurology.[360] *Despite different clinical manifestations, the occipital paroxysms are similar – also activated by the elimination of central vision and fixation (left of the vertical bar, symbol of eyes with glasses) and inhibited by fixation (right of the vertical bar, symbol of eyes without glasses).*
Modified from Panayiotopoulos, 1980 and 1981[599] *with the permission of the editor of Neurology.*

ized discharges of small spike and slow waves are frequently recorded usually late in the evolution of the EEG and also during sleep.[277,313,605,606]

The occipital spikes of the BOS are activated by sleep in more than half of the patients.[277] There are also reports of children with the Panayiotopoulos syndrome where occipital spikes are detected only in sleep EEGs.[150,272]

However, there are children for whom the diagnosis of BOS is based only on the characteristic clinical evidence, as series of EEGs during alert and sleep stages may be entirely normal,[608,793] or others where the occipital spikes may appear long after the onset of clinical manifestations.[368] Seven (5.3 per cent) of 113 children with the Panayiotopoulos syndrome had the typical clinical features without occipital spikes.[277]

It should be emphasized that posterior EEG paroxysmal activity attenuating on eyes-open should never be equated with the occipital paroxysms of BOS. Polyspikes, tiny spikes intermixed with slow waves, scattered occipital spikes like those seen in photosensitive patients or slow waves that happen to attenuate on eyes-open, all these are not occipital paroxysms and should not be confused with BOS. Furthermore, fixation-off sensitivity has also been reported in other than BOS epileptic conditions, some of which are severe generalized epilepsies.[8,646]

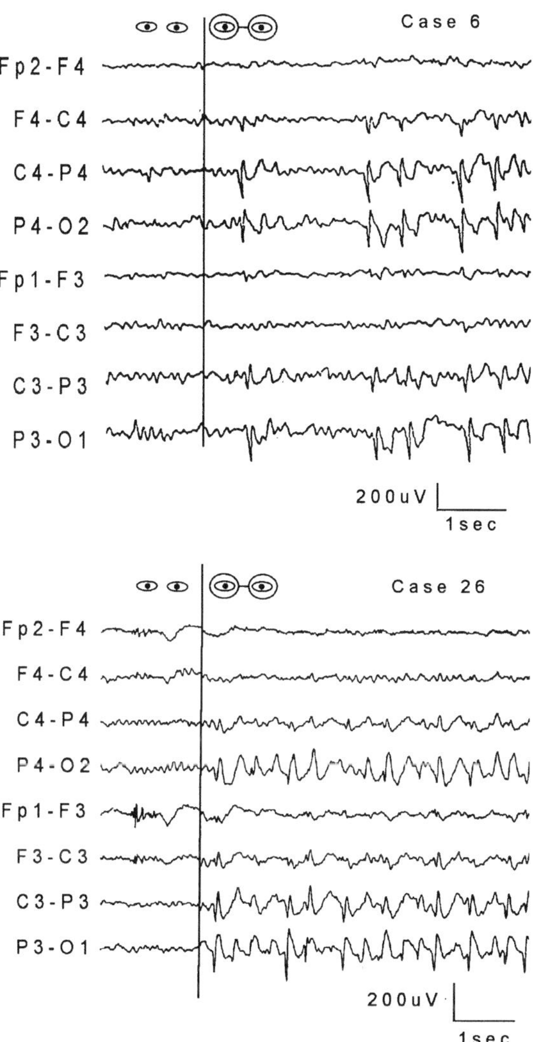

Fig. 10.1b. Occipital paroxysms of case 6 (Table 13.1) with EBOS (upper) and case 26 (Table 13.3) with LBOS (lower).
Note the similarities of the occipital paroxysms, despite remarkably different clinical manifestations and the fact that the upper trace was recorded in 1977 with an eight channel ink-pen EEG while the lower trace is extracted from a recording in 1992 on a multichannel modern video-EEG machine.
Also, for both children, the occipital paroxysms are activated by the elimination of central vision and fixation (right of the vertical bar, symbol of eyes with glasses) and inhibited by fixation (left of the vertical bar, symbol of eyes without glasses).

Occipital paroxysms in EEGs should raise the possibility of BOS but they are not diagnostic of them as they may also occur in children who do not even suffer from seizures[83,327,386,438] or in more severe forms of cryptogenic/symptomatic epilepsies.[18,180,287,568] Occipital spikes are even less significant than occipital paroxysms for the diagnosis of BOS and this has been known for many years.[324,326,327,331, 333,440,464,487,702] In this respect the words of the Gibbses may act as a reminder:

'During infancy and early childhood a focus of spike activity in the occipital area is the most common type of spike focus; it is rare in adults. In only two-thirds of cases are clinically recognisable seizures present; thus it is one of the least epileptogenic of the spike foci. This finding is likely to be associated with eye defects such as strabismus and congenital cataracts. It is especially common in cases of retrolental fibroplasia. Although prematurity and perinatal injury are important causal factors, occipital spikes can also result from encephalitis and postnatal trauma. With increasing age occipital spiking tends to disappear or shift to the midtemporal area'. *Gibbs and Gibbs, 1967* p. 50 [331]

Interictal EEG in benign childhood occipital seizures: literature review

There is unanimous agreement regarding the EEG findings in benign childhood occipital seizures (BOS).[74,146,150,192,213,270,277,302,304,308,313,344,367,386,443,484,514,517,599,600,604–606,608,626,636,750,797] BOS is an idiopathic condition and therefore, the background activity in all children is normal except in post-ictal recordings.

Abbreviations

BOS =	Benign childhood occipital seizures (to include EBOS and LBOS)
EBOS =	Early onset benign childhood occipital seizures or Panayiotopoulos syndrome
LBOS =	Late onset benign childhood occipital seizures or Late onset idiopathic childhood occipital epilepsy
RS =	Rolandic seizures
CTS =	Centrotemporal spikes
FOS =	Fixation-off sensitivity
IPS =	Intermittent photic stimulation
VER =	Visual evoked responses
CSWS =	Continuous spikes and waves during slow sleep
GTCS =	Generalized tonic–clonic seizures

Occipital spike-slow wave complexes and occipital paroxysms

The individual occipital spike complexes of BOS are morphologically similar to the centrotemporal spikes of the Rolandic seizures (RS). They are recorded in more than 90 per cent of the patients either during the awake or slow wave sleep stage (Figs. 10.1a and 10.1b). They show a diphasic spike component with a sharp, surface negative peak followed by a small-amplitude surface-positive peak and a surface-negative slow wave component. The spike component is of higher amplitude than the slow wave, often exceeding 200 μV and reaching 300 μV. The duration of the spike component is often more than 70 ms. They can occur singularly or in brief clusters but usually they are continuous rhythmical repetitive occipital paroxysms from 1 to 3 Hz which may last for as long as the eyes remain closed. They are bilateral and synchronous with usually a constant voltage asymmetry, or predominantly unilateral, more on the right. They focus on the occipital electrodes, but some location shifting limited to the posterior areas is not uncommon (Figs. 10.1a and 10.1b).

van der Meij *et al.*, 1997[780] found that the dipole sources of the occipital spikes in idiopathic BOS are located superficially within the cortical layers while symptomatic occipital spikes may have a deeper location. They suggested that a superficial dipole source location of the occipital spikes in BOS has a 67 per cent sensitivity and 74 per cent specificity.

Reactivity of the occipital spikes

In routine EEGs in an illuminated room, the occipital spikes are mainly or exclusively seen when the eyes are closed; they are totally or partially inhibited when the eyes are open (Figs. 10.2, 10.3a and 10.3b). If occipital spikes or paroxysms persist with eyes open, these can be eliminated by asking the child to fixate on a visual target (the tip of a pencil will do) (Fig. 10.3a).

Panayiotopoulos (1980,1981,1998)[599,600,620] documented that the effect of eyes-closed on the occipital spikes is due to the elimination of central vision and fixation, a phenomenon for which he coined the

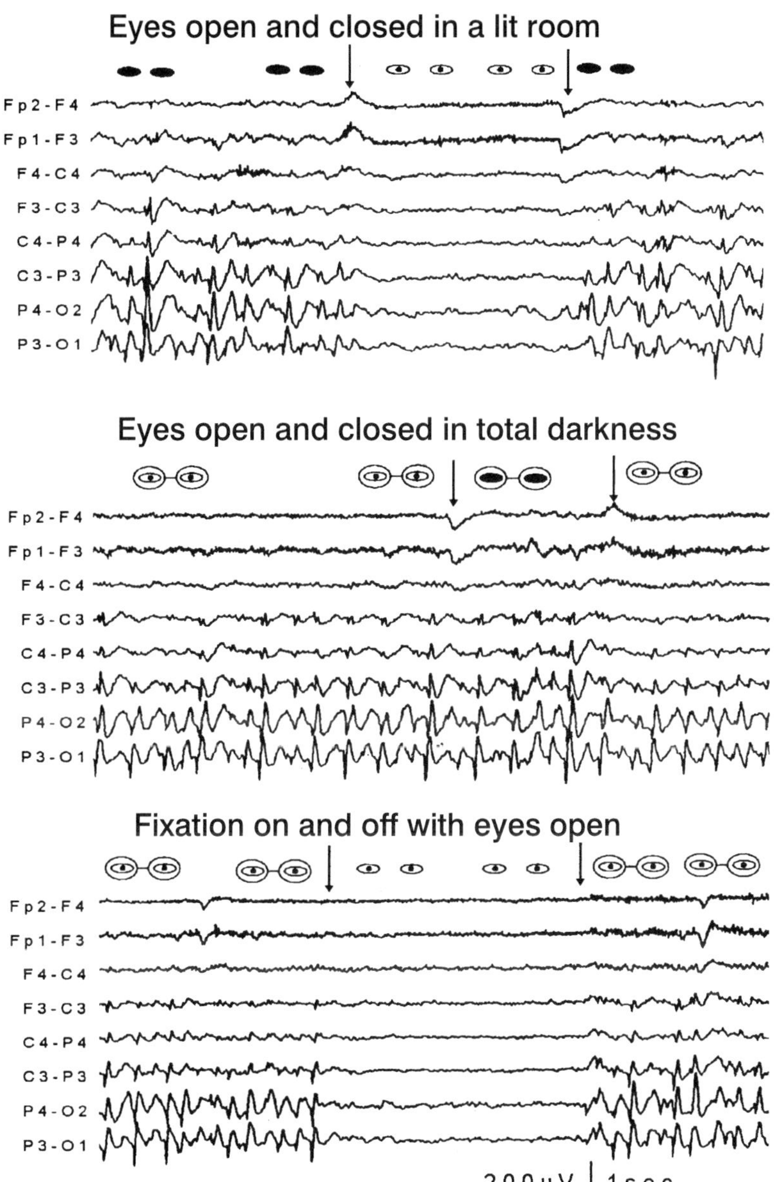

Fig. 10.2. From video-EEG recording of patient 26, described in Chapter 9 (page 166).
Occipital paroxysms occur as long as fixation and central vision are eliminated by any means (eyes closed, darkness, + 10 spherical lenses, Ganzfeld stimulation). Under these conditions, even in the presence of light, eyes-opening is not capable of inhibition. Conversely, occipital paroxysms are totally inhibited by fixation and central vision.
Symbols of eyes open and closed without glasses denote that fixation is possible when eyes are open (routine EEG recordings in a lit room).
Symbols of eyes with glasses indicate elimination of central vision and fixation, in the middle by complete darkness and at the bottom by other means detailed in the text.

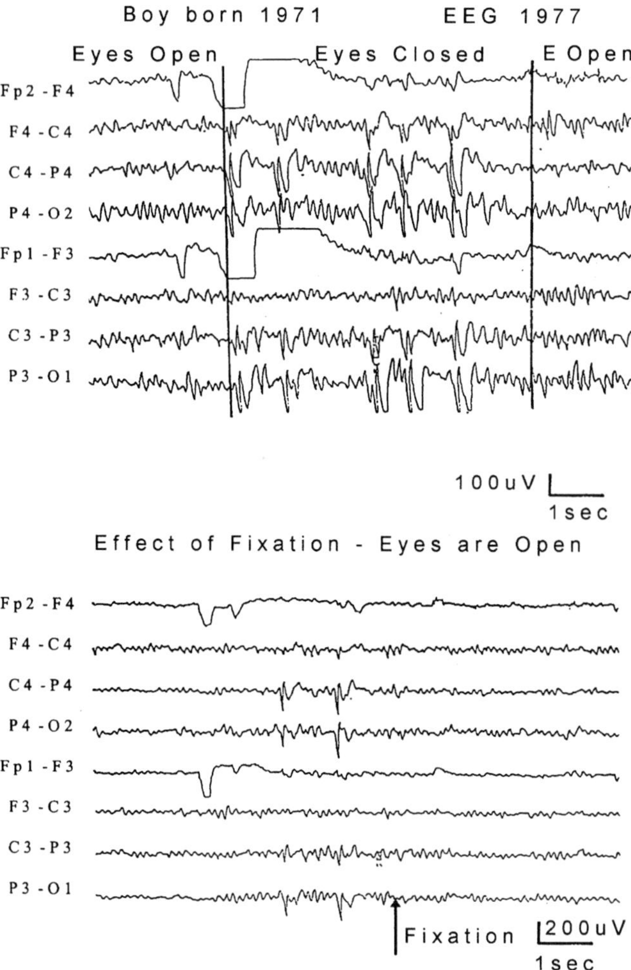

Fig. 10.3a. Routine EEG of case 6[606] of Table 13.1 in a lit room. Occipital paroxysms occur when eyes are closed (upper). Occasionally, they may appear when eyes are open but are immediately inhibited by fixation (in this occasion, asking the child to look at the tip of a pen).
From Panayiotopoulos, 1989[606] with the permission of the editor of the Journal of Child Neurology.

term fixation-off sensitivity. Activation and inhibition of the occipital paroxysms is usually immediately or within a second after closing or opening of the eyes.

Fixation-off sensitivity

Fixation-off sensitivity (FOS) refers to the forms of epilepsy, EEG abnormalities or both that are elicited by elimination of central vision and fixation.[599,600,620]

Fixation-off sensitivity is a relatively newly described specific mode of precipitation of seizures and paroxysmal EEG abnormalities.[599,600,616,620,626] Elimination of central vision and fixation, even in the presence of light, induces high amplitude occipital or generalized paroxysmal discharges. FOS is suggested in routine EEG by abnormalities which consistently occur as long as the eyes are closed but not when eyes are open. The model example of FOS is EBOS and LBOS as I have described it.[599,600,616,620,626] Idiopathic and cryptogenic generalized epilepsies with FOS have been de-

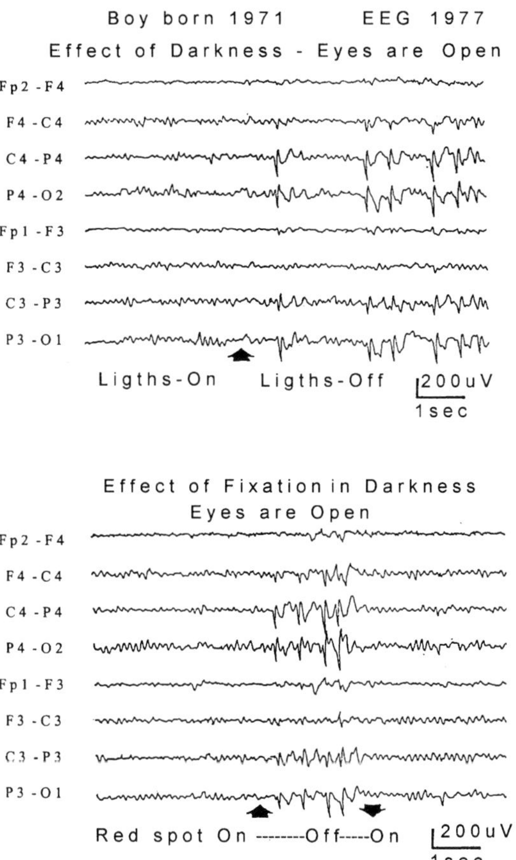

Fig. 10.3b. Same case as in Fig. 10.3a. Eyes are continuously open. The occipital paroxysms are activated by darkness (upper) and inhibited by fixation on a spot of red light (lower).
From Panayiotopoulos, 1989[606] with the permission of the editor of the Journal of Child Neurology.

scribed.[8,620] Scotosensitive epilepsy[620] implies seizures and EEG abnormalities elicited by complete elimination of any retinal light stimulation and most cases described as scotosensitive are probably FOS. FOS has the opposite characteristics of photosensitive epilepsies but conversion from one to the other or even co-existence in the same patient may rarely occur.[616,620]

The underlying mechanisms of FOS are not known but they may be related to an abnormality of the alpha rhythm generators.[8,256,620]

Fixation-off sensitivity can be better understood in reviewing the steps I followed for their detection and study.[595,596,598–600,602,604–606,620,626]

Between 1973 and 1978, I saw children who clinically had either nocturnal seizures with tonic deviation of the eyes and vomiting (EBOS) or partial visual seizures (LBOS). They had identical interictal EEG abnormalities consisting of continuous high amplitude occipital paroxysms as long as the eyes were closed and disappearing for as long as the eyes were open (Figs. 10.1a, 10.2 and 10.3a). These children were not photosensitive. Instead, illumination of the closed eyes with a strong light or high frequency intermittent photic stimulation (IPS) sometimes had a partial inhibitory effect on the occipital paroxysms (Fig. 10.4).

I considered that these children might be scotosensitive because their occipital paroxysms would appear on eyes-open by switching-off the lights of the recording room but this effect, with some light coming through closed doors and windows, was variable. It was only in complete darkness, eliminating any possible light sources, that the occipital paroxysms were invariably activated when the eyes were opened and became continuous whether eyes were open or closed. In complete darkness with the eyes open, the reactivity of the occipital paroxysms could be controlled by turning the light on and off and not by opening or closing of the eyes. Thus light was inhibiting and darkness was activating the occipital paroxysms (Fig. 10.3b). The next step was to find out the characteristics of a light source responsible for such marked inhibition. A small spot of low intensity red light, initially produced by the light of an ophthalmoscope shown through my finger from a distance of approximately 3 m, totally inhibited the occipital paroxysms as long as the patient was fixating on it. Thus, in complete darkness with the eyes open, occipital paroxysms were inhibited by fixation and activated by the absence of fixation (Fig. 10.3b).

Scotosensitivity or fixation-off sensitivity?

The behaviour of the occipital paroxysms indicated that they were reactive to fixation-on and off rather than to the presence of light or its intensity. This was documented by testing the effect of central vision and fixation in a normally-lit room. Central vision and fixation were eliminated with +10 spherical lenses or underwater goggles covered with semitransparent tape. Under these conditions of fixation-off in the presence of light, the occipital paroxysms showed the same reactivity as in complete darkness: it was continuous whether the eyes were open or closed (Fig. 10.2). Occipital paroxysms would disappear again if central vision and fixation were restored either binocularly or monocularly (Fig. 10.2). I concluded that the excitatory effect of darkness was in fact due to the elimination of central vision and fixation and that darkness was not a prerequisite for the activation of the occipital paroxysms. I thus coined the term fixation-off sensitivity to distinguish this from scotosensitivity.

Fixation independent of visual cues is not important. There was no inhibition of occipital paroxysms if a patient 'looked' at his/her finger in complete darkness.[601]

Furthermore, occipital paroxysms could not be modified by any eye movement or stimulation other than those involving central vision and fixation, suggesting that input from extraocular muscles or other ocular sensory or proprioceptive impulses did not contribute to FOS. Also, the fact that the occipital abnormalities could be inhibited or activated with eyes opened by fixation-off or on was against such a proposition.

FOS is probably more often associated with benign childhood occipital seizures than with any other epileptic condition.

The prevalence of FOS in BOS is unknown. FOS was not specifically studied in many reports of this condition. Lugaresi *et al.* (1984)[514] and Cirignotta *et al.* (1987)[167] were the first to confirm FOS in nine children with BOS and noted that 'central vision represents the critical factor, not only in the appearance of the spike and wave discharges of benign occipital epilepsy...but also in the triggering of the alpha and slow alpha variant rhythm and of the ictal occipital discharges provoked by darkness'. However, contrary to my results a delay of 1–6 s was found from the onset of fixation -off to the appearance of occipital paroxysms in light conditions and of 2–18 s in darkness. Like my results, fixation on a spot of red light immediately suppressed the spikes.

In a recent multicentre collaborative study of Panayiotopoulos syndrome, FOS was confirmed in 24 out of 28 children tested for it.[277]

Beaumanoir (1981,1983,1987)[74,82,83] described epileptic children, many with early onset BOS, and non epileptic children mainly with amblyopia, whose occipital paroxysms were inhibited by visual perception. Other authors have described a great variety of EEG abnormalities recorded with the eyes closed and suppressed with eye opening.[18,180,753] These include slow waves, multiple spikes, small spikes and slow waves, which are not necessarily the characteristic occipital paroxysms of BOS,

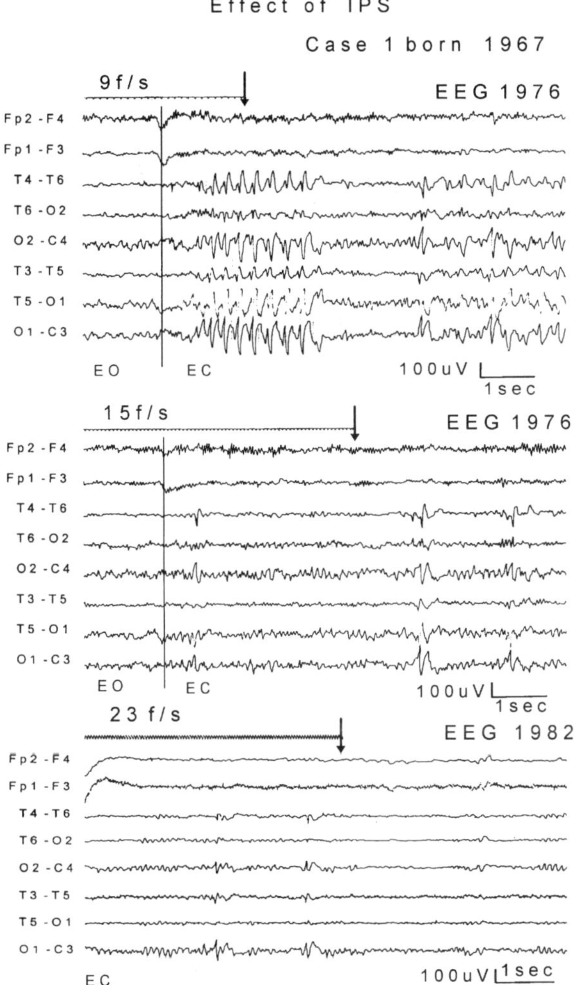

Fig. 10.4. Effect of IPS in case 1 of EBOS, described in Chapter 8, page 146. IPS at high frequencies had an inhibitory effect (middle) on the occipital paroxysms at their active period in 1976. Some small occipital spikes were elicited by IPS, six years later (1982) when no more spontaneous occipital spikes occurred.

associated with both benign and intractable epilepsies. FOS has not been studied in these conditions. It is possible that FOS may be associated more with idiopathic than with symptomatic epilepsies but this has yet to be properly assessed.

However, not all children with occipital paroxysms have FOS. Figure 10.5 is an example of this. This patient (case 11, Table 13.1) is also the only one who had infrequent GTCS as an adult. Coincidence cannot be excluded.

Scotosensitivity

Scotosensitivity (skotos in Greek means darkness) denotes forms of epilepsy, seizures, or EEG abnormalities which are elicited by the complete elimination of retinal stimulation by light. All patients with FOS will be sensitive to complete darkness because of the loss of central vision and

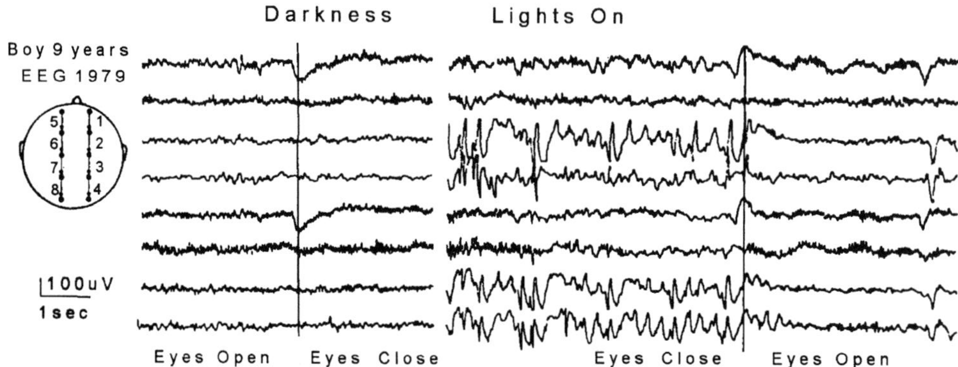

Fig. 10.5. Occipital paroxysms of a patient with EBOS. They are inhibited instead of activated by darkness. From Panayiotopoulos, 1989[605] with the permission of the editor of Annals of Neurology.

fixation. Therefore, the term scotosensitivity should be reserved only for those patients who do not have FOS.

Complete darkness, in which the retina is completely deprived of light stimulation, can be difficult to achieve. Even a small spot of red light on which the eyes may fixate can totally inhibit occipital paroxysms induced by complete darkness. All possible light sources such as small indicators on the EEG machine and other equipment or light coming through doors or window openings must be excluded: if not, central vision and fixation may not be eliminated during the testing and the results jeopardized. Switching off the lights in the EEG recording room is not adequate and this may explain conflicting results in the literature. Complete darkness may be produced with underwater goggles covered completely with opaque tape.

Clinical and EEG manifestations of scotosensitive patients

Scotosensitive epilepsy was rarely reported in the literature before the recent papers on FOS. Pazzaglia *et al.* (1970)[646] reported a 14-year-old boy with seizures mainly in darkness, because of which he would sleep with the lights on. The seizures consisted of tonic deviation of the eyes to the left with concomitant clonic movements and left hemianopia. Elementary visual hallucinations consisting of geometric shapes and brilliant colours occurred in the hemianopic field. There sometimes was mild impairment of consciousness. Secondary complex partial seizures with *déjà vu* phenomena or generalized tonic–clonic convulsions could occur. A seizure was recorded after 55 s in darkness. It consisted of mainly right sided occipital spikes with increasing frequency to 14–16 Hz followed by high amplitude bioccipital spike and slow wave activity.

Beaumanoir *et al.* 1989[81] reported nine patients with at least 'one reflex scotosensitive seizure recorded with EEG'. Seizures were elicited when passing from light conditions to darkness, and in at least four patients it was confirmed that the eyes did not close during this procedure. Age at onset was from 3 to 7 years and eight patients appeared to have a good prognosis. CT brain scan was normal in eight patients who 'fulfilled the accepted criteria for a diagnosis of benign epilepsy with occipital focus'. All patients had parieto-occipital spike or multiple spike foci which were inhibited by IPS at frequencies higher than 6 Hz. In five of them the occipital discharges were also induced as an off-response to IPS, i.e. they occurred immediately after the end of a train of IPS. Also, five patients developed photosensitivity during the course of the disease. Three different electroclinical types of scotosensitive seizures were recorded:

(a) Less than 5 s episodes of 'dazzle or flash' often associated with an unpleasant feeling. Ictal

EEG showed unilateral or bilateral accelerating multiple occipital spikes often followed by a slow wave.

(b) Seizures of 8–32 s duration with a 'flash' followed by impairment of consciousness, 'complex absences' and falls. An EEG illustrating such a seizure shows generalized multiple spikes with posterior amplitude predominance.

(c) Complex behaviour described above without the preceding dazzle or flash.

Whether these interesting patients had FOS or true scotosensitive epilepsy cannot be deduced.

One of the cases (No. 1) reported by Mancia *et al.*[519] is of particular interest as he started having at age 6 years ictal symptoms similar to early onset occipital seizures (right-side frontal headache accompanied by pallor, sweating and loss of touch with his surroundings but not vomiting). He later, at age 12 years, developed 'visual troubles of seeing a yellow spot entering his visual field and accompanied by slight impairment of consciousness'. Such episodes occurred more frequently after passing from a dark environment into a well-lit one and again into darkness. Ictal EEG documented that these were epileptic seizures. The interictal EEG shows a right occipital spike and slow wave. The seizure starts abruptly with generalized fast activity which predominates in the occipital regions bilaterally while the child complains of visual 'yellow spots'. This after 2 s is followed by mainly fast spikes more prominent in the bi-occipital regions which last for 1 min and it is clinically associated with 'blindness and impairment of speech'. The seizure ends again abruptly followed by a relative EEG normalization. Whether this patient had idiopathic or cryptogenic occipital epilepsy is not clear. However, the frequent and the intractable character of his seizures as well as the ictal EEG would rather favour a cryptogenic/symptomatic nature of his seizures.

Do true cases of scotosensitive epilepsy exist? That is, are there patients in whom the excitatory role of darkness is not due to FOS? I have not found a convincing case so far, although some patients with FOS certainly have a graded response, i.e. darkness may be more effective than +10 spherical lenses. Genuine cases of scotosensitivity may exist but their documentation would require exclusion of FOS.

Intermittent photic stimulation (IPS) in benign childhood occipital seizures

Patients with EBOS are not photosensitive and therefore IPS does not elicit photoparoxysmal abnormalities. On the contrary, because of FOS, IPS has a tendency to cause inhibition, particularly at high flash rates (Fig. 10.4).[604,606,620] However, this inhibitory effect is not constant in all patients and for the same patient in the same or other EEG sessions. It is interesting, in that two of my patients with spontaneous occipital paroxysms and FOS consistently recorded for years (cases 1 and 2 of Panayiotopoulos,1989),[606] IPS evoked occipital spikes at an older age and at a stage of EEG evolution when 'spontaneous' occipital spikes were no longer recorded (Fig. 10.4).[606]

Cases with clinical photosensitivity and EEG photoparoxysmal discharges included by Gastaut and Zifkin[313] and Terasaki *et al.* (1987)[763] in LBOS probably belong to idiopathic photosensitive occipital seizures or other syndromes with photosensitivity, and these are dealt with in Chapter 12B.

Four of the seven patients of Terzano *et al.* 1993[766] with 'intercalated seizures' and 'occipital paroxysms attenuated by eyes open' (that is FOS) also had marked photosensitivity which is an unusual combination of FOS and photosensitivity.

Photosensitivity versus fixation-off sensitivity

Photosensitive epilepsy appears to have opposite mechanisms of excitation and inhibition from those of FOS:[604,616,620,626] (a) The resting EEG of photosensitive patients frequently shows 'eye-closure' (not eyes-closed) EEG abnormalities which are inhibited by total darkness and probably by elimination of central vision and fixation (Fig. 10.6). (b) Photosensitivity is mainly mediated through central vision and fixation. Photoconvulsive responses are induced only if the patient 'looks' at the centre of the stroboscope. (c) Occipital spikes induced by photic stimulation are elicited when IPS is combined with patterns (Fig. 10.7).[631,632] The occipital spike appears to emerge from the negative component

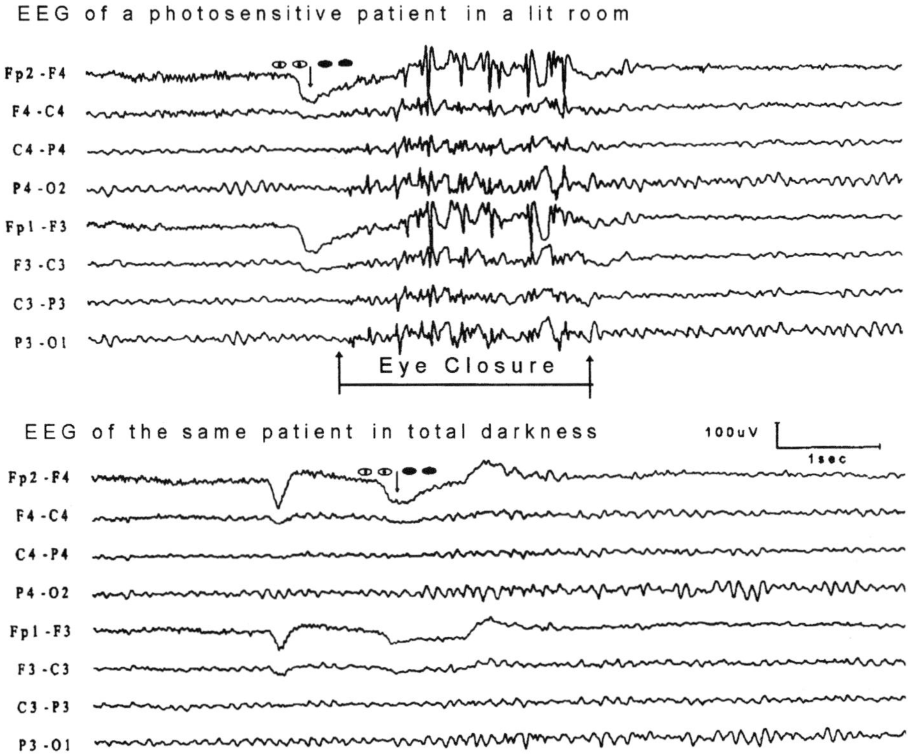

Fig. 10.6. Eye-closure induced generalized discharges (upper) in a photosensitive patient that are inhibited in darkness (lower).
Note that the discharge lasts for a few seconds and does not continue in the remaining period when the eyes are closed. Symbols of eyes indicate when these are open or closed. Arrows indicate the time of eye-closure.

of a triphasic P100 visual evoked response (Fig. 10.8) and caused us to postulate that an increase in sensitivity of the occipital cortex is implicated in the pathophysiology of photosensitive epilepsy.[593,631,632] This well documented view of a regional or lobar (the term regional or lobar is introduced for the epilepsies in which there is a bilateral sensitivity restricted to cerebral lobes subserving a certain function) occipital lobe sensitivity has recently been well established.[805]

Hyperventilation in benign childhood occipital seizures

Hyperventilation does not appear to activate the occipital spikes. Only Terasaki *et al.* (1987)[763] reported that they were activated by hyperventilation in nine (60 per cent) of 15 cases.

Sleep EEG in benign childhood occipital seizures

Sleep appears to facilitate occipital paroxysms of BOS though the results of relevant studies are conflicting, probably because of selection criteria.

Gastaut and Zifkin[313] found that in 13 (59.1 per cent) of 22 patients, the occipital paroxysms disappeared with drowsiness and were not seen during the following slow wave sleep. In five (22.7 per cent) patients occipital paroxysmal activity was recorded only during sleep. Five patients also had apparent electrographic seizures over the occipital regions during slow wave sleep, with no clinical accompaniment. In six patients, bursts of generalized bilaterally synchronous spike and wave complexes were recorded.

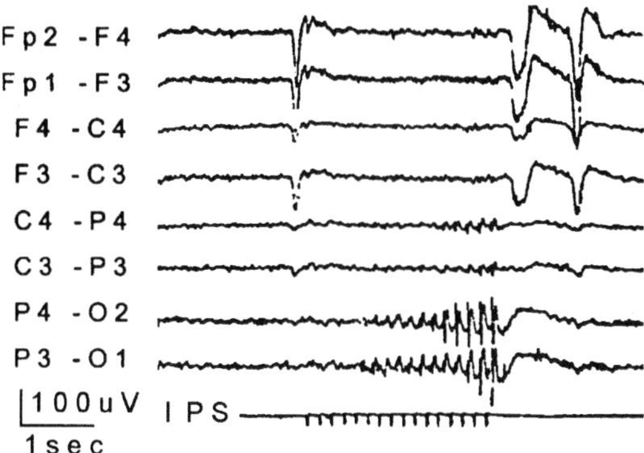

Fig. 10.7. Occipital spikes that are time-locked to photic stimuli in a photosensitive patient. These are elicited with combined patterns and IPS.
Modified from Panayiotopoulos et al, 1972[632] *with the permission of the editor of Electroencephalography and Clinical Neurophysiology.*

In all 18 patients with BOS of Beaumanoir (1983)[74] slow sleep increased the occipital paroxysms or 'brought them into evidence'. They disappeared or became less evident during REM sleep.

Terasaki *et al.* (1987)[763] found that occipital discharges of BOS were activated by sleep in only 4 (23.5 per cent) of the 23 cases and were suppressed in 6 of BOS (35.3 per cent).

Dalla Bernardina *et al.* (1993)[192] found that occipital spikes increased during sleep in approximately half of the patients irrespective of whether they were idiopathic (51.5 per cent) or cryptogenic/symptomatic (42 per cent).

In all 18 children of Guerrini *et al.*, 1993[367] EEG abnormalities were recorded during awake state and activated during slow wave sleep.

Ferrie *et al.*[277] in their study of a homogeneous group of children with EBOS found that occipital spikes were activated by sleep in 84 per cent, decreased in 2 per cent and were not altered in 12 per cent.[277] There are also reports of children with EBOS where occipital spikes appeared only in sleep EEGs.[150,272]

Centrotemporal, frontal and giant somatosensory evoked spikes in benign childhood occipital seizures

That children with occipital paroxysms may also have in the same EEG or mainly subsequent EEGs centrotemporal spikes has been emphasized in many reports[25,87,277,308,326,386,603,605,608,793] from the times of Gibbs *et al.* 1954[326] (see details in historical aspects, Chapter 11). This has also been illustrated in this book on many occasions.

Gibbs *et al.* (1954)[326] reported 45 children with occipital foci who were restudied after the age of nine years. In 18 per cent of them 'the pure occipital spike-focus had disappeared and had been replaced by an occipito-temporal focus and in 14 per cent the focus had shifted to the midtemporal area and of these about one third were seizure free'.

A similar association between centrotemporal spikes and occipital spikes was described by Beaussart (1972)[87] in children with Rolandic seizures.

Lerman and Kivity,1981[485] found that 14 per cent of 100 children with EEG focal spikes but without seizures had both occipital and centrotemporal foci.

Gastaut and Zifkin[313] found that 19 of 50 children with LBOS had either 'centrotemporal spikes or generalized discharges of spike and wave or polyspike and wave complexes without any clinical evidence of this type of seizures'. They commented that 'the association of centrotemporal spikes and occipital paroxysms mainly occurred in children with hemiclonic seizures'.

One of the 18 patients of Beaumanoir[74] also had 'Rolandic seizures prior to the onset of the occipital ones' and two patients had one brother each with Rolandic seizures.

This association of BOS and Rolandic seizures was also noted by Herranz Tanarro *et al.* (1984)[386] who concluded that 'this benign occipital epilepsy is related to childhood epilepsy with Rolandic paroxysms' on the basis that 13 (41.9 per cent) of 31 children with occipital paroxysms also had 'functional spike-wave focus of temporo-Rolandic localization'. Clinically, 10 children were seizure-free with minimal brain dysfunction in eight of them and two were diagnosed as having basilar migraine. Only four patients suffered from febrile convulsions while the other 17 patients had visual, motor or vegetative partial seizures, and even generalized fits.

Aso *et al.* (1987)[52] reported five cases where the occipital focus 'migrated to central, temporal and frontal areas'.

Amit (1987)[28] reported a 10-year-old girl with a single GTCS and EEG with two independent, occipital and centrotemporal, foci. Also, a 10-year-old boy evaluated for headaches showed typical centrotemporal spikes while his 8-year-old asymptomatic sister had 'occipital-temporal spikes'.

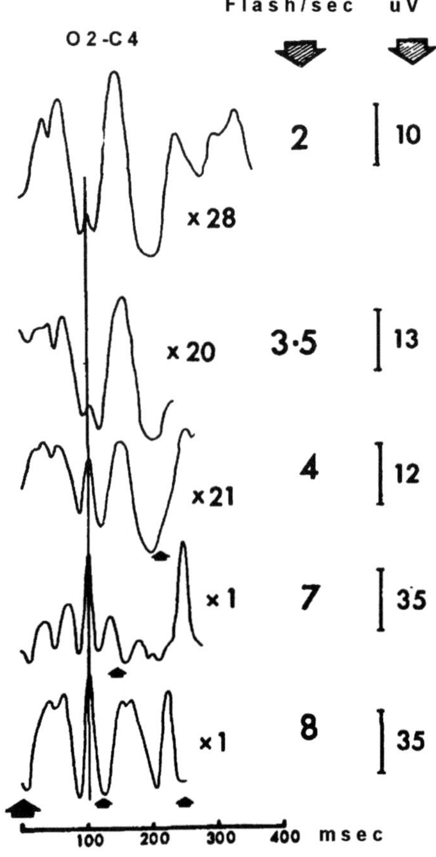

Fig. 10.8. The relation of the time-locked IPS elicited occipital spikes and visual evoked responses (VER) in a photosensitive patient.
Average evoked response (times are indicated by X) at 2, 3.5, 4, 7 and 8 flashes per s. Note that with increasing rate of stimulation, a negative component (the occipital spike) emerges from the positive P100 complex of the VER. Also note the much higher amplitude of the spike in relation to VER.
Modified from Panayiotopoulos et al., 1970[631] with the permission of the editor of Nature.

Regarding EBOS, four of the 16 children with EBOS that I reported[603,605] also had 'centrotemporal spikes either in the same or subsequent EEG and one showed additional frontal spikes'.[603] Furthermore, three other children had Rolandic seizures with occipital and centrotemporal spikes.[605] It was also apparent that some children initially have seizures typical of EBOS and later develop Rolandic seizures.[605,608] Panayiotopoulos[608] described a girl with a nocturnal partial status epilepticus of EBOS at age 7 and a nocturnal Rolandic seizure one year later (case 14, page 146). Series of EEG showed occipital paroxysms, centrotemporal and frontal spikes as well as giant somatosensory evoked spikes (Fig. 8.5).[608] Her EEG normalized at the age of 12 years. She was seizure free, with a normal EEG and no treatment in her last follow-up at age 16 years. These findings have also been confirmed by Vigevano and Ricci[793] who reported 14 children with EBOS, six of whom had centrotemporal spikes together or independently of the occipital spikes. One of nine cases of Kivity and Lerman (1992)[443] also had centrotemporal spikes.

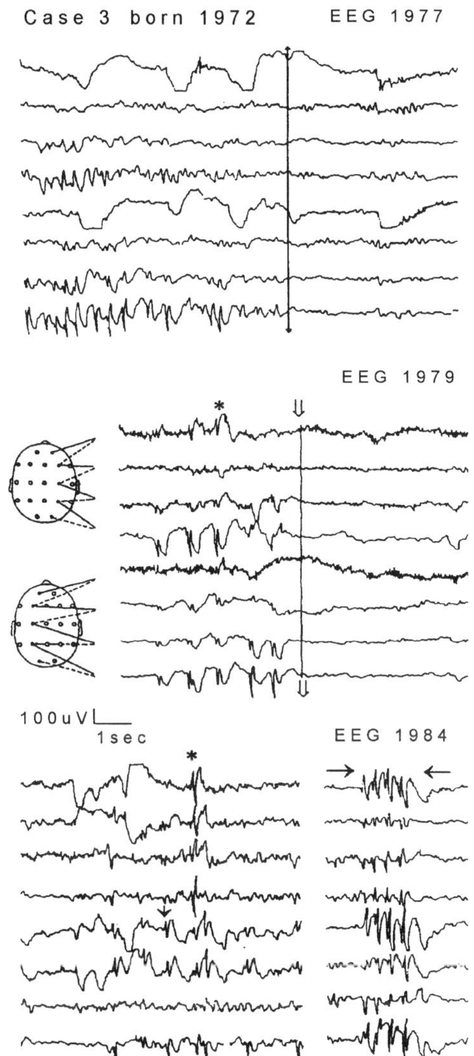

Fig. 10.9. Serial EEG of case 3 (Table 13.1) with EBOS. Initial EEGs showed occipital paroxysms only (upper), but later these occurred simultaneously with right (asterisk) or left (arrow) frontal spikes (middle and bottom). That the frontal spikes, in this case, were probably driven by the occipital ones is indicated by their reactivity to fixation-off. The EEG on the left of the vertical bars is with elimination of central vision and fixation. All spikes are inhibited by fixation (right of the vertical bars). Also, note bi-synchronous occipital and frontal spikes (bottom, in between the horizontal arrows).
Despite the marked deterioration in her EEG, this girl had only three Panayiotopoulos type of seizures from age 4 to 6.

Nagendran *et al.*, 1990[557] reported siblings with LBOS and occipital paroxysms while an asymptomatic brother had centrotemporal spikes in the EEG.

Ferrie *et al.* 1997[277] found that from 113 children with EBOS 29 (25 per cent) had centrotemporal spikes, eight (7 per cent) had frontal spikes, three giant somatosensory spikes and 14 (12 per cent) diffuse discharges. The incidence of giant somatosensory spikes may be underestimated as not all of their patients were tested for this. Four children developed RS after remission of the EBOS.[277] Similar association has also been found by others.[368]

Fejerman, 1996,[270,271] 1997[272] and his associates (Caraballo *et al.*, 1997)[150] reported nine children fulfilling 'clinical and EEG criteria for the concomitant diagnosis of benign partial epilepsies in childhood with centrotemporal spikes and Panayiotopoulos type BOS. These patients had Rolandic seizures and ictal vomiting with head deviation independently during the course of the disease, and showed centrotemporal or Rolandic spikes and occipital spikes in the same interictal EEG.'

Ricci and Vigevano (1993)[677] described a 10-year-old normal boy with normal MRI who had febrile and afebrile seizures at age 1 year old. He later had brief, spontaneous or TV-induced seizures of 'sudden right sided headache followed by vision of a bright spot of light in the right visual field, deviation of the eyes to the right and unresponsiveness'. Interictal EEGs showed 'bilateral centrotemporal spikes, giant somatosensory evoked spikes and generalized photoparoxysmal responses to IPS that were associated with massive myoclonic jerks. IPS elicited his habitual seizure of right sided elementary visual hallucinations and ipsilateral deviation of the eyes with no post-ictal deficit'. The ictal EEG starts with a high amplitude generalized discharge of polyspikes and slow waves with eyelid blinking. These discharges appear in a repetitive fashion during the whole duration of the ictus and cause eyelid blinking. A few seconds from onset there is also a left occipital discharge of fast spikes that appear in between the generalized discharges.

That occipital spikes may also occur with spikes

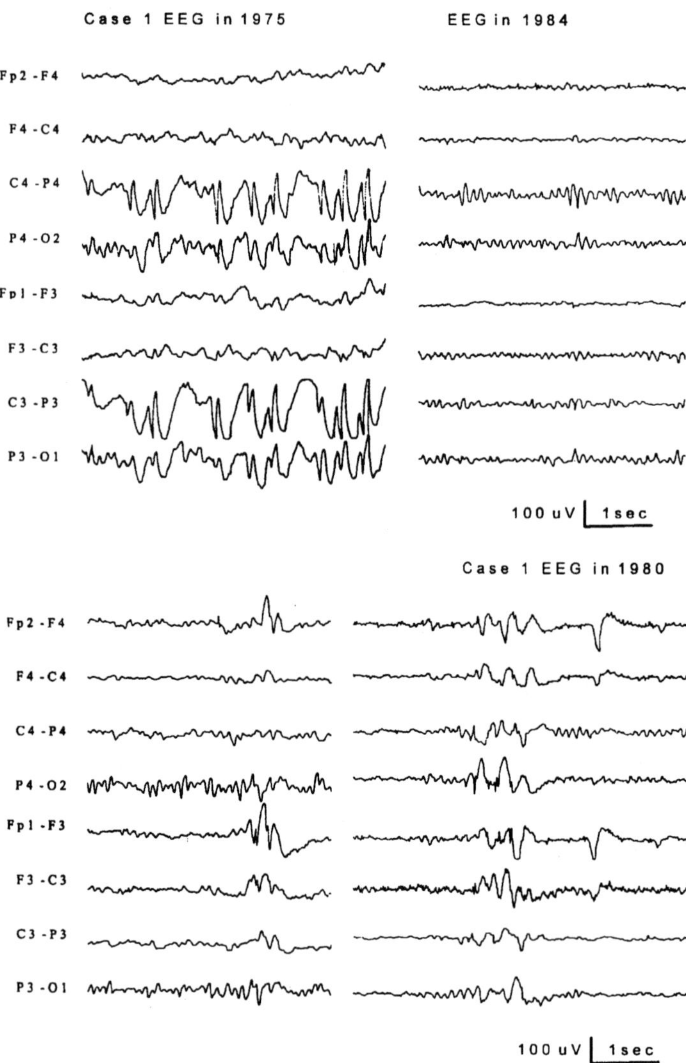

Fig. 10.10. Evolution of EEG of case 1 (Chapter 8) with EBOS also illustrated in Figs. 10.1 and 10.4. Brief generalized discharges occurred when occipital spikes were not very active.

in other locations is illustrated in Fig. 8.2 and Fig. 10.9.

Generalized discharges in benign childhood occipital seizures

Generalized discharges occur in 10–50 per cent[277,313,443,606] of patients with BOS. They usually consist of brief, 1–3 s, atypical or typical spike and slow wave complexes with a tendency to appear late during the EEG evolution (Figs. 10.10 and 10.11). They are usually infrequent, brief and are not associated with clinical manifestations.

Gastaut and Zifkin[313] found that 'generalized bilaterally synchronous spike and wave or polyspike and wave complexes, characteristic of primary generalized epilepsy; and Rolandic spikes, typical for benign partial epilepsy of childhood, were recorded in 19 of the 50 children (38 per cent) who had no clinical evidence of either of these forms of epilepsy. The coexistence of Rolandic spikes and typical

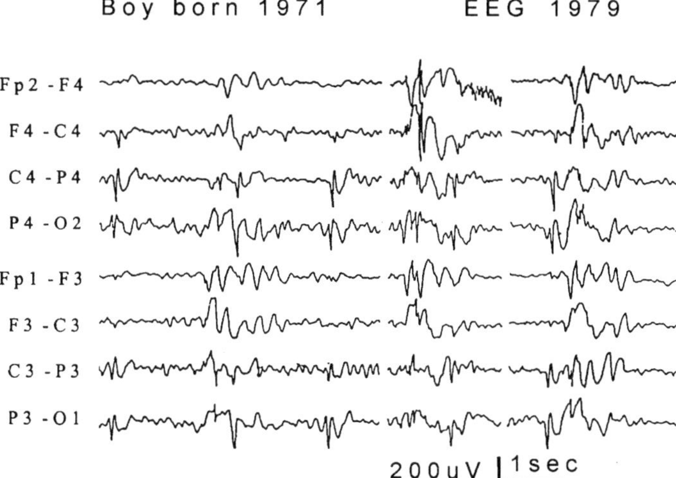

Fig. 10.11. Evolution of EEG of case 6, Table 13.1. Three brief generalized discharges occurred at age 8 years, 3 years after his last seizure. In some of them secondary generalization from the occipital regions is apparent. Compare this with previous EEG in Figs. 10.3a and 10.3b.
From Panayiotopoulos (1989)[606] with the permission of the editor of the Journal of Child Neurology.

occipital paroxysmal activity was seen principally in patients with hemiclonic seizures. It is noteworthy that a similar association was described by Beaussart (1972)[87] in children with benign partial epilepsy and nocturnal hemiclonic seizures.'[313]

This view reflects the selection criteria of Gastaut and Zifkin.[313] Figure 10.12 is from one of my patients, a 10-year-old girl, with intractable and severe typical absence seizures who also has occipital paroxysms in her EEG. Her mother and her maternal uncle are also amongst my patients with severe absences and GTCS that continue in adult life and are resistant to treatment. Based on my experience with a few other similar cases (Figs. 10.12, 11.1a and 11.1b), I am of the opinion that these are the most resistant cases of a syndrome of typical absence seizures with occipital involvement which is severe and cannot be considered as part of benign occipital seizures.

Beaumanoir 1983[74] found asymptomatic generalized discharges of polyspike or spike and slow wave in three of 11 patients with BOS who had 24 h EEG monitoring. One patient had also absence seizures.

Dulac *et al.* 1986[254] described 19 patients who had onset of partial seizures but later developed GTCS, myoclonic jerks, absences alone or in combination. Fourteen of these patients had a mean onset of seizures at 10 years with motor partial seizures, frequently secondary generalization and 'eventually associated absences or generalized myoclonias'. Their EEG showed spontaneous generalized discharges in all, generalized photoparoxysmal responses in 11 and centrotemporal spikes in 12 patients. The other five patients had a median onset at 4 years with 'visual illusions of micropsia or frightening visual hallucinations'. Three developed GTCS, myoclonic jerks or absences. Spontaneous discharges that were accentuated with IPS occurred in all and four had centrotemporal spikes. The authors concluded that sodium valproate was more effective than other drugs that are considered specific for partial seizures. They constitute an exceptional group of patients for whom we do not know much about the underlying cause, evolution and treatment.

Panayiotopoulos[606] reported that four of eight children with EBOS had brief discharges of generalized spike and slow wave with a tendency to appear late during the EEG evolution. Two of nine cases of Kivity and Lerman (1992)[443] also had brief generalized discharges. Ferrie *et al.* (1996)[277] found that only 14 (12 per cent) of their patients had diffuse generalized discharges.

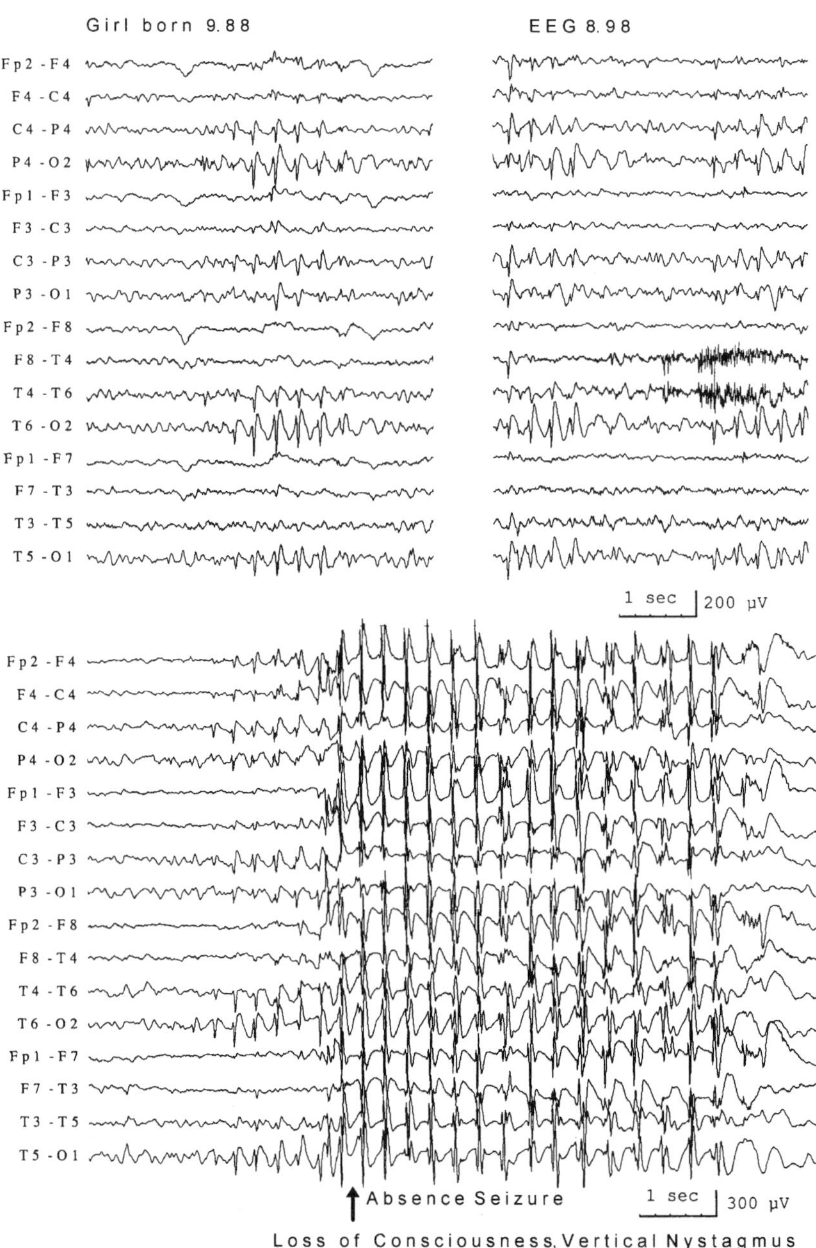

Fig. 10.12. Video-EEG of a 10-year-old girl, with intractable and severe typical absence seizures who also has occipital paroxysms. Her mother and her maternal uncle are also amongst my patients with severe absences and GTCS that continue in adult life and are resistant to treatment. Based on my experience with a few other similar cases I am of the opinion that these are the most resistant cases of a syndrome of typical absence seizures with occipital involvement which is severe and cannot be considered as part of benign occipital seizures. This case may be comparable from the EEG point of view with the case of Gastaut, 1950[300] (see Fig. 9 of Gastaut[308]) which is probably erroneously considered as the first reported case of benign childhood occipital seizures.

Late onset BOS and continuous spikes and waves during slow wave sleep (CSWS)

Only three cases are reported in the literature with BOS that later developed CSWS with or without clinical and mental deterioration.[52,762] They all had LBOS or the Gastaut type of BOS. Aso *et al.* (1987)[52] reported a normal boy who at the age of 7 had occipital seizures with visual hallucinations of flickering lights and non-visual symptoms of tachypnea, pale face, generalized motor symptoms and unresponsiveness and an EEG with occipital paroxysms. This later evolved to continuous spike-waves during sleep without psychomotor change or atonic seizures. Tenenbaum *et al.* (1977)[762] reported an atypical and rather aggressive seizure and behaviour evolution of a 'Gastaut type'-like LBOS. These were two boys with clinical and EEG features of the late onset childhood epilepsy with occipital paroxysms (visual hallucinations and occipital spikes) who experienced severe cognitive deterioration associated with continuous spike wave activity during slow wave sleep. Neurological examination and brain imaging were normal but both children had some learning difficulties, probably before or at the onset of seizures. One child showed global improvement in behaviour and partial restoration of cognitive functions after control of seizures and normalization of the EEG. The authors concluded that 'their findings suggest a spectrum ranging from a benign course for most children with idiopathic partial epilepsies to the syndrome of Continuous Spikes and Waves During Slow Wave Sleep' (see Chapter 17).

Evolution of occipital spikes in benign childhood occipital seizures

The presence or absence of occipital paroxysms does not predict clinical outcome. Occipital spikes may persist years after clinical remission and are usually 'resistant' to drug treatment although some temporary suppression may be seen initially. However, there is a tendency for the occipital spikes to decrease in amplitude and abundance with progressive age. They usually disappear within 2–6 years (median 5 years) from onset of seizures but in others they may be recorded only once in a series of EEGs or persist and consistently be recorded up to the age of 16 years.

Other types of EEG abnormalities such as centrotemporal spikes or generalized discharges may appear when occipital spikes are active or more often later as the children become older and occipital spikes have remitted.

Cumulative results from four longitudinal studies of 70 children with BOS[74,367,605,750] with long clinical and EEG follow-up indicate that the 'life-span' of occipital paroxysms is long (Fig. 10.13). The mean age at first EEG with occipital paroxysms was 5.8 ± 2.5 years (range 2–14 years), and they persisted in regularly taken EEGs over years before their disappearance at a mean age of 11.4 ± 4.3 years (range 4–26 years). This means that they persisted for a mean of 5.7 ± 3.8 years (median 5 years and range 2 months to 20 years). The rate and degree of attrition varied significantly between patients irrespective of clinical course. In 19 per cent the EEG normalized within the first 2 years after the first demonstration of occipital paroxysms, in another 23 per cent within 2–4 years, 27 per cent within 4–6 years, 15 per cent within 6–8 years, 7 per cent within 8–10 years and in the remaining 9 per cent in the next 10–20 years (Fig. 10.13). Most of these patients were treated with anti-epileptic medication which did not appear to influence the occipital spikes.

These findings are qualitatively similar but quantitatively different from the attrition rate found by Kellaway[438] in children with occipital spikes irrespective of cause, with or without clinical seizures. In these children there was an initial period of one to two years of a high attrition rate, with 50 per cent to 60 per cent of them losing their focus within 12 months of its first demonstration. Within five years, only about 15 per cent to 22 per cent of the foci were still present. The trend was similar for all such foci, irrespective of location (occipital, frontal, centrotemporal). In children who did not have seizures and who were not treated, the attrition curves for occipital spikes were essentially similar to those of the group as a whole. The attrition rate had an L-shaped curve which made Kellaway[438] 'suggest the possibility that the steep and the flatter parts of the curves may represent two disparate aetiological or functional patient categories; this idea is given some credence by the fact that the attrition curve for spike foci consequent to deprivation or aberration of visual input dating from infancy

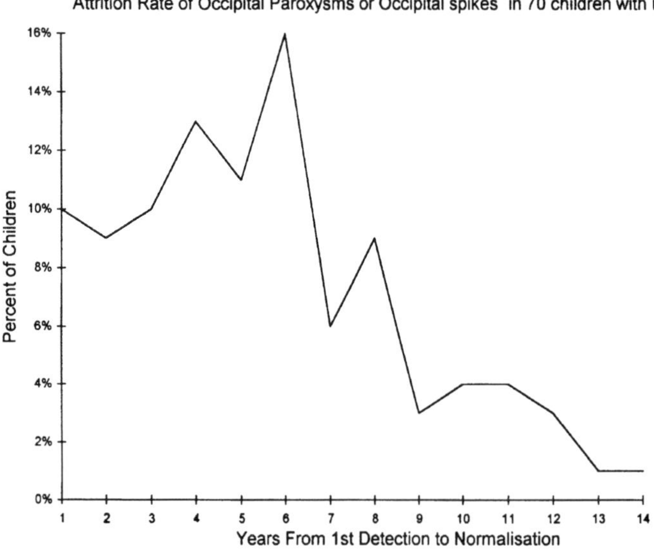

Fig. 10.13. Attrition rate of occipital paroxysms and occipital spikes in 70 children with benign occipital seizures estimated from four studies.[74,367,605,750] *See text for details.*

tends to persist into adult life. A large subgroup of temporal foci also shows a strong tendency to persist'.

He concluded that 'The important inference of the high incidence of spike foci in early and middle childhood, as compared to later life, the particular distribution of foci according to age, and the tendency for foci to disappear with increasing age, is that ontogenetic factors play an important role in their natural history and possibly in their genesis'.

However, occipital spikes do not have a long life span for all children. I have demonstrated in this book that occipital spikes may occur only once (see for example case 26 in Chapter 9), may not be seen in the first EEG (Fig. 10.14) and that they may have a short life span.

Occipital spikes in normal children, in children with congenital or early acquired defective vision, unselected children with or without seizures referred for EEG, and other cryptogenic or symptomatic occipital epilepsies

Occipital spikes in normal children

From extensive studies in normal children regarding detection and localization of spikes, two significant conclusions can be drawn:

(a) Centrotemporal spikes mainly occur in school-age children with a peak age at discovery around 8–9 years and they are 9.7 times more frequent than the occipital spikes.

(b) Occipital spikes mainly occur in pre-school-age children with a peak age 4–5 years.
Frontal and spikes at other locations occur much less frequent and do not have any particular peak of occurrence.

In four main studies[154,260,331,586] of 6392 normal children aged mainly from 5–6 to 12–15 years, the prevalence of occipital spikes varied from 0–0.3 per cent (median 0.1 per cent) while in the same age group the prevalence of centrotemporal spikes varied from 0.7 to 3.5 per cent (median 2.2 per cent) and of frontal spikes from 0 to 0.6 per cent (their higher prevalence in one study[260] is because they were found in three children who also had centrotemporal spikes together with the frontal ones).

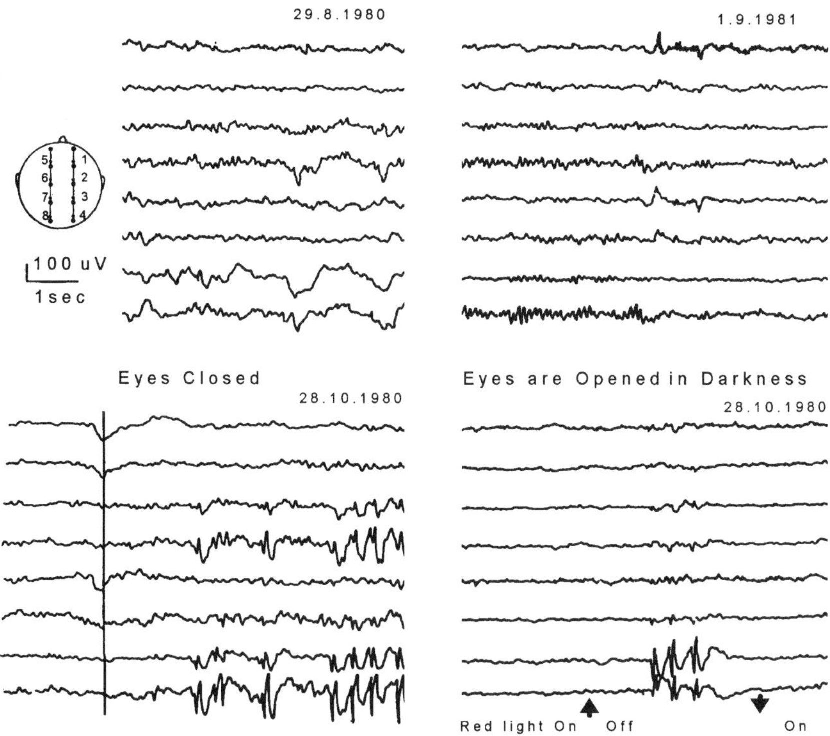

Fig. 10.14. Serial EEGs of a girl with a single, one and a half hour prolonged, nocturnal seizure of the Panayiotopoulos type. Slow delta waves are seen in the posterior regions mainly on the left with unilateral poverty of alpha-rhythm and scattered small occipital spikes two days after the fit (upper left, 29.8.80). A second EEG (lower traces, 28.10.80), two months later, demonstrated high amplitude occipital paroxysms which were seen on eyes-closed and in darkness. Fixation on a red spot of light inhibited the abnormalities (lower–right). One year later, her EEG was normal (upper right, 1.9.81) and has remained normal up to her last follow-up many years later.
From Panayiotopoulos, 1989[605] by permission of the editor of Annals of Neurology.

However, in younger normal children aged 2–4 years the prevalence of occipital spikes increases to 0.9 per cent while that of centrotemporal spikes is low at 0.3 per cent (see Table 10.1). Thus overall, children aged 1–16 years of age have a 2.0 per cent median prevalence for centrotemporal spikes and 0.6 per cent for occipital spikes. Therefore, centrotemporal spikes are 9.7 times more frequent than the occipital spikes in normal children from 1 to 16 years of age.

Table 10.1. EEG spike foci in normal children

	Number	CTS (%)	OS (%)	FS (%)	GD (%)
From age 5 and 6 years to 12 and 14 years: cumulative results of four studies[154,260,331,586]					
	6392	2.2	0.1	0.1	1.0
From age 1 and 2 years to 4 and 5 years: cumulative results of two studies[260,331]					
	936	0.3	0.9	0.1	0.3

CTS = Centrotemporal spikes; FS = Frontal spikes; OS = Occipital spikes; GD = Generalized discharges.

Gibbs and Gibbs, 1967[331] found that amongst the EEGs of 1802 normal children aged 2–14 years the prevalence of occipital spikes was 0.4 per cent which was slightly less than the 0.53 per cent for centrotemporal spikes and much higher than the 0.03 per cent for frontal spikes. These results are compatible to those of Eeg-Oloffson *et al.*, 1971[260] who amongst 743 well defined normal children aged 1 to 15 years found 14 (1.9 per cent) children who had definite focal spikes. Two (0.3 per cent) children aged 2 and 5 years had right sided occipital spikes. Centrotemporal spikes alone (nine children) or with frontal spikes (three children) occurred in 1.6 per cent. More precisely, occipital spikes were found in two (0.95 per cent) of 210 children aged 1–5 years and none amongst 533 children aged 6–15 years. Conversely, centrotemporal spikes were found in only one (0.48 per cent) of the 210 children aged 1–5 years and in 11 (2.6 per cent) of the oldest group. The mean age of children with centrotemporal spikes was 8.6 ± 2.8 (median 8) years. The median age of children with occipital spikes was 4 years. It is also interesting that two of the children with centrotemporal spikes developed paroxysmal activity during IPS which was localized in the posterior regions.

That the prevalence of occipital spikes is reduced at older age is also shown by the results of Cavazzutti *et al.*[154] and Okubo *et al.*[586] who found a prevalence of 0.1 per cent of occipital spikes in children older than 6 years (Table 5.2).

Occipital spikes in children with congenital or early acquired defective vision

Many studies[83,324,325,333,438,440,464,487] have demonstrated that EEG occipital spikes develop in children with congenital or early acquired defective or deranged vision (retrolental fibroplasia, optic nerve lesions, anophthalmia, amblyopia, cataracts, strabismus) provided that this defect exists from birth or develops during the early maturation process of the visual cortex probably up to the age of 4 years.[438] Occipital spikes first appear towards the end of the first year of life or within 7–10 months from the onset of the visual defect. Initially, the occipital spikes are very fast (needle spikes), singular or polyspikes often recorded only during slow wave sleep. However, their amplitude, frequency and duration tend to increase with age, finally taking the form of spike and slow wave complexes. This evolution of the needle spikes is similar regardless of pathological cause of the visual defect. It is attributed according to Kellaway[438] 'to increased synchronization of the activity of involved neurones and increase in the size of the involved neuronal aggregate'. Furthermore, Kellaway[438] highlights the significance of this as follows: 'The demonstration that spike foci may arise as a consequence of a pathological process acting peripherally (on the sense organ) is the first evidence we have that such foci, which have classically been considered a sign of a palpable brain lesion, may be engendered by an agent that does not act directly at the site of the focus. Clearly, spike foci elsewhere, for which no aetiologic cause can now be specified, might also have their origin in defects of afferent input or other pathophysiological mechanisms presently unidentified. The recognized causes of focal electrical abnormalities (trauma, tumour, infection, etc.) may in fact account for a minority of the EEG spike foci seen in children.'[438]

Occipital spikes in unselected children with or without seizures referred for EEG

The age-dependent prevalence of occipital and centrotemporal spikes in normal children should be expected in view of the similar age-dependent distribution in unselected EEG referrals of children with or without seizures.[331,438] Kellaway[438] reported that the overall prevalence of spike foci, at single or multiple locations, in a cohort 35,458 children referred for EEG for various reasons was 10.7 per cent. Occipital spikes had a peak at age 4 years and approximately 50 per cent of children with occipital foci were younger than age 5 years. Centrotemporal spikes had a peak at 8 years and only one-third of children with this localization were younger than 5 years. Frontal spikes were equally distributed though all ages. Centrotemporal spikes (63 per cent) were twice as frequent than the occipital spikes (29 per cent) while frontal spikes (8 per cent) were unusual.[438] This age-dependent distribution and prevalence of occipital, centrotemporal and frontal spike foci is also apparent in relevant histograms provided by Gibbs and Gibbs[331] based on 19,350 consecutive EEG referrals with spike discharges. Furthermore, Gibbs and Gibbs[331] amongst 38,082 routine, consecutive EEG referrals of children and adults, found occipital spikes in 974 (2.56 per cent), mid-temporal spikes in 1003 (2.63 per cent), frontal spikes in 322 (0.85 per cent), parietal in 390 (1.02 per cent), anterior temporal spikes in 3358 (8.82 per cent) and multiple spike foci in 1655 (4.35 per cent) compared with 'petit mal' discharges in 1688 (4.4 per cent) or all types of generalized spike wave discharges in 2197 (5.77 per cent).

The results of Trojaborg[776] in another classical study of 'Focal spike discharges in children, a longitudinal study' were similar.

There are also many other reports on occipital and centrotemporal spikes in children without seizures, the best known being Fois *et al.*, 1968[286] and Lerman and Kivity,1981.[485]

Fois *et al.*[286] from 3000 children's EEG referrals found 110 (3.7 per cent) children who had unequivocal focal spikes without 'clinical signs for what is usually considered epilepsy'. Hyperactivity, nervousness, sleep disturbances, headache, abdominal pain, speech retardation, enuresis, vomiting, fainting spells and rage attacks were the main problems of these children. It is interesting that 12 children had 'paroxysmal vomiting'. According to the table provided 106 children had spike foci during sleep but only 56 of them also showed these foci in the awake record. In sleep, occipital foci were found in 36 (34 per cent or 1.2 per cent of the total 3000 EEGs) being bilateral in 18 children (occipital paroxysms are well illustrated in their figures) while 'parietal spikes' were recorded in 50 (47.2 per cent and 1.7 per cent), midtemporal in six (5.7 per cent and 0.2 per cent) , frontal in four (3.8 per cent and 0.1 per cent) and multiple foci in nine (8.5 per cent and 0.3 per cent). Fifteen children (15.1 per cent) also had associated generalized spike and wave discharges during sleep only. In awake EEG, occipital spikes were found in 11, parietal in 32, midtemporal in one, frontal in five and multiple foci in five children. Thus, parieto-temporal foci were 1.55 times more frequent than the occipital ones and sleep mainly facilitated the parietal and occipital spikes. The age of these children ranged from 2 to 16 years with the majority being between 5 and 9 years.

Lerman and Kivity,1981[485]studied 100 children (64 were boys) who did not have seizures but in EEGs showed centrotemporal spikes (78 children), occipital spikes alone (five children) or combined with centrotemporal spikes (14) and centrotemporal spikes with generalized spike wave discharges (three). Their age at discovery of the spikes ranged from 3 to 15 years (mean 7.7 years). The main reasons for referral were behaviour problems, headache, trauma, endocrine problems, nocturnal enuresis and abdominal pain. In follow-up studies of 1–16 years the EEG foci disappeared within months to as long as after 10 years but mainly within 1–2 years. None of these children who it was possible to review developed epileptic seizures.

Interictal EEG in cryptogenic/symptomatic occipital epilepsies

In symptomatic occipital epilepsy the interictal EEG may be normal. However, more often it may show unilateral occipital slowing ipsilateral to the lesion and this may be associated with asymmetrical physiological rhythms such as alpha, lamda waves, photic following and positive occipital sleep transients. An occipital focus of unilateral or bilateral spikes or sharp wave and slow wave complexes is more likely to be seen in children than adults. However, in symptomatic occipital epilepsy, asymmetries of physiological rhythms should be noted but interpreted with caution. These asymmetries are rather non-specific particularly in children for whom the alpha rhythm is higher in the non-dominant hemisphere, frequently lambda waves and positive occipital sleep transients are asymmetric, and photic following is usually higher in the 'epileptogenic' side of the brain.

Occipital spikes are rarely seen in adults with symptomatic occipital seizures, more often there are runs of slow waves or sharp and slow waves in the posterior temporal and occipital regions. Salanova *et al.*[700] reported for patients with severe occipital epilepsy that surface EEGs showed posterior temporal-occipital epileptiform discharges in 46 per cent of patients. Only 18 per cent had electronegative spiking limited to occipital electrodes. The results in these neurosurgical series of symptomatic occipital epilepsy[131,700,811] indicate that interictal EEG abnormalities are rarely strictly occipital. The most common localization is in the posterior temporal regions and less than one-fifth show occipital spikes. Also, most of the EEGs have an abnormal background and focal posterior slow activity depending on the extent, nature and progression of the structural abnormality. Kuzniecky[459] suggested that there might be a correlation between the type of underlying pathology and the electrographic abnormalities. During his recent experience with colleagues,[457] patients with occipital lobe developmental malformation would present with frequent interictal spiking or low-amplitude, fast, sharp activity almost resembling ictal activity. In contrast, patients with polymicrogyria or destructive lesions, such as porencephaly, have a paucity of interictal epileptiform discharges over the occipital lobe. There were 10 patients with occipital lobe cortical developmental malformations and epileptic seizures.[457] The interictal EEGs usually showed unilateral abnormality in the posterior regions with occipital preponderance. Only one of 10 patients had a normal EEG and only three had normal alpha rhythm. Three patients had exclusively focal 'occipital epileptogenic abnormality' consisting of almost continuous occipital spikes (similar to those of occipital sharp waves of BOS) which were associated with 'fast spiking activity during sleep' (similar to that of ictal fast spike activity of BOS). Surface ictal EEG of eight patients showed localized occipital onset in two, regional parieto-occipital onset in three, posterior diffuse low voltage fast activity in one and bilateral temporal theta in the last two patients.

One of the most cited reports is that of Ludwig and Marsan,1975[513] on clinical ictal patterns in epileptic patients with occipital EEG foci. Most of the patients had cryptogenic/symptomatic epilepsies. Few statistically significant differences in clinical or ictal patterns were found between subjects with purely focal occipital involvement and those with temporal and temporo-parietal spread or minor additional independent foci. On the other hand, cases with bilateral synchronous occipital spike activity (eight patients) appeared to reflect a different type of epileptic disorder. The EEG in these eight patients consisted of 'synchronous sharp slow complexes at 1–2 Hz of rapid spikes and waves interspersed with polyspikes. Most had abnormal neurological examinations, three had encephalopathies, three had miscellaneous disorders and the cause was unknown in two. Clinically, this group had the lowest incidence of visual aura, the highest percentage of non focal seizures "primarily generalized or non motor" and the highest incidence of metabolic abnormalities'.

Gilliam and Wyllie, 1995[335] reported seven patients with onset of occipital seizures in childhood and abnormal MRI findings in six of them. Ictal symptoms with amaurosis as the prominent feature as well as post-ictal migraine-like symptoms had striking clinical similarities with LBOS of the Gastaut type. Furthermore, six had occipital spikes often appearing with eyes-closed and one patient had 'independent bilateral central-temporal spikes'. The authors rightly concluded that 'the constellation of ictal amaurosis, occipital paroxysms, and post-ictal migrainous symptoms does not necessarily signify a benign, nonlesional epilepsy; MRI is recommended for such patients'. However, there is no information regarding other EEG abnormalities, particularly as three of these children had abnormal neurological state, and therefore this conclusion should not be considered to apply to BOS, which is idiopathic, i.e. normal neurological examination is needed.

Symptomatic occipital epilepsy in coeliac disease is probably the most likely of all to imitate clinically and in EEGs the LBOS of the Gastaut type.[338,343–345,409,516,821] This interesting association between occipital seizures, bilateral occipital calcifications and coeliac disease has been well documented mainly due to the Italian Group on coeliac disease and epilepsy.[343,345,409] The age at onset is 2–14 years (mainly around 6 years) with clinical and EEG manifestations indistinguishable from late onset BOS.[344,409] Thus, awake EEGs particularly at the early stages of the disease are indistinguishable from those of BOS with occipital paroxysms that attenuate with eyes-open. However, sleep EEG polyspike discharges and clinical or EEG photosensitivity may be seen in this symptomatic form of occipital lobe seizures and this may differentiate them from the idiopathic form of the late onset BOS. Some of these children with coeliac disease may progress to more severe forms of seizures and EEG abnormalities of symptomatic generalized epilepsies and develop severe learning difficulties (see Chapter 7).

Comparison of occipital spikes in idiopathic and cryptogenic/symptomatic occipital epilepsy of children

That occipital spikes are more frequent in idiopathic than symptomatic occipital epilepsies in children is well documented in many studies as shown in the reports of Terasaki *et al.* (1987)[763] and Dalla Bernardina *et al.* (1993).[192]

Terasaki *et al.* (1987)[763] compared 26 idiopathic and nine symptomatic cases of occipital seizures. The idiopathic compared with the symptomatic group had:

(a) More frequent occipital spikes (52.2 per cent versus 11.1 per cent, $P < 0.02$).

(b) Less frequent multiple spike (39.1 per cent versus 66.7 per cent). Centrotemporal spikes were found in six of 23 idiopathic patients.

(c) Occipital discharges were more frequently suppressed by eye opening (in all seven cases tested) and increased by hyperventilation (nine of 15 cases examined). Conversely, in the symptomatic group occipital spikes were not suppressed by eye opening in any of three cases and were activated by hyperventilation in two cases (28.6 per cent).

(d) Occipital spikes were less often activated (23.5 per cent) and more often reduced (35.3 per cent) by sleep. In symptomatic cases, 'these were easily induced by sleep'.

Photosensitivity was found in one third of each group.

The results of Dalla Bernardina *et al.* (1993),[192] who compared the clinico-EEG manifestations of 64 children with idiopathic (33 patients), cryptogenic (12) and symptomatic (19) occipital epilepsies are different. From the EEG point of view, idiopathic occipital epilepsy was more frequently characterized by occipital spike and slow waves (66.5 per cent versus 5 per cent in the symptomatic group), while occipital spikes were equally increased during sleep for both groups (51.5 per cent versus 42 per cent) and equally attenuated on eyes-open (42.5 per cent versus 31.5 per cent). Dalla Bernardina *et al.* (1993)[192] also highlighted a significant EEG differentiating factor that is almost characteristic of symptomatic occipital epilepsy. These are fast spikes and polyspikes, polymorphous slow waves, brief electrical suppression following the spikes and morphological modifications of the paroxysmal abnormalities during sleep that were seen only in the symptomatic and the cryptogenic groups.[192]

What are occipital paroxysms?

Erroneous arguments against the existence of benign occipital seizures at any childhood age are based on populations of children who have any type of EEG abnormality (spikes, multiple spikes, slow waves with abortive small spikes) in the posterior regions that appear mainly with eyes-closed and attenuate with eyes-open (Fig. 10.15). These, in accordance with the definitions applied by all authors who described benign childhood occipital seizures and their EEG accompaniments, are not occipital paroxysms. Polyspikes, tiny spikes intermixed with slow waves, scattered occipital spikes as seen in photosensitive patients or slow waves that happen to attenuate with eyes-open, are not occipital paroxysms and should not be confused with benign childhood occipital seizures. See the definitions and clarifications regarding occipital spikes and occipital paroxysms at the beginning of this chapter.

Ictal EEG of benign childhood occipital seizures:

Brief description

Surface ictal EEG[18,52,57,63,74,76,82,212,213,215,284,304,313,370,371,561,568,648,649,651,677,700,751,763,811] in occipital seizures, irrespective of cause, usually manifests paroxysmal fast activity, fast spiking or both, localized in the occipital regions with occasional gradual anterior spreading and generalization with irregular spike wave discharges or monomorphic spike and wave activity (Fig. 10.16). A brief occipital flattening may be seen before the fast rhythmic pattern.[57]

There are many reported cases of ictal EEG recordings of benign childhood occipital seizures.[18,52,74,76,77,212,277,312,519,568,763,793] The most common ictal EEG pattern of visual hallucinations is sudden onset of paroxysmal fast activity or fast spikes, 10–12 Hz, packed together or a mixture of

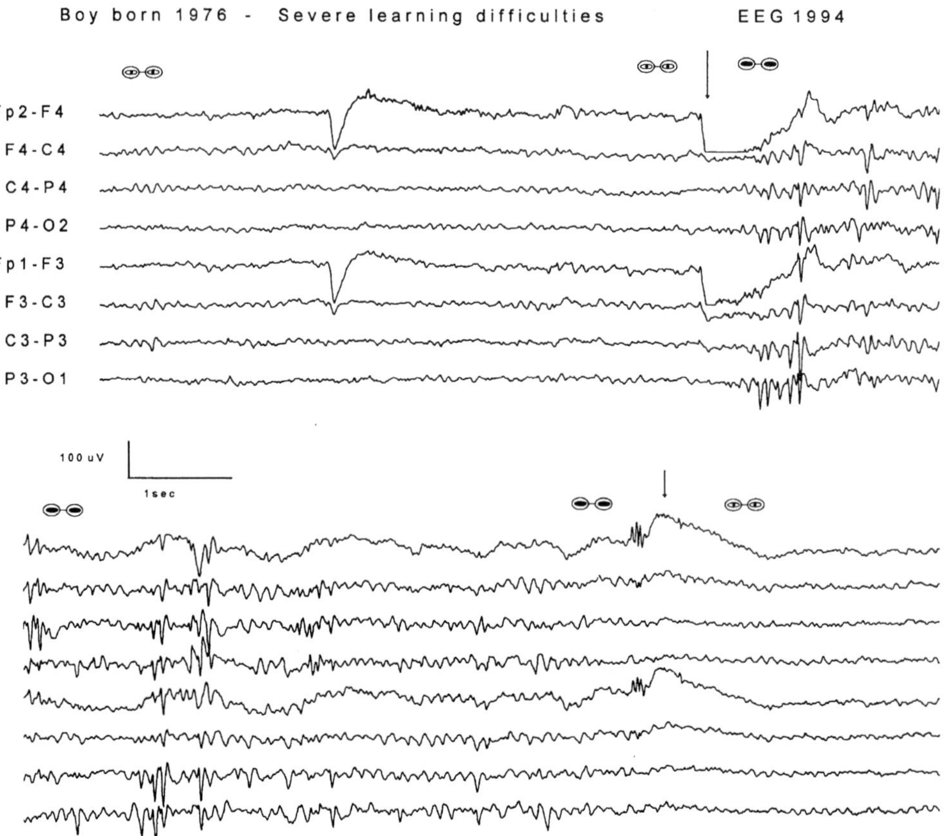

Fig. 10.15. Occipital spikes in a boy with severe learning difficulties, white matter lesions in MRI and a ring chromosome. He has spontaneous and photically induced GTCS, absences and eyelid myoclonus. His EEG persistently showed these bilateral occipital spikes which occur only when eyes are closed but not in darkness or any other condition of elimination of central vision and fixation. This child would be erroneously included in studies of the so-called 'reactive occipital epileptiform activity', a meaningless term invented only to confuse.

both fast activity and fast spikes. This starts from one or both occipital electrodes often spreading to more anterior regions. The amplitude of fast rhythms or spikes is initially small (10–30 μV) and certainly much smaller than that of the interictal occipital paroxysms which stop a few seconds before the onset of the ictal discharge. Ictal localized fast activity and spikes increase in amplitude and frequency and progress to higher amplitude spikes intermixed with slow waves. Visual hallucinations usually occur during the paroxysmal fast and spike activity. Blindness may also occur during that EEG stage but in other occasions it may appear during a subsequent relative flattening of the EEG. The EEG ictal occipital discharge and associated clinical symptoms may last for seconds but it may also be prolonged for minutes to more than half an hour. Secondary spreading with symptoms from other cortical areas and unilateral or generalized convulsions may follow. The EEG during ictal vomiting (Fig. 10.17) appears to be more diffuse, mainly right sided but certainly it can also be left sided only, with high amplitude sharp slow waves intermixed with fast rhythms and spikes. post-ictally, if the seizures are brief, the EEG shows a relative normalization with some arrest of the occipital paroxysms. Usually, there is no post-ictal localized slow activity unless the seizure is prolonged or progressed to secondary GTCS.

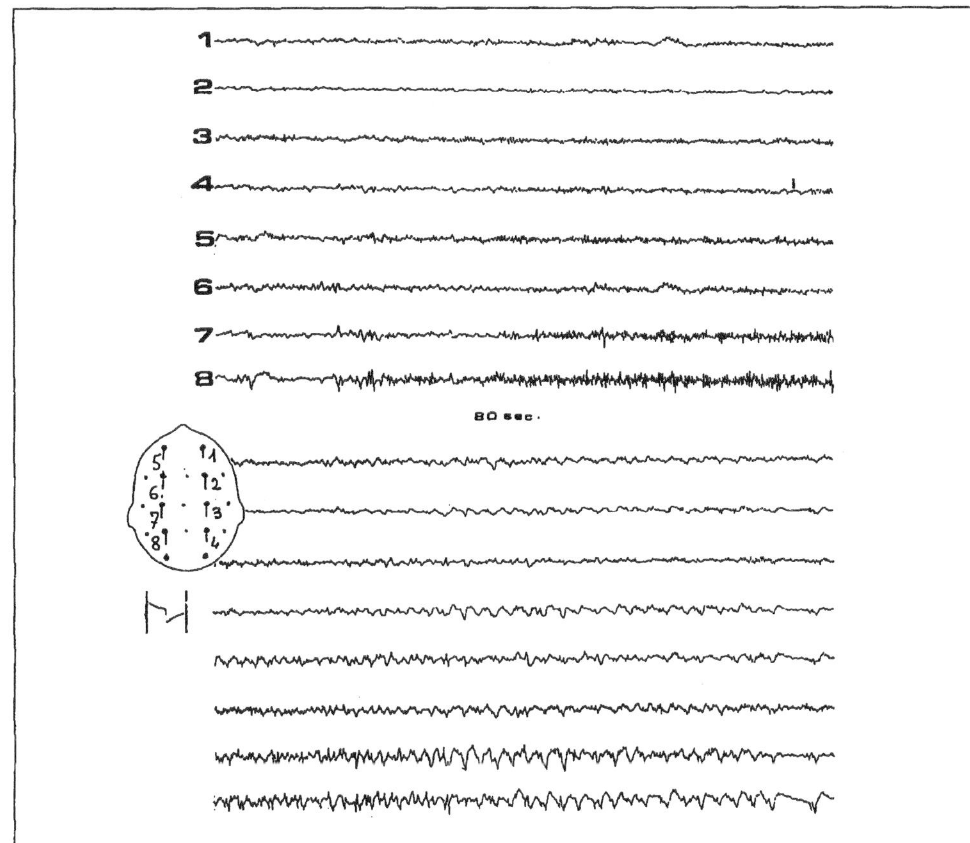

Fig. 10.16. Ictal EEG of a boy aged 6 years with visual seizures, from Beaumanoir, 1993.[77]
The seizure started from the left occipital region with fast rhythms associated with 'scintillating phosphenes'. 4 s later this spread to the parietal regions and the child saw 'a bundle of coloured balloons swinging in his right hemifield'. This lasted for 40 s followed by slow waves, progressively becoming slower and diffuse over the whole brain. At this stage he complained of clouded vision.
This boy was normal physically and intellectually and also had a normal CT brain scan. At age 3 years he had a nocturnal left hemi-convulsion. His first EEG showed occipital paroxysms with FOS. Since the age of 4 years he started having frequent, brief visual seizures (simple coloured visual hallucinations) provoked by sudden darkness.
[With the kind permission of A. Beaumanoir and the publisher John Libbey.]

Ictal EEG of benign childhood occipital seizures:

Literature Review

The main contribution in this field comes from Beaumanoir alone or with her associates[74,76,77,82,84] and De Romanis and colleagues.[212,213,215]

Beaumanoir (1983)[74] reported one patient with diurnal and nine with nocturnal seizures who had ictal EEG confirmation. The diurnal seizure showed a discharge of focal occipital rapid spikes becoming progressively slower. All nocturnal seizures started with a discharge of unilateral occipital spikes at 10 Hz with a remission of the interictal occipital spikes. This phase of unilateral sided spikes was followed, after 10–20 s, by slow monomorphic activity of spikes and waves localized in one or both the posterior areas. In some seizures the occipital discharge of 10 Hz spikes spread to the parietal regions of one or both hemispheres before the appearance of the monomorphic spikes and slow waves. None of the seizures lasted for more than 2 min.

In another report Beaumanoir, 1993[77] presented three cases of ictal recordings during visual ictal manifestations of children with interictal occipital paroxysms and reached the following conclusion which we should remember: 'Simple partial occipital seizures with positive signs are characterized by fast spike activities which, when slowing down, can reach neighbouring regions of the scalp. While the amplitude of the ictal activity increases, the frequency of repetition lessens. In oculoclonic seizures, spikes and spike and waves are typical of the last part of the discharge. There are usually no post-ictal abnormalities. Phosphenes are related to the fast spike activity, often quickly involving the two hemispheres; on the contrary, when the discharge is slower complex hallucinations may take place. In oculoclonic seizures, a localized ictal fast spike rhythm may be observed before the deviation of the eyes.'[77] Furthermore, she also concluded that the ictal EEG during 'temporary blindness is characterized by pseudoperiodic slow waves and spikes which are different from those of positive visual hallucinations'. See Figure 10.16.

Beaumanoir (1993)[76] also stressed the importance of the post-ictal EEG, emphasizing that *'Contrary to the prolonged post-critical EEG abnormalities of migrainous attacks, the post-ictal EEG of occipital seizures frequently returns quickly to the preictal state'.* I have italicised this significant conclusion of Beaumanoir[76] because it is a very important point in the EEG differentiation between occipital seizures and aura of migraine.

De Romanis *et al.*, 1988,[215]1991[213] provided us with most impressive, excellent ictal EEGs in patients whose interictal EEG had occipital paroxysms. Clinically, these patients had occipital seizures similar to those of LBOS of the Gastaut type though the authors[213,215] felt that they also had migraine with aura or basilar migraine. Most interesting is the ictal EEG of a patient 'during the phase of positive and negative ictal visual symptoms'. The seizure starts with rapid occipital spikes when the patients reports bright coloured spots in both hemifields for 23 s. This is followed by amaurosis with simultaneous flattening of the EEG for about 20 s. Subsequently, the 'EEG showed the reappearance of low amplitude sharp waves for 90 s, in the above-mentioned areas, with higher voltage on the right side and a pseudorhythmic pattern followed by a normal activity for 4 min. After that, sharp waves gradually increased in frequency and amplitude, prevalent on the right side for 5 min, and were followed by interictal activity. The above phenomena were followed by nausea, vomiting and photophobia, lasting for about 8 h. A left homonymous hemianopsia, that disappeared after 24 h, was detected by visual field examination'. The same patient, at the age of 24 years, had ictal EEG 'characterized by 50–60 μV sharp-waves and tiny spikes of the same pattern of temporal localization and evolution during the occurrence of "phosphenes".'

Another patient of De Romanis *et al.* (case 14),[213,215] was a 12-year-old boy with ictal EEG at age 10, during a 'migraine attack' with a 2 Hz high voltage activity in the left hemisphere and spike-wave complexes in an almost continuous sequence. This was followed by a secondary generalized seizure. My view is that this was an occipital seizure progressing to secondary GTCS but De Romanis *et al.* 1988,[215] 1991[213] are experienced physicians in this field and their interpretation should also be respected. See also page 218 and 221–222.

De Romanis (1993)[212] also presented seven children who had interictal unilateral or bilateral occipital paroxysms. All had ictal EEG that 'showed diffuse high voltage delta activity associated with spikes and sharp waves or diffuse delta activity which could be recorded from 1–7 days'. Figures of ictal EEGs show that they are mainly dominated by spikes and clusters of rapid spikes superimposed onto slow waves.

Newton and Aicardi (1983)[568] and Aicardi and Newton (1987)[18] presented ictal records for three patients. These 'comprised a rhythmic discharge of spikes at about 10 Hz, starting on the side of the maximal abnormality, spreading to the opposite hemisphere while becoming progressively slower. In a fourth case, very little paroxysmal EEG activity was seen during seizures, although the interictal complexes disappeared several seconds before the onset of the attacks'.

Gastaut and Zifkin,1987[313] recorded spontaneous electro-clinical seizures in six patients. Electrical seizures during sleep were recorded in another five. An ictal EEG of case 2 shows bilateral paroxysmal fast activity, 16–18 Hz for 8 s, while the child sees stars. In another case (no. 5), the seizure starts with fast occipital spikes predominating on the left and a visual hallucination of the number 57. This is followed after 30 s by bilateral fast activity mainly in the posterior regions with fast spikes on the left and ictal blindness. In their case no. 4 the visual hallucination 'here it comes, I see yellow' starts with a high amplitude singular generalized sharp and slow wave (higher in the right occipital and posterior temporal regions) followed by a 3–4 s normalization before the appearance of sharp slow waves with posterior paroxysmal fast activity followed by sharp theta waves and generalized fast activity. Gastaut and Zifkin[313] concluded that 'The EEG showed occipital ictal activity of spikes or paroxysmal fast activity originating from an occipital lobe and often spreading to adjacent areas and to the other hemisphere'.

Aso *et al.* (1987)[52] presented ictal EEGs for three patients. One child with idiopathic occipital seizures had 'ictally rhythmic slow waves' and inter-ictally 'sporadic slow waves'. In two of their cryptogenic/symptomatic cases this started with low voltage, unilateral occipital paroxysmal fast activity 'followed by rhythmic occipital spikes of increasing amplitude and decreasing frequency, spreading to other areas and finally followed by generalized irregular spikes and waves'. Ictally one of these children had blinking and blurring of vision.

Terasaki *et al.* (1987)[763] reported that the ictal EEGs in five cases 'showed repetitive occipital spikes or bursts of paroxysmal fast activity from occipital regions, occasionally with gradual generalization followed by irregular spike wave discharges'.

Mancia *et al.* (1986)[519] in their review of the possible associations of migraine and epilepsy described four interesting patients with occipital seizures and migrainous-like symptoms who all had ictal EEG recording. Two of their cases were symptomatic. One of their cases (No. 1) is of particular interest, and this is detailed on page 183.

Kivity and Lerman, 1992[443] reported an EEG recorded during a prolonged seizure of the EBOS that 'showed continuous bilateral spike and wave complexes, more prominent on the left side'. In seven patients the EEG was obtained within 24 h post-ictally. The commonest finding was occipital slow activity with occipital paroxysms in subsequent not post-ictal EEG. One third of these patients showed occipital paroxysms in their first post-ictal EEG.

Vigevano and Ricci (1993)[793] reported ictal EEG during vomiting and deviation of the eyes in a prolonged seizure of EBOS (Fig. 10.17). The EEG is dominated by unilateral, *left* sided diffuse but with posterior preponderance, high amplitude (200 μV) rhythmic sharp slow waves at around 2 Hz intermixed with fast rhythms and spikes during vomiting and autonomic symptoms.

Beaumanoir 1993[77] presented a 9 min duration nocturnal seizure of an 8-year-old girl characterized by vomiting, other autonomic disturbances and mild impairment of consciousness with probably 'disturbed vision'. The ictal EEG starts with remission of the occipital paroxysms and the appearance of occipital sharp rhythms, progressing to monomorphic theta activity in the bi-occipital regions. The frequency of the slow activity becomes lower with the progress of the seizure and ends without post-ictal abnormalities.

Ferrie *et al.*,1997[277] reported ictal EEG in four patients with EBOS. An illustrative example of their cases is that of Vigevano and Ricci[793] described above.

Ictal EEG of idiopathic versus symptomatic occipital seizures

I am not certain that idiopathic can be differentiated from symptomatic occipital seizures on the basis of isolated ictal EEG recordings if other symptoms, signs and interictal EEG are not considered. However, surface ictal scalp EEG recordings in patients with symptomatic occipital lobe epilepsy

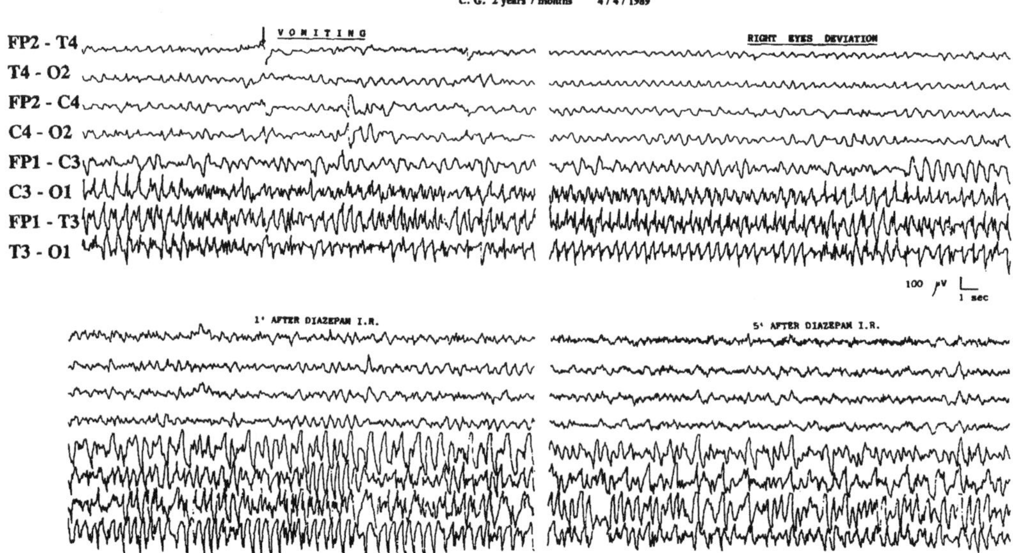

Fig. 10.17. Ictal EEG of an early onset benign childhood occipital seizure during vomiting and deviation of the eyes. The EEG is dominated by unilateral, left sided diffuse but with posterior preponderance, high amplitude (200 µV) rhythmic sharp slow waves at around 2 Hz, intermixed with fast rhythms and spikes during vomiting and autonomic symptoms.
[From Vigevano and Ricci (1993)[793] with the kind permission of the authors and the publisher John Libbey.]

often demonstrate epileptiform activity that is more widespread (regional) rather than having a precise occipital localization. Salanova *et al.*[700] reported that 50 per cent of the patients in the Montreal series exhibited mainly regional involvement while occipital localization was found in only 17 per cent of patients. This was also emphasized by Williamson *et al.*[808,811] who reported that often the ictal discharge appeared to involve the posterior temporal and parietal regions. In patients with focal destructive lesions, the ictal discharge tends to be confined to one occipital lobe at least for several seconds before spreading to the contralateral side.

Depth electrode studies[700,808,811] also confirmed that most ictal discharges are widespread rather than focal, localized to the occipital lobe, though this may also occur. Simultaneous discharges in the occipital-temporal regions can be seen. However, in most of these cases, there is no independent temporal lobe onset.

Babb *et al.*, 1981[57] performed neuronal recordings at the occipital cortex and hippocampus during a seizure originating in the right occipital lobe of a patient with an occipito-temporal tumour. They demonstrated that the visual aura resulted from neuronal activation of medial peristriate and possibly other occipital lobe neurones. Conversely, the psychomotor automatisms which followed 10–20 s later were caused by recruitment of hippocampal neurones bilaterally. This confirmed that the complex seizure symptoms were caused by propagation from an occipital lobe focus. The visual hallucinations consisted of 'flashing coloured lights that the patient referred to as butterflies'. They appeared to move from right to left and persisted for 10 to 20 s before a complex partial seizure occured after the invasion of the temporal lobe. The surface ictal EEG showed a brief occipital flattening before the fast rhythmic small spikes.

Benign Childhood Partial Seizures and Related Epileptic Syndromes. C P Panayiotopoulos
©1999 John Libbey & Company Ltd., pp. 203–228.

Chapter 11

Benign childhood occipital seizures and related epileptic syndromes: Historical aspects and literature review

Historical aspects

Gibbs and Gibbs (1952)[327] were the first to document that EEG 'seizure foci in one or both occipital lobes are most commonly found in young children... Occipital foci tend to disappear in adult life, and the subsidence of the electroencephalographic abnormality is usually accompanied by a cessation of seizures.'[327] They also described amongst the 'atypical seizures of 38 patients with a spike focus in the occipital area' syncope (4 per cent), strabismus and diplopia (1.5 per cent), staring (2.2 per cent), fortification figures (1.5 per cent), formed visual hallucinations (0.7 per cent), pressing hands to eyes (1.5 per cent), vomiting (1.5 per cent), headache (0.7 per cent) and blindness (0.7 per cent).[327]

In 1954 Gibbs, Gillen and Gibbs[326] also published their results of follow-up studies on children with occipital and mid-temporal spikes. 'Forty-five children who were known to have had occipital foci of seizure activity were restudied after they had reached nine years of age. In 40 per cent of these cases the focus had disappeared and the electroencephalogram had become entirely normal. All of this group with normal electroencephalograms were seizure free. Twenty three per cent still had their occipital spike focus; of these about one quarter were seizure free. In 18 per cent the pure occipital spike-focus had disappeared and had been replaced by an occipito-temporal focus; of these about one quarter were seizure free. In 14 per cent the focus had shifted to the mid-temporal area and of these about one third were seizure free. Five per cent had developed 14 and 6 per s positive spikes which we believe are presumptive-evidence of epileptic disorder in thalamus or hypothalamus, and of these one third were seizure free. None of the 45 patients who had an occipital focus developed diffuse seizure activity or an anterior temporal focus but in larger series it is likely that such cases could be encountered.'[326] Twenty per cent of these patients had clinical evidence of non-progressive brain damage (symptomatic epilepsy) and their occipital foci changed in the same manner as those of the idiopathic epilepsy. Thus, 56 per cent of these children were seizure free by the age of 9 years. This was as good as that of 98 patients with mid-temporal spikes where 68.5 per cent were seizure free when re-examined after the age of 15 years.

Relevant to this chapter is a boy initially reported by Gibbs and Gibbs,1952 (plate 203 on page 281)[327] and later by Gibbs *et al.*, 1954[326] in more detail (their Fig. 4).[326] I present him because he demonstrated symptoms of early onset benign childhood occipital seizures (EBOS) and later developed centrotemporal spikes (CTS) and probably Rolandic seizures. He was 12 years and had serial EEG from age 7 years.

> He had 'four episodes of prolonged unconsciousness without convulsive movements but with choking, gagging, vomiting and cyanosis. The first attack occurred at one year of age; the second with measles at 2 years; the third at 6 years; and the fourth at 7 years. Strabismus of left eye turned in. No other neurological signs. High intelligence. Phenytoin treatment'. His EEG at age 7 years showed 'focus of sharp spikes and slow waves in the right occipital area, showing also in the left occipital area'. In the following year he had 'one choking spell and three tonic–clonic convulsions. On phenytoin therapy. The EEG at age 8 years showed 'fewer spike seizure discharges in the right occipital area, none in the left; the spikes are slower than previously; however independent foci of spike seizure activity are now evident in both mid-temporal areas spreading as a positive spike to both frontal areas'. His next EEG was at age 10 years. He had 'no further seizures but complained of dizzy spells and headaches'. The EEG during slight sleep showed that 'the negative spike foci in the right occipital and temporal area had disappeared. However, the negative spike focus in the left mid-temporal area persists and 14-per-s positive spikes are now evident in the right hemisphere'. At age 12 years 'no more clinically evident seizures or dizzy spells but patient complained of headache. Still on phenytoin'. The EEG during slight sleep showed '14-per-s positive spikes in the right and left hemisphere (suggesting epileptic foci in the thalamus and hypothalamus). The spike discharges are of lower voltage than in the previous record. There were no more occipital or mid-temporal spikes'.

Another boy of Gibbs and Gibbs, 1952[327] probably represents late onset benign childhood occipital seizures (LBOS).

> He was 8 and a half year and had 'onset of attacks two months before the recording, consisting of blindness followed by holding both hands to eyes, rolling up of eyes, and loss of consciousness. Severe headache after attack. No convulsions at any time'. The EEG showed independent bilateral spike foci in occipital areas (plates 205 and 206, pages 283–284).[327]

Although no prognosis or further details were given, these two cases of Gibbs and Gibbs are probably the first reports of the early and late onset BOS also exemplifying the relation between childhood occipital spikes and occipital seizures with centrotemporal spikes and Rolandic seizures.

In fairness, though, the report of Gastaut, 1950[300] on 'the electrographic evidence of subcortical mechanisms on certain partial epilepsies' is often cited as the first publication on 'several cases of benign childhood epilepsy with visual seizures and occipital spike and wave complexes'.[36,313] I do not think that this is so. In that paper, Gastaut[300] described a 12-year-old girl with onset of visual seizures at age 7 years. These consisted of 'sparkling flashes throughout her visual fields for several seconds, sometimes followed by a typical petit mal absence'. The EEG showed interictal right sided 'high amplitude occipital spike and wave complexes which repeated rhythmically at 2–3 Hz and appeared with eye closure or photic stimulation'.[313] Furthermore, she also had brief ictal 3 Hz spike and polyspike generalized discharges associated with typical absence seizures. The same case was included by Gastaut[308] amongst the benign partial epilepsy of childhood with occipital spike-waves with no additional information regarding prognosis. In my experience (see Figs. 10.12 , 11.1 and 11.2) this combination of symptoms and EEG findings herald rather a bad than good prognosis.

Sorel and Rucquoy-Ponsar (1969)[735] reported on 'functional epilepsies of maturation'. Of 2303 patients with onset of seizures before the age of 15 years, 171 children (7.4 per cent) had 'occipital, Rolandic or temporal spikes'. Rolandic spikes were twice as frequent as occipital spikes. They also emphasized the different spike localization of 28 cases in the same or successive EEGs. Twenty six per cent of the patients had attacks with 'viscero-vegetative' symptoms, 16 per cent paroxysmal headaches, and 2 per cent 'colores' paroxysmal. One third of the seizures were nocturnal. Sorel and Rucquoy-Ponsar (1969)[735] were probably the first to propose that this is a 'functional epilepsy of maturation' which is very much similar to the 'benign childhood seizure susceptibility syndrome'[609] that I proposed 25 years after them.

Delwaide *et al.* (1971)[220] described 13 patients with occipital seizures and emphasized that they are more frequent in children (nine of 13 were younger than 15 years old with four below the age of 10 at onset), visual hallucinations were mainly coloured and amaurosis was common. Seizures were

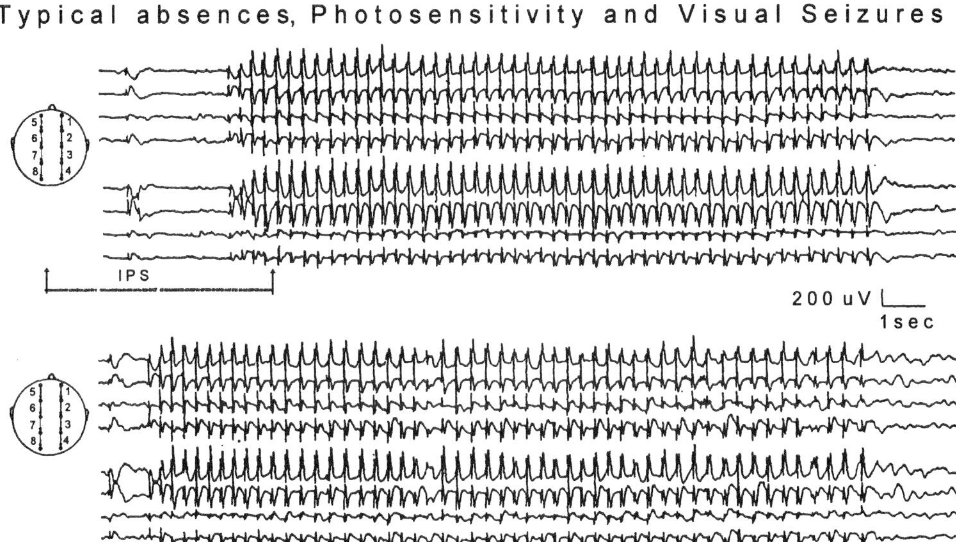

Fig. 11.1. Video-EEG of a 9-year-old boy with typical absence seizures, spontaneous (bottom) or IPS-induced (top). He also has photically (TV and video-games) induced seizures during which he complains of headache, may vomit and becomes 'vacant and not with it'. He also has complex visual hallucinations and fear. There is a strong family history of epileptic disorders from both parents. This, the next patient of Fig. 11.2 as well as the case of Fig. 10.12 in this book cannot be considered as benign childhood occipital seizures. On the contrary, they appear to be severe and resistant to medication. IPS = intermittent photic stimulation.

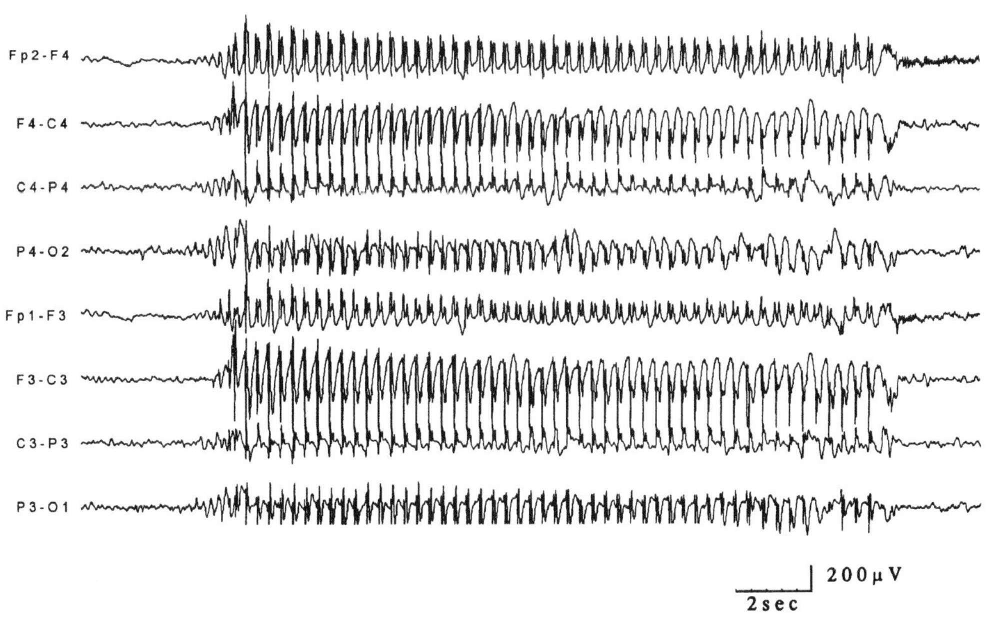

Fig. 11.2. Video-EEG of an 8-year-old boy with a history of prolonged febrile convulsions and intractable childhood typical absences. Afterwards he reports visual illusions. On this illustrated occasion, he said that the shoes of his mother who was in front of him looked different and they were covered with flowers.

frequently associated or followed by headache and vomiting. Three children were also photosensitive and in one of them a fit provoked by IPS was recorded. Some patients had a good prognosis.

Huott *et al.* (1974)[404] described five interesting cases of occipital lobe epilepsy. Relevant to the topic in this section is their second case, a 14-year-old boy with an 'ictal' EEG that had all the features of the 'interictal' EEG of benign occipital seizures (BOS). This was associated with blurring of vision for 9 min. This child had at the age of 9 years an episode of agitated and automatic behaviour that lasted for 30 min and he subsequently developed frequent seizures of blindness with a complex visual hallucination of female faces. The other three patients had symptomatic occipital epilepsy with a combination of ictal symptoms such as blindness, complex visual hallucinations, somnolence, vomiting and urine incontinence. The remaining patient had visual seizures preceded by severe diffuse headaches during pregnancy only.

Despite these important contributions suggesting and often documenting the existence of idiopathic occipital seizures with good prognosis, the identification of their clinico-EEG features was delayed for many years. Even today, expert reviews on the subject lack clear descriptions and commitments on this important subject, children with these disorders are erroneously diagnosed as having migraine or severe neurological disorders or they are given the general statistical predictions regarding relapses after the first epileptic seizure. Furthermore, interest in benign childhood occipital seizures came from a report by Camfield *et al.* (1989),[146] renowned epileptologists, who probably erroneously suggested that this was a form of basilar migraine causing secondary epileptogenic brain abnormalities. Therefore, I feel that it is important to detail chronologically the work and reports of authors who contributed to the identification and recognition of EBOS and LBOS. This is also because this is still considered as a developing subject, not yet entirely settled and resolved.

Abbreviations

EBOS =	Early onset benign childhood occipital seizures (Panayiotopoulos syndrome)
LBOS =	Late onset benign childhood occipital seizures
BOS =	Benign occipital seizures
CEOP =	Childhood epilepsy with occipital paroxysms
BNCOE =	Benign nocturnal childhood occipital epilepsy
RS =	Rolandic seizures
CTS =	Centrotemporal spikes
ROEA =	Reactive occipital epileptiform activity
IGE =	Idiopathic generalized epilepsy
GTCS =	Generalized tonic–clonic seizures
AED =	Anti-epileptic medication
IPS =	Intermittent photic stimulation

Literature review

Conclusions and explanations

From an extensive literature review detailed in this chapter, I reached the following conclusions:

(a) EEG occipital paroxysms or occipital spikes may be seen in a wide variety of conditions from normal children to those with visual problems (congenital or acquired in early life) but no seizures, benign occipital seizures or severe forms of symptomatic and cryptogenic partial or generalized epilepsies. Therefore, they are not pathognomonic of benign occipital seizures without sound clinical evidence. They comply with what I emphasized elsewhere in this book: Though not a substitute for the clinical examination, the EEG is an integral part of the diagnostic process in epilepsies provided that it is properly interpreted in a well described clinical setting.

(b) Amongst the idiopathic childhood occipital epilepsies with good prognosis EBOS or Panayiotopoulos syndrome are by far more frequent and more benign than LBOS, as established by Gastaut.

(c) There are some rare cases with a plethora of bizarre ictal and post-ictal symptoms which may last for hours. These may be extreme cases combining features of both EBOS and LBOS and these are the more likely to cause differential diagnostic problems. The occipital lobes can generate long lasting partial seizures, spontaneous or evoked, with sometimes peculiar symptomatology as documented with ictal EEG recordings.

(d) It is difficult to deduce what some authors call migraine. Visual hallucinations, headache, vomiting alone or in combination, which may be visual seizures, are often equated with migraine aura, basilar and acephalgic migraine. Therefore, I often cite the relevant paragraphs in quotation marks as published by these authors.

Literature review

Camfield, Metrakos and Andermann (1978)[146] reported four adolescents diagnosed as 'basilar migraine, seizures and severe epileptiform EEG abnormalities'. These patients from the age of 7–11 years started having mainly prolonged episodes of visual hallucinations often followed by blindness, vomiting and headache. The duration of the visual hallucinations and blindness was more than 10–15 min and sometimes lasted for hours. In a patient, blindness was preceded by severe dizziness and persistent vomiting lasting from 1 to 2 h to as long as several days. All patients also had infrequent focal or generalized convulsive seizures in the course of these events or independently. The EEG of all patients showed continuous 'rhythmic temporo-occipital sharp and slow wave discharges, or generalized spike and wave complexes' which occurred when the eyes were closed and blocked when the eyes were opened. The rare seizures seemed to be readily controlled with anticonvulsant medication. The clinical course was benign, with normal personality, mentation and neurologic examination. Camfield *et al.* (1978)[146] attributed the prolonged episodes of visual hallucinations, headache and vomiting to basilar migraine and considered that the EEG abnormalities and the convulsive seizures resulted from ischaemic changes caused by migraine attacks in the territory of the basilar migraine.

Manzoni and colleagues (1979)[525] described a 28-year-old man with migraine with aura occasionally progressing to occipital seizures. They coined the term intercalated seizures to denote epileptic seizures occurring between the migrainous aura and the headache phase of migraine.

Panayiotopoulos (1980)[599] questioned the diagnosis of basilar migraine in 'Basilar migraine*?* Seizures, and severe epileptic EEG abnormalities'[599] (note the question marked after basilar migraine which is often erroneously omitted when this paper is cited). He reported a boy who had brief, for seconds, episodes of visual hallucinations later followed by headache. The patient also had independent episodes of blindness and the visual hallucinations on a few occasions progressed to a convulsive seizure. The EEG showed occipital paroxysms on eyes-closed which were eliminated by central vision and fixation. This was also the first time that fixation-off sensitivity (FOS) was documented in these cases with occipital paroxysms. This case is detailed in Chapter 9, page 164–165, case 24.

Panayiotopoulos and Siafacas (1980)[636] reported 10 children with occipital paroxysms and documented fixation-off sensitivity. Clinically, seven children had what is now known as EBOS with 'nocturnal prolonged episodes of tonic deviation of the eyes sometimes followed by tonic–clonic seizures'. Three other patients had diurnal seizures with elementary visual hallucinations.

Panayiotopoulos (1981)[600] documented in detail fixation-off sensitivity in four patients with occipital paroxysms. Also, this was the first report in which prolonged, non visual occipital nocturnal seizures with deviation of the eyes were associated with occipital paroxysms. This EBOS type of ictal presentation was described in two cases. The other two patients had LBOS (case of reference no. 599) and symptomatic occipital epilepsy demonstrating the clinical heterogeneity associated with occipital paroxysms.

[Note: Though published in *Neurology*, in 1981[600] these clinical observations escaped the attention of authors who subsequently described childhood epilepsy with occipital spike and waves.]

The two cases with EBOS are detailed in Chapter 8 with more than 20 years follow-up. I had initially dismissed ictal vomiting as a coincidence and did not make reference to it in the tight format of the report,[600] but later it became apparent to me that ictal vomiting was one of the most consistent clinical symptoms of these children.[602,603,605,606]

Lugaresi *et al*. organized in 1981 in Bologna an International Symposium on 'Migraine and Epilepsy' which was subsequently published, with additional significant contributions,[18,31,33,34,82, 84,120,121,132, 313,763] in 1987 by F. Andermann and E. Lugaresi.[39] One session, chaired by H. Gastaut, the great French epileptologist, is of particular interest. F. Andermann presented the views of the Canadian group[146] in favour of basilar migraine. Panayiotopoulos supported his thesis that these are occipital seizures, not basilar migraine, and reported the 'difficulties in differentiating migraine and epilepsy based on clinical and EEG findings'.[602] Gastaut supported Panayiotopoulos that this was most likely an occipital epilepsy rather than a form of basilar migraine. That should be the end of the debate, particularly in view of the reports of Gastaut that followed.[302–306] It was not.

Gastaut (1981, 1982) [302–306] retrospectively identified 36 patients with occipital paroxysms from the department of clinical neurophysiology in Marseilles which he extensively reported in French, English and German.[302–306] These reports dominated our attitude towards benign childhood occipital seizures as clearly illustrated by recent reviews.[36,43] Though selection criteria are not defined, these appeared to be children and adolescents with occipital paroxysms and seizures.

All 36 patients (61 per cent girls) had EEG occipital paroxysms. All had '"almost" normal neuropsychiatric, ophthalmological and neuroradiological status' and the 'visual symptoms were the inaugural events of most if not all seizures, although purely related by the younger child'. Mean age at onset was 6 years and family history of epilepsy was found in 47 per cent and migraine in 19 per cent. The prognosis in this relatively homogeneous group was excellent with 'full remission of seizures in 92 per cent of them before the age of 19 years'. Also response to anti-epileptic drugs was excellent. 'Institution of treatment suppressed seizures in 53 per cent compared to 65 per cent in patients with Rolandic seizures'.

However, in two subsequent publications of cumulative results by **Gastaut,**[308] and **Gastaut and Zifkin**[313] an additional 27 patients were added to the original 36 patients. The selection criteria were different in these[308,310,313] from the original study.[302–306] I detail them because this is a significant matter to understand. Of the 63 patients in the final report by Gastaut and Zifkin:[313]

(a) Seven had occipital sharp and slow waves only during photic stimulation. Thus, these had evidence of photosensitive occipital seizures only.

(b) Six had abnormal neurological examinations (all were developmentally delayed and three had hemiparesis), one post-traumatic subdural heamatoma, one skull fracture, one hemi-atrophy, hemiplegia epilepsy syndrome. Seven other patients had prematurity of mild perinatal distress or both. Five (8.3 per cent) had abnormal brain scan. Thus, these patients had symptomatic, not idiopathic, occipital seizures.

(c) Seven patients had occipital paroxysms in the resting EEG with IPS inducing generalized discharges of spike or polyspike and slow wave often associated with myoclonic jerks. Thus, these patients had superimposed generalized photosensitivity.

Furthermore, there are three illustrative cases (cases 11,12 and 13) which were included because of ictal visual symptoms prior to generalized seizures mainly evoked by photic stimuli.

Thus, it appears that inclusion criteria for this later study[308,313] were for patients who had seizures and occipital paroxysms as well as for patients with any form of visual seizures irrespective of EEG abnormalities. Therefore, this was a heterogeneous group of patients including photosensitive, symptomatic and generalized epilepsies. This may explain the initial impression of Gastaut that this was a relatively common form of benign childhood epilepsy and that the prognosis was worse in this than in the first homogeneous group of 36 patients.

Gastaut (1985)[308] **and Gastaut and Zifkin (1987)**[313] divided these 63 patients into:

(a) 33 patients representing the complete syndrome with visual hallucinations and occipital paroxysms;

(b) 17 patients having the incomplete syndrome with either the visual hallucinations or the occipital paroxysms absent; and

(c) 13 patients with the complete syndrome but also associated with other forms of idiopathic generalized epilepsy, Rolandic seizures and symptomatic generalized or cryptogenic epilepsy.

There were 33 boys and 30 girls. Age at onset varied from 15 months to 17 years with a mean age of 7 years and 5 months. A family history of epilepsy was found in 36.6 per cent and of migraine in 15.9 per cent. Fourteen per cent had febrile convulsions.

Neuropsychological examination was normal in 90 per cent and the other 10 per cent had developmental retardation. Three cases had hemiparesis. All had normal ophthalmological examination and 91.7 per cent had normal CT brain scan.

It has been emphasized on many occasions in this book that normal brain CT scan does not exclude cryptogenic or symptomatic occipital lobe epilepsy. High resolution MRI would probably reveal malformations of cortical development or other structural abnormalities that CT brain scan is not sensitive to detect. Also, some patients, such as their case 5, may have been just patients with cryptogenic/symptomatic occipital epilepsies, which would explain the bad prognosis and the intractable seizures. In one of their patients there was a consistent left occipital focus of spike and seizures which were initially adversive and giratory on the right side before the appearance of a numeral visual hallucination.

Seizures mainly consisted of brief visual symptoms which occurred in more than 75 per cent of the patients. 'All patients old enough to answer questions about their attacks reported visual phenomena. In others, behaviour during their seizures often suggested visual symptoms that they could not describe or remember. Several different visual experiences might be reported by the same patient as part of one or several seizures'.

Partial or complete visual loss was the commonest visual symptom, noted by 33 of 63 patients (52 per cent). It was almost always associated with other phenomena but could occur alone. It could be preceded by simple or complex visual hallucinations and be followed by convulsions, automatic behaviour, or headache. The visual loss typically lasted up to several minutes and the entire visual field was eventually affected, although an initial hemianopia sometimes occurred. In one patient blindness (case 3)[308] 'lasted for 45 min followed by a 2 min dysphasia and a major convulsion'. Elementary visual hallucinations occurred in 29 of 63 subjects (46 per cent). 'Generally taking the form of moving multicoloured flashing spots occupying only one homonymous visual field in one-third of these cases, such hallucinations could begin in the visual field either ipsilateral or contralateral to the discharging focus before filling the entire visual field in the remaining two thirds. These phenomena could be either isolated or associated with other symptoms. If isolated, they usually occurred in flurries, each hallucination lasting up to 10 s. Longer lasting teichopsia might be followed by seizures, visceral sensations such as nausea, or headache. They did not have similarities to the migraine visual aura'.

Complex visual hallucinations were described by nine patients (14 per cent). They could occur alone or followed by further symptoms. The most unusual hallucination – a 1- or 2-digit number – was noted by three patients.[312,313]

Of the 63 patients, nine (14 per cent) reported visual illusions, including micropsia, metamorphopsia and palinopsia.

Visual ictal seizures were often followed by other, non-visual ictal symptoms such as hemiconvulsions (43 per cent) and complex partial seizures (14 per cent). Eight patients had GTCS, three bilateral clonic attacks and two had tonic seizures. Seven patients had adversive seizures, seven ocular movements, six fluttering of the eyelids at the time of the visual hallucinations, eight ictal dysphasia, five unilateral dysaesthesia and three elementary auditory hallucinations.

Headache: 'diffuse headache, only rarely hemicranial' occurred only post-ictally in 33 per cent of the patients and migraine-like nausea and vomiting sometimes with headache in 17 per cent. That the headache was post-ictal was also showed by the absence of any ictal discharge in the 13 cases in which the EEG was recorded during this phase.

Frequency and precipitating factors: 'Seizures varied in frequency from many per day and for several months to only occasional seizures with seizure-free intervals of several years. Although there were no clear precipitating factors, ambient light and the menstrual cycle contribute to their occurrence. Seizures that were apparently precipitated by light were reported by 16 patients. Some occurred on going from a dark area into a brighter one, or, conversely, from a well-lit area into a darkened one. Three occurred while on a sunlit beach or at sea, or while watching television. In five of 12 pubescent girls, seizures began with puberty and continued to occur with menstruation'.

Prognosis was 'usually good but not as good as Rolandic seizures. Complete seizure control was achieved in 60 per cent of the patients with any type of antiepileptic medication. In none of the cases have the seizures persisted into middle adulthood, and other types of recurring seizures in adulthood were seen in only three patients'. The prognosis, as expected, was poorer in patients with other evidence of cerebral disturbance such as mental retardation or abnormal CT scans, or whose EEGs showed an additional secondary epileptiform disturbance. Complete seizure control with anti-convulsant drugs was achieved in 38 patients (60 per cent), and seizures persisted in three patients followed beyond age 19. Seizure control could be achieved, although the epileptiform EEG could persist for several months or years after the seizures had ceased.

'Almost all available anticonvulsants have been tried without any one being the obvious drug of choice. The rapid response to clobazam was noted in seven of nine patients in whom it was used, both seizures and interictal spikes ceased after only several days of treatment.'

Beaumanoir (1983)[74] published a careful and influential report on 18 patients with EEG occipital paroxysms and seizures of good prognosis. Criteria of selection were: EEG occipital paroxysms with normal background, seizures in remission for at least three and a half years, and normal neurological and neuroradiological examinations, although half of the patients were amblyopic.

The age at seizure onset was from 2 to 8 years with a peak between 4 and 8 years.

Three patients had only diurnal seizures, 10 had only nocturnal seizures and five had both diurnal and nocturnal seizures. The ictal clinical manifestations were different between diurnal and nocturnal fits.

Diurnal seizures. The diurnal seizures were 'most often sensorial and rarely motor'. Seven patients had visual ictal symptoms consisting of micropsia (four patients), macropsia occasionally associated with photopsia (one patient), visual eclipse (two patients) and hallucinations (three patients). Non-visual sensorial symptoms consisted of a strong pain in the eyes (one patient) or unilateral dysaesthesia of the face and occasionally of the ipsilateral upper limb. These sensorial symptoms were often followed by 'an oculo-clonic seizure with tonic deviation of the eyes and then clonia of the eyeballs'. In one case the seizure ended with loss of consciousness and in another one with GTCS. Automatic behaviour following the visual or motor symptoms occurred in three patients.

Nocturnal seizures. All seizures were motor and started with 'eyes opening followed by their tonic deviation with sometimes a tonic deviation of the head and then ocular clonia'. Clonic convulsions of the upper or lower extremity, mainly the proximal parts, could follow.

post-ictal headache: Two patients experienced post-ictal headache.

Other seizures: One patient also had Rolandic seizures prior to the onset of the occipital ones, and two patients had typical absences with EEG confirmation of the absences and occipital paroxysms before the onset of the occipital seizures.

Frequency of seizures: The frequency of the seizures varied but generally did not appear to be frequent and could occur in clusters. In untreated patients the second seizure could occur within minutes, months or one and a half year from the first fit.

Prognosis: By definition of selection criteria all patients had a good prognosis. They were free of seizures for more than three and a half years to a maximum of 14 years (average 7 years and 4 months). All patients had received anti-epileptic medication. Four were still on treatment, the other 14 were free of seizures from 3 to 11 years with no medication.

The duration of the active seizure phase was between 3 and 7 years, average 4 years and 7 months. The duration did not appear to be related to the age of onset or the frequency of the seizures.

Family history. Two patients had a brother each with Rolandic seizures. In two other families there were instances of idiopathic generalized epilepsy (IGE), the father of another patient had oculoclonic seizures in childhood and in another case the sister had febrile convulsions.

Newton and Aicardi (1983)[568] and Aicardi and Newton (1987)[18] studied retrospectively the clinical manifestations of 21 children, 11 were girls, selected because of occipital paroxysms. Idiopathic, cryptogenic and symptomatic cases were grouped together.

The onset of seizures occurred between the ages of 4 months and 12 years (mean: 6 years 1 month). In seven patients, 'there was a history of periodic headache and vomiting prior to the onset of the seizure disorder, consistent with a diagnosis of migraine'. In only two cases was there a family history of convulsive disorder in second-degree relatives. Another child had a father with migraine.

The seizure patterns were described as follows:

Migrainous features: 'Transient loss of consciousness was regularly preceded by headache in five patients. In four of these the headache was bilateral, usually frontal, and in the fifth it was unilateral, on the same side as the EEG abnormality. The headache was associated with nausea in four patients, and two others experienced nausea and vomiting before a seizure but had no headache'.

Visual phenomena: Of the 21 children, nine experienced visual symptoms at the onset of their seizures. In addition, four patients experienced transient loss of vision, four saw brightly coloured discs in the visual field contralateral to the side of the EEG abnormality, and another described distortion of the visual image.

Non-visual phenomena: All but one of the children had transient loss of consciousness with maintenance of posture, often accompanied by fluttering of the eyelids. In three of the children, these bouts were at times prolonged, lasting up to 45 min. Two children had only generalized tonic–clonic seizures. One was only 13 months old at presentation, the other had a single seizure at age 9 years 10 months. In two patients, this transient loss of consciousness was not accompanied by other seizure phenomena.

Unilateral tonic–clonic movements, contralateral to the EEG abnormality, sometimes accompanied the transient loss of consciousness in five cases. Of these children, four had transient paresis of the affected limb or face contralateral to the side of the EEG abnormality on at least one occasion. Adversive movement of the head away from the side of the EEG abnormality accompanied the seizures in three patients.

Psychomotor phenomena were seen in five children. Two experienced fear during attacks, one in conjunction with auditory hallucinations; one child frequently laughed aloud; and another experienced a feeling of 'derealization' prior to attacks. In eight cases, bilateral tonic–clonic movements sometimes accompanied the seizures, and in another child the tonic–clonic movements were either unilateral or bilateral.

There were two patients who frequently experienced myoclonic movements of all four limbs shortly after waking each morning; one child developed myoclonic–atonic seizures at age 10, 8 years after the start of the seizure disorder. In five of the children seizures occurred predominantly at night, though in one case this lasted for only a few weeks at the beginning of the seizure disorder.

Duration of the seizure disorder: In seven of the 20 patients treated, treatment was stopped after the seizures had abated. In these seven patients the seizure disorder lasted from 1 month to 11 years (mean: 3.1/7 years). In three patients, the response to medication had always been poor before the eventual remission of the seizure disorder. These three cases experienced learning difficulties at school which required remedial education.

Despite being medically treated for periods of 6 months to 13 years (mean: 5 years 4 months), the seizure disorder persisted in the other 14 children. Of these, six required remedial education; four others were mildly mentally handicapped.

However, it is deduced from their table that seven of nine children of the idiopathic group (cases 5, 8, 11, 12, 13, 15, 17, 19, 21) had a good prognosis. Age at onset of seizures for these nine children was 4 to 11 years (mean 7.1 ± 2.4 years). Two children had single seizures and the duration of the disease (seizures) was less than one year in all but two children. Conversely, in all but one of the 12 cryptogenic/symptomatic cases the prognosis was poor.

These important reports by Newton and Aicardi (1983)[568] and Aicardi and Newton (1987)[18] are often misinterpreted as indicating bad prognosis of benign occipital seizures. Newton and Aicardi[18,568] did not study the prognosis of idiopathic occipital epilepsy but the clinical conditions associated with the EEG pattern of occipital spikes. They made this very clear by concluding that these *'cases illustrate the wide range of clinical disorders that may accompany this EEG abnormality and indicate that the prognosis associated with this EEG pattern is not necessarily benign'.*

Herranz Tanarro *et al.* (1984)[386] reported that from 15,000 EEGs, 31 (0.21 per cent) EEGs of children had 'runs of high amplitude and variable frequency spike-and-wave discharges on the occipito-posterio-temporal regions when eyes were closed'. They estimated an incidence of 1.4 per 1000. Thirteen (41.9 per cent) of the 31 children also had additional centrotemporal spikes. Clinically, 10 children had mainly minimal brain dysfunction but no seizures and four suffered febrile convulsions. The remaining 17 other patients were treated for visual, motor or vegetative partial seizures, and even generalized fits. The prognosis was good with phenobarbital therapy in almost all cases. The authors concluded that 'this benign occipital epilepsy is related to childhood epilepsy with Rolandic paroxysms'.

Gil *et al.* (1984)[334] reported a woman who started having 'classic migraine' from the age of 14 years. Ten years later she had onset of epileptic seizures with blurring of vision and loss of consciousness with or without secondary GTCS. Other infrequent attacks were characterized by blindness lasting 15 min which progressed to a left adversive seizure with secondary GTCS or blindness, decreased hearing, dysarthria lasting 15 min and followed by headache and vomiting. EEG showed left sided occipital spikes inhibited on eyes-open. Neuroradiological investigations were normal.

Lugaresi *et al.* (1984)[514] and Cirignotta (1987)[167] were the first to confirm the findings of Panayiotopoulos (1980, 1981)[599,600] regarding the activating effect of the elimination of central vision and fixation on occipital paroxysms and other eyes-closed related EEG abnormalities. They concluded that 'scotosensitive epilepsy and benign partial epilepsy of childhood with occipital spike-waves may represent the same clinical entity'.

Deonna *et al.* (1984)[223] reported that of 195 children with idiopathic partial or generalized epilepsy 14 children with visual seizures and an additional four also had migraine. There was only one child (0.5 per cent) who the authors considered to have benign partial occipital epilepsy (phosphenes, moving lights, headaches and occipital high voltage biphasic spike-waves blocked by eye opening on the EEG) while all others had other types of epilepsy. Furthermore, of 30 different children selected because of migraine with aura 'migraine accompagnee' EEGs showed a centrotemporal focus in one and generalized spike-waves in two children. The authors concluded that this 'new' type of benign partial occipital epilepsy 'can be distinguished from symptomatically resembling entities but its place needs to be further defined'.

Deonna *et al.* (1986)[225] also reported a clinical and EEG study of 107 neurologically normal children with partial seizures. Sixty-three children had simple partial seizures, 39 had complex partial seizures, and five children were unclassifiable. Thirty eight (35.5 per cent) had 'the syndrome of benign partial epilepsy of children with Rolandic spikes that was clearly identified and its uniformly benign final prognosis was confirmed even if some of these children had at times severe or poorly controlled seizures'. The authors were unable to find a homogeneous clinical or electroclinical subgroup among 25 children with simple partial seizures (after excluding the Rolandic seizures) and 39 cases of complex partial seizures. There were only two children with benign partial epilepsy and myoclonic-astatic seizures ('atypical benign partial epilepsy of childhood') and one child with 'benign epilepsy with occipital spike-waves'. Seventy four per cent of children with complex partial seizures had a 1-year seizure-free interval, and many children with simple partial seizures (outside the Rolandic seizures group) had no more than two seizures. Deonna *et al.* (1986)[225] concluded that 'a benign course is thus not limited to the Rolandic seizures but is difficult to predict. Prospective studies are necessary to confirm the existence of well-defined benign syndromes among the idiopathic partial epilepsies of childhood, which appear quite rare outside the Rolandic seizures'.

Giroud *et al.* (1986)[340] reported on 'epilepsy with occipital spike waves' and on its place among the benign epilepsies.

Gallet *et al.* (1986)[296] found nine cases of benign epilepsy with occipital paroxysms amongst 244 children with partial epilepsy. They commented on the diagnostic procedures to 'address secondary occipital epilepsy and migraine with ocular symptoms'.

Terzano *et al.* (1986)[768] presented a girl who at the age of 11 years had three episodes 'beginning with an odd sensation on the eyes and bilateral scintillating scotomata. The latter changed shortly after, into red, yellow and green coloured spots over the entire visual field. After a few minutes, this visual phenomenon started to migrate laterally and was followed by loss of vision. Witnesses then reported staring eyes and impairment of consciousness. Within 60 s, the seizure disturbances cleared, but were replaced by a severe throbbing frontal headache lasting about 36 h and accompanied by nausea and vomiting'. The EEG showed typical right sided occipital paroxysms. Flunarazine controlled both the migraine attacks and the seizures.

The girl had another three sisters and a brother. The younger sister had from the age of 7 recurrent episodes of common migraine and an EEG at age 10 showed right sided occipital paroxysms. An older sister suffered from occasional attacks of migraine with aura 'scintillating scotomata preceded by frontal throbbing headache. Her first EEG at age 20 years was normal'. Their mother suffered from migraine with aura 'scintillating scotomata' from the age of 8 to her menopause. Her first EEG at age 48 years was normal.

The authors proposed that the EEG occipital focus was a functional one, not caused by presumed ischaemic changes of the migraine. They suggested that 'the intense neuronal excitation preceding Leao's cortical spreading depression (migraine aura) might play a triggering role on the occipital epileptogenic focus, changing the interictal activity into seizure activity'.

Mancia *et al.* (1986)[519] reviewed the possible associations of migraine and epilepsy and described four interesting patients having occipital seizures and migrainous-like symptoms. They all had ictal EEG recordings. Two patients had symptomatic occipital seizures. Another patient with occipital seizures after passing from a dark environment into a well-lit one and again into darkness has been detailed in Chapter 10, page 183 on scotosensitive seizures.

Mancia *et al.*[519] concluded that the EEG and clinical features of these 'patients demonstrated that migraine and epilepsy are two distinct pathophysiological entities which may occur associated or even intertwined with each other, often posing problems of differential diagnosis'.

Aso *et al.* (1987)[52] studied 21 children (11 boys) suffering from visual seizures. Nine were symptomatic/cryptogenic, nine idiopathic childhood epilepsy with occipital paroxysms and three (all girls) had idiopathic photosensitive occipital seizures. In the 18 non-photosensitive children, visual hallucinations manifested with 'visual loss in seven, blurring of vision in five, flickering lights in five and figurative hallucinations in three. Only one complained of coloured hallucinations – involving red or yellow'. Visual seizures tended to appear in clusters, several daily or several per month. 'Visual seizures were usually followed by non-visual signs. Of these, the commoner were eye deviation (13 cases), vomiting (10 cases), generalized motor seizures (eight cases) and automatisms (seven cases). Adversive seizures occurred in six and always in association with eye deviation. Five patients had attacks of blinking and four facial pallor. Eight children had nausea and two vertigo ictally. Nine children had ictal severe headache. Aso *et al.* (1987)[52] also reported a normal boy who at the age of 7 had occipital seizures with visual hallucinations of flickering lights and non-visual symptoms of tachypnea, pallor, generalized motor symptoms and unresponsiveness. EEGs showed occipital paroxysms. This later evolved to continuous spike-waves during sleep without psychomotor change or atonic seizures. In five other cases the occipital focus 'migrated to central, temporal and frontal areas'.

Beaumanoir and Grandjean (1987)[82] selected 41 patients, 23 males and 18 females, aged 17 to 27 at the time of their last EEG, according to the following EEG criteria: (1) the most recent EEG showing no spike discharges and obtained at least 6 years after the first recording; (2) background activity normal for their age; and (3) presence in at least one EEG of a unilateral or bilateral parieto-occipital focus of pseudorhythmic spikes and/or spike and wave complexes. The characteristic paroxysmal discharges were inhibited by visual perception. They generally increased during slow-wave sleep and disappeared during rapid-eye movement (REM) sleep. They did not correlate with ocular movements.

'The mean age at discovery of this EEG pattern was 6½ years, with extremes ranging from 3½ years to 11 years. The age at which this activity first appear cannot be inferred from these data. In most cases it is discovered in the first EEG, recorded at a time when clinical findings already suggest some functional or structural disturbance of the central nervous system. The mean age at disappearance of this pattern is 12½ years, with extremes ranging from 8 to 19 years. This was determined by follow-up EEGs every 6 to 12 months'.

The first EEG was usually performed for one of four indications: (1) behavioural disturbances or learning disability; (2) disturbances of visual function; (3) migraine; or (4) epileptic seizures. In many cases these symptoms were combined: 26 patients (63.4 per cent of cases) had epilepsy, which was associated in 12 cases with a deficit in visual function, in five with migraine, and in five with a behavioural or learning disorder. In addition, eight patients (19.5 per cent of cases) had migraine, which was associated in five with epilepsy, in five with visual function deficit, and in one with behavioural problems. Finally, 12 patients (29.3 per cent of cases) were free of both seizures and migraine; six of these children had behavioural disturbances, associated in two cases with a deficit in visual function and six had disturbances of visual function alone.

Thus, 22 patients (53.6 per cent) had disturbances arising from congenital deficit of visual function and 11 (26.8 per cent) had behavioural or learning problems; 21 (51.2 per cent) had epilepsy but no migraine, five (12.2 per cent) suffered from both migraine and epilepsy, and only three had migraine.

Epilepsy: 26 patients had seizures. These were of variable frequency but usually occurred rarely. Of those patients over age 15, 10 had not had a seizure since age 13. When the seizures ceased, the EEG abnormalities also disappeared, with one exception. The EEG abnormality was still present after age 13 in only two patients.

Seizures were diurnal in five patients, diurnal and nocturnal in 14, and exclusively nocturnal in seven. The diurnal attacks always presented with sensory and visual symptoms, often also with associated oculoclonic twitching. One patient described episodes of left orbital pain either alone or followed by brief palinopsia. Nocturnal seizures were characterized by partial motor seizures involving the eye and face in all but one case. Sometimes the arm was also involved. One patient seemed to have additional alternating hemiconvulsions and another had a generalized seizure.

Migraine: Migraine occurred in eight patients, five of whom also had epilepsy; a sixth suffered an episode of febrile convulsions at age 18 months. EEGs showed a Rolandic focus in addition to the occipital paroxysms in two cases. Of these two patients, one had nocturnal seizures typical of benign Rolandic epilepsy which were independent of his diurnal visual seizures and migraine. The other had typical absences as well as diurnal visual seizures and episodes of basilar migraine.

Migrainous attacks were always characteristic of either classical or basilar migraine.

The three patients with migraine only had strange and prolonged episodes described as 'a feeling of general discomfort, perspiration, and blurred vision lasting 5 h', 'right visual field scotoma followed by diffuse headache and marked photophobia, and lasted about 10 h', 'violent posterior headaches associated with abdominal discomfort, vomiting, vertigo, and perhaps also diplopia. These lasted for a couple of hours', 'occipital headaches lasting 7 and 12 h were preceded by brilliant flashes in the entire visual field, followed by blindness and then by retro-orbital pain, both lasting a few minutes'.

The five patients with epilepsy and migraine had Rolandic seizures or occipital seizures with visual hallucinations (elementary or complex-micropsia, blindness) , hemiconvulsions and one had absences. The 'migrainous episodes' were prolonged and consisted of: 'dazzling flashing lights followed by blindness, agitation, vomiting, vertigo, bilateral paresthesia of the hands and diffuse headache mainly posterior', 'dazzling lights evolving to a red spot, hemianopia and blindness, paresthesia of both hands with reduced awareness fluctuating for some hours after the headache stopped', 'altitudinal hemianopia followed by diffuse headache lasting 5–24 h and associated with marked photophobia, abdominal discomfort and intermittent vomiting or a marked confusional state with agitation and ataxia', 'agitated, complaining of a feeling of heat in the back of the head lasting for ¾ h, and then of headache over the calvarium lasting a few more hours. Three hours after onset she lost consciousness while standing. Her face was very pale. There were no abnormal movements. Migrainous episodes recurred every two months, usually starting with a glittering scotoma in the right visual field, sometimes followed by hemianopia or complete blindness. Bilateral occipital headaches, abdominal discomfort, diarrhoea, vomiting, and anxious agitation were constant features of her attacks', 'He suddenly saw the landscape becoming very bright and appearing as though he was looking at it "through a broken mirror". Blindness followed after a few seconds, lasting 15 min. The child was ataxic and felt paresthesiae in both hands. He was agitated, and talked continuously, but his father could not understand what he was saying. Occipital headache, lasting several hours, started once vision had returned. Vomiting was present in a few similar episodes'.

The authors also noted that 'In our small group of five patients who had basilar migraine and epilepsy with interictal EEG occipital epileptogenic abnormalities, migraine always started many months or years after the first epileptic attack. On the other hand, in four patients the EEG focus was already present before the first migrainous attack and disappeared before migraine stopped'.

Terasaki *et al.* (1987)[763] retrospectively studied 23 children with idiopathic occipital epilepsy (Group 1) and compared them with nine children who also had neurological deficits, CT brain scan abnormalities or both (symptomatic Group 2).

Idiopathic occipital seizures showed 'a remarkable age-dependent mode of onset with a peak at 7 to 9 years of age, whereas no age characteristic was observed in the symptomatic group. The girls/boys ratio was 1.6 in the idiopathic group; and 1/2 in symptomatic cases. A strong family history of convulsive disorders was found in Group 1 (43.5 per cent) versus only one case (11.1 per cent) in Group 2. Predisposition to headache was high in Group 1 (39.1 per cent) , but only 11.1 per cent in Group 2. All five cases (15.6 per cent) with familial predisposition to both convulsions and headaches were in Group 1.

Clinical Seizure Manifestations: Overall, visual seizures predominated (90.6 per cent). They consisted of blurred vision, blindness or both (71.9 per cent); phosphenes described as round, coloured, flickering luminous shapes (34.4 per cent); complex visual hallucinations of human faces, eyes, square patterns and figures (18.8 per cent); and visual illusions such as distortion of ceilings or floormats (15.6 per cent). Oculoclonic seizures were less frequent (9.4 per cent). All children were able to respond accurately during visual seizures, whereas three patients had impaired consciousness during oculoclonic seizures.

There was no difference between Groups 1 and 2 regarding incidence of visual seizures and oculoclonic attacks.

Visual seizures and oculoclonic attacks were followed by partial seizures with hemifacial involvement and/or hemiconvulsions (25 per cent), generalized tonic–clonic convulsions (13.6 per cent), and automatism (12.5 per cent). Seventeen patients (53.1 per cent) went on to another seizure pattern, and this was slightly more frequent in Group 2. Among these patients, alteration of consciousness (76.5 per cent) and loss of consciousness (29.4 per cent) occurred in those who developed secondary GTCS. In Group 1, seizures evolved predominantly into partial motor whereas complex partial seizures with automatism or generalized tonic–clonic convulsions predominated in Group 2. Therefore, impairment of consciousness during the course of the seizures was less frequent in Group 1 (63.6 per cent) than Group 2 (100 per cent) and this was statistically significant ($P < 0.02$).

Autonomic symptoms such as headache, nausea, vomiting, and vertigo 'during and/or after visual seizures' occurred in 24 cases (75.0 per cent). Headache occurred in 16 patients. It was described mainly as a heavy feeling (11 cases), pulsative migraine-like headache (four) and occipital pain (one). In two cases every visual seizure was accompanied by headache. The duration of headache was rather short and lasted 10 min or less in 10 cases (62.5 per cent) and 1–2 h in only two cases. Four children fell asleep after every headache. There was no difference in the incidence and features of the headache between Groups 1 and 2.

Terasaki *et al.* (1987)[763] emphasized that 'The headaches observed in our cases were different from migraine, especially basilar artery migraine, because of their characteristics: the headaches were rarely pulsatile and considered primarily of a heavy feeling (68.8 per cent); localization was mainly diffuse and rarely localized to the occipital region; duration was generally short; and they were rarely followed by sleep'.[763]

Other type of seizures. Febrile and/or afebrile GTCS preceded occipital seizures in nine patients (28. 1 per cent). Nine patients had a combination of occipital seizures with GTCS or complex partial seizures and this mainly occurred in Group 2 ($P < 0.005$) which included a patient with the Lennox–Gastaut syndrome.

Prognosis. Twenty one patients were followed for more than 2 years. Prognosis was favourable in Group 1, in which 10 cases (71.4 per cent) were seizure-free for over two years and no case was uncontrolled. Group 2 had a poor prognosis. Only one case (14.3 per cent) was seizure-free for over two years and four cases (57.1 per cent) showed no change or only a slight decrease in seizure frequency. All four cases that were free of epileptic discharges for over 1 year were in Group 1.

Terzano *et al.* (1987, 1993)[765,766] found that from 450 patients with migraine, 16 (3.6 per cent) also had seizures. In four of these 16 patients the two conditions, migraine and epilepsy, appeared to be coincidental. In another five patients 'the two types of attacks were quite distinct but often an epileptic seizure was followed by a migraine attack and vice versa'. The remaining seven patients had 'intercalated seizures'. These seven patients had a family history of migraine and two also had relatives with epilepsy. They all had visual seizures consisting of 'highly stylized contours of plain figures, or single or multicoloured spots that often rotated. They lasted for 1–2 min and came out of a scintillating scotoma slowly developing in the visual field and evolving into unilateral or bilateral hemianopia. The change of visual perception from negative to positive corresponded to the beginning of the epileptic seizure which was later followed by migraine headache. The visual epileptic symptoms were considered different from the migraine aura by the patients themselves'.

In EEG, these seven patients had occipital paroxysms attenuated with eyes open. Four patients exhibited marked photosensitivity. The EEG abnormalities tended to disappear before the third decade. Seizures remitted before the age of 20 years in six of the seven. Migraine continued but the attacks became increasingly less frequent and responded to antimigraine treatment.

Panayiotopoulos (1987)[602] reported 'a new syndrome of benign occipital seizures with nocturnal seizures, tonic deviation of the eyes and vomiting' and detailed the 'difficulties in differentiating migraine and epilepsy based on clinical and EEG findings'. I quote: 'The syndrome has been recently recognized in eight out of 20 patients with "occipital lobe epilepsy" seen by the author in a 10 year period. The syndrome is characterized by a clinical triad of nocturnal seizures, tonic deviation of the eyes and vomiting. In all eight children, vomiting occurred during the ictal phase of the seizures when the eyes were deviated and always preceded other partial epileptic manifestations and generalized tonic–clonic seizures which may have followed. Consciousness is usually, but not always, disturbed. The duration of the seizures varies from a few minutes up to 3 h. The frequency of the seizures is remarkably low; in all eight children only 29 seizures were witnessed and two children suffered only solitary ones. Non-nocturnal seizures are extremely rare. The age of onset varies from 2- to 6-years-old with a peak at age 4. The prevalence of this syndrome appeared to be higher than that of "childhood epilepsy with migrainous phenomena and occipital paroxysms"; only two patients were seen with the latter syndrome in the same period. The prognosis is excellent, with all children free of seizures in a 1 to 10 year follow-up. The duration between onset and remission of seizures does not exceed 2 years. Remission occurs before age 7. There is no family history of epilepsy or migraine, both sexes are equally involved and no definite causative factor has been detected'.

'Electroencephalography reveals abnormalities identical to those previously reported (Panayiotopoulos, 1980, 1981).[599,600] In physiological terms they suffer from "fixation-off sensitive" epilepsy'. In the same report Panayiotopoulos (1987)[602] also argued against 'a causal relationship between migraine and a secondary "autonomous epilepsy": There is no evidence that clinical and EEG manifestations of epilepsy deteriorate progressively as would be expected from the frequent "epileptogenic" insults of migrainous attacks to the brain, recurring sometimes throughout life. It is possible that the link suggested between migraine and epilepsy may reflect differential diagnostic difficulties between the two diseases' and concluded that:

(a) Migraine and epilepsy are two entirely different disorders although some symptoms are common for both;

(b) Most of the cases presented as a migraine-epilepsy syndrome reflect problems in differential diagnosis or pure coincidence;

(c) There is no evidence that migraine, secondary, causes epilepsy, as this would be expected to result in multiple epileptic foci and a bad prognosis; and

(d) There is a strong possibility that epileptic discharges may trigger migrainous phenomena, particularly in children, and to describe this disorder the term 'childhood epilepsy with migrainous phenomena and occipital paroxysms' is proposed.

Kuzniecky and Rosenblatt (1987)[458] reported three siblings with 'benign occipital epilepsy' and a fourth with EEG abnormalities. The first sibling had two motor partial seizures that had good prognosis. The second sibling had a single seizure similar to the EBOS at age 5 years. 'He complained of diffuse headache and nausea and went to sleep. Two hours later he woke up confused and vomiting which was followed by left sided clonic movements for 1 min'. The third sibling had her first nocturnal seizure at age 6, two years after an occipital spike was detected in her EEG. 'The episode was initiated by staring followed by tonic deviation of the eyes to the left and confusion and had several episodes of staring the following week'. The fourth sibling had a normal EEG at age 18 months and occipital spikes at age 4 years with no seizures. A 'typical EEG occipital abnormality' was found in 26 per cent of 25 relatives examined. These EEG changes were more evident in younger members. The authors suggested an autosomal dominant pattern for the EEG abnormalities with age-dependent expression and variable penetrance of the seizure disorder in BOS.

Fois *et al.* (1988)[287] evaluated associated symptoms and patient outcome in 293 children selected because of occipital paroxysms in their EEG. Patients had a variety of clinical problems such as mental retardation (74 patients), neurological symptoms, headache or migraine, paroxysmal abdominal pain, vomiting or sleep disturbances (57), behaviour problems (46), ocular symptoms (30), and 'convulsions of various types were present'. Only eight patients had ictal visual phenomena consistent with the diagnosis of benign epilepsy with occipital spike and wave. Clinical symptoms in these patients were quite heterogeneous and frequently not ictal. In the 141 children with at least 6 months follow-up, 58 had other types of convulsions. Clinical and EEG normalization was observed in 25 and clinical normalization only in 17. The use of anti-epileptic drugs did not seem to influence the outcome although seizure control was obtained in 26 patients. In all the cases where follow-up was 9 or more years, clinical normalization was observed. The disappearance of the occipital paroxysms with increasing age was rightly interpreted as 'not lesional' in origin.

Niedermeyer (1988)[574] described six cases with 'benign occipital lobe epilepsy'. However, three cases are rather atypical for BOS despite EEG occipital spikes. For example, no. 2 is a 32-year-old woman with 'atypical absences' since age 7 years, no. 3 is a 22-year-old man with mainly attacks of blindness and intractable nocturnal GTCS and no. 5 is a 19-year-old woman with attacks of flashing lights and spots since age 18 years.

De Romanis *et al.* (1988)[215,214] reported twenty children with EEG 'temporo-parieto occipital or temporo-occipital spikes or spike-wave complexes suppressed by eye-opening'. Patients showed different neurological syndromes: classic migraine, vertebrobasilar migraine, visual phenomena, epilepsy and psychomotor retardation. Thirteen patients had epileptic seizures. These 'were preceded by visual phenomena in 12 cases. In six cases, a combination of classic migraine, visual phenomena and seizures was found. In one case of vertebrobasilar migraine, seizures occurred 5 years after the first episode of migraine. Follow-up data indicate a non-benign evolution of occipital epilepsy: partial or generalized seizures persisted in 13 treated cases. Moreover, the EEG finding of occipital spike-wave complexes seems to extend to different neurological syndromes'.

Note: The patients with occipital paroxysms of De Romanis *et al.* in these two[214,215] and subsequent reports[212,213] are well studied, often with ictal EEG and very long follow-up. However, it is likely that most of their patients suffered from childhood occipital seizures and this may also be the case for their 14 patients reported as 'migraine and epilepsy with infantile onset and EEG findings of occipital spike-wave complexes'.[213] For the majority of the patients visual hallucinations were described as bright rings, bands, red or other-coloured discs lasting for a few seconds to 1–2 min. These were often followed by amaurosis which lasted longer for about 5–10 min. Visual phenomena could be an isolated event or could precede headache or convulsions. The ictal EEGs with repetitive fast occipital spikes or slow waves and spikes favour the view that these are epileptic seizures rather than migraine attacks.

Panayiotopoulos (1988)[603] reported on 'vomiting as an ictal manifestation of epileptic seizures and syndromes'. Twenty-four out of 900 adult and child patients with epilepsy were found to have vomiting during an ictus. All the 24 patients were children before puberty with a similar clinical pattern consisting of partial seizures which were mainly nocturnal. Ictal vomiting was always concurrent with other epileptic manifestations, more often deviation of the eyes and impairment of consciousness. The initial part of the ictus was short for minutes or prolonged for hours with frequent 'marching' to hemi-convulsions and generalized seizures. Seventeen of the 24 children suffered from benign childhood epilepsies with complete remission in long follow-up. A significantly higher association was found between ictal vomiting and the syndrome of EBOS ($P < 0.001$) but not with centrotemporal spikes. He concluded that the recognition of this association may have important theoretical implications and on clinical grounds, it may prevent unnecessary investigations and undue concern.

Beaumanoir *et al.* 1989[81] reported nine patients with at least 'one reflex scotosensitive seizure recorded with EEG'. Eight of them 'fulfilled the accepted criteria for a diagnosis of benign epilepsy with occipital focus'. Seizures were elicited when passing from light conditions to darkness and in at least four patients it was confirmed that the eyes did not close during this procedure. Age at onset was from 3 to 7 years and eight patients appeared to have a good prognosis. CT brain scan was normal in all but one. All patients had parieto-occipital spike or multiple spike foci which were inhibited by IPS at frequencies higher than 6 Hz. In five of them the occipital discharges were also induced as an off-response to IPS, i.e. they occurred immediately after the end of a train of IPS. Also, five patients developed photosensitivity during the course of the disease. Three different electroclinical types of scotosensitive seizures were recorded:

(a) Less than 5 s episodes of 'dazzle or flash' often associated with an unpleasant feeling. The ictal EEG consists of recruited unilateral or bilateral multiple occipital spikes often followed by a slow wave.

(b) Seizures of 8–32 s duration with a 'flash' followed by impairment of consciousness, 'complex absences' and falls. An EEG illustrating such a seizure shows generalized multiple spikes with posterior amplitude predominance.

(c) Complex behaviour described above without the preceding dazzle or flash.

Whether these interesting patients had FOS or true scotosensitive epilepsy cannot be deduced and this is discussed in detail in Chapter 10, page 180.

Nalin *et al.* (1989)[560] studied 13 children 'treated for ictal visual episodes'. In 10 cases visual symptoms (amaurosis, hallucinations, and illusions) started between 6 and 14 years, associated with occipital EEG abnormalities (sharp-waves, slow waves, spikes, spike-waves) which disappeared in six after eyes-opening. All were of normal intelligence and behaviour and there was no significant antecedent in the history of half of these cases. One patient had on CT scan bilateral occipital calcifications. In nine, visual ictal symptoms disappeared after anti-epileptic treatment. They also commented that three of these nine cases with visual seizures 'did not show the typical EEG picture of benign occipital epilepsy, and must be diagnostically distinguished from psychiatric disorders, basilar migraine, and other partial epilepsies'.

Panayiotopoulos (1989)[606] described in detail the 'benign nocturnal childhood occipital epilepsy: a new syndrome with nocturnal seizures, tonic deviation of the eyes, and vomiting'. I quote: 'An epileptic syndrome of benign nocturnal childhood occipital epilepsy with excellent prognosis is described. The syndrome is characterized by a clinical ictal triad of nocturnal seizures, tonic deviation of the eyes, and vomiting. There may be marching to involve the head and limbs, ending with a generalized tonic–clonic seizure. Consciousness is usually, but not invariably, disturbed. Infrequent daytime fits may develop one to two years after remission of the nocturnal seizures. Age of onset is usually from 3 to 5 years. Both sexes are involved. There is no family history of epilepsy or migraine. No definite causative factor was detected. The frequency of the seizures is very low with two children having only solitary ones. The interictal electroencephalographic features consist of repetitive occipital spike and slow wave complexes that are induced by closed eyes and darkness and are inhibited by open eyes and fixation with visual cues. It is proposed that this is a new idiopathic age-related-onset syndrome of the localization-related epilepsies'.

[Note: The difficulties of publishing these reports are well illustrated here. This report was completed in 1985 but was rejected by a major neurological journal. It was submitted in December 1986 to the *Journal of Child Neurology* but was finally published 2 years later in January 1989. Furthermore, acceptance would probably have been impossible without the strong recommendations of one of the assessors, with whom I had shared details of these patients and copies of my medical and EEG reports.]

Panayiotopoulos (1989)[605] reported the results of a 15-year prospective study on 'benign childhood epilepsy with occipital paroxysms'. Eighteen of 418 children who had onset of epilepsy before the age of 13 years showed clinical and electroencephalographic evidence of benign childhood epilepsy with occipital paroxysms. They represented one-fifth of all benign age- and localization-related idiopathic epilepsies. Some patients were followed for as long as 15 years. There was a preponderance of females and peak age at onset of epilepsy was 5 years. In 16 children, the seizures were infrequent and sometimes prolonged and consisted mainly of tonic deviation of the eyes and vomiting, often with evolution to unilateral or generalized convulsions. Seizures were only nocturnal in 11 and nocturnal and diurnal in another five children. Prognosis was excellent; five children had only one fit. Remission usually occurred 1–2 years after onset and no seizures occurred after the age of 12 years. The remaining two children had frequent diurnal episodes consisting of visual hallucinations, post-ictal headache, and occasional nocturnal hemiconvulsions. Their prognosis was less favourable. Electroencephalographic abnormalities in all 18 patients consisted of repetitive spike and slow-wave discharges confined to the occipital regions and attenuated when the eyes were open. These outlasted clinical remission for many years, sometimes up to the age of 16. Fixation-off sensitivity was demonstrated frequently. Based on these findings, a unifying definition for benign childhood epilepsy with occipital paroxysms was proposed.[605]

Kivity and Lerman (1989)[442], (1991)[484] and (1992)[443] reviewed BOS and confirmed with their own cases the reports of Panayiotopoulos[600,602,636] of partial status epilepticus which they vividly called 'stormy onset with prolonged loss of consciousness in benign childhood epilepsy with occipital paroxysms'. Amongst 62 children with BOS, 18 had visual symptoms, 24 adversive seizures, 24 headache and 15 vomiting.[442] In nine (seven were boys) of these 'the onset was stormy and alarming'. 'The first and often only seizure was characterized by prolonged loss of consciousness lasting up to 12 h, suggesting an acute cerebral insult. In all but one case there was a tonic aversion either of eyes alone or of both head and eyes which was interpreted as conjugate deviation. The other accompanying ictal motor phenomena were either partial or generalized convulsions. In five patients the seizure was heralded by headache, and in five cases was accompanied by vomiting. The seizure began with visual symptoms in only one patient. The seizure occurred while awake in seven and during sleep in two'. The age at onset was from 3 ¼ to 10 years (mean = 6.7 years, median 8 years). Interictal EEGs showed occipital paroxysms, and the clinical course was benign. In four cases a few partial or complex partial seizures recurred during subsequent anticonvulsant therapy, but in five cases seizures were solitary. Anticonvulsants were discontinued in five patients who remained free from seizures for 1 to 11½ years after withdrawal of treatment. The authors concluded that 'sudden coma in a child associated with focal features such as tonic deviation of the head or eyes or both may represent a benign seizure disorder'.

Vigevano *et al.* (1989),[794] Ricci *et al.* (1991),[676] and Vigevano and Ricci (1993)[793] also confirmed in their reports the existence of partial status epilepticus in the Panayiotopoulos syndrome with prolonged seizures and autonomic symptoms. In their most recent publication[793] they presented six boys and eight girls with prolonged nocturnal seizures which like the patients of Panayiotopoulos[602] were 'characterized in sequence by nausea, vomiting, lateral deviation of the eyes, impaired consciousness and hemiconvulsions'. Four patients also had sporadic diurnal seizures. Age at onset was from 2 to 6 years (mean 3.8 ± 1.2 and median 4 years). Total number of seizures varied from one (four children), two (five children), three (three children) to a maximum of four (one) or six (one). The duration of seizures varied from 15 min to 2 h. Prognosis was excellent for all with a follow-up from 1 year and 4 months to 9 years. In EEG, all but three children had occipital spikes and three of them also had centrotemporal spikes. Three children had normal EEG. All had normal CT brain scan. Ictal EEG unequivocally documented the ictal character of the autonomic symptoms (Fig. 10.17). Four children had simple febrile convulsions. Three had a family history of epilepsy, one of epilepsy and febrile convulsions and three of febrile convulsions alone. The authors also emphasized the frequent occurrence of febrile convulsions and centrotemporal spikes in patients with Panayiotopoulos syndrome.

Nagendran *et al.* (1990)[557] reported a family with benign occipital seizures. The youngest boy had at age 7 years visual hallucinations of 'seeing coloured spots' lasting 5–10 min and followed by several hours of drowsiness. Seizures occurring twice per day were abolished with sodium valproate. His youngest sister had at age 6 years two GTCS in one night. She admitted seeing brightly coloured spots and later her attacks comprised visual loss for some 30 s. Her seizures were difficult to control. Both brother and sister had EEGs with occipital paroxysms. Their middle brother had centrotemporal spikes in the EEG and was asymptomatic. The oldest brother had occipital slow waves at age 11 years. The mother said that she had 10 attacks of visual disturbances between the ages 10–20 years. The father had some major convulsions at age 31 years which did not recur. Both parents had normal EEGs.

Takaishi *et al.* (1991)[750] studied 25 idiopathic epileptic children with occipital EEG foci for more than 3 years. They were categorized into two groups:

Group A with visual symptoms, probably corresponding to LBOS of Gastaut and Group B without visual symptoms but mainly with ictal tonic deviation of the eyes and probably corresponding to EBOS of Panayiotopoulos.

In all patients, interictal EEG consisted of spikes or spike and wave complexes in the occipital regions but foci in frontal and centrotemporal regions were also recorded particularly in group A.

Group A consisted of 12 children (three were boys) with onset of seizures at a mean age of 8 ± 2 years (range 5 to 13 years). Visual symptoms consisted of micropsia or macropsia (23 per cent), 'phosphenes'(50 per cent), amaurosis (25 per cent) and rarely 'change in distance or dysmorphia.' Other symptoms such as auditory hallucinations, dizziness and vomiting and headache could occur and usually followed the visual symptoms but could also precede them. In particular, nausea and vomiting occurred in 67 per cent either preceding or following other symptoms. The duration of the active seizure period was 4 ± 2 years. Remission was obtained after the age of 15 years in 82 per cent and 80 per cent of the patients had EEG epileptiform discharges after that age. Seizure control with treatment was good in only two children. There was a family history of convulsive seizures in 50 per cent and three (25 per cent) children also had febrile convulsions.

Group B consisted of four boys and seven girls with onset of seizures at a mean age of 5 ± 1 year (range from 3 to 8 years). Seizures consisted of tonic deviation of the eyes (62 per cent), nausea and vomiting (31 per cent), headache (8 per cent) and GTCS (46 per cent). The active duration of seizures was 11 ± 11 months and five children had solitary seizures in long follow-up. Remission was obtained after the age of 15 years in 10 of the 11 children (91 per cent) and only two (18 per cent) had EEG epileptiform discharges after the age of 15 years. Seizure control with treatment was good in nine of the 11 children. There was a family history of convulsive seizures in 15 per cent and 6 (54.5 per cent) children also had febrile convulsions. The difference between the two groups regarding age at onset, good control, duration of the active seizure period and remission of seizures was statistically significant ($P < 0.05$).

De Romanis *et al.* (1991)[213] reported 14 very interesting patients as 'migraine and epilepsy with infantile onset and EEG findings of occipital spike wave complexes'. All patients had EEG occipital paroxysms attenuated with eyes open, visual symptoms interpreted as migraine aura and all but one also had convulsions. For the majority of the patients visual symptoms and convulsions were followed by long lasting severe headache, often associated with vomiting.

'Eight were females, whose age presently ranges between 12 and 24 years (present mean age: 17.3 years). Patients were first seen shortly after the onset of the symptoms; at that time patients' ages ranged from 3 to 9 years (mean age 5.4 years). The clinical and EEG follow-up ranged from 4 to 16 years (mean 11.2 years). All patients had normal neurological, ophthalmological and brain CT scan examinations. The psychometric evaluation revealed a low score in one subject only. A family history of migraine was present in six subjects and of epilepsy in one'.

Visual phenomena were described as bright rings, bands, red or other-coloured discs, in both visual fields or in the visual hemifield opposite to the hemisphere where spike-wave complexes were recorded. In all subjects but two (cases 4 and 11), amaurosis followed the appearance of these phosphenes, and lasted longer (about 5–10 min) than the phosphenes (which lasted only from a few seconds up to 1 or 2 min). Two patients had complex visual hallucinations, probably terrifying, occurring in the dark.

'Visual phenomena could be an isolated event over a variable period of time, and then later on come to precede headache or convulsions in five patients. In four patients visual phenomena followed by headache were present 1–2 years before the onset of convulsions. In one patient only, convulsions appeared before migraine (case 9), the latter appearing four years after the onset of seizures. Visual hallucinations and convulsions appeared simultaneously in three subjects'.

[Note: The description of the visual symptoms and their duration are more in favour of visual occipital seizures than migrainous visual aura.]

The ictal EEG of a patient is probably unique as it clearly documents that the visual hallucinations were epileptic and illustrates well the sequence of electrical events during the phase of positive and negative ictal visual symptoms. The seizure started with rapid occipital spikes when the patient reported bright spots in both hemifields for 23 s. This was followed by amaurosis with a simultaneous flattening of the EEG for about 20 s. EEGs then showed the reappearance of low amplitude 'sharp waves' for 90 s, in the above-mentioned areas, with higher voltage on the right side and a pseudorhythmic pattern followed by a normal activity for 4 min. After that, sharp waves gradually increased in frequency and amplitude, prevalent on the right side for 5 min, and were followed by interictal activity. 'The above phenomena were followed by migraine accompanied by nausea, vomiting and photophobia, lasting for about 8 h. A left homonymous hemianopsia, that disappeared after 24 h, was detected by visual field examination'. This ictal EEG was of a woman with onset of symptoms at the age of 9 years. 'She reported visual phenomena lasting for 5 min and consisting of bright spots on the left side, rapidly spreading to the right and followed by amaurosis. These symptoms recurred for three years, either isolated or followed by migraine. At age 12 the patient experienced two seizures with secondary generalization, preceded by the above visual phenomena and migraine lasting 12 h. Seizures disappeared following treatment with Sodium Valproate (600 mg) and Clobazam (30 mg); however the visual phenomena continued to recur once per month. Twice a year they were followed by a throbbing headache accompanied by nausea, vomiting, photophobia and usually lasting 5 to 6 h and occasionally up to 72 h. The patient was followed up for 15 years. EEGs showed occipital high voltage 'sharp waves', mostly on the right, suppressed by eye-opening, during the first three years, later replaced by slow activity (0.5 Hz) in the temporo-occipital regions, the amplitude of which was higher in the right hemisphere.

In another patient (case 14), 'a 12-year-old boy, an EEG during a migraine attack followed by a generalized seizure could be recorded. At the age of 3 years, this patient suffered from febrile convulsions. At 6, seizures characterized by complex visual hallucinations representing people in movement, occurred before sleeping; they disappeared whenever the light was turned on. At 7, one episode of the same visual phenomena was followed by four hemiclonic seizure attacks in the same day. Treatment with phenobarbital (150 mg) and Phenytoin (200 mg) reduced the frequency of attacks from 4 to 1 per year. Throbbing headache then appeared immediately before complex or elementary visual hallucinations and amaurosis. Headache was accompanied by nausea and/or vomiting and photophobia. Migraine attacks lasted 12 to 24 h and were followed by generalized or left hemiclonic seizures. The patient was followed up for about 9 years. EEGs constantly revealed high voltage spike-waves complexes in the left temporo-occipital region, suppressed by eye opening. At the age of 10, an EEG recorded during a migraine attack showed a 2 Hz high voltage activity in the left hemisphere and spike-wave complexes in an almost continuous sequence. This finding was followed by a generalized seizure'.

Anti-epileptic treatment reduced the frequency of migraine attacks in most of the patients. I quote: 'In four subjects migraine attacks completely disappeared; a 75 per cent reduction was obtained in three subjects, and a 50 per cent reduction was observed in two. In one patient only was no improvement obtained. In three subjects, chronic treatment with Pizotifen (1.5 mg/day) induced a complete remission of migraine attacks. Seizures completely disappeared in two subjects; seizures occurred from the age of 5 to the age of 8 years and at the age of 21 the patient was still attack-free after having discontinued the antiepileptic treatment at the age of 13; in the other patient, seizures disappeared at the age of 12 and the patient was still attack-free at the age of 16 two years after medications were discontinued. In the remaining 11 subjects affected by epilepsy, a 50 per cent reduction in the frequency of seizures was obtained after treatment was begun'.

Cooper and Lee (1991)[180] retrospectively studied EEG occipital epileptiform activity that was almost continuous and reactive to eye opening (ROEA) in order to evaluate its prognostic value. The EEG and hospital record of patients with ROEA were reviewed with an observation period of 6 months to 8 years. The patients were divided into good and poor outcome groups based on response to treatment. Of 33 patients, 12 (36.4 per cent) had complete seizure control; 21 (63.6 per cent) continued to have poorly controlled seizures. Only three (9.1 per cent) patients were able to discontinue anti-epileptic drugs without seizure recurrence. Analysis of clinical and EEG variables showed that a history of perinatal difficulties, abnormal neurologic findings, and abnormal EEG background activities occur significantly more frequently in the poor outcome group. The authors concluded that ROEA is not uniformly associated with a benign course and that other factors are involved in determining prognosis of the epilepsy.

[Note: It is interesting and significant that in these retrospective reports,[180,753] children with Panayiotopoulos syndrome, the next common after Rolandic seizures benign childhood partial seizure syndrome, are entirely absent. This is most likely because EEG referrals are poor and medical records incomplete, causing doubts about the significance of such retrospective studies.]

Likewise, **Talwar *et al.* (1992)**[753] studied EEG and clinical features of 30 children and young adults with EEG occipital paroxysms. Prolonged occipital paroxysms (greater than 6 s) occurred only in children with seizures ($P < 0.001$). Brief discharges (1–6 s) appeared immediately after eye closure. Generalized spike wave discharges (11 patients, 37 per cent) and background abnormalities (17 patients, 57 per cent) were common. Photic activation of occipital paroxysms was not observed. Twenty-four patients (80 per cent) manifested paroxysmal phenomena seizures (20 patients, 67 per cent) and 'migraine (12 patients, 40 per cent, four alone and eight with seizures)'. Fifteen patients (75 per cent) had partial seizures, and five (25 per cent) had absence seizures. In seven patients with partial seizures, an aetiology was evident. Neurologic examination was more often abnormal in patients with secondary partial seizures than in those with idiopathic partial seizures ($P < 0.05$) and absence seizures. Conversely, migraine was more often associated with idiopathic partial seizures than with secondary partial seizures ($P < 0.05$) and absence seizures. Six children (20 per cent) had no paroxysmal events. Generalized spike wave discharges were uncommon in patients with idiopathic partial seizures. The authors concluded that occipital paroxysms are a non-specific epileptiform abnormality that may occur in children with (a) idiopathic partial, (b) symptomatic partial, and (c) absence epilepsies, but it may also occur in patients with no evidence of seizures.

Panayiotopoulos and Igoe (1992)[630] described 'cerebral insult-like partial status epilepticus in the early onset variant of benign childhood epilepsy with occipital paroxysms'. They all had EEG occipital paroxysms and protracted, 'cerebral insult-like, ictal episodes of impairment of consciousness, vomiting, tonic deviation of the eyes and hemi-convulsions or generalized tonic–clonic seizures. Long term follow-up confirmed that this is an entirely benign epileptic condition despite partial status epilepticus.

Beaumanoir and Thomas (1992)[86] gave an excellent review on 'benign epilepsy of childhood with occipital paroxysms'.

Beaumanoir *et al.* organized an International Symposium in Milan, March 1992, on occipital seizures and epilepsies in children. In this informative and constructive meeting Beaumanoir,[76,77] Dalla Bernardina *et al.*,[192] Guerrini *et al.*[367] and Vigevano and Ricci[793] reported their studies on benign childhood occipital epilepsies which also offered unequivocal evidence in support of the early onset BOS of Panayiotopoulos who also reviewed his experience and presented new illustrative cases.[608] Details of these reports were published the following year, 1993, by John Libbey & Co. Limited in a book on 'Occipital seizures and epilepsies in children' edited by Andermann *et al.*[38]

Dalla Bernardina *et al.* (1993)[192] compared the clinico-EEG manifestations of 64 children with idiopathic (33 patients), cryptogenic (12) and symptomatic (19) occipital lobe epilepsy. In children with idiopathic occipital epilepsy, seizures were more often 'pure occipital' (63.5 per cent versus 31.5 per cent of the symptomatic group), more frequently spreading to the motor (30.5 per cent versus 10.5 per cent) than temporal regions (9 per cent versus 42 per cent), associated with ictal vomiting (63.5 per cent versus 21 per cent) of more than 30 min duration (30.5 per cent versus 16 per cent),and infrequent or rare (91 per cent versus 26.5 per cent). Polymorphous seizures occurred only in the symptomatic or cryptogenic groups. Headache was equally reported in idiopathic (30.5 per cent) and symptomatic (31.5 per cent) occipital epilepsy.

On the basis of clinico-EEG features these authors proposed that idiopathic occipital epilepsy consists of three groups:

(a) Fourteen cases 'with partial visual seizures with focal occipital spike wave often suppressed by eye-opening, more or less increased in frequency during sleep. Headache is relatively frequent; vomiting less frequent. These cases appear very similar to those described by Gastaut,[303,304,308] Nalin *et al.*,[560] Giroud *et al.*,[340] and some of those described by Beaumanoir'.[74]

(b) Eight 'cases with long-lasting seizures frequently appearing during sleep characterized by tonic deviation of the eyes and vomiting and, in some cases only, with focal occipital spike-wave complexes suppressed by eyes-opening. These cases are very similar to those described by Panayiotopoulos (1988,1989),[603,605] Vigevano *et al.* (1989)[794] and Dalla Bernardina *et al.* (1992)'.[195]

(c) Eleven 'cases with partial occipital seizures often spreading to motor areas and frequently associated with Rolandic or hemiconvulsive seizures and with EEG focal spike-wave complexes similar to those of the Rolandic epilepsy, dramatically increasing in frequency during sleep. These last cases evoke some of Beaumanoir's (1983)[74] cases and the electroclinical picture described by Dalla Bernardina *et al.* (1984,1991)[190,194] under the name of benign partial epilepsy with occipital spikes'.

Guerrini *et al.* (1993)[367] reported the 'outcome of idiopathic childhood epilepsy with occipital paroxysms'. They studied 18 patients (11 were boys) with CEOP aged 4½ years to 18½ years (mean 11½ years). The most frequent ictal pattern was tonic deviation of the eyes which occurred without other signs in four patients and was accompanied by ictal vomiting in another four. Both these and unilateral seizures could last as long as 30 min in some children. Age at onset ranged from 3 to 14 years (mean 7 years) with a peak at around the third year. Eleven patients had one seizure type only, six patients two types and one patient three types. 'Six patients had visual symptoms and some of them had excellent outcome'. Four had ictal headache. 'Clinical presentation and outcome coincided partially with those reported both by Gastaut (1985)[308] and Panayiotopoulos (1989)'.[605,606]

Six patients (33 per cent) suffered an isolated seizure and three others (16 per cent) had two attacks. 'This seemed the case in patients presenting with the seizure pattern of tonic deviation of the eyes and vomiting, even when prolonged, or when typical occipital EEG paroxysms are only captured in post-ictal recordings'. In other patients clusters of seizures were frequent, especially at the beginning of the disease, and did not seem to be influenced by treatment.

The authors concluded 'that none of the antiepileptic drugs seems to be more effective than the others. Relapses do not seem to be predictable on a clinical basis because patients with more than a 2-year seizure remission under treatment can relapse at drug withdrawal. On the other hand, long spontaneous remissions could be not definitive. Seizure duration and age of onset were not indicators of disease severity'. However, contrary to their statement that 'relapses do not seem to be predictable on a clinical basis' they found that 'the ictal pattern of tonic deviation of the eyes and vomiting more often occurred in patients who suffered isolated seizures'. Clusters of seizures appeared in five patients (27 per cent), two of whom were under treatment. In no patient could epilepsy be considered so severe as to influence school achievement or social adjustment. The treatment was successfully withdrawn before the age of 16 in 33 per cent of patients but the authors did not differentiate between EBOS and LBOS.

Panayiotopoulos (1993)[608] reported a 19 year prospective study of 22 children with benign childhood epilepsy with occipital paroxysms who are detailed elsewhere in this book (see Chapters 8, 9 and 13) and there is no need to repeat this work here. See also the illustrative cases in Chapters 8 and 9.

De Romanis (1993)[212] presented seven children, five were girls, diagnosed as suffering from 'basilar migraine with EEG findings of occipital spike-wave complexes'. Neurological, ophthalmological and CT brain examinations were normal. 'Migraine headache was heralded in most of the patients by 'unilateral or bilateral visual distortions represented by circles, triangles or coloured bands lasting for seconds to minutes. Throbbing headache was localized in the occipital region or was diffuse and lasted from 5 to 12 h. Eight to 12 h of sleep or drowsiness followed'. The sequence of the neurological symptoms (given in a table) during these episodes is not clear. Neurological symptoms such as ataxia, nystagmus and dysarthria alone or in combination occurred in all patients, probably during the long headache phase of the attacks as deduced by three case reports in a previous publication of the same group of authors.[215]

Age at onset was from 3 to 8 years (mean = 5.4 years). The interictal EEG in all patients had unilateral or bilateral occipital paroxysms. Ictal EEGs were recorded from all patients and 'showed diffuse high voltage delta activity associated with spikes and sharp waves or diffuse delta activity which could be recorded from 1 to 7 days.' However, the sample of the ictal EEG provided is dominated mainly by spikes and clusters of rapid spikes superimposed on slow waves.

During a long, 8–16 years, follow-up 'basilar migraine attacks disappeared within 1 year in all subjects'. However, in four patients 'migraine with aura' started 2–4 years after remission of basilar migraine attacks. The migraine aura was similar to that preceding the basilar migraine. In two patients these migraine aura episodes progressed to complex partial seizures in one and hemiconvulsions in the other. A fifth patient later developed absences and GTCS (whether these were true absences is not deducible from the details provided for the same patient in a previous report of the authors).[215]

'In all seven patients the final outcome was excellent with complete remission of seizures and migraine symptoms. Some patients were treated only with flunarazine which had a beneficial effect on the headaches'.[212]

Niedermeyer (1993)[569] in a report on 'migraine-triggered epilepsy' studied 'eight young adult patients, referred because of generalized tonic–clonic seizures with unsatisfactory treatment response. All of them had migraine. The major convulsions were preceded by a typical visual prodroma in six out of eight patients, and a full-blown migraine attack followed the convulsion in all patients. Clinical findings were unremarkable, the EEG was mostly normal or slightly abnormal without typical paroxysmal findings, and CT scan and MRI were normal. All patients also had independent migraine attacks without convulsions; all of them had a positive family history of migraine. The response to anti-migrainous and/or antiepileptic medication was sluggish or disappointing in most cases. A correction of the patient's life style proved to be the most effective approach'.

Fonseca and Tedrus (1994)[289] studied EEGs of 24 patients (aged 3 to 25 years) with 'reactive occipital epileptiform activity'. In addition, the EEG showed generalized discharges in eight, centro-temporal spikes in four and background abnormalities in four cases. Eighteen (75 per cent) patients had epileptic seizures. Non febrile seizures (16 cases) were partial (nine cases), generalized (six cases) and unclassified (one patient). Two children had neurological examination or CT brain scan abnormalities. Clinical and EEG data allowed for the following epileptic syndrome diagnosis: CEOP, seven cases; benign childhood epilepsy with centrotemporal spikes, one case; CEOP or benign childhood epilepsy with centrotemporal spikes, one case; partial symptomatic/cryptogenic epilepsy, four cases; generalized idiopathic, two cases; febrile convulsions, two cases. The authors concluded that 'reactive occipital epileptiform activity' may be observed in cases with different types of idiopathic partial, cryptogenic/symptomatic and idiopathic generalized epilepsies and may also occur in patients with no seizures'.

Aicardi (1994)[15] reviewed 'epilepsy with occipital spike-wave complexes suppressed by eye opening' (pp. 151–154)[15] in his excellent monograph on 'Epilepsy in children'.[15] He illustrated (Fig. 21–4, page 371) an EEG of occipital paroxysms that blocked on eyes open. They were consistently recorded between the ages of 4 and 10 years from 'a 15-year-old boy that had five partial clonic seizures between the ages of 4 and 15 years. Since age 7 he also had attacks of classical migraine with visual auras'.

Genton and Guerrini (1994)[319] reviewed the 'idiopathic localization-related epilepsies: the non-Rolandic types' and concluded that 'Occipital epilepsy with onset in childhood may correspond to a variety of clinical, aetiological and prognostic entities. Some of these patients do have an idiopathic type of epilepsy, but the clinical presentation is very variable even in these cases; the existence of a bimodal distribution of the ages of onset even suggests the possibility of two different clinical entities... There are no reports of a genetic overlap with Rolandic seizures... It clearly appears that the classical criteria of idiopathic localization related epilepsies cannot be applied in benign CEOP. Given the great variability of clinical and EEG patterns and of prognosis, benign CEOP should be called "idiopathic occipital epilepsy", as the term benign is inappropriate and the reference to the EEG changes may be misleading.[367] Perhaps there is a subset of patients, as suggested by Panayiotopoulos (1989)[605] that does fulfil the criteria of both idiopathicity and benignity.'[319]

Deonna and Ziegler (1994)[222] reviewed 'so-called benign epilepsies in children' and expanded on 'practical diagnostic, prognostic and therapeutic implications of this concept of benign'.

Maher and colleagues (1995)[517] reported on the 'variability in clinical and seizure manifestations in children with occipital paroxysmal discharges suppressed by eye opening'. They reviewed 5291 EEG reports made in 5½ years in the only tertiary paediatric centre in Newfoundland and Labrador of Canada. They identified 31 children who had one or more EEGs with occipital spike/sharp waves showing suppression of discharges with eye opening and normal background activity. Two of these 31 children did not have seizures, five had symptomatic epilepsy and four had only provoked mainly generalized seizures. From the remaining 20 children, only one had CEOP with visual symptoms (corresponding to LBOS of Gastaut), 10 had only nocturnal seizures (corresponding to EBOS type of Panayiotopoulos), and five had symptoms of both EBOS and LBOS (with visual hallucinations). The other three children with 'unusual complex partial seizures' most likely had diurnal seizures of the EBOS type. Their seizures consisted of 'episodes of prolonged alteration in the level of consciousness, during which the child was poorly responsive, immobile, and stared straight ahead for periods of up to 30 min. Seizures were frequently associated with vomiting and post-ictal headache'. Age at onset was 2.6, 3 and 4 years and two were free of seizures for more than one year. One of these three children also had nocturnal seizures 'with tonic deviation of the head and eyes and vomiting'. In this group of 20 children, 11 were boys and age at onset of seizures varied from 2.6 to 14.9 years with a mean at 5.8 and median 5.7 years. The prognosis was good for the 13 children with EBOS (10 with only EBOS without visual hallucination and three with the above described prolonged diurnal episodes), the majority having no seizures for 1–2 years follow-up. However, the only child with LBOS as well as two of the five with a combination of EBOS and visual hallucinations continued to have 'at least two seizures per week'.

Watanabe (1996)[797] published a detailed and well balanced review on benign partial epilepsies.

Dermirbilek *et al.* (1996)[228] presented an 'electroclinical survey on benign epilepsy with occipital paroxysms' in 33 idiopathic children. Age at onset was from 2 to 14 years. Motor (39 per cent), visual (33 per cent), autonomic (30 per cent) and complex partial (21 per cent) were the main seizure types. Secondary GTCS occurred in 70 per cent of the children. Headache, nausea, vomiting and dizziness were noted in 36 per cent before or during the seizures and 24 per cent post-ictally. Centrotemporal (27 per cent) and generalized discharges (24 per cent) could occur with the occipital paroxysms which had a mainly right sided preponderance.

Fejerman (1996,[270,271] 1997[272]) and his associates (Caraballo *et al.*, 1997)[150] reported their well performed prospective studies on 'idiopathic partial epilepsies with occipital paroxysms'. They confirmed 'the existence of two variants: the "Gastaut" type and the "Panayiotopoulos" type of benign occipital seizures'. They also confirmed that the Panayiotopoulos type was more frequent and more benign than the Gastaut type. In more detail, they prospectively analysed the electro-clinical characteristics of 74 patients seen between January 1990 and June 1996 who fulfilled the diagnostic criteria of benign occipital seizures. Follow-up ranged from 6 months to 6.5 years. They identified two groups:

> Group I (corresponding to Gastaut type LBOS) of 18 patients had visual seizures and post-ictal migrainous symptoms, with or without motor fits. Age at onset was 8.7 years and seizures were predominantly when awake. EEG occipital paroxysms reacted to eyelid opening.
>
> Group II (corresponding to Panayiotopoulos syndrome of EBOS) of 56 patients had attacks of vomiting followed by oculocephalic deviation. Age at onset was 4.9 year and the seizures were predominantly during sleep. EEG occipital spikes had identical morphology to that of the Rolandic spikes.

Two, and later in another report, 'seven additional children fulfilled clinical and EEG criteria for the concomitant diagnosis of benign partial epilepsies in childhood with centrotemporal spikes and Panayiotopoulos type EBOS. These patients had Rolandic seizures and ictal vomiting with head deviation independently during the course of the disease, and showed centrotemporal or Rolandic spikes and occipital spikes in the same interictal EEG'.

For comparison, at the same time 130 children were found to have Rolandic seizures.

Based on their experience, Fejerman (1996,[270 271] 1997[272]) and (Caraballo *et al.*, 1997)[150] emphasized the differentiation of the new variant of EBOS of 'Panayiotopoulos type' from the classic LBOS of 'Gastaut type'. Fejerman[272] concluded that 'a distinctive idiopathic epileptic syndrome occurring in children and featuring ictal vomiting, partial motor seizures, and occipital spikes has been so clearly delineated that I think it will be included in future classifications as a separate epileptic syndrome. The main differences between this new "Panayiotopoulos type" and the "Gastaut type" CEOP are: onset of seizures occurs earlier (2 to 8 years of age), usually during sleep and ictal manifestations include vomiting, which adds a peculiar and rarely mentioned type of seizure associated with head deviation, impaired consciousness and in some cases hemiconvulsions. In our experience, EEG is also different from the Gastaut type CEOP because we usually find occipital spikes during sleep instead of spike-wave occipital paroxysms reactive to eye opening while awake'.

Commending on the atypical evolution of CEOP Fejerman[270,271] stated that 'Concerning Panayiotopoulos type of CEOP, motor partial status is not rare, it has been repeatedly reported and it does not seem to be correlated with unfavourable prognosis'. He also reported two cases of Gastaut type CEOP that developed serious seizures, electrical status and cognitive impairment. These two cases have been detailed in a subsequent report by Tenenbaum *et al.* (1977).[762]

Tenenbaum *et al.* (1997)[762] reported an atypical and rather aggressive seizure and behaviour evolution of a 'Gastaut type' LBOS. These were two boys with clinical and EEG features of the late onset childhood epilepsy with occipital paroxysms (visual hallucinations and occipital spikes) who experienced severe cognitive deterioration associated with continuous spike wave activity during slow-wave sleep. Neurological examination and brain imaging were normal but both children had some learning difficulties probably before or at the onset of seizures. One child showed global improvement in behaviour and partial restoration of cognitive functions after control of seizures and normalization of the EEG. The authors concluded that 'their findings suggest a spectrum ranging from a benign course for most children with idiopathic partial epilepsies to the syndrome of Continuous Spikes and Waves During Slow Wave Sleep'.

Guerrini *et al.* (1997)[368] reported the 'delayed appearance of interictal EEG abnormalities in early onset childhood epilepsy with occipital paroxysms'. They carried out a close clinical and EEG follow-up (range, 2–12 years; mean, 6 years 7 months; median, 7 years) of 24 patients (age range,

4–19 years; mean, 11 years 8 months; median, 11 years). In five children with early seizure onset and particularly benign prognosis without any treatment, EEG abnormalities appeared 3–10 months after the first seizure. Four of them exhibited the ictal patterns of EBOS. Their findings confirm that in EBOS interictal EEG abnormalities may be lacking at the beginning of the disorder.

Gobbi and Guerrini (1997)[344] reviewed extensively 'childhood epilepsy with occipital spikes and other benign localization-related epilepsies'.

Ahmed Sharoqi *et al.* (1997)[12] reported a few more cases of 'early onset benign childhood occipital seizures' for which they proposed the name of 'Panayiotopoulos' syndrome.'

Yalcin *et al.* (1997)[826] reported the seizure manifestations and EEG features of 21 cases with childhood epilepsy with occipital paroxysms (CEOP) and benign nocturnal childhood occipital epilepsy (BNCOE). 'Nine patients had BNCOE, six had CEOP, four had CEOP and BNCOE and the remaining two belonged to the incomplete syndrome because of no paroxysmal discharges in EEG. When the patients with BNCOE awoke from sleep, they had tonic deviation of the eyes and could describe visual symptoms. Patients with CEOP had seizures beginning with visual symptoms followed by loss of consciousness but no generalized convulsions. In three cases, in addition to the occipital spikes, independent centrotemporal spikes were recorded and in another three cases generalized spike-wave discharges were recorded'.

Ferraro *et al.* (1997)[275] found 18 (2.5 per cent) patients with 'Panayiotopoulos type BCOS' amongst 707 patients mainly children with epilepsy (87 per cent were younger than 18 years) and also reported three new cases having both BOS of Panayiotopoulos type and Rolandic seizures.[274]

Panayiotopoulos *et al.* (1997)[625] reviewed the differentiating clinical symptoms of migraine with aura and reported two cases of LBOS imitating acephalgic migraine (see illustrative cases in Chapter 9).

Ferrie *et al.* (1997)[277] reported the results of a multicentre study on 'early-onset benign occipital seizure susceptibility syndrome'. Participating investigators from England, Greece, Japan, Italy and Israel 'submitted details of patients with idiopathic occipital seizures characterized by ictal head or eye deviation and vomiting'. One hundred and thirteen patients were recruited. Seizures began in early childhood (mean, 4.6 years) and occurred infrequently (mean total seizures, three); 30 per cent of patients had only a single seizure. Two thirds of seizures were nocturnal. Ictal eye deviation occurred in 79 per cent, vomiting in 70 per cent, and head deviation in 35 per cent. Seizures were predominantly complex partial in type. Partial status epilepticus occurred in 44 per cent of patients. Seventy-four per cent of patients had occipital interictal EEG epileptiform activity, predominantly right sided, with fixation-off sensitivity. Extra occipital EEG abnormalities such as centrotemporal spikes occurred in 35 per cent of patients. Prognosis was excellent: the mean duration of active seizures was 1 year.

They concluded that 'although the two groups (EBOS and LBOS) shared identical EEG features, the distinct clinical symptoms probably justify separate classification. Early-onset benign occipital seizure syndrome (EBOS) is suggested as an appropriate name for the variant group'.

Fejerman (December 1998), Chairman of the Commission on Classification and Terminology of the International League Against Epilepsy, proposed the official recognition by the Commission of 'Panayiotopoulos type EBOS'.

Benign Childhood Partial Seizures and Related Epileptic Syndromes. C P Panayiotopoulos
©1999 John Libbey & Company Ltd., pp. 229–239.

Chapter 12A

Epilepsies characterized by seizures with specific modes of precipitation (reflex epilepsies): General aspects

Introduction

Epileptic seizures can arise in a 'spontaneous' unpredictable fashion without detectable precipitant factors, or they can be provoked by certain recognisable stimuli.

Stimuli which contribute towards the initiation of a seizure are provided by the internal and external environment of the subject. Hormones, electrolytes, state of consciousness and body temperature are examples of internal factors which alter the epileptogenic threshold. External stimuli may be sensory, electrical or biochemical. A complex interaction between external and internal stimuli may explain why the effectiveness of a well-defined seizure-precipitating stimulus may vary and why a patient may experience both 'spontaneous' and 'stimulus-induced' seizures.

Epileptic seizures which are consistently elicited by a specific stimulus are called stimulus-sensitive, or reflex, triggered or sensory-evoked epileptic seizures. They have a 4–7 per cent prevalence amongst patients with epilepsies. The Commission on Classification and Terminology of the International League Against Epilepsy[177] has named these stimulus-sensitive seizures of epilepsies 'Epilepsies characterized by seizures with specific modes of precipitation (reflex epilepsies)'. They classified them amongst 'generalized epilepsies and syndromes' though they recognized that 'certain partial seizures may also occur following acquired lesions, usually involving tactile or proprioceptive stimuli'.[177] The Commission[177] has probably undermined that:

(a) In most of the idiopathic photosensitive epilepsies the EEG discharge originates from the occipital lobes,[377,421,593,631,632] and that

(b) There are an increasing number of reports of idiopathic photosensitive seizures with clinical and EEG manifestations entirely confined to the occipital lobes (which is the main subject of Chapter 12B).

The stimulus evoking an epileptic seizure is specific for a given patient and may be simple (i.e. flashes of light, elimination of visual fixation, tactile stimuli) or complex (coloured pictures, eating). Stimuli may be extrinsic, as in the above examples, proprioceptive (i.e. movements), or involve higher brain function, emotions and cognition (i.e. thinking, music, arithmetic).

The seizures may be generalized such as typical or atypical absences, myoclonic jerks and generalized tonic/tonic–clonic, or they may be partial such as visual, motor or sensory. Generalized tonic–clonic seizures may be either primary or secondary to a partial, simple or complex partial seizure, or may follow a cluster of absences or myoclonic jerks. Myoclonic jerks are by far the most common type of stimulus-elicited seizures. They may be manifested in the limbs and trunk or localized in a specific muscle group, such as in the jaw muscles (reading epilepsy) or the eyelids (eyelid myoclonia with absences).

Table 12.1. Stimulus-sensitive epilepsies and the responsible stimuli

I.	**Somatosensory stimuli**
1.	***Exteroceptive somatosensory stimuli:***
a.	Benign childhood epilepsy with somatosensory evoked spikes
b.	Sensory (tactile) evoked idiopathic myoclonic seizures in infancy
c.	Tapping epilepsy
d.	Tooth-brushing epilepsy
2.	***Proprioceptive somatosensory stimuli:***
a.	Seizures induced by movements
b.	Seizures induced by eye closure and/or eye movements
c.	Paroxysmal kinesiogenic choreoathetosis
3.	***Complex proprioceptive stimuli:***
a.	Eating epilepsy
II.	**Visual stimuli**
1.	***Simple visual stimuli:***
a.	Photosensitive epilepsies
b.	Pattern-sensitive epilepsies
c.	Fixation-off sensitive epilepsies
d.	Scotogenic epilepsy
e.	Self-induced photosensitive epilepsy
f.	Self-induced pattern-sensitive epilepsy
2.	***Complex visual stimuli and language processing:***
a.	Reading epilepsy
b.	Graphogenic epilepsy
III.	**Auditory, vestibular and olfactory stimuli**
a.	Seizures induced by pure sounds or words
b.	Musicogenic epilepsy (and singing epilepsy)
c.	Olfactorhinencephalic epilepsy
d.	Eating epilepsy triggered by tastes
e.	Seizures triggered by vestibular and auditory stimuli
IV.	**High-level processes induced seizures (cognitive, emotional, decision-making tasks and other complex stimuli)**
a.	Thinking (noogenic) epilepsy
b.	Reflex decision-making epilepsy
c.	Epilepsia arithmetica (mathematica)
d.	Emotional epilepsies
e.	Startle epilepsy

EEG is fundamental in establishing the provocative stimulus in reflex epilepsies because it allows subclinical EEG, or minor clinical ictal events to be reproduced repeatedly and on demand with application of the appropriate stimulus. However, there are cases in which the stimulus-seizure relation is difficult to prove. An example is video game-induced seizures.[116,278,279,356,377,436,616] Intermittent photic stimulation elicits photoconvulsive responses in 70 per cent of these patients, demonstrating that the epileptic seizures of these subjects were due to photosensitivity. The provocative factors in the other 30 per cent remain unknown and speculative; sleep deprivation, mental concentration, fatigue, excitement, minimal photosensitivity, fixation-off sensitivity, proprioceptive stimuli (praxis) or more complex visual or auditory stimuli, alone or in combination, are all possibilities.[278,279] There are also epileptic syndromes in which EEG 'epileptogenic activity' is consistently elicited by a specific stimulus but its provocative relevance to the clinical situation is difficult to prove. This is for example the case in early onset benign childhood occipital seizures. Elimination of fixation and central vision elicits continuous EEG abnormalities of occipital spike and slow wave activity, though clinically these children appear to have 'unprovoked' seizures. The situation in children suffering from benign partial seizures with extreme somatosensory evoked spikes is similar. It is even more difficult to prove that complex, emotional and cognitive stimuli can elicit seizures.

Table 12.1 lists simple and complex stimuli which have been reported in association with reflex epilepsies: some of these are well known and common (photosensitive epilepsies), others are extremely rare in humans but may be common in animals (audiogenic epilepsy). Some other forms are only recently described (fixation-off sensitive epilepsies). Seizures induced by visual stimuli from flickering lights and patterns are by far the commonest. There is a good number of comprehensive reviews on photosensitive epilepsies[119,437] which I have recently detailed[616] and the book by Jeavons and Harding,1975[421] with a new edition in 1994[377] remains an excellent reference. I will provide a relatively brief review of photosensitive epilepsies.

Photosensitive epilepsies

It should be emphasized that 'photosensitive epilepsy' is a broad term comprising all forms of epilepsies in which seizures are triggered by photic stimulation, and does not correspond to a particular epileptic syndrome. Thus, patients with syndromes of idiopathic generalized epilepsies such as juvenile myoclonic epilepsy, or patients with symptomatic epilepsies such as Lafora's disease, may have seizures elicited by photic stimulation. Even amongst the pure forms of photosensitive epilepsies there may be subdivisions, as for example those manifested with generalized or occipital epileptic seizures. Eyelid myoclonia with absences is probably the only well-defined syndrome of a form of photosensitive epilepsies.[256] Although photosensitivity is usually classified amongst the generalized epilepsies,[177] there is evidence that photosensitivity in humans is mainly generated in the occipital lobes and is therefore regional (occipital lobar) epilepsy.[391,593,616,632,707,805] In many cases both clinical (visual hallucinations, obscuration of vision and blindness, deviation of the head and eyes) and EEG features show a clear-cut occipital onset (see Chapter 12B on idiopathic occipital epilepsy). It is also possible that in other forms of photosensitivity (eyelid myoclonia with absences may be an example) the onset is in the frontal regions, as is the case in the photosensitive baboon Papio papio.[533]

Photosensitivity, the propensity to seizures induced by light, is a genetically determined trait, which may be asymptomatic throughout life or manifest with epileptic seizures. Photosensitivity is best demonstrated in EEG with appropriate intermittent photic stimulation (IPS) techniques.[377,435,437,616]

An historic review of photosensitive epilepsy and relevant literature before 1970 can be found elsewhere.[377,593]

EEG and clinical photosensitivity

The abnormal responses in their mildest form consist of posterior abnormalities which do not spread into the anterior regions. These are occipital spikes which are often time-locked to the flash with a latency of approximately 100 ms, coinciding with the positive P100 of the visual evoked response

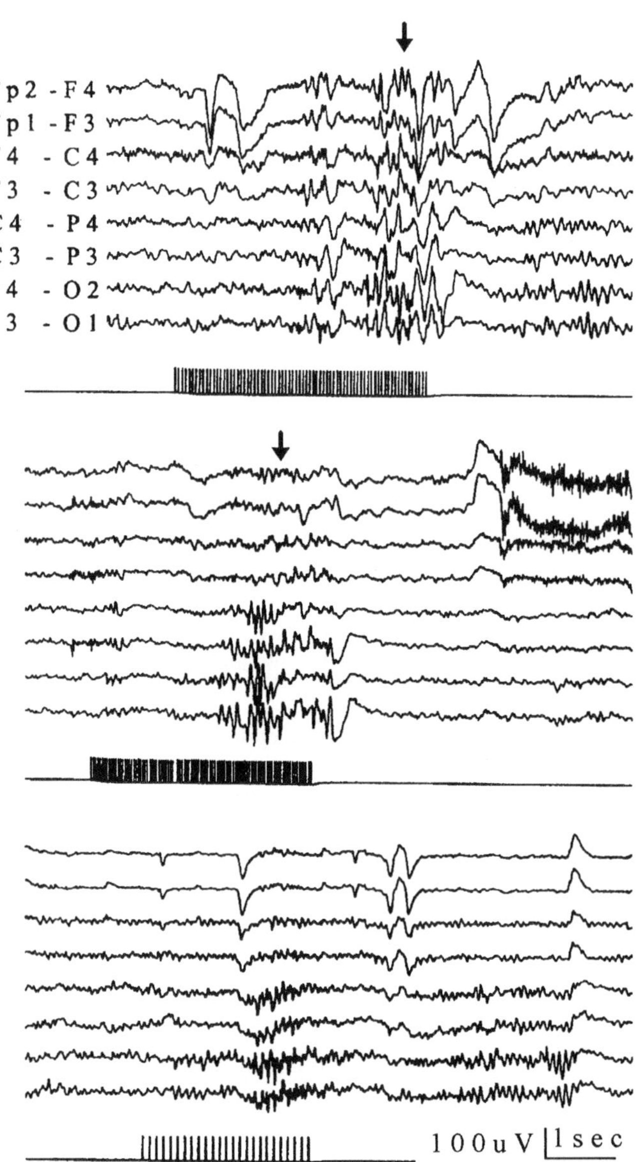

Fig. 12.1. From video-EEG of case 12.2 (upper), case 12.1 (middle) and 32 (Table 13.3) (bottom). All had visual seizures that in cases 35 and 36 were also photically induced. Case 32 had visual seizures that occurred only spontaneously after awakening.
IPS is indicated by the horizontal bars. At arrows the patients had eyelid fluttering.

(Figs. 10.7 and 10.8),[632] or slow waves intermixed with small, larval spikes (Figs. 12.1 and 12.3).[377,391,421,437,593] Half of the subjects demonstrating posterior abnormalities also have clinical epileptic seizures.[377]

However, it is the photoconvulsive discharges which are significantly (90–95 per cent) associated with clinically evident epileptic disorders.[377,435,437,616] Video-EEG and close questioning of the patients reveal that clinical manifestations, such as mild localized or generalized jerks and/or impairment of cognition or subjective sensations, occur in more than 60 per cent of the photoconvulsive responses.[437] Subjects who, for employment reasons, have an EEG showing photoconvulsive responses but do not have clinical evidence of epileptic seizures should be re-examined with video-EEG recording and appropriate testing for cognition or other minor ictal symptoms such as eyelid or perioral symptoms. This may reveal clinical manifestations during otherwise silent photoconvulsive responses.

The photoconvulsive responses consist of generalized spikes or multiple spike and slow wave discharges which are of higher amplitude in the anterior regions but their onset, particularly if patterned IPS is employed, often consists of occipital spikes. IPS in order to be provocative has to imply all potent physical characteristics of the stimulus (intensity, frequency, contrast), combine flash with patterns (a linear grid, not a chequerboard, in front of the stroboscobe may be sufficient), central vision is mandatory (the patient should look at the centre of the stroboscope), and IPS on eye-closure should be tested.[377,421,437,616] Photosensitivity increases after sleep deprivation.

Prevalence of photosensitive epilepsies

Photosensitive epilepsy affects one in 4000 of the population (5 per cent of patients with epileptic seizures), two thirds are women (video-game induced seizures occur more often in men) and the onset has a peak age at 12–13 years.[377] The prevalence of EEG photosensitivity is 5 per cent amongst patients with clinically evident epileptic seizures. Amongst patients with photoconvulsive responses and seizures, 42 per cent have only photically induced without spontaneous seizures (pure photosensitive epilepsy), 40 per cent have spontaneous and photosensitive seizures and the remaining 18 per cent have spontaneous seizures only. In a recent demographic study by Quirk *et al.*,1995[667] the overall annual incidence of cases with a newly presenting seizure and unequivocal photosensitivity in Great Britain was 1 per 100,000 (5.7 per 100,000 in the age group from 7 to 19 years). This means that photosensitivity is found in 2 per cent of patients of all ages presenting with seizures and 10 per cent of patients presenting with seizures in the age range 7–19 years.[667] Photosensitivity was found in 48 (0.35 per cent) of 13,625 healthy male candidates, aged 17–25 years, for Royal Air Force crew training.[357]

Precipitants of seizures

Television, video-games, visual display units of computers, discotheques and natural flickering light (across the trees or reflecting from the sea waves) are in that order common precipitants of seizures.[377,435,437,593] Video-game induced seizures are increasingly more frequent but should not always be equated with photosensitivity from which only 70 per cent of them suffer.[278,279,356]

Pure photosensitive epilepsy

Pure photosensitive epilepsy is a term used only for patients whose seizures are always photically induced without spontaneous, unprovoked seizures.[377,421] Pure photosensitive epilepsy has a prevalence of 42 per cent amongst the photosensitive epilepsies. Generalized tonic–clonic seizures are reported by far more commonly (87 per cent) than absences (6 per cent), partial seizures (2.5 per cent) and myoclonic jerks (1.5 per cent). However, my experience with video-EEG recordings is that many patients categorized as having only GTCS, frequently have mild myoclonic jerks or absences elicited by lights either independently or preceding a GTCS. The common problem in epilepsies is that minor epileptic phenomena like jerks and absences are not usually reported or detected by history unless they are severe. The resting EEG is normal in half of the patients with pure photosensitive epilepsy, abnormal photoconvulsive responses occurring only during IPS. Approximately 20 per cent of them show generalized discharges on eye-closure during the resting EEG. The seizures are usually infrequent and the prognosis is often excellent. Avoidance of precipitating factors may be the only treatment.

Photosensitivity and epileptic syndromes

A quarter of patients with spontaneous seizures and EEG photosensitivity belong to a variety of epileptic syndromes of idiopathic generalized epilepsy, such as juvenile myoclonic epilepsy. Absences with onset in childhood are associated with a higher prevalence (18 per cent) of photosensitivity than absences appearing in the second decade of life (7.5 per cent). Absences combined with photosensitivity have worse prognosis than those of childhood absence epilepsy.[617] A high prevalence of photosensitivity is also found in certain forms of symptomatic generalized epilepsies like severe myoclonic epilepsy in infancy (70 per cent), Baltic–Mediterranean myoclonus (90 per cent) and progressive myoclonic epilepsies.[684]

Eyelid myoclonia with absences (EMA)

This is a syndrome not yet recognized by the Commission on Classification and Terminology of the International League Against Epilepsy[177] although vividly described by Jeavons as we have detailed in a recent book on this interesting condition (Duncan and Panayiotopoulos, 1996).[256]

We have reasonable evidence to propose the following definition for EMA:[617] 'Eyelid myoclonia with absences is an idiopathic epileptic syndrome manifested with frequent (pyknoleptic) seizures, consisting of eyelid myoclonia often associated with absences. Onset is usually in the early childhood. The seizures are brief (3–6 s) and occur mainly after eye closure. They consist of eyelid myoclonia which persists through the attack with or without absences but absences without eyelid myoclonia do not occur. The eyelid myoclonia consists of marked, rhythmic and fast jerks of the eyelids, often associated with jerky upward deviation of the eyeballs and retropulsion of the head. There is probably an associated tonic component of the involved muscles. If the seizure is prolonged, impairment of consciousness occurs. The latter is mild or moderately severe without associated automatisms. Milder seizures of eyelid myoclonia without absences are common, particularly in adults and treated patients and this may occur without EEG accompaniments. All patients are highly photosensitive in childhood but this declines with age. Infrequent GTCS, either induced by lights or spontaneous, are probably inevitable in the long term and are likely to occur after sleep deprivation, fatigue and alcohol indulgence. Myoclonic jerks of the limbs may occur but are infrequent and random. The eyelid myoclonia of EMA is resistant to treatment and may be life-long. However, clinical absences may become less frequent with age.

The EEG ictal manifestations consist mainly of generalized polyspikes / slow waves at 3–6 Hz which are more likely to occur after eye closure in an illuminated room. Total darkness abolishes the abnormalities related to eye closure. Photoparoxysmal responses are recorded from all untreated young patients.'

Self-induced seizures

Self-induction has been well established as a mode of precipitation but prevalence is disputed from a small number to as high as 30 per cent of photosensitive patients.[256,377,435,437,628] Self-induction is employed not only by the mentally handicapped as it was initially reported but also by patients of normal or above average intelligence. Techniques of self-induction vary from hand-waving the abducted fingers in front of a bright light source, to eyelid blinking, making the television screen roll or viewing geometric patterns. Whether eyelid blinking or compulsive attraction to television or bright sun is mainly an attempt for self-induction or part of the seizure is presently debated, although both may be true.[256,628] Absences and myoclonic jerks are the commonest types of seizures in self-induction. A GTCS may be induced after a series of absences or jerks.

Stimulus-sensitive typical absences

Typical absences may be induced by flickering lights (photosensitive), patterns (pattern sensitivity), elimination of central vision and fixation (fixation-off sensitivity), somatosensory and probably other stimuli.[617] Absences are common in self-induced seizures. These stimulus-sensitive typical absences are seen either independently or within the broad framework of certain epileptic syndromes.

Pattern sensitive epilepsy

Pattern sensitive epilepsy is a term used for epileptic seizures and EEG abnormalities induced by patterns.[45,119,377,593,616,805–807] Pattern sensitive epilepsy is closely related to photosensitivity; nearly all pattern sensitive patients are also photosensitive, 30 per cent of photosensitive patients are sensitive to stationary continuously illuminated and 70 per cent to appropriately vibrating patterns of stripes. Pattern sensitivity depends on the spatial frequency, orientation, brightness, contrast and size of the pattern. Adding a quadrille pattern of small squares (2 mm x 2 mm) of fine black lines (1/3 mm) in front of a stroboscope increased photoconvulsive range in all patients.[420] An optimally epileptogenic pattern consists of black and white stripes of equal width and spacing. Pattern sensitivity without photosensitivity, patients sensitive to non-geometric patterns and self-induced pattern sensitivity have been described but are rare.[143,377,597,616]

Treatment of generalized photosensitive epilepsies

In patients with pure generalized photosensitive epilepsies, avoidance of and protection from the provocative stimulus may be effective. In TV photosensitivity and for 70 per cent of patients with video-game epilepsy the patient: (a) should maintain the maximum comfortable viewing distance from the TV screen which is 4–5 times the diagonal measurement of the screen i.e. 2.5 m for a 19" screen; (b) use the telecontrol and not be close to the screen when changing channels, or switching on and off; (c) avoid prolonged watching, particularly if sleep deprived and tired; and (d) watch in a well lit room with a table lamp close to the screen to reduce the relative intensity of the light from the screen. Polaroid sunglasses may be used to protect against flickering sunlight. Monocular occlusion of one eye should be advised either when watching TV or when the subject is suddenly exposed to flickering lights, i.e. in discotheques. The drug of choice is sodium valproate which controls all types of generalized seizures induced by light in more than 80 per cent of the patients. Clonazepam may control absences but mainly jerks. Ethosuximide is effective in absences only. Ethosuximide or clonazepam or Lamotrigine (in doses smaller than used as monotherapy) added to the therapeutic doses of sodium valproate may be needed, particularly in resistant cases like eyelid myoclonia with absences.

Reading epilepsy

Reading epilepsy is a distinctive form of idiopathic reflex epilepsy that has been extensively reviewed by Wolf, 1992[814] and Rasmani,1998.[670] The most recent and comprehensive study is by Koutroumanidis *et al.*, 1998.[451]

In reading epilepsy, seizures are elicited by silent or aloud reading and consist of brief myoclonic jerks mainly restricted to the masticatory, oral and perioral muscles. They are described as clicking sensations and occur a few minutes to hours after reading, particularly the reading aloud of texts that are difficult or unusual. Jaw myoclonus is by far the commonest manifestation of reading epilepsy. One quarter of the patients may also have similar jaw jerks provoked by talking (particularly if this is fast or argumentative), writing, reading music or chewing. If the patient continues reading despite jaw jerks, these may become more violent, spread to trunk and limb muscles or generate other seizure manifestations before a generalized tonic–clonic seizure develops. This is usually the first and last GTCS in their life because the condition is effectively treated with clonazepam and the patient learns to stop reading or talking when oral/perioral jerks occur. The sister of one of my patients with reading

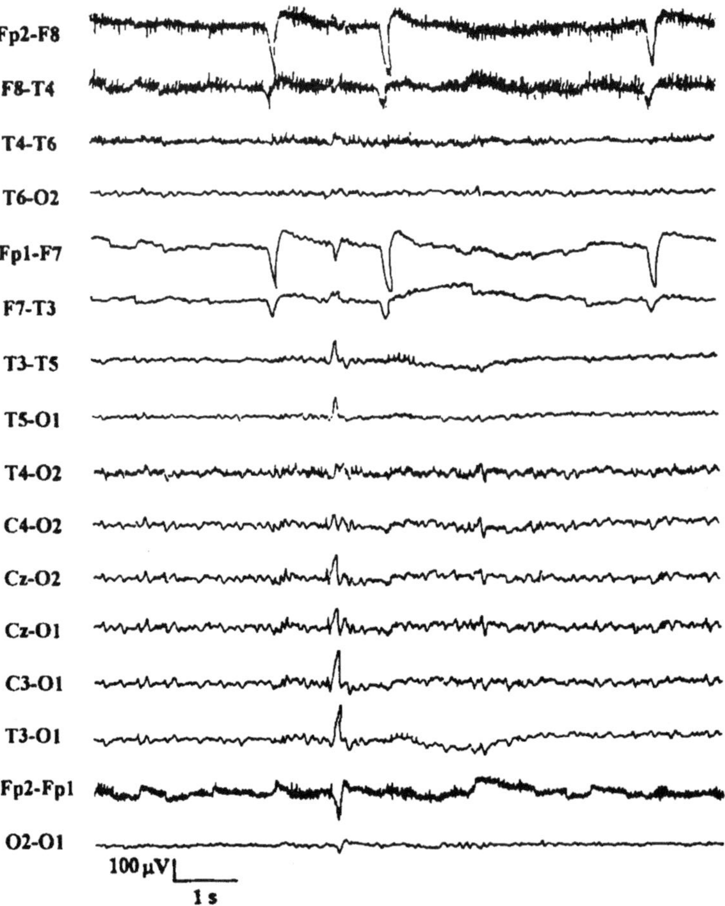

Fig. 12.2a. Ictal EEG of a woman with myoclonic type reading epilepsy. Her sister also had similar symptoms when involved in argumentative talk. The patient's jaw jerks are entirely controlled for 8 years with clonazepam 0.5 mg nocte. Phenytoin prescribed elsewhere was totally ineffective.
Modified from Koutroumanidis et al. (1998)[451] *with the permission of the authors and the editor of Brain.*

epilepsy, who has never asked medical advice for her condition and never had a GTCS, controlled her condition by modifying her way of reading and talking. It is extremely rare for patients with reading epilepsy to have more than 1–5 GTCS, either when reading, or spontaneous, not related to reading, or triggered also by other means of precipitation (talking, reading numbers or music, chewing or writing). The majority of the patients have one GTCS which is usually self-inflicted because of their curiosity to see what will happen if they continue reading despite jaw jerks or other manifestations. It is also rare for reading epilepsy to present with other types of ictal manifestations (mainly visual hallucinations) in addition to the jaw myoclonic seizures. Hand myoclonic jerking is common amongst those with writing precipitation of seizures. Age at onset is usually 12–19 years with a peak in late teens, i.e. long after reading skills have been acquired. There is a male preponderance of 1.8/1. Reading epilepsy is probably genetically determined and has been reported in identical twins and amongst first degree relatives. The inter-ictal EEG is usually normal. Ictal EEG manifestations may be inconspicuous and difficult to detect because of muscle activity from the jaw muscles and head but more

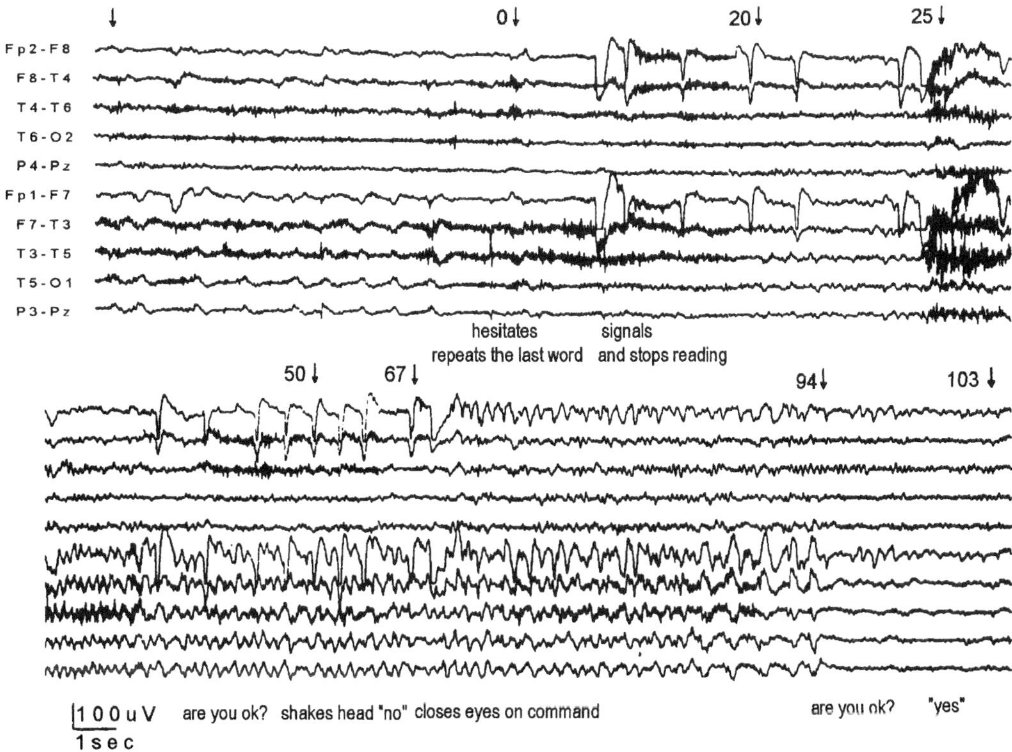

Fig. 12.2b. Ictal video-EEG of a young man with partial seizures of mainly alexia during reading. Note the exclussive EEG discharge mainly around T3–T5.
Numbers indicate seconds from onset of clinical symptoms.
Modified from Koutroumanidis et al. (1998)[451] with the permission of the authors and the editor of Brain.

frequently they consist of a brief burst of sharp waves which is bilateral with a left sided preponderance in the temporo-parietal regions (Fig. 12.2a). The prognosis of reading epilepsy appears to be good because seizures are usually minor and they are related to a precipitant stimulus which can be avoidable or modified. Clonazepam (0.5 mg nocte), which is my preference, is highly effective.

Koutroumanidis *et al.*, 1998[451] presented clinical and electrographic data of 17 patients with reading-induced seizures documented with ictal video-EEG studies during provocation with language related tasks. The median age at onset was 15 years (range 11–22 years) and the male to female ratio was 2.4. Fourteen patients had no spontaneous seizures of any type while the remaining three had infrequent generalized tonic–clonic seizures during nocturnal sleep. Two distinct electroclinical ictal patterns were confirmed on video EEG analysis: (i) Fifteen patients had reading-induced jerks which invariably involved the region of the jaw but also included the upper limbs in five of them. Ictal EEG discharges were noted in 12 patients; these were brief but varied in terms of morphology and spatial distribution, with a clear tendency for left-sided predominance. All but one of these patients had similar myoclonic seizures induced by linguistic activities other than reading, the phenomenon probably justifying the term 'language-induced epilepsy'. Some patients had evidence of transient cognitive impairment associated with the reading-induced jaw or limb jerks. Three patients had a sibling with reading epilepsy but there was no other family history of epileptic seizures. (ii) Two patients had reading-provoked paroxysmal alexia without motor symptoms, associated with prolonged focal ictal EEG abnormalities. Reading provoked a subclinical, continuous and reproducible EEG activation over the left posterior temporal area (Fig. 12.2b).

Koutroumanidis *et al.*[451] also proposed that 'ictogenesis in reading or language-induced epilepsy is based on the reflex activation of a hyperexcitable network that subserves the function of speech and extends over multiple cerebral areas on both hemispheres. The parts of this network responding to the stimulus may, secondarily, drive the relative motor areas producing the typical regional myoclonus. This network hyperexcitability can be genetically determined and its clinical expression is age-related'.

Reading epilepsy is of particular interest as this is the only other type of 'epilepsy' that is classified together with the benign childhood partial seizures in the international classification.[177] Thus, reading epilepsy is the third syndrome after 'childhood epilepsy with centrotemporal spikes' and 'childhood epilepsy with occipital paroxysms' in the idiopathic, age and localization-related (partial) epilepsies in this classification.[177] I could never understand this categorization of reading epilepsy which is characterized by reflex seizures elicited by silent or aloud reading. The best position for reading epilepsy should be amongst epilepsies characterized by seizures with specific modes of precipitation (reflex epilepsies). These like photosensitive epilepsies may be partial or generalised, idiopathic or symptomatic.

Koutroumanidis *et al.*[451] commenting on the classification of reading epilepsy stated: 'The present classification of reading epilepsy among the localization-related idiopathic epilepsies with age-related onset (Commission on Classification and Terminology of the ILAE, 1989)[177] is based on the assumption that the regional myoclonus, as always developing in clear consciousness, is the clinical expression of a simple motor partial seizure. Further arguments include the relationship to a specific cortical area (the angular region of the language-dominant hemisphere), the age-related onset and the relatively benign course, in the sense that seizures remain strictly bound to the precipitating factor. Generalized spike-and-wave discharges, when present, are attributed to a genetic trait.[814] Conversely, Radhakrishnan *et al.* (1995)[668] expressed the view that the age at onset, the anti-epileptic drugs to which it is more responsive, the natural history and the EEG findings are distinct features from those of benign epilepsy with centrotemporal or occipital spikes. These authors emphasized the overlap between reading epilepsy and epilepsies with seizures precipitated by language-related activities other than reading and high cognitive processes; they stressed the electroclinical and therapeutic similarities and proposed the classification of reading epilepsy amongst the idiopathic generalized epilepsies with seizures precipitated by specific modes of activation. In his critical review, Ramani (1998)[670] emphasized the inadequacy of the distinction between primary and secondary types as a classification tool, and pointed out that the clinical heterogeneity of reading epilepsy defies its position in any single category of the present classification schema of the ILAE.[177] This author proposed that the different subtypes (of the myoclonic form) can be categorized separately into the groups of idiopathic generalized (age-dependent), idiopathic localization-related and symptomatic localization-related epilepsies, depending on clinical and EEG features, while Bickford's secondary reading epilepsy can be included in the group of symptomatic generalized epilepsies (Ramani, 1998).[670] Our present findings confirm that, apart from the myoclonic reading- or language-induced epilepsy which represents a valid entity, given its relatively uniform clinical semiology (Ramani, 1998),[670] a second variant also exists with clearly partial seizures manifested by prolonged episodes of dyslexia. These observations, along with the recent description of a patient with reading-induced absence seizures, indicate that the electroclinical spectrum of reading epilepsy is much wider than currently believed. We concur that there is no reason for splitting reading epilepsy into separate syndromes that share the same precipitating factors and pathophysiology, and in this sense reading epilepsy cannot fit into any given category of the present classification system of the ILAE with the dual dichotomy between 'generalized' and 'focal' or 'partial' for seizures, and 'generalized' and 'localization-related' for syndromes. Even if a separate categorization was pursued, it would present no difficulty regarding the clearly partial and absence subtypes, but would result in obvious inconsistencies regarding the myoclonic variant. Although the demonstration, with functional neuroimaging, of the bilateral hyperexcitable parts of the neuronal network which integrate speech is a reasonably sufficient argument for positioning myoclonic reading epilepsy among the localization-related syndromes (Commission on Classification and Terminology of the International League Against Epilepsy),[177] the fact that it is manifested in at least two out of three of the patients with generalized seizures (in which the first clinical changes indicate initial involvement of both hemispheres and the ictal encephalographic patterns are initially bilateral[175]) makes such a classification more confusing than informative. From the clinician's point of view, reading- or language-induced myoclonic seizures are neither partial nor generalized, but bilateral and synchronous focal motor resulting from the simultaneous activation of parts of the speech network that expands over both hemispheres, with a potential for rapid spread and secondary generalization if exposure to the stimulus is not interrupted. Further electrophysiological and functional neuroimaging studies in epilepsies with seizures precipitated by specific modes of activation are expected to facilitate understanding of epileptogenesis, and any future classification system should encompass ongoing developments. Until then, an effective definition of reading- or language-induced epilepsy should be based largely on clinical semiology, and any attempt to position the syndrome in the current classification system of the ILAE would be premature.'[451]

Koutroumanidis *et al.*[451] proposed the following definition for reading epilepsy:

'Reading epilepsy is a distinct form of reflex epilepsy in which all, or almost all, seizures are precipitated by the act of reading. In many patients, clinically identical seizures can also be provoked by the other linguistic activities to the extent that the term language-induced epilepsy should be justified. The clinical spectrum of reading- or language induced epilepsy is wide. Regional myoclonic jerks that most often involve the masticatory muscles and the tongue, but may also extend to the upper extremities, are the most frequent and remarkably uniform seizure pattern. Some patients have prolonged, clearly partial, seizures manifested with alexia and possibly dysphasia, while occasionally absences may occur. Seizures usually evolve into GTCS if reading persists. Ictal EEG changes show considerable heterogeneity in terms of discharge morphology and scalp topography. In the myoclonic variant, discharges are brief, bilateral synchronous or focal, while in the partial variant they are prolonged and focal. There is a clear tendency for left hemisphere predominance. Reading or language epilepsy is most often idiopathic and rarely symptomatic. Ictal functional neuroimaging studies show multiple cortical hyperexcitable areas that are part of the neuronal network which subserves the function of speech. Secondary excitation of the relevant motor areas may produce the typical regional myoclonus and the underlying physiological mechanism may relate to cortical reflex myoclonus. This network hyperexcitability can be genetically determined, and its clinical expression is age-related. Reading or language epilepsy is non-progressive and optimal treatment relates to the electroclinical variant; patients with the myoclonic form are usually best treated with clonazepam or sodium valproate, whereas those with the partial variant respond to anti-epileptic drugs that are effective for partial seizures.'

Benign Childhood Partial Seizures and Related Epileptic Syndromes. C P Panayiotopoulos
©1999 John Libbey & Company Ltd., pp. 241–256.

Chapter 12B

Idiopathic photosensitive occipital seizures

Definition

Idiopathic photosensitive occipital seizures (IPOS) are a rare manifestation of occipital seizure susceptibility to external visual , mainly photic, stimuli. This may be an expression of a childhood seizure susceptibility syndrome or occur in predisposed individuals under the activating effect of visual stimuli such as flickering lights, video-games and television. The cardinal features of the IPOS are infrequent occipital seizures with visual and other occipital ictal symptomatology which may remain localized or progress to other manifestations from more anterior spread and secondary generalization. The EEG is characterized mainly by posterior occipital spikes elicited by intermittent photic stimulation (IPS) but spontaneous occipital spikes and generalized discharges may also co-exist (Figs. 12.1 and 12.3). Onset of ictal EEG consists of paroxysmal fast activity and fast occipital spikes. Prognosis of these cases varies from excellent with 1–2 provoked fits to relatively bad with a persistent liability to seizures.

Onset of seizures is between 5 and 19 years of age with visually induced occipital seizures often after watching television, computer screens or video-games.[370,616]

Note: There are some singular cases, mainly children, having elementary or even bizarre complex visual hallucinations and other strange ictal semiology. These may be spontaneous, photically induced or both and EEG is dominated by spontaneous and IPS elicited generalized multiple spike and wave discharges. These are of unknown classification and prognosis.

A typical case of IPOS with good prognosis

There is probably no typical case of IPOS as by definition there is a great variability from cases of isolated occipital seizures exclusively induced by photic stimuli to more complex cases of spontaneous and evoked occipital as well as generalized seizures. Examples can be found in the following literature review (page 248). However, a typical case of IPOS with a benign course is of a child that at age 11 years had two visual seizures while playing video-games for a long time. On both occasions there were elementary visual hallucinations of multi-coloured circular patterns, headache, and tendency to become sick which on one occasion progressed to secondary GTCS. EEG showed some spontaneous occipital spikes which were also activated by IPS. By following appropriate advice regarding avoidance of precipitating factors, no further seizures occurred in the next 3 years and EEG normalized. No drug treatment was prescribed.

Introduction

Patients, mainly children and adolescents, of normal physical and mental state and brain imaging may suffer from occipital seizures precipitated by photic stimuli.[51,52,278,313,356,369,370,535,616,677,761]

These by definition are idiopathic photosensitive occipital seizures (IPOS) which should be categorized amongst the partial or regional 'epilepsies characterized by seizures with specific modes of precipitation (reflex epilepsies)'[177] though some of them may well be 'situation-related seizures'.[177] According to the Commission of ILAE:[177] 'Epilepsies characterized by seizures with specific modes of precipitation (reflex epilepsies)' are classified under 'Generalized epilepsies and syndromes'. This has probably been overlooked as it is well known that localization-related (focal, partial, local) seizures and epilepsies may well be characterized by specific modes of precipitation (reading epilepsy may be an example). Furthermore, most of the photosensitive generalized epilepsies have a 'regional, lobular onset' in the occipital lobes.[616]

Guerrini *et al.* 1995[370] proposed that IPOS constitute an idiopathic age and localization-related epilepsy syndrome,[370] while Gastaut and Zifkin, 1987[313] included and studied IPOS together with late onset benign childhood occipital seizures (LBOS).

Historical aspects

It is interesting that the first scientific evidence of photosensitive epilepsy by Gowers (1881)[351] refers to occipital seizures induced by bright light. This was a man, with 'bright blue lights, like stars – always the same', subject to GTCS that were elicited 'at any time by looking at a bright light, even a bright fire. The relation is intelligible since the discharges apparently commenced in the visual centre'.

In 1927 Gordon Holmes[396] wrote that 'Some men subject to epileptiform attacks commencing with visual phenomena owing to gunshot wounds of the occipital region, have told me that bright lights, cinema exhibitions and other strong retinal stimuli tend to bring on attacks'. He attributed this 'reflex epilepsy' to an enhanced excitability of the visual cortex.

With the advent of EEG it was discovered that the majority of patients with photosensitivity have generalized discharges and suffer mainly from idiopathic generalized epilepsies and these have dominated the relevant literature.[616]

Photically induced EEG abnormalities confined or starting from the occipital regions, occipital foci driven or activated by IPS, and visual seizures with or without secondary generalization[109,182,198,220,284,309,311,391,421,494,593,631,632,648] have attracted less attention. However, reports with ictal EEG recording showed that the onset of photically induced seizures could be with rapid spikes and fast rhythms starting or limited in one or both occipital regions. Ictally seizures start with elementary or

Fig. 12.3 (facing page). From video-EEG recordings of illustrative case 12. 1 (upper), 12.2 (middle) and 12.3 (bottom).

Upper: *From video-EEG of case 12.1 (page 254).*

Left: High voltage spontaneous occipital spikes that are often associated with eyelid fluttering. They mainly occurred when eyes were closed but they were not activated by fixation-off.

Middle: Generalized discharge of spike and slow waves at 3–3.5Hz with impairment of cognition and eyelid fluttering.

Right: IPS evoked occipital spikes associated with eyelid fluttering.

Middle: *From video-EEG of case 12.2 (page 254).*

Left and middle: Spontaneous occipital spikes, mainly when eyes were closed. There was no FOS.

Right: IPS with generalized sharp waves at 10–12 Hz with posterior emphasis intermixed with a few occipital spike-wave complexes. Eyelid fluttering could occur.

Bottom: *From video-EEG of case 12.3 (page 255).*

Left: Small random spontaneous occipital sharp waves.

Middle: Generalized discharges of spike/polyspikes and waves on IPS associated with an eyelid myoclonic absence.

Right: IPS evoked discharge with posterior spikes associated with eyelid fluttering.

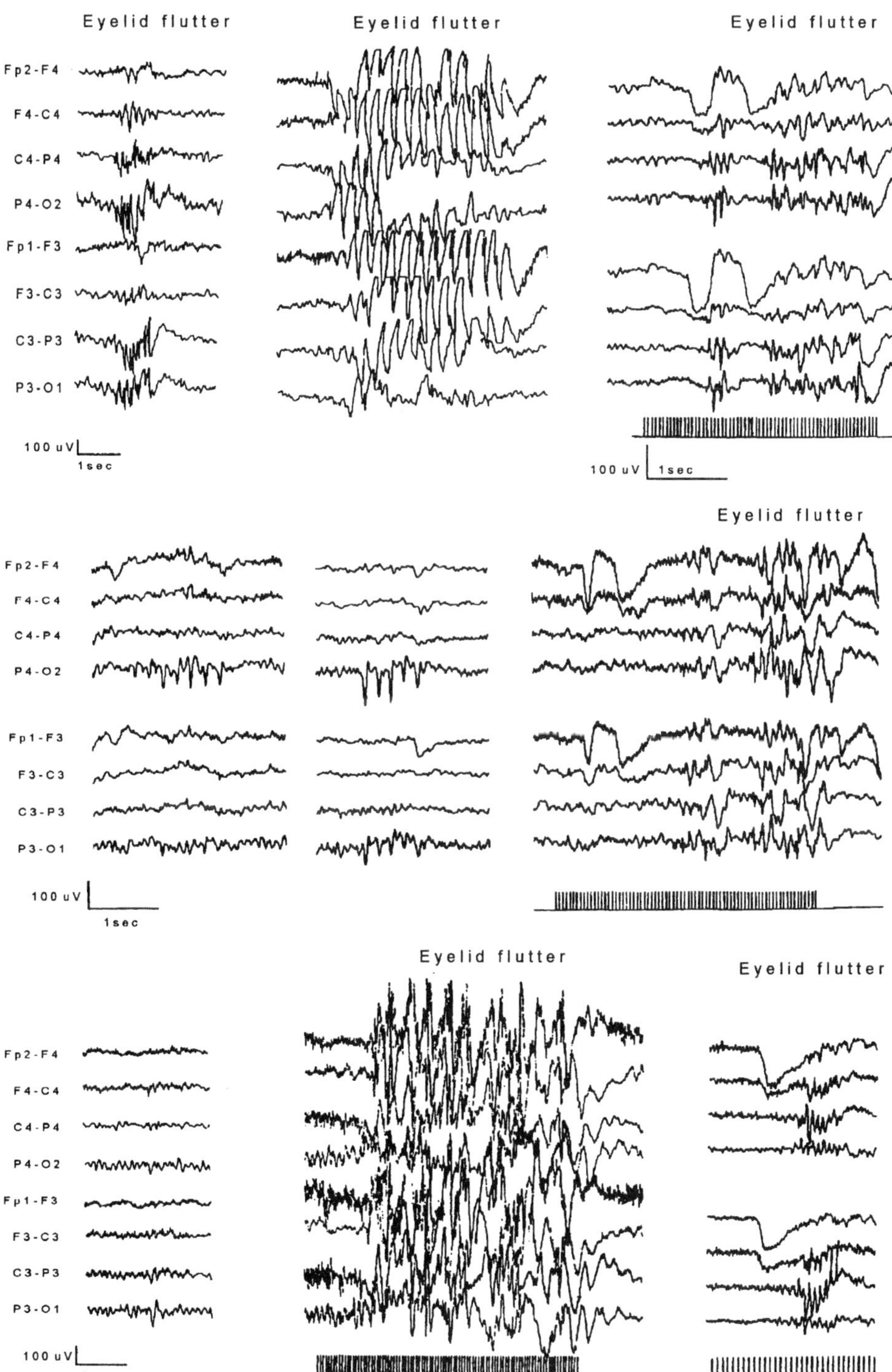
Eyelid flutter
Eyelid flutter
Eyelid flutter
Fp2-F4
F4-C4
C4-P4
P4-O2
Fp1-F3
F3-C3
C3-P3
P3-O1
100 uV
1sec
100 uV
1sec
Eyelid flutter
Fp2-F4
F4-C4
C4-P4
P4-O2
Fp1-F3
F3-C3
C3-P3
P3-O1
100 uV
1sec
Eyelid flutter
Eyelid flutter
Fp2-F4
F4-C4
C4-P4
P4-O2
Fp1-F3
F3-C3
C3-P3
P3-O1
100 uV
1sec

complex visual hallucinations, hemianopia or blindness often followed by tonic deviation of the head and eyes with secondary GTCS.[51,198,284,370,561,648] Bizarre and prolonged 16 min seizures of complex visual hallucinations with nausea, belching, confusion and additional 'psychoneurotic-like' symptoms induced by IPS were recorded in a middle aged woman who had infrequent spontaneous and photic seizures and 'so-called migraine for 20 years'.[284] Extensive neuroradiological investigations were normal and the patient was well in a 13 year follow-up.[284]

Delwaide *et al.* (1971)[220] described 13 patients with occipital lobe epilepsy. Three children were also photosensitive and in one of them a fit provoked by IPS was recorded. Ictally this patient had 'obnubilation, deviation of the head to the left and left hemiclonic convulsions'. Some of their patients had a good prognosis.

Prevalence

It appears that prevalence is small, less than 0.5 per cent amongst adult and child patients with epilepsies. Guerrini *et al.*[370] found 10 (0.41 per cent) patients with IPOS amongst 2447 adults and children with epileptic seizures. In the same group there was one patient with reading epilepsy, 53 with Rolandic seizures and 22 with other benign childhood occipital seizures. This prevalence is remarkably similar with 0.45 per cent in my study of 1360 patients with seizures (see personal experience in Chapter 13)

Sex and age at onset

Of 39 reported patients[51,369,370,535,729] with IPOS that I reviewed, 18 are boys and 21 are girls. Age at onset ranges from 5 to 19 years with a mean at around 12 years of age.

Clinical manifestations

Clinical ictal manifestations

Seizures start with visual hallucinations, blurring of vision or blindness. Visual hallucinations are usually elementary multi-coloured and circular spots, circles or spheres[278,369,370] but other shapes (square, triangular)[535] may occur. They may be stationary, flashing, moving or expanding, appearing to one side or at the centre of the visual field. Metamorphopsia and sensations of objects moving around are rarely reported.[535] Blurring of vision and blindness may be the first ictal symptom reported by almost one fifth of the patients.[51,515,535,704] More often they appear after the visual hallucinations.[369,370] Visual may be the only ictal manifestations[370] usually lasting for seconds, frequently 1–3 min and rarely longer, from 5 to 15 min.[370] Consciousness is not impaired during the phase of visual symptoms but visual hallucinations frequently progress to tonic deviation of the eyes and head and secondary generalized tonic–clonic seizures.[370,761] In other patients, the visual symptoms may progress to ictal epigastric discomfort or nausea, followed by vomiting with or without impairment of consciousness.[370] These seizures usually last for 2–5 min but they may also be prolonged up to 2 h.[370] Headache in the form of 'sharp' or 'piercing' pain, often localized in the eyes, may occur during or before the ictus.[370] These ictal symptoms frequently end with secondary GTCS.

Post-ictal symptoms

Visual simple partial seizures are more likely than any other type of partial seizures to be followed by headache, nausea and vomiting. The headache is usually mild and diffuse but it may also be severe and throbbing, occurring 10–20 min after the end of the visual hallucinations.[370] Post-ictal headache and vomiting with fatigue, malaise and drowsiness occur in more than two thirds of patients after secondary GTCS.

Other type of seizures

Patients may have exclusively occipital seizures which are only photically induced. Others may also have spontaneous occipital seizures with or without secondary GTCS. In some cases secondary GTCS occur only during sleep (see illustrative cases, pages 253–256). Patients with IPOS may also have other types of seizures that are spontaneous, photically induced or both. These may vary from eyelid flickering to myoclonic jerks, absences and GTCS which occur independently of the occipital seizures. There are also patients with Rolandic seizures who may later develop IPOS[369] (see illustrative cases, pages 253–256).

Precipitating factors

By definition, all patients with IPOS are sensitive to flickering lights. Depending on the severity of photosensitivity, in some patients seizures may be elicited by minimal photic provocation, in others combined pattern and photic or prolonged exposure may be needed and for others (probably the majority of IPOS) photic stimuli are effective only if combined with other precipitating factors such as excitement or frustration, hunger, fatigue and sleep deprivation.

Frequency of seizures and prognosis

This varies according to the severity of the individual occipital seizure sensitivity and exposure to the offending visual stimuli. There are reported cases that have only 1–2 occipital seizures in their life despite cautious exposure to precipitating factors and no drug treatment. Others, particularly those also having spontaneous seizures, needed medication for 1–3 years together with strict avoidance or precautions regarding insulting stimuli, and did well with only a few age-related fits. However, other patients have frequent spontaneous and elicited occipital fits alone or in combination with other types of seizures which may be myoclonic jerks, often of the eyelids, infrequent absences and GTCS.

They may be three groups of idiopathic occipital seizure photosensitivity:

a. Patients with low occipital epileptogenic threshold who may have situation-related seizures. Accidental provocation of single occipital seizures in normal young persons or patients with migraine during IPS are most likely due to a low threshold to such events and may not happen again. This may also be the case for those who have one or two visual seizures triggered while watching television from close distance or playing video-games for long hours particularly when other well documented seizure-precipitating factors such as sleep deprivation, fatigue, hunger, thirst, excitement and others cluster together.[279] That a seizure may be accidentally elicited during IPS is of no surprise particularly with patterned IPS at 14–20 Hz in long bursts[561] or continuous provocation,[51] which sometimes is used and may also continue despite the appearance of EEG epileptiform paroxysms. This practice of EEG provocation should be firmly discouraged.

Ferrie *et al.*[278,279] reported cases with video-game seizures in which partients were not photosensitive under 'near-natural' conditions of IPS (maximum 5 s trains of IPS on eyes-closed, eyes-opened and eye-closure). Because of lack of evidence for laboratory photosensitivity, these patients cannot be classified in IPOS. However, more aggressive photic stimulation (which is by no means advised) may have induced EEG abnormalities and probably seizures.

b. Patients with idiopathic pathological occipital epileptogenicity demonstrated with the existence of occipital spikes in the resting EEG. This may or may not be sufficient by itself to cause spontaneous occipital seizures which occur as the result of activation by visual, mainly photic stimuli, These make up the majority of patients with IPOS.

c. Patients with idiopathic diffuse and occipital cortical excitability demonstrated with spontaneous and photically evoked GTCS and absences who also have occipital seizures. These are often difficult cases to classify, treat and assess prognosis.

Electroencephalography in IPOS

Interictal response to intermittent photic stimulation

By definition, all these IPOS patients are photosensitive and IPS elicits abnormal EEG paroxysms of spikes or polyspikes that may be entirely confined to the occipital regions or generalized photoparoxysmal responses of spikes or polyspikes and slow waves that predominate in the posterior regions (Fig. 12.3).

Resting interictal EEG

This may be normal but more frequently, in two thirds of the patients, there are unilateral or bilateral, random and infrequent occipital spikes.[278,369,370,535,677,761] Occasionally, there are occipital polyspikes that occur after closing of the eyes and rarely persist while the eyes are closed. These spikes do not demonstrate fixation-off sensitivity (Fig. 12.3). Four IPOS children with centrotemporal spikes in EEGs at an earlier age have been reported.[369,370,704]

Ictal EEG during IPS or TV and video-game stimulation

In all relevant reports[51,369,370,535,677] the ictal EEG discharge consists of occipital paroxysmal fast activity (recruiting response) and runs of fast spikes (the spikes are so fast that they imitate sudden muscle contraction artefacts). These may be unilateral or bilateral, and may be sustained in the occipital regions, frequently spreading to other anterior regions of one, often both hemispheres before secondary generalization to a GTCS. Focal lateralized theta at onset,[677] generalized fast spike-wave[729] and bioccipital spike and wave discharge before spreading to secondary GTCS[535] have been reported. Terasaki *et al.* (1987)[763] reported one patient who had a visual seizure during photic stimulation that showed a diffuse spike wave burst with occipital predominance.

Figure 12.4 is from the ictal EEG of a patient of Guerrini *et al.*, 1995.[370]

We often detect, with video-EEG, other types of seizures such as eyelid flickering and myoclonia, limb, head, body or fingers myoclonic jerks, and brief absences that are sometimes mild and may escape detection (Fig. 12.3).

Treatment

Advice regarding avoidance of precipitating factors is essential. This is similar for those with any type of photosensitivity. Particular emphasis is needed regarding video-games and television. Some may have to do without video-games. Others may have to exercise strenuous caution, playing for only brief intervals, avoiding sleep deprivation or tiredness, and probably using an eye-patch (this may be sufficient to discourage them from playing completely). Precautions regarding television are well known: watch from a distance of at least 3 m with lights of the room on, and use tele-control for switching TV on or off and changing channels. These are described in the preceding Chapter 12A on photosensitive epilepsies – general aspects.

Though in generalized photosensitive epilepsies, sodium valproate is the drug of choice, it is not

Fig. 12.4 (facing page). A prolonged occipital seizure induced by IPS recorded by Guerrini et al.[370] *The seizure begins with an ictal discharge initially recognisable over the O2–Oz channel. At 19 s, the patient sees 'three rainbow-coloured spots surrounded by a dark shadow' in the left visual field which roll to the left. Seizure activity spreads progressively over the right occipitoposterior temporal area while transmitted waves are present contralaterally (from 2' to 5'); the patient reports that the spots have slowly faded while the shadow progressively covers the left visual field, producing left hemianopia. At 12', seizure activity involves both occipitoposterior temporal areas but still predominates on the right; the patient reports complete blindness, as confirmed by visual field assessment. At 15', slow waves appear on the right and the patient's eyes deviate tonically to the left. At 17', the ictal discharge progressively slows to rhythmic spike and slow waves on the right while it persists on the left. The patient's head deviates toward the left, and he remains completely responsive. At 18', the patient's head returns to midline; he complains of sudden headache and epigastric discomfort and, at 20', retches. Ictal activity ceases on the right hemisphere 18 min after seizure onset (18'), but continues 2 min longer on the left (20'). Continuous clinical testing showed a gradual post-ictal improvement of visual blurring. The patient fully recovered vision 3 min after the end of the seizure but remained agnosic, beginning to identify objects 6 min later.*

[From Guerrini et al.1995[370] *with the kind permission of the authors and the editor of Epilepsia.]*

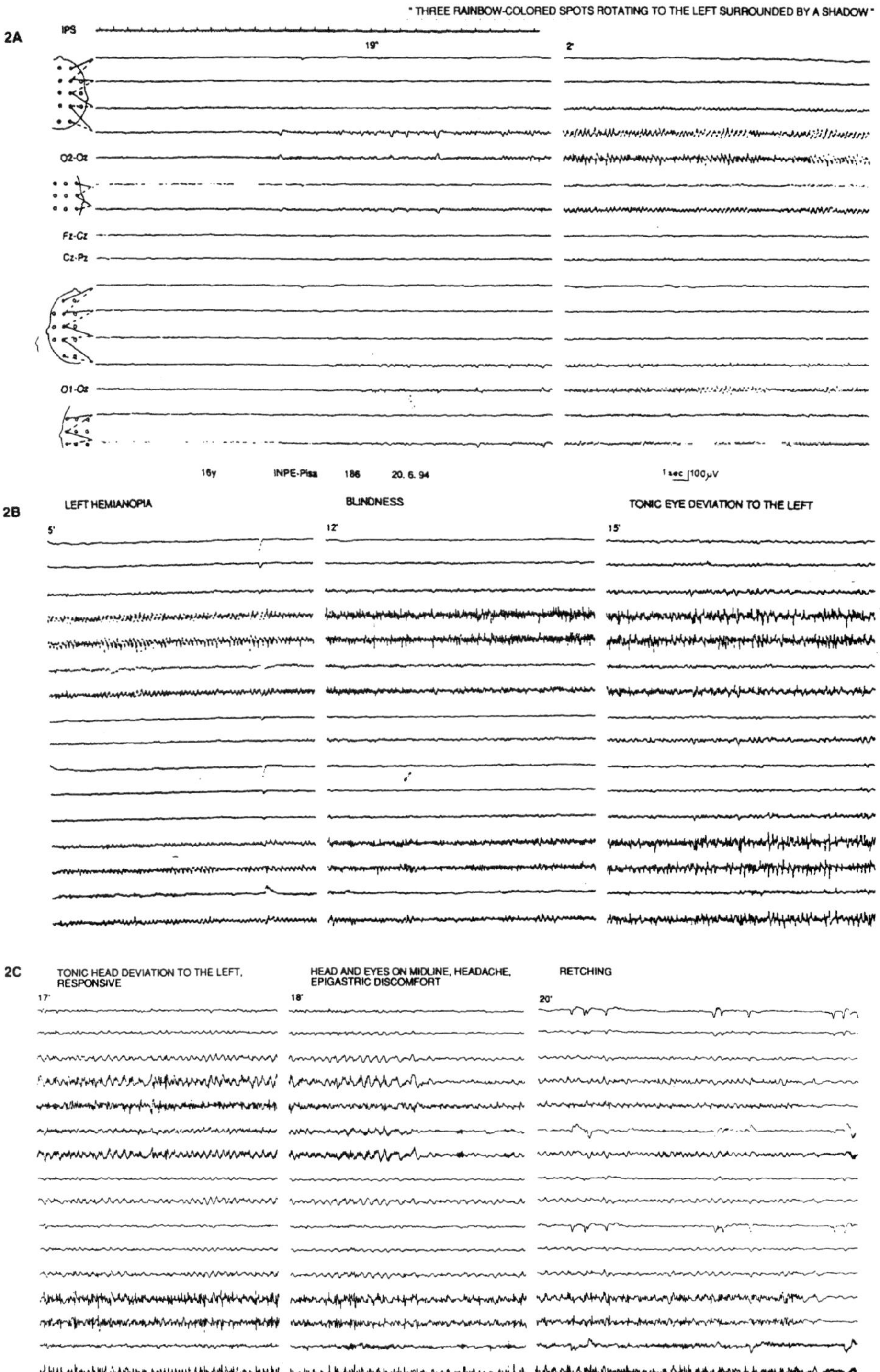
2A
" THREE RAINBOW-COLORED SPOTS ROTATING TO THE LEFT SURROUNDED BY A SHADOW "
IPS
19"
2'
O2-Cz
Fz-Cz
Cz-Pz
O1-Cz
16y
INPE-Pisa
186
20. 6. 94
1 sec 100μV
2B
LEFT HEMIANOPIA
5'
BLINDNESS
12'
TONIC EYE DEVIATION TO THE LEFT
15'
2C
TONIC HEAD DEVIATION TO THE LEFT, RESPONSIVE
17'
HEAD AND EYES ON MIDLINE, HEADACHE, EPIGASTRIC DISCOMFORT
18'
RETCHING
20'

certain that this is also the case for IPOS. I have seen cases of IPOS where seizures were not controlled until carbamazepine was added to sodium valproate (see illustrative cases, pages 253–256). Clobazam may be an alternative. We simply do not know yet.

Video-game induced occipital seizures

Media reports in the early 1990s highlighted the risk of seizures precipitated by video-games and again in December 1997 when 700 children in Japan developed 'vomiting and convulsions' while watching a TV popular animated cartoon programme called 'Pokemon' (Pocket Monsters). The offending scene according to Takahashi was repeated 'flickering of red lights' (personal communication). An extensive review of the literature regarding video-game induced seizures is by Graf *et al.* (1994)[356] and Ferrie *et al.* (1994)[278] reporting 28 new patients.[278,356] The majority of the 49 reported patients suffer from various syndromes of idiopathic generalized epilepsy. However, 15 (30.6 per cent) had partial seizures with 11 of them (22.4 per cent) having onset with visual symptoms (elementary visual hallucinations, blurring of vision, multiple scotomata) with or without secondary GTCS. Though most of these 11 patients with visual seizures had random, mainly unilateral occipital spikes in the resting EEG, only four (8.2 per cent)[278,294,356,515] had evidence of EEG photosensitivity to comply with the diagnosis of IPOS.

Quirk *et al.* 1995[667] identified 118 patients who had a first seizure while playing an electronic screen game during two 3-month periods through active surveillance by virtually all electroencephalographic departments in Great Britain. Patients were divided into Group A (46 patients) – those for whom there was thought to be a definite causal relationship (type 4 photoparoxysmal response); Group B (25 patients) – those for whom there was a probable causal relationship (types 1–3 photoparoxysmal response, clinical evidence of photosensitivity, subsequent recurrent seizures on repeat exposure to electronic screen games, and/or occipital spikes in the resting electroencephalogram); and Group C (47 patients) – those for whom there was no apparent causal relationship. Most (103/118) of the patients were in the age range of 7 to 19 years. Within this age group the annual incidence of first seizures triggered by playing electronic screen games (Groups A and B combined) was estimated to be 1.5/100,000. From the 71 patients of groups A and B, there were only two patients with 'partial seizures', the majority had GTCS (64 patients). Three patients had absences and two myoclonic jerks. There was only patient with occipital spikes in the resting record. As in all community based studies, minor events such as visual seizures either alone or preceding GTCS may have escaped attention. Furthermore, in Great Britain paediatricians do not require an EEG after a first seizure and it is likely that children with infrequent visual seizures, particularly if associated with headache and vomiting, would be diagnosed as having migraine rather than epilepsy.

Literature review of idiopathic photosensitive occipital seizures

Recent interest in idiopathic photosensitive occipital seizures (IPOS) mainly induced by television and video-games has been accumulating.[51,200,236,254,278,279,313,356,369,370,515,535,616,677,729,761] There are rare case reports of normal young people[198,677] or patients with migraine[200,236,677] having an occipital seizure during IPS but these are exceptions. Some of these patients would never have been reported as having a seizure if an EEG with IPS had not been performed. See for example the normal young man reported by Davidoff and Johnson,1963[198] or the migraine suffering woman of Ricci and Vigevano, 1993.[677] However, idiopathic photosensitive occipital seizures mainly occur in children and teenagers who have occipital seizures elicited by television and video-games [51,278,356,369,370,515,535,677,729,761] or patients with idiopathic generalized epilepsy, mainly with typical absences that have during IPS photoconvulsive responses started from the occipital regions often with clinical manifestations implicating the occipital lobes.[182,677] The largest studies of IPOS are those of Ricci and Vigevano[677] with five patients having ictal EEG documentation of occipital seizures induced by IPS, Michelucci and Tassinari[535] with 12 patients and Guerrini *et al.*[370] with 10 patients.

In seven of 63 patients of Gastaut and Zifkin[313] with 'benign epilepsy of childhood with occipital spike and wave complexes', occipital sharp waves, not seen in the resting EEG and 'unrelated to eye opening and closing', were evoked by IPS. This response occurred several seconds after the beginning of IPS and was not related to the frequency of IPS. It was suggested that 'the resulting bursts are related to an induced hyperexcitability of the occipital cortex rather than being a response locked to the photic stimuli'. In seven other patients with typical occipital paroxysms, IPS evoked generalized bursts of spike or polyspike and slow wave activity, at times with associated myoclonus. Amongst their illustrative cases (no. 11) there is a 13-year-old girl who had typical absence seizures from age 6 years. In addition, on three occasions she had seizures induced by television. These started with 'phosphenes in all visual fields, followed by right sided hemiclonic convulsions with post-ictal headache and vomiting that lasted several hours. Seven EEG showed only 3 Hz spike and wave discharges associated with absences during hyperventilation'.[313]

Terasaki *et al.* (1987)[763] in their study of occipital lobe epilepsy in childhood found that photosensitivity occurred in 31.3 per cent of their patients without significant difference between idiopathic and symptomatic patients; one patient had a visual seizure during photic stimulation associated with a diffuse spike wave burst with occipital predominance.

Tassinari *et al.* (1989)[761] reported that of 30 consecutive patients with TV induced GTCS, six had occipital seizures preceding secondary GTCS. In their subsequent updated report[535] there were 35 consecutive patients with TV or video-games induced GTCS. Twelve of them had focal symptoms at the beginning of the seizures. Visual seizures consisted of little bright flashes or triangular geometric patterns (three cases), metamorphopsia (one), blurring of vision or blindness (four), and sensation of objects moving around (one). Deviation of head and eyes occurred in three. All patients had secondary GTCS. Seizures were induced by TV in all cases, two also with video-games and two also had spontaneous fits. Three patients had a single seizure. All others had infrequent fits that were easily controlled with sodium valproate and carbamazepine. Mean age at onset was 14 years, ranging from 7 to 18 years and eight patients were male. Three patients had a family history of epilepsy and all had normal brain imaging. The interictal EEG was normal (two), showed generalized spike wave discharges (two), posterior paroxysmal abnormalities (two), generalized spike wave discharges and posterior paroxysmal abnormalities (four). Spontaneous EEG paroxysms increased with IPS and 'became clearly predominant over the occipital regions in eight patients'. Three patients had ictal EEG with seizures elicited by IPS. In two patients there was a 5 min spike wave discharge over both occipital regions associated with elementary visual hallucinations before spreading to secondary GTCS. The third patient had an initial paroxysmal fast activity in the left occipital region followed by diffuse spike wave.

Santanelli, 1989[704] reported an unusual case of 'idiopathic partial epilepsy with reflex visual seizures and both multifocal and generalized EEG discharges'. This was a 13-year-old girl with a strong family history of epilepsy. At the age of 15 months she started having seizures, occurring only when entering her bathroom which had bright white walls and shiny chromed plumbing. Each seizure, lasting for 1 min, manifested with cessation of her activities, head and eyes turning to the left and jerks of the eyelids. EEG had interictal right occipital spikes and IPS induced her habitual seizures associated with high amplitude 10 Hz rhythmic discharge in the right occipital regions. No further seizures occurred with phenobarbitone but the EEG showed from age 2 to 5 years right occipital and centrotemporal spikes with spontaneous and IPS induced generalized spike wave discharges. At the age of 11 years she had numerous daily visual occipital seizures of amaurosis (5–15 s) with left eyelid jerking which were elicited by changes of light illumination and TV. EEG showed multifocal and bilateral synchronous spikes and IPS induced bursts of left occipital spikes. One year later she developed seizures typical of eyelid myoclonia with absences.

Silvestri *et al.*, 1989[729] reported a 12-year-old girl who had at age 11 years an episode of 'blurred and blunted vision without impairment of consciousness' while watching TV. One year later a similar episode progressed to secondary GTCS. She also had myoclonic jerks in the morning and while watching TV. IPS induced high amplitude generalized polyspikes with a significant posterior, right more than left, preponderance. A 1-min seizure induced by IPS consisted of head rotation to the left associated with EEG 'generalized fast spikes and wave complexes with hypersynchronous delta waves'.

Aso *et al.* (1987)[52] reported three girls with idiopathic television induced occipital seizures (visual loss, flickering lights, colours) followed by eye deviation, blinking, unresponsiveness and GTCS. 'Nausea or vomiting occurred in all cases, and two complained of severe post-ictal headache'. They all had generalized irregular discharges of spike, polyspike-waves during IPS. The resting EEG showed small anterior temporal (two) or centrotemporal spikes (one). Two of these girls are described in more detail by the same authors (Aso *et al.*, 1988).[51] The first is a 14-year-old girl who at the age of 10 had two secondary GTCS preceded by 'abnormal visual sensations' and followed by post-ictal headache. Spontaneous and TV-induced seizures with blindness followed by secondary GTCS occurred at age 12. Interictal EEGs showed small spikes in the right temporal area during sleep and consistent photoparoxysmal responses. These were either bilateral occipital polyspikes or generalized irregular spike-waves. An IPS induced seizure was recorded at age 13 years after 100 s 14 Hz IPS that also continued 20 s from the onset of the seizure. The seizure started with low voltage paroxysmal fast activity in the right occipital electrode spreading to other regions and ending in 2 min with generalized irregular spike and slow wave discharges. Clinically, 'she complained of flickering lights, nauseated and became mute responding only to simple commands'.

The other case of Aso *et al.* (1988)[51] is a girl who at the age of 11 years 'vomited and fell asleep' while watching TV. EEG showed generalized photoparoxysmal responses of polyspikes. One year later a seizure was recorded during 6 Hz IPS which induced generalized discharges of spikes/polyspikes, maximum in the posterior regions, followed by episodic high amplitude fast activity mainly in the right occipital region 7 s before a secondary GTCS. During the occipital discharge her 'eyelids began to twitch' followed by eye opening and GTCS.

Ricci and Vigevano (1993)[677] reported that of 30,000 patients of all ages who had an EEG in their department, five patients had an occipital seizure provoked by IPS. Their ages ranged from 10 to 32 years and none had demonstrable occipital lesions. Three patients had occipital epilepsy with visual seizures and interictal EEG with occipital foci (two) or bilateral spontaneous and evoked centrotemporal spikes as well as generalized discharges (one). The first is a 10-year-old boy with febrile and afebrile seizures at 1 year of age. He later had brief, spontaneous and TV-induced seizures of 'sudden right sided headache followed by vision of a bright spot of light in the right visual field, deviation of the eyes to the right and unresponsiveness'. Interictal EEG showed bilateral centrotemporal spikes, giant somatosensory evoked spikes and generalized photoparoxysmal responses that were associated with massive myoclonic jerks. IPS elicited his habitual seizure of right sided elementary visual hallucinations and ipsilateral deviation of the eyes with no post-ictal deficit. The ictal EEG starts with high amplitude generalized discharges of polyspikes and slow waves with eyelid blinking. These discharges appear in a repetitive fashion during the whole duration of the ictus and cause eyelid blinking. A few seconds from onset there is also a left occipital discharge of fast spikes that appears in between the generalized discharges. The boy is of normal neurological state with normal MRI.

The second is a 15-year-old normal boy who had two TV-induced seizures at ages 8 and 10 years. The first started with amaurosis followed by confusion and vomiting for 5 min. The second started again with amaurosis, progressive loss of consciousness and left side hemiconvulsions that were stopped after 30 min with intravenous diazepam. Subsequently, he had brief photically induced visual partial seizures consisting of 'little stars in the left hemifield' and one of them was recorded during IPS. Interictally, there were random right sided occipital spikes. Ictally, the seizure starts with fast rhythms and small spikes in the right occipital region, progressing with irregular theta activity intermixed with tiny spikes in the right posterior regions for 80 s.

The third case of Ricci and Vigevano[677] is a 17-year-old boy who from age 14 had only photically induced seizures of 'visual hallucinations of horizontal colour bands' in the left hemifield followed by vomiting, loss of consciousness, deviation of the eyes and mouth to the left and purposeless limb movements. Following treatment with sodium valproate he continued having brief, photically induced seizures of a very bright spot of 'white, but with all colours of the rainbow' in the left hemifield followed by post-ictal hemianopia. The interictal EEG had rare right sided occipital spikes. Two seizures were elicited by IPS, one lasting for 11 min. They both started with 'a bright spot of light on the left; the spot appearing in a blue area with a well defined contour involving the entire left visual field, and vision through the blue area was impossible'. This progressed, in the longer seizure, to left sided parasthesia and 'visual hallucinations related to memory flash backs'. The ictal EEG started with low amplitude fast rhythms and small spikes in the right occipital regions before increasing in amplitude and spreading with rhythmic spikes and theta waves in more anterior regions.

The fourth patient of Ricci and Vigevano[677] is a 16-year-old girl with brief absences and 3–4 Hz generalized polyspike and slow wave. Following treatment with valproic acid she had photically induced (TV or bright lights) seizures of 'palpebral myoclonias'. Several EEG from 9–15 years showed generalized photoparoxysmal responses preceded by brief occipital rhythms. The ictal EEG consisted of low amplitude bi-occipital fast spikes rapidly spreading with increasing amplitude to more anterior regions. Clinically, the seizure started with 'repeated palpebral myoclonias' followed by complex visual hallucinations (objects like TV sets coming at her) and fear ending after 2 min with loss of consciousness without convulsions.

The fifth patient of Ricci and Vigevano[677] is a rare but certain example of a patient with migraine having an occipital seizure evoked from a prolonged intermittent photic stimulation in an EEG examination. This normal woman had from age 24 years episodes of common migraine, with alternating side, without visual or other sensory aura. At age 28 years she had the only seizure of her life elicited by 22 Hz IPS of 45 s duration. This started with bi-occipital fast spikes, which were of higher amplitude on the left, progressing to left posterior rhythmic theta activity intermingled with spikes. Clinically, the seizure consisted of 'multicoloured spots moving quickly from the extreme right of the centre of the visual field followed by tonic deviation of the eyes to the right with a post-ictal complete right sided hemianopia'.

The authors concluded that occipital seizures provoked by IPS probably constitute a rare type of photosensitivity, sometimes appearing in occipital epilepsies, generalized epilepsies, and migraine.

Graf *et al.* (1994)[356] **and Ferrie *et al.* (1994)**[278] in an extensive literature review on video-game induced seizures found 21 patients and reported another 28 new cases.[278,356] The majority of the 49 patients suffer from various syndromes of idiopathic generalized epilepsy. However, 15 (30.6 per cent) had partial seizures with 11 of them (22.4 per cent) having onset with visual symptoms (elementary visual hallucinations, blurring of vision, multiple scotomata) alone or progressing to secondary GTCS. Though most of these 11 patients with visual seizures had spontaneous and random mainly unilateral occipital spikes in the resting EEG, only four (8.2 per cent)[278,294,356,515] had evidence of EEG photosensitivity to comply with the diagnosis of IPOS. These were:

1. A 6-year-old boy (case 1 of Maeda *et al.*)[515] with video-game seizures of scotomata followed by loss of consciousness. He also had spontaneous GTCS. His resting EEG had an occipital slow wave focus and IPS elicited photoconvulsive responses.
2. A 12-year-old normal boy reported by Fukusako *et al.*, 1990[294] who had attacks of 'binasal visual field defects' when playing a family computer game. EEG showed right sided occipital spike and slow wave activated by chequerboard pattern reversal stimuli.
3. A 13-year-old boy (case 1 of Graf *et al.*)[356] with video-game seizures described as 'blurring of vision followed by dizziness, headache and jerking of the right hand'. He also had spontaneous unprovoked seizures. His resting EEG showed generalized discharges, 3–4 Hz spike-wave with right sided preponderance, and IPS provoked photoparoxysmal responses.
4. A 15-year-old girl (case 10 of Ferrie *et al.*)[278] who is detailed below as case 12.1.

Guerrini *et al.* (1995)[370] offered a complete study of 10 neurologically normal patients (eight females, two males) aged 8–30 years (mean 17 years) with recurrent visually induced occipital seizures. Seizure onset occurred between the ages of 5 and 17 years (mean 11 years). In all patients, seizures were triggered by television, video-games or both. Computer screens, sudden transitions from darkness to bright light or flickering sunlight represented less frequent triggers. Reflex activation was obvious at referral in seven patients, but this became evident only after repeated questioning of the other three. The initial ictal manifestation for all patients was a 'bright', 'colourful', or 'multicoloured' ring or spot which was fixed or flashing in the periphery of the visual field, or moving slowly. Seven patients also experienced blindness or blurring as late ictal manifestations. In three patients, the attacks would cease after visual symptoms, but in five patients visual seizures were followed by 'conscious' head or eye deviation. Seven patients experienced epigastric discomfort or nausea, followed in six by vomiting, sometimes accompanied in four by unresponsiveness. Five patients reported brief paroxysms of 'sharp' or 'piercing' pain localized either in one head region or in one orbit. In seven patients, one or more seizures became secondary generalized. Headache was a constant post-ictal phenomenon in four of the five patients who also reported cephalic pain during seizures. Headache occurred after both generalized and partial seizures, beginning 15–30 min post-ictally. It was reported as pulsating or pounding, lasting up to several hours. Two patients reported occasional post-ictal vomiting. No patient had self-induced seizures. These cases 'because of the clustering of visual aura, vegetative symptoms, and cephalic pain, had frequently been misdiagnosed as having migraine before adjunctive clinical and EEG evidence of epilepsy was obtained.'[370]

Background EEG activity was normal in all patients. Resting EEGs were normal in two patients and showed bilateral synchronous and asynchronous occipital spikes or spikes and waves in eight, associated with isolated generalized spike-wave in four. Paroxysmal abnormalities were enhanced both on eye closure and with the eyes closed. Three patients also exhibited centrotemporal spikes that were independent of the occipital discharges. IPS induced occipital photoparoxysmal response in all patients and was accompanied by generalized discharges in six. The photosensitivity range was between 5 and 40 Hz. Several seizures were triggered in the EEG laboratory, by television in one patient and by IPS in two. Duration of recorded seizures varied from 20 s to 25 min. The ictal discharges remained localized to the occipital regions, shifting from side to side while the patients were experiencing visual symptoms, and could eventually spread slowly over the temporal regions with the appearance of autonomic symptoms; these were only minor, and there was no clouding of consciousness. In two patients, the Oz electrode was critical in demonstrating the ictal discharge associated with the elementary initial visual symptomatology (Fig. 12.4).

All patients were of normal neurological development, average intelligence, regular schooling, and normal development. Three patients had a history of uncomplicated febrile convulsions. At age 5 years, one patient had a focal motor seizure accompanied by EEG findings typical of Rolandic seizures and was treated with phenobarbital until age 11, with no relapse.

Three patients had a first-degree relative with migraine. Three others had a first-degree relative with seizures, one each with febrile seizures, Rolandic epilepsy, and idiopathic generalized epilepsy.

Complete seizure control was achieved in most patients with monotherapy, although occasional stimulus-related seizures occurred in three patients who showed a wider range of photosensitivity. The authors[370] concluded that these patients have an idiopathic localization-related epilepsy with age-related onset and specific mode of precipitation and emphasized the difficulties of differentiating this clinically from migraine or from non-reflex childhood idiopathic occipital epilepsy.

Guerrini *et al.* (1997)[369] also reported that two of 33 patients with Rolandic seizures developed IPOS after remission of their Rolandic seizures. These were two 19-year-old women. They both had clinico-EEG features of Rolandic seizures with onset at age 4 and 5 years. At age 12 years they both had onset of occipital seizures precipitated by TV or bright lights. The first patient's seizures consisted of 'phosphorescent multicoloured spots moving in the visual field, slow sustained head version to the left, headache, unresponsiveness and vomiting with secondary GTCS twice per year. Seizures with visual hallucinations lasting 10–15 min without secondary GTCS occurred monthly. Visually induced seizures ceased when valproate was added to carbamazepine. At age 17 years the EEG showed bilateral occipital spike and wave complexes and IPS induced paroxysmal driving. A habitual visual seizure was induced by IPS with EEG fast (needle-like) occipital spikes, more prominent on the right and spike-slow wave occipital complexes. The second patient had only two visually induced seizure (TV or bright light) with blurring of vision or moving multicoloured spots and amaurosis followed by nausea, vomiting, headache and unresponsiveness. The EEG showed spontaneous and IPS evoked occipital spikes. No further seizures occurred from age 12 years (she was receiving vigabatrin between age 12 and 14 years).

Illustrative cases of the variability of idiopathic photosensitive occipital seizures are presented in the following section, from my personal studies and experience on IPOS.

Personal experience and illustrative cases

My experience with photosensitive epilepsy started in 1969 with the wise and friendly guidance and support of P.M. Jeavons and G.F.A. Harding in Birmingham whose book on photosensitive epilepsy[377,421] is a classic reference. They supervised my PhD Thesis on 'A study of photosensitive epilepsy with particular reference to occipital spikes induced by IPS' (1972).[593] Amongst 50 patients with clinical and EEG photosensitivity there were three patients relevant to this Chapter 12B. Case 11 of the thesis was a 12-year-old girl who had two television-induced seizures starting with 'visual disturbances of not been able to see' which progressed to loss of consciousness without convulsions. The resting EEG showed small left sided occipital spikes and generalized discharges on eye closure. Time-locked occipital spikes were induced by IPS from 4.5 to 8 Hz. IPS at higher rates, 8–59 Hz, induced generalized photoparoxysmal responses preceded by occipital spikes. Another patient, a 12-year-old girl (case 23), had spontaneous and TV induced GTCS that were preceded by stomach pain and vomiting. The resting EEG was slower on the left side and she had generalized spike and slow wave discharges. IPS elicited generalized photoparoxysmal discharges without occipital spikes. Finally, another 12-year-old girl (case 18) had attacks of 'feeling sick and becoming pale' that were induced by TV, rotation of the turntable of record players or moving escalators. Her resting EEG showed eye-closure generalized discharges of spike and wave. IPS induced time-locked occipital spikes alone at 5–7 Hz IPS or preceding generalized photoparoxysmal responses at 7–50 Hz.

Amongst 418 patients of my subsequent Athens study[603] with onset of seizures before the age of 13 years, there were 13 patients with photosensitive epilepsy and an additional patient had self-induced pattern sensitive epilepsy also with photosensitivity.[597] From the 13 (3.1 per cent) patients with clinical and IPS photosensitivity, five had self-induced photosensitivity (three were of entirely normal neurological, intellectual and developmental state), five had one or more GTCS induced by television (two were brother and sister) and one started with photosensitivity which converted to scotosensitivity (FOS) and to photosensitivity again.[598,620] None of these 13 patients had evidence of spontaneous or evoked occipital seizures.

Finally, amongst 930 patients that I saw in St. Thomas' Hospital there were six with clinical and EEG evidence of IPOS. The mildest case was a child with Rolandic seizures who had a single TV-video game visual seizure followed by GTCS. Details of these patients follow. Note, however that no one single case is like another.

The first patient, briefly reported by Ferrie *et al.*,1994[278] is of great interest. She has early onset photosensitive visual seizures that have continued for more than 10 years despite appropriate medication. Mild eyelid fluttering is associated with spontaneous and IPS evoked occipital spikes as documented with serial video-EEG over the years (Fig. 12.3). In addition, she had brief absences that remitted later.

> Case 12.1 (case 35 of Table 13.3). This 15-year-old girl had three febrile convulsions at the age of 1 year. There is a strong family history of febrile convulsions. Her maternal grandmother had migraine. Her mother had two episodes of migraine with aura in her late thirties.
>
> Aged 5 she started having infrequent visual simple partial seizures that started with bright, multicoloured, stationary lights in small squares in her right temporal hemifield lasting 3–5 min followed by sleep for 2

h. Rarely these visual seizures would progress to secondary generalization. At the age of 13 years, the elementary visual hallucinations were followed by complex visual hallucinations lasting 2–3 min with small faces of people superimposed on the colours (Fig. 9.2). post-ictally she was drowsy, nauseous and occasionally she had mild headache.

Nearly all of her seizures occurred after awakening while watching television, playing video-games and on one occasion while toasting a bun in front of a fire. They rarely occurred spontaneously. Infrequent, very mild brief absences accompanied by eyelid fluttering were reported during her early childhood.

Treatment commenced with sodium valproate, 600–1000 mg/day. Absences stopped and the occipital seizures reduced to 1 per year.

EEGs at the age of 7 years showed single and runs, 1–3 s duration, of high voltage occipital spikes/polyspikes and slow waves frequently associated with eyelid fluttering (Figs. 12.1 and 12.3). They occurred with the eyes closed and on eye-closure. They attenuated in complete darkness thus excluding fixation-off sensitivity. There was also a single, brief, spontaneous generalized discharge of spike and slow waves at 3–3.5 Hz accompanied by mild impairment of cognition and eyelid fluttering (Fig. 12.3).

Subsequent serial video-EEG consistently showed occipital discharges that were often associated with eyelid fluttering as above. Also, IPS at 13–30 Hz consistently evoked occipital spikes and polyspikes (Fig.12.3). CT brain scan and MRI are normal.

The next patient is also very interesting. She started with Rolandic seizures and centrotemporal spikes. Spontaneous and photically induced seizures appeared nearly simultaneously with the Rolandic seizures. She also has the rare ictal symptom of 'white blindness' and seizures appear drug-resistant.

Case 12.2 (case 36 of Table 13.3). This 13-year-old normal girl had six nocturnal Rolandic seizures with fast secondary generalization at age 10. These nocturnal seizures were not preceded by visual symptoms. Her mother finds her with generalized convulsions sometimes preceded by right eye twitching. On one occasion the seizure was witnessed from onset. She tried to say 'mum', made 'funny breathing noises' and progressed to GTCS. The EEG showed centrotemporal spikes independently right and left. IPS at 11 Hz elicited a singular brief generalized spike-wave discharge after eye-closure. At approximately the same age, she started having visual seizures within 2 min of watching television or occasionally with video-games. They consisted of bright, multi-coloured lights like a pattern on a football (Fig. 9.2), lasted for 10 s, and were followed by hemianopia and frontal non throbbing headache for 1 h. She described them well: 'Lights appear above my eyes. There are very bright colours. Usually yellow, red, orange and bright green. They usually appear 2 min after I watch TV close to it. They last for about 10 s and then I could see only from one eye for 5–10 s. This is followed by bad, pressing frontal headache for an hour'. On one occasion at age 12 years TV-elicited visual seizures were followed by generalized convulsions despite treatment with carbamazepine that started at age 10 years. She subsequently developed frequent nocturnal generalized convulsions preceded by elementary visual hallucinations which wake her up. The visual hallucinations consist of a multi-coloured chequerboard that fills her whole visual field; she cannot see through them, she is scared, she calls her mother and has a GTCS within a minute from onset. On other occasions she wakes up from sleep with white blindness, 'all white', before a GTCS. Sodium valproate was added which stopped the nocturnal, but she continues to have TV-induced occipital seizures, also probably having subtle myoclonus of her arms.

Serial video EEGs showed spontaneous single and short runs (1 s) of bi-occipital sharp waves (Fig. 12.3). They occurred mainly when the eyes were closed and disappeared in complete darkness irrespective of whether the eyes were closed or opened. Occipital spikes also occurred with the eyes opened during TV activation. IPS elicited occipital spikes. Also on eye closure during IPS there were brief, 0.5–2 s, discharges of generalized sharp theta waves with posterior emphasis intermixed with a few occipital spike-wave complexes (Fig. 12.3). These were occasionally associated with eyelid fluttering. On one occasion, they were preceded by low voltage occipital fast activity. High resolution MRI at age 13 is normal.

The next case studied with Dr A. Parker and Dr A. Agathonikou is an example of a patient who starts with what may be interpreted as a pure form of television-induced generalized seizures but later visual seizures, spontaneous and photically induced, became more apparent and they are drug-resistant.

Case 12.3 (case 37 of Table 13.3). This 17-year-old girl, at the age of 9 years started to have television/computer screen evoked generalized convulsive, predominantly tonic, seizures with loss of consciousness lasting for 2–3 min. These were followed by blindness, vomiting and headache. She was often 'drawn' to the screen in a trance-like state. Treatment with sodium valproate was commenced with initial improvement, followed by further seizures. Aged 12 she complained of 'orbs' of brightly coloured lights in the left upper quadrant of her visual field, associated with shaking of her upper limbs triggered by fluorescent lights and television. Lamotrigine was added to the sodium valproate. She continues to have eyelid fluttering with jerking of her arms on exposure to fluorescent lighting.

EEG at age 12 years showed a few occipital sharp waves. IPS at 16 and 20 Hz elicited brief, 3 s, generalized discharges of spike/polyspikes and waves associated with eyelid fluttering and impairment of consciousness. At the age of 14 years, IPS at 10–14 Hz provoked posterior discharges of spikes associated with eyelid fluttering and subtle head jerking (Fig. 12.3).

The next case demonstrates spontaneous and evoked visual occipital seizures. He also has secondary GTCS which occur only during sleep. Seizures were controlled only when carbamazepine was added to sodium valproate which was not effective.

Case 12.4 (case 38 of Table 13.3). This normal 16-year-old boy started having brief photically induced visual seizures at age 9 years. They consist of flashing light, 'like a flash of a camera switching on and off' in the left visual field. This lasts for seconds and it may be associated with giddiness which make him sit down. They are always elicited when watching black and white TV from close distance. He never had these with coloured TV, computers or video-games. In addition, from the same age he has 3–4 nocturnal secondary GTCS every year. Once he had three such seizures in one night. These are stereotyped. He wakes up with the same visual hallucination of a flashing light on the left, he calls his parents and within a minute he has the convulsions.

He has six routine and sleep EEG that are normal except for one at age 12 years in which IPS, delivered on awakening, provoked brief generalized discharges of spikes and occasionally multiple spikes that occurred after eye closure.

Phenytoin 200 mg daily and later sodium valproate 1500 mg daily did not make any change. At age 15 years, carbamazepine 600 mg daily was added to sodium valproate. He did not have any other, spontaneous or evoked seizures, in the next 16 months of follow-up. High resolution MRI at age 16 years was normal.

The next patient is the best example I have to demonstrate that Rolandic seizures may co-exist with a seizure susceptibility of the occipital cortex to visual stimuli.

Case 12.5 (case 39 of Table 13.3). This 20-year-old man had 15 nocturnal Rolandic seizures from age 11 to 14 years: 'there was a noise like grunting or moaning, his eyes widely opened and deviated to the left and then he would go stiff with no clonic convulsions'. Next morning he would have headache and vomiting. EEG showed right sided centrotemporal spikes. At age 14 years he had a single diurnal seizure the day after his grandfather died. He was playing a television video-game when he had visual hallucinations on the left of his visual field. These consisted of small multi-coloured concentric circles of mainly blue, green and yellow (Fig. 9.2) which gradually within seconds multiplied, not allowing him to see through them. These were within half a minute followed by a generalized tonic–clonic seizure. On recovery he had post-ictal headache. Treatment with carbamazepine was initiated after this seizure. He had one more nocturnal Rolandic seizure in the same year. Subsequently, in the next 6 years he was well, studying at the University and without medication from age 16 years.

The last patient with IPOS that I have, demonstrates late onset, after the age of 16 years, of infrequent photically induced occipital seizures with secondary GTCS. Medication for an obsessive disorder may have facilitated these seizures.

Case 12.6. This is a 19-year-old otherwise normal woman who has a severe obsessive-compulsive disorder treated with clomipramine 150 mg nocte. Two photically induced seizures occurred at age 18 years. They both occurred while watching TV from close distance. The first started with the eyes and head deviating to the right, the second with 'rounded, yellow and blue, flickering fireworks in the centre of the vision'. On both occasions a secondary GTCS occurred within 3–5 s from outset. post-ictally she was confused, with severe headache and nausea. EEG showed brief bursts of generalized theta waves sometimes with intermixed larval spikes. IPS evoked mainly posterior discharges with bilateral occipital spikes.

Benign Childhood Partial Seizures and Related Epileptic Syndromes. C P Panayiotopoulos
©1999 John Libbey & Company Ltd., pp. 257–277.

Chapter 13

Benign childhood occipital seizures and related epileptic syndromes: Personal studies

Introduction

I often refer in this book to the results of my studies on the subject. The methods, the patients, the background and some of the results of these studies from 1973 to date are described in this chapter.

In 1971, having finished my PhD Thesis on photosensitive epilepsy[593] in Birmingham, England, I returned to Athens, Greece. There in 1973, I first saw children with benign childhood occipital seizures. They were private patients referred to me for clinical or EEG evaluation. Both the occipital seizure manifestations and the EEG occipital paroxysms fascinated me, particularly as the subject appeared largely unknown. Therefore, I initiated a prospective study on occipital epilepsies that occupied 25 years. Having studied the effect of darkness on eye-closure related generalized discharges of photosensitive patients,[593,594] it was natural for me to investigate this on occipital paroxysms which could last as long as the eyes were closed. This is how fixation-off sensitivity was discovered.[599,600] As a clinician I had a more difficult task. One of the children, a colleague's son, had symptoms that would qualify him for migraine with aura or basilar migraine but a number of other features did not fit this diagnosis which I questioned in favour of occipital seizures in 1980.[599] At the same time, nearly all other children with occipital paroxysms had rather prolonged, mainly nocturnal seizures, with deviation of the eyes and vomiting before secondary generalized tonic–clonic seizures (GTCS). This is the early onset benign childhood occipital seizures or Panayiotopoulos syndrome as some authors[12,150,270–275] honoured me by terming it lately. I detailed the clinico-EEG features of these children in (*Neurology*, 1981).[600] Subsequent publication became more difficult, after the reports of Gastaut in 1982, establishing 'benign partial epilepsy of childhood epilepsy with occipital spike-waves'.[303–306] They are all detailed in the relevant chapters.

Methods

My studies divided into two periods, the first in Athens from 1973 to 1983 and the other in London from 1989 which continues today. In both studies, I personally evaluated all patients clinically and with EEG. Combining clinical and EEG data is the most powerful tool in the diagnostic process of epilepsies.

Athens study

This started in 1973, mainly based on a modest private practice outside my commitments to the Department of Neurology, Athens University where I was primarily assigned to the evaluation of neuromuscular disorders. Private practice is well accepted and encouraged in Greece for University physicians.

In this private practice, from 1973 to 1983, I examined 900 patients with definite epileptic seizures. Their ages varied from 6 months to 80 years. There was a wide spectrum of personal referrals covering all aspects of mainly adult but also child neurology. The sources included physicians, paediatricians, neurologists and, to a lesser extent, relatives of the patients. All patients were examined clinically and with EEG which I also interpreted and which was usually performed on the same day as the examination. Sleep EEG were rarely performed. Though I continued to see some of these patients, no new cases were added in the period 1984–88 when I served as Head and Professor of Neurology, King Khalid University Hospital, Riyadh, Saudi Arabia.

Prospective study: This prospective study was for all patients with epileptic events related to the occipital lobes. My particular interest was for idiopathic occipital seizures and EEG occipital spikes.[599,600,605,606] Patients with these conditions were exhaustively interrogated clinically and thoroughly studied with EEG. Whenever possible these patients are still followed-up mainly through correspondence, telephone calls and contacts, either personal or through their families or physicians. Though the primary motivation for initiating this prospective study was the responsiveness of occipital paroxysms to light and darkness, fixation and central vision that I documented and named fixation-off sensitivity,[595,598–600,604] it was soon apparent to me that occipital lobe epilepsy was a rather neglected chapter in epileptology, as I have detailed,[596] and that there was significant confusion regarding the differentiation of visual seizures from migraine aura, as I have reported.[599,602,611] These areas were also explored in this prospective study, limited by means, funds and probably experience.

Having documented in this prospective study that:

(a) Early onset benign childhood occipital seizures (EBOS) were the main and the most benign representative amongst otherwise normal children with occipital paroxysms;[600,602,605,611]

(b) Children with late onset benign childhood occipital seizures (LBOS) were of a rare occurrence and did not have basilar migraine;[599,602,605] and

(c) Ictus emeticus was a main seizure manifestation in EBOS;[603–606]

I was naturally interested to find:

(i) the relevant prevalence of EBOS in relation to other benign childhood partial epilepsies and

(ii) the incidence and symptomatology of ictus emeticus in other epilepsies.

This I did with the following retrospective studies.

Retrospective studies: The clinical and EEG records of 900 patients with definite epileptic seizures were retrospectively evaluated for ictus emeticus, that is vomiting during the ictal phase of the seizures.[603] Cases with vomiting occurring after a seizure or with a symptom-free interval between vomiting and a subsequent fit were not included.

Twenty four of the 900 patients had ictal vomiting and all were children.[603] Only three had evidence of symptomatic partial seizures. From the other 21 children with idiopathic partial seizures, 12 had EBOS.[603,604] The remaining nine children had unilateral central spikes that were also elicited with somatosensory stimuli (two), midline spikes (two), frontal spikes (one), ill sustained photoparoxysmal response (one) or consistently normal EEG (three).[603,622]

Furthermore, of these 900 patients 418 had onset of their first afebrile seizure before the age of 13 years. These were studied retrospectively and classified in accordance with the International League Against Epilepsy recommendations.[177] Ninety four patients fulfilled the criteria of benign idiopathic age and localization related epilepsies. They did not have evidence of structural brain abnormality and their neurological examination was normal. They were further classified according to the main

EEG spike localization into 72 (76.6 per cent) with centrotemporal spikes, 18 (17 per cent) with occipital paroxysms, 2 with frontal and 2 with midline spikes.[603,605]

London study

This started in 1989 in a new clinic for epileptic disorders in St. Thomas' Hospital, London. This is the major general teaching hospital for patients of all ages within the National Health Service. Supported by a Special Trustees of St. Thomas' Hospital grant for 'a prospective study on the syndromic classification of the first 1000 patients with epilepsies' a clinic for epilepsies was established in February 1989 within the department of clinical neurophysiology. There are 942 patients evaluated from 1989 to March 1998. Their mean age is around 30 and only 10 per cent are between the ages of 4 and 14 years.

Referral pattern: Most of the patients, mainly adolescents and adults, are National Health System (NHS) referrals from general practitioners, neurologists, paediatricians, other specialists and the accident and emergency department of St. Thomas' Hospital. Approximately 20 per cent of the patients are tertiary referrals from outside the catchment area of the hospital or private patients.

We also enrol in the clinic, with the permission of their physicians, those patients referred for EEG only, whose EEG, clinical manifestations or both are of particular interest for the purposes of our studies. Thus, there may be a bias towards patients with idiopathic generalized epilepsies, fixation-off sensitivity or occipital seizures with visual hallucinations.

Clinical evaluation: All patients are examined personally either alone or together with the clinical and research fellows of the department who are all qualified neurologists or paediatricians trained in paediatric neurology. Patients, relatives and witnesses are interrogated through either free-form or semi-structured interviews regarding clinical manifestations, major or minor seizures, circadian distribution, precipitating factors, possibly causative factors and family history. We previously detailed the emphasis we give and the methods we apply for the detection of minor seizures, such as myoclonic jerks,[610] absences,[617] and simple or complex partial seizures preceding or occurring independently of major fits.[613] The clinical information is often additionally supplied with written accounts of the seizures and related factors and when possible, with home-made videos of the clinical events. Patients with IGE and absences often have additional semi-structured written or verbal interviews with us and with our EEG technologists which are frequently video-taped. More recently, all patients are requested to complete a detailed structured questionnaire.

Patients with recent onset of seizures are prospectively studied, while those with the established condition are also retrospectively investigated from the time of presentation to the onset of the disease with scrutinization of old medical and EEG records which are systematically sought. All patients have at least one follow-up per year.

EEG evaluation: All patients have at least one EEG or video-EEG and if this is not conclusive, an EEG during sleep and awakening is performed. In view of my particular interest in IGE and typical absences,[617] all patients with IGE also have serial video-EEG recordings and video-EEG after partial sleep deprivation followed by at least 30 min recording on awakening, especially when prolonged routine video-EEG studies fail to record ictal phenomena. Cognitive impairment during 3–4 Hz spike-wave discharges is routinely tested by asking the patients to count their breaths during hyperventilation.[322,627]. Optional IPS is performed without endangering the patient to have a major convulsive seizure.[594,616] Video-EEGs are appropriately tailored for patients with precipitating factors such as photosensitivity, pattern sensitivity, reading, menstruation, awakening and sleep. Fixation-off sensitivity is tested for those with EEG abnormalities occurring on eyes-closed and the effect of darkness is evaluated for patients with eye-closure related paroxysms.[620,626]

Brain imaging: High resolution MRI is obtained for all patients with partial and late onset seizures and it is often performed for patients with IGE, particularly with seizures resistant to treatment, or focal elements in the EEG or the seizures. Positron emission tomography is acquired for patients with intractable partial or cryptogenic/symptomatic generalized seizures.

Diagnostic aim: Our prospective aim for all patients is to establish a syndromic diagnosis according to strict clinical and video-EEG criteria;[613] when this is not possible, a seizure-symptom categorization is attempted. With this approach, we were able to show that some unclassified patients have a non-fortuitous clustering of clinico-EEG features indicating that they belong to epileptic syndromes previously unrecognized by the ILAE such as eyelid myoclonia with absences, perioral myoclonia with absences, IGE with phantom absences, GTCS and frequently absence status.[612,617,633]

Data storage: All data are stored in a detailed database system.

Prospective study of occipital epilepsy in St.Thomas' Hospital

Patients with occipital seizures are prospectively evaluated and followed up as in the Athens study.[605] Additionally, patients with visual seizures are also asked to complete a purposely structured questionnaire and draw their visual experiences (Appendix 13.1, page 277). MRI is requested for all patients. There were only eight children with EBOS, probably because of the pattern of referral which is mainly of adult patients. It is of interest that three of them were referred by physicians in Athens. The other five were local referrals from paediatric neurologists jointly working in our department (two), because of occipital paroxysms in EEG after a second seizure (two) and because a junior paediatrician in our hospital asked for an EEG after the first afebrile seizure (one).

In addition, there was only one child with LBOS and occipital paroxysms.[630] A prevalent idiopathic group is of patients with visual seizures of LBOS but without occipital paroxysms or occipital spikes (12 patients). This is entirely missing from my studies in Athens probably as a result of selection and diagnostic criteria. Most of these cases were specially referred because of their similarities to migraine aura which we have published extensively.[611,625] Photically induced visual seizures is another interesting group of six patients which is largely heterogeneous and also conspicuously absent from the Athens study.

Patients with occipital seizures and epilepsy in the two studies

Of 1360 patients with epileptic seizures in the two studies, 63 patients had incontrovertible clinical evidence of occipital seizures with or without secondary generalization. These, listed in order of relative homogeneity are:

(a) Twenty four children with early onset benign childhood occipital seizures. Sixteen of these patients have been previously reported,[605] and eight more were seen in St. Thomas' Hospital.

(b) Seventeen patients with cryptogenic or symptomatic occipital epilepsy. Three of these patients were initially categorized as idiopathic occipital epilepsy because routine MRI were normal. However, in two of them recent high resolution 3D MRI showed definite abnormalities. I have also included in this group a normal child with intractable visual seizures but persistent and marked lateralized focal occipital slow waves in EEG, despite normal MRI.

(c) Sixteen patients with definite or possible idiopathic occipital epilepsy who had spontaneous visual hallucinations as the inaugural symptom of their occipital seizures. All were of normal neurological and mental state.

(d) Six children and adolescents with idiopathic photosensitive occipital epilepsy, that is photically elicited occipital seizures.[278,370] No one was like another and one was older than 16 years at first seizure.

In addition, three patients with idiopathic generalized epilepsies had visual hallucinations amongst other ictal symptoms of generalized epilepsy and EEG generalized discharges of 3–4 Hz spike and slow wave.

Thus, from these 63 patients the largest and most homogeneous group was that of 24 patients with EBOS or Panayiotopoulos syndrome. The second largest group was of 17 patients with symptomatic occipital epilepsy of various causes including cortical developmental malformations and neonatal insults.

Inclusion criteria for benign childhood occipital seizures

Inclusion criteria are to justify idiopathic occipital partial seizures with onset from 1 to 16 years of age.

(a) Idiopathic. All patients are of normal physical and mental state and development. Brain imaging with CT brain scan, preferably high resolution MRI, or both is normal.

(b) Occipital partial seizures. Partial seizures with onset of symptoms unequivocally originating from the occipital cortex. Ictal vomiting may not be an occipital symptom, but it is accepted in the inclusion criteria because it is mainly reported in patients, predominantly children, with EEG evidence of primarily occipital involvement.[605]

(c) EEG confirmation of occipital spikes and paroxysms is optional. However, 18 patients (case 1–16, 24 and 25, Tables 13.1 and 13.3) of the initial study were selected because of occipital paroxysms in their EEG.

(d) Age at onset is between 1 and 16 to match the age limits of other benign childhood partial epilepsies.

Exclusion criteria for benign childhood occipital seizures

These are to exclude patients with symptomatic/cryptogenic epilepsies, generalized epilepsies, complex or simple partial seizures of extra-occipital origin, patients with onset of idiopathic occipital epilepsy after the age of 16 years, and patients who do not strictly meet the inclusion criteria.

The following 23 of the 63 patients with occipital seizures are excluded:

(a) Seventeen patients with cryptogenic or symptomatic occipital epilepsy in order to comply with the idiopathic definition.

(b) Three patients with idiopathic occipital epilepsy starting after the age of 16 years as follows: A 25-year-old man who had at that age four seizures of elementary visual hallucinations with secondary GTCS. High resolution MRI, routine and sleep EEG are normal. Treatment with carbamazepine started. An 18-year-old normal man with one single GTCS preceded by unilateral palinopsia that started flashing for 2 s followed by visual illusions of the surroundings coming on him and ending within 5 s with GTCS. Routine EEG, sleep deprivation EEG and MRI arc all normal. No medication was prescribed. Two years later he remained well with no further visual or other seizures. A 19-year-old woman with a severe obsessive-compulsive disorder and two photically induced occipital seizures at age 18 years.

(c) Three children with typical seizures of elementary visual hallucinations because brain imaging was not performed.

Three additional patients are also excluded who have visual hallucinations amongst other ictal symptoms of generalized epilepsy and EEG generalized discharges of 3–4 Hz spike and slow wave associated with typical absence seizures.

Results

1. Early onset benign childhood occipital seizures

Tables 13.1 and 13.2 provide chronological and clinical data of 23 out of 24 children with early onset benign childhood occipital seizures. An additional case of EBOS was seen just after these tables had been compiled for statistical evaluation. This boy of West Indian origin was seen at the end of March 1998 because of two prolonged seizures typical of EBOS within one year at age 5. EEG had occipital paroxysms.

Physical, mental state and brain imaging

All patients by selection criteria have normal neurological and mental state. Cases 1–16 have normal brain CT scan and cases 17–23 normal MRI. None have visual deficits. Five had mild to moderate myopia and two strabismus. All patients attended main stream schools and most of them were good students. Three patients probably had mild learning or concentration difficulties with low grade school records.

Sex, age at onset and last follow-up (Table 13.1)

These are 12 girls and 11 boys. Age at onset of first afebrile seizure is 2–12 (mean = 5 ± 2.1, median = 5) and age at last seizure is 2–25 (mean = 7.1 ± 4.6, median = 6) years.

All but three patients were first seen within the first year from onset of seizures. The other three (cases 1, 20 and 21) were seen between 2 and 6 years after their first seizure.

Table 13.1. Chronological data of Panayiotopoulos syndrome

Case no.	Sex	Age (years)			Number of seizures	Life span of seizures (years)	Seizure free (years)
		Last follow-up	Onset of seizures	Last seizure			
1	F	29	5	9	11	4	20
2	F	25	6	6	2	1	19
3	F	14	4	6	3	2	8
4	F	18	5	5	1	1	13
5	M	16	3	5	4	2	11
6	M	16	5	6	12	1	10
7	F	13	2	2	1	1	11
8	M	7	4	4	4	1	3
9.	F	6	5	5	1	1	1
10	F	14	7	7	1	1	7
11*	M	27	3	25	3*	22*	2
12	F	15	6	6	1	1	9
13	M	8	4	5	3	1	4
14	F	16	7	8	2	1	8
15	M	14	6	6	3	1	8
16	F	7	6	6	2	1	1
17	F	8	6	6	1	1	2
18	M	6	4	5	2	1	1
19	M	7	5	6	2	1	1
20	M	7	2	6	6	4	1
21	M	13	5	12	4	7	1
22	F	14	12	12	1	1	2
23	M	6	3	4	5	1	2
Mean		13.3	5	7.1	3.3	2.5	6.3
SD		6.7	2.1	4.6	3	4.5	5.7
Min.		6	2	2	1	1	1
Max.		29	12	25	12	22	20
Median		14	5	6	2	1	4

*This is the only patient who later developed infrequent GTCS.

Clinical manifestations (Table 13.2)

There is a remarkable similarity for all patients with mainly nocturnal seizures (21 patients), characterized by vomiting (19), deviation of the eyes (19) or both (13) which may last longer than 30 min to hours (12) before progressing to hemiconvulsions or GTCS (15). In a typical nocturnal seizure, the child is found vomiting but responding, eyes deviate to one side, impairment of consciousness occurs and this state, usually lasting for 1–3 h, ends with convulsions.

Table 13.2. Ictal manifestations, duration of seizures, circadian distribution, and EEG findings in EBOS

Case no.	Vomit	EDev	Other symptoms	Hemi-GTCS	Duration (min)	Nocturnal (number)	Diurnal (number)	EEG
1	Y	Y	ED,V,Ap	N	> 15–20[1]	3[1]	8[1]	OP,IPSOS
2	Y	Y	ED,V	Y	60–180	2[2]	0	OP,IPSOS
3	Y	Y	ED,V	N	10–45	2	1	OP,F
4	Y	Y	V,ED	Y	> 30	1	0	OP
5	Y	Y	V,ED	Y	> 120	4	0	OP
6	Y	Y	C,ED,LOC	N	> 7	12[3]	0	OP
7	Y	Y	V,ED,IU,LOC	N	> 10	1	0	OP
8	Y	Y	V,ED	N	> 10	4	0	OP
9	Y	N	V,EO	Y	> 10	1	0	OP
10	Y	N	V,LOC	Y	> 10	1	0	OP
11	N	N	R,Ap,EO	Y	> 10	3	12GTCS[3]	OP[3]
12	N	Y	ED	Y	> 30	1	0	OP
13	Y	Y	V,ED	Y	> 10	1	2	OP,CTS
14	Y	Y	V,ED,OPM	Y	> 30	2[4]	0	O,F,CT,GSS[4]
15	N	Y	OPM,ED	Y	> 10	2	1	OP,CTS
16	N	Y	C,ED	Y	> 30	2	0	OP,CTS
17	Y	Y	V,ED,P,Ag,ED,IU	Y	> 30	0	1	OP,FOS
18	Y	Y	V,ED,P,Ag	N	> 30	0	2	OS
19	Y	Y	V,ED,P,LOC	N	> 30	1	1A	OP,F
20	Y	Y	V,ED,P,OPM	Y	> 30Y	6	0	OS
21	Y	Y	V,P,ED	Y	120–180[5]	1[5]	3[5]	OS,CTS
22	Y	Y	V,ED	Y	> 15	1	0	OS
23	Y	N	AO,P,V,LOC	N	> 15	5	0	NORMAL

Y = Yes; N = No; Vomit = Ictal vomiting; EDev = Ictal horizontal deviation of the eyes; EO = Eyes widely open and in midline; VH = Visual hallucinations; LOC = Loss of consciousness without convulsions; R = Retching; OPM = Oropharynolaryngeal movements; Ag = Agitated behaviour; IU = Incontinence of urine; D = Diurnal; N = Nocturnal; A = On awakening; OP = Occipital paroxysms; OS = Clusters or random occipital spikes; F = Frontal spikes; CTS = Centrotemporal spikes; GSS = Giant somatosensory spikes; IPSOS = Occipital spikes evoked by IPS.

[1] She later developed eight seizures of visual illusions (see text).

[2] Previously reported attacks at age 11 were vasovagal episodes.

[3] He is the only patient with infrequent, around 12, GTCS, without focal signs in adolescence and adulthood. Last one at age 25 when he was also taking Anafranil for obsessive neurosis. He remains on carbamazepine 800 mg daily. Despite occipital paroxysms in his EEG, this was not FOS.

[4] She had a prolonged nocturnal seizure with ictal vomiting, impairment of consciousness, deviation of the eyes and hemiconvulsions at age 7 years. One year later, she had a nocturnal Rolandic seizure. EEGs from age 7 years were dominated with occipital, centrotemporal, frontal spikes and giant somatosensory evoked spikes before normalization at age 13 years.

[5] He had two prolonged (more than 1–2 h) diurnal seizures at age 5 years, which started with feeling sick, vigorous vomiting, gradual impairment of consciousness, deviation of the eyes and hemiconvulsions. At age 7 years he had a typical nocturnal Rolandic seizure for 2–4 min. At age 12, when phenobarbitone was gradually withdrawn, had a prolonged 2–3 h seizure on awakening with orofacial movements, dysarthria, unilateral deviation of the eyes and impairment of consciousness which ended with diazepam intravenously.

Ictal vomiting and deviation of the eyes. Vomiting, mainly vigorous but sometimes mild, is often the first symptom attracting attention in nocturnal seizures but may also occur later before the convulsions. Unilateral deviation of the eyes may co-exist, precede or follow it. The deviation is usually slow, more of a shifting of the eyes to one side, which horizontally move often to their extreme and are barely seen in the corner through the open eyelids. This is not associated with any other convulsive features of the eyes or eyelids though the head may also turn axially towards the same side. These oculotonic symptoms may be brief for minutes or prolonged for hours, continuous or less often intermittent with eyes returning into midline and tonically deviated again towards the same side. The eyelids remain open, but may be semi- or widely open without any clonic movements or jerks. There are no hemifacial spasms or dystonic movements of any type at this stage.

Eyes widely open without deviation to one side are reported by three patients.

Other ictal symptoms. Retching (two patients), coughing (one) incontinence of urine (one) are extremely rare (Table 13.2) and oropharyngolaryngeal movements occurred in two patients (nos. 14 and 15) with occipital and centrotemporal spikes in their EEG. Patients may be very pale (six) during the ictus and some may show an agitated behaviour (two).

Level of consciousness. Consciousness may be impaired either from the onset or more commonly during the course of the seizure. This may be mild or moderate with the child retaining some ability to respond to verbal commands but often unable to speak. Severe disturbance of consciousness with complete unresponsiveness is uncommon at the beginning of the seizure. In three patients consciousness is preserved throughout the ictus.

Convulsions. The phase of vomiting, deviation of the eyes and other ictal symptoms, with or without impairment of consciousness, ends with convulsions in 15 patients. These are unilateral clonic seizures of the face and the extremities, alone in six patients and followed by GTCS in another four patients. GTCS without preceding hemiconvulsions occur in five patients. In all patients hemiconvulsions or GTCS are always preceded by the ictal symptoms described above and never occur independently with the exception of case 11 who later developed infrequent GTCS.

Visual hallucinations. None of the children, whether younger or older with nocturnal or diurnal seizures, have any visual hallucinations during the ictus. One patient (no. 1), with three nocturnal seizures typical of the EBOS at age 5, had 2 years later eight diurnal, less than a minute, episodes of 'dizziness' in which the environment seemed to move away from her and return to her with increasing speed.[600] Two of them progressed to automatisms and loss of consciousness without convulsions. Two patients (nos. 10 and 15) revealed on questioning that they saw a diffuse coloured light when concentrating with closed eyes.

Duration of seizures and partial status epilepticus. Twelve patients have partial status epilepticus as their seizures last for more than half an hour, usually 1–2 h. In the other 11 patients the duration is of more than 6–10 min. Shorter seizures are not reported.

Febrile convulsions and other seizures. Two patients had febrile convulsions prior to onset of other seizures. Patient no. 12 had two febrile convulsions at ages 2 and 3. A prolonged nocturnal seizure of vomiting, unresponsiveness and tonic deviation of the eyes for 3–4 h prior to hemiconvulsions occurred at age 7. One year later, she had another nocturnal seizure characterized by symptoms of Rolandic epilepsy with oropharyngolaryngeal movements and aphemia lasting for 10 min. Patient no. 21 had two prolonged, more than 1–2 h, diurnal seizures at age 5 years which started with feeling sick, vigorous vomiting, gradual impairment of consciousness, deviation of the eyes and hemiconvulsions. At age 7 years he had a typical nocturnal Rolandic seizure for 2–4 min. At age 12 when phenobarbitone was gradually withdrawn, he had a prolonged 2–3 h seizure on awakening with oropharyngolaryngeal movements, dysarthria, unilateral deviation of the eyes and impairment of consciousness which ended with diazepam intravenously. Patient no. 11 is the only one with infrequent, around 12, GTCS without focal signs in adolescence and adulthood. The last GTCS occurred at age 25 when he was also taking

Anafranil for obsessive neurosis. He is the only patient who continues on anti-epileptic medication, carbamazepine 800 mg daily.

Circadian distribution. Nocturnal seizures are by far the commonest (21 patients), alone (14 patients) or together with diurnal fits (seven). There are only two patients with diurnal seizures only. The clinical manifestations of the diurnal did not appear to be different from the nocturnal seizures either for the same patient or for the whole group of these 23 patients.

Precipitating factors. There are no obvious precipitating factors. Case 1 thought that daily seizures may be precipitated by darkness. Two patients (nos. 10 and 15) revealed on questioning that they saw a diffuse coloured light when concentrating with closed eyes.

post-ictal symptoms. Headache and other migraine-like features. post-ictal headache is not a prominent symptom for any of the patients who usually went to sleep after their convulsive seizures. Two patients (nos. 19 and 23) had minor headache after non-convulsive seizures.

Migraine symptoms. None of the patients has or developed migraine with aura, basilar or acephalgic migraine. Six patients have frequent but unspecified headaches that are not associated with neurological symptoms.

Electroencephalographic findings (Table 13.2)

All but one patient (no. 23) had in their interictal EEG occipital paroxysms (17 patients) or clusters of occipital spikes (five). Patient no. 23 had consistently normal awake and sleep EEG. When tested, fixation-off sensitivity was demonstrated in all but one (case 11) patients with occipital paroxysms. Five patients had additional centrotemporal spikes in the same or subsequent EEG. Three patients also had frontal spikes which sometimes appeared synchronously with the occipital spikes. Brief and infrequent, asymptomatic, generalized discharges of spike and wave sometimes appeared in EEG at an older age. The EEG normalized in all patients who had long follow-up. IPS, usually at high frequencies, had an inhibitory rather than excitatory effect on the occipital paroxysms. Two patients in their early teens, long after the active clinical stage, had occipital spikes that were time-locked to IPS flashes but these were not consistent or sustained and never spread anteriorly, also disappearing in follow-up EEG.

Family history of migraine and epilepsy

None of the patients have any family history of similar seizures occurring in other relatives. Six patients have a family history of migraine and four of epilepsy.

Diagnosis, treatment and outcome (Table 13.2)

All of the first 16 patients were treated, sometimes for years, with mainly cyclohexyl-2-methylamino-propranol-phenylethyl barbiturate and less frequently with phenobarbitone or carbamazepine. Four (cases 17–19 and 22) of the other seven patients were not treated. The other three received phenobarbitone or carbamazepine.

The prognosis is excellent for all but one (case 11) patient. The median number of seizures is two, seven had a singular seizure, nine 2–3, three had 4, and the other four patients from 5 to a maximum of 12 seizures. At a median age of 14 years at last follow-up only case 11 had infrequent GTCS. All others are free of seizures for a median follow-up of 4 years after their last seizure (range 1–20 years).

2. Idiopathic occipital epilepsy with visual seizures

There were 22 patients (34.9 per cent of the 63 patients with occipital epilepsy) with definite (normal high resolution MRI) or possible idiopathic occipital epilepsy with visual seizures. They all had normal neurological examination and intelligence. Those who also had normal high resolution MRI were considered definite cases of idiopathic occipital epilepsy with visual seizures while those who only had normal CT brain scan or did not have brain imaging were considered as possibily idiopathic.

Table 13.3. Chronological and treatment data of the LBOS

Case no.	Sex	Age (years)				Lifespan of seizures	Treatment				Seizure free (years)
		Last follow-up	First seen	Onset of seizures	Last seizure		Age at onset (years)	Drug	Seizures after treatment	Age at withdrawal	
24	M	30	11	11	23	12	12	Brb	5	24	7
25	F	22	13	9	15	6	14	Cbz	0	20	7
26	M	17	11	10	11	1	11	Cbz	0	14	6
27	M	16	14	8	16	8	11	Cbz	Few VS	Cnt	0
28	M	14	13	7	12	5	12	Cbz	Few VS	Cnt	2
29	F	24	18	12	20	8	14	SV-Cbz	0 after Cbz	Cnt	4
30	M	17	16	14	17	3	17	Cbz	0	Cnt	0
31	M	21	21	12	21	9	16	SV-Cbz	0 after Cbz	Cnt	0
32	F	25	25	11	25	14	13	Cbz	0	15*	0
33	M	55	54	13	54	41	14	Phen-Prim	VS	54**	1
34	F	9	9	9	9	0	None	None	–	None	0
35	F	15	7	5	15	9	7	SV	VS	Cnt	0
36	F	12	10	10	10	2	11	Cbz-SV	Ineffective	Cnt	0
37	F	17	16	12	17	5	12	SV-Ltg	Ineffective	Cnt	0
38	M	16	14	9	15	5	10	Phen, SV-Cbz	0 after Cbz	Cnt	1
39	M	21	13	11	14	0	12	Cbz	3	15	7
Mean		20.7	16.6	10.2	18.4	8.2	12.3			23.8	2.2
SD		10.5	11	2.3	10.5	9.6	2.4			15.7	2.9
Min.		9	7	5	9	0	7			14	0
Max.		55	54	14	54	41	17			55	7
Median		17	13.5	10.5	15.5	5.5	12			17.5	0.5

*Treatment stopped at 15 years, despite various seizures. No GTCS until age 25, when they relapsed. Treatment restarted.
** Treatment stopped at 54 years, despite persistent visual seizures. GTCS relapsed. Treatment restarted, Cnt = Treatment continues.
Cbz = Carbamazepine; SV = Sodium valproate; Phen = Phenytoin; Ltg = Lamotrigine; Prim = Primidone; Brb = Cyclohexyl-2-methylamino-propranol-phenylethyl-barbiturate; VS = Visual seizures.

Table 13.4. Clinical and laboratory data of LBOS

No.	EVH	CVH	Illus	DEH	EFlut	Blind	TLS	Hemic	GTCS	LOC	HMA	PIHead	Indep.S	CircD	FH	Imaging	EEG	Dur.	Freq.
24	Y	–	–	–	–	Y	–	1	1	–	–	S	Y	D/NGTCS	M	CT,MRI	OP	s<1–3 m-one 20 min	w
25	Y	–	–	Y	–	–	–	6	–	–	–	Mod	–	D/N	–	CT,MRI	OP	s<3m	d
26	Y	Y	Y	–	–	Y	–	–	–	Y	Y	–	Y	D	–	CT,MRI	OP	s<3m	w
27	Y	–	–	Y	–	–	–	4	–	–	Y	S	–	D	–	CT,MRI	N	s<3m	w
28	Y	–	–	–	–	Y	–	–	–	–	–	–	–	D	M-E	CT,MRI	N	s<2m	d
29	Y	–	–	–	–	–	–	–	12	–	–	S	–	N	M-E	CT,MRI	BOS,IPSOS	s<2m	m
30	Y	–	–	–	Y	–	–	–	7	–	–	S	–	D/A	M?E?	MRI	GP	s-1–10 min	d
31	Y	–	Y	–	Y	–	F	–	12	–	Y	S	–	D/NGTCS	–	MRI	N	1–5 min	dw
32	Y	Y	–	–	–	–	–	–	7	–	–	–	–	A	–	CT	GP,IPSOS	<1m	w3
33	Y	–	–	Y	–	–	–	–	4/yr	–	–	–	–	D	–	CT	N	<1–3m	wm
34	Y	–	–	Y	–	–	–	2	–	–	–	–	–	D	M-E	CT,MRI	N	s<10m	d-w
35	Y	Y	–	–	Y	Y	–	–	–	Y	Y	–	Y/Abs	A/D	F-M-E	MRI	BOS,SW,IPSOS	3–5 m, 20m	my
36	Y	–	–	–	Y	Y	–	Y	6/yr	–	Y	Mod	Rolandic	D/NGTCS	–	MRI	BSO,IPSOS,CTS	s-2mi	m
37	Y	–	–	–	Y	–	–	–	4/yr	–	?	–	MJ/GTCS	D	–	MRI	BOS,IPSOS,SW	s-4m	my
38	Y	–	–	–	–	–	–	–	3–4/yr	–	–	–	–	D/NGTCS	–	CT,MRI	PPR	s-1m	my
39	Y	–	–	–	–	–	–	–	1*	–	–	–	Rolandic	D	–	MRI	CTS	1m	one

EVH = Elementary visual hallucinations; CVH = Complex visual hallucinations; Illus = Illusions; DEH = Deviation of eyes and head; EFlut = Eyelid fluttering or eyelid closures; Blind = Blindness; TLS = Symptoms of temporal lobe seizures; Hemic = Hemiconvulsions; GTCS = Generalized tonic–clonic seizures; LOC = Sudden loss of consciousness without preceding visual hallucinations, and not associated with convulsions; HMA = Hemianopia; PIHead = post-ictal headache; S = Severe; Mod = Moderate; Indep.S. = Seizures independent of those with EVH; CircD = Circadian distribution; D = Diurnal; N = Nocturnal; A = Awakening; FH = Family history; M = Migraine; E = Epilepsy; F = Febrile convulsions; Y = Symptom present; – = Symptom is not present; yr = Year; NGTCS = GTCS occurred only during sleep; Abs = Absences; MJ = Myoclonic jerks; CT = normal brain computer tomography; MRI = normal brain magnetic resonance imaging; OP = Occipital paroxysms; BOS = Bilateral occipital spikes; IPSOS = Occipital spikes induced by IPS; ROS = Right occipital spikes; SW = Generalized discharges of spike and slow wave; GP = Non-specific paroxysmal activity; CTS = Centrotemporal spikes; PPR = Photoparoxysmal response; N = Normal; w = weekly; d = daily; m = monthly; y = yearly. Numbers denote total numbers of seizures.
* This patient also had 15 nocturnal Rolandic seizures.

Sixteen patients (25.4 per cent of the 63 patients) had spontaneous visual seizures and most of them are detailed in the illustrative cases of Chapter 9, while another six patients had idiopathic photosensitive seizures (9.5 per cent) and their history is detailed in the illustrative cases of Chapter 12B.

These are heterogeneous patients with spontaneous or photically induced visual seizures. Only three (0.48 per cent) of them (cases 24–26, Tables 13.3 and 13.4) would meet the diagnostic criteria of 'childhood epilepsy with occipital paroxysms' as defined by the Commission on Classification and Terminology of the International League Against Epilepsy.[177] Conversely, most of them would have been included in the relevant studies of Gastaut[308] and Gastaut and Zifkin[313] who applied wider criteria. Thus, those prospectively studied patients offer the opportunity to study late onset benign childhood occipital epilepsy as defined by Gastaut[308] and Gastaut and Zifkin[313] by applying similar criteria of selection to theirs.

Late onset benign childhood occipital seizures (including idiopathic photosensitive occipital seizures)

I have emphasized before that the definition of 'childhood epilepsy with occipital paroxysms'[177] or late onset benign childhood occipital seizures, is based entirely on a well performed retrospective study of Gastaut (1981,1982,1985,1987)[302–306,308,310] and an update by Gastaut and Zifkin (1987).[313] An accurate description of LBOS may not be possible at this stage of our knowledge. In order to get a better insight into this interesting condition I selected 16 of my 63 patients from my prospective study on the basis of similar criteria applied by Gastaut and Zifkin.[313] Their criteria were very broad (see details in Chapter 11) probably including any patient with visual seizures, occipital paroxysms or both, irrespective of whether idiopathic or symptomatic, generalized or partial, photosensitive or not photosensitive epilepsies. Age at onset ranged from 17 months to 17 years. Therefore, this was a heterogeneous group of patients including photosensitive, symptomatic and generalized epilepsies.

I have narrowed these criteria, by excluding patients with generalized epilepsies, so as to comply with the localization related epilepsies. From the 63 patients with occipital seizures/occipital epilepsy I have also excluded 17 patients with symptomatic epilepsies so as to comply with the idiopathic definition, and 24 patients with Panayiotopoulos syndrome as these cases are not illustrated in the reports of late onset benign childhood occipital seizures of Gastaut.

From the remaining 22 patients with definite or possible idiopathic occipital seizures/epilepsy I have also excluded three patients who did not undergo CT scan or brain MRI, and three patients with onset of seizures after the age of 16 years, so as to comply with the age limitations of benign childhood partial seizures. These were one patient with onset of spontaneous visual seizures at the age of 25 years, one woman with onset of photosensitive occipital seizures after the age of 16 years and a man with a single visual seizure progressing to GTCS at age 17 years (see page 261).

The remaining 16 (25.4 per cent) of the 63 patients with occipital epilepsy would comply with similar, though more restrictive criteria to those applied by Gastaut[308] and Gastaut and Zifkin[313] for LBOS.

Tables 13.3 and 13.4 show chronological, clinical and other data for these 16 patients who had definite or probable idiopathic occipital epilepsy with spontaneous or photically induced visual seizures that started before the age of 16 years. Occipital paroxysms, occipital spikes and photosensitivity were optional.

Physical, mental state and brain imaging

By selection criteria all patients have normal neurological and mental state and brain MRI, CT or both (Tables 13.3 and 13.4). None has visual deficits. Four have mild or moderate myopia. Case 35 has mild comitant strabismus. Case 28 has borderline normal learning disability with visual less well developed than verbal memory skills (low average normal). Case 35, despite normal intelligence, has a specific difficulty with coding tasks often related to hand writing skills.

Sex, age at onset and last follow-up (Table 13.3)

These are nine men and seven women. Age at onset of first seizure is 5–14 years (mean = 10.2 ± 2.3, median = 10.5) and age at last follow-up is 9–55 (mean = 20.7 ± 10.5, median = 17).

Clinical manifestations (Tables 13.3 and 13.4)

Elementary visual hallucinations alone, without other ictal symptoms or impairment of consciousness, are by far the commonest and most frequent type of seizure. They infrequently progress to other non-visual symptoms, impairment of consciousness and convulsions.

Elementary visual hallucinations

In all but one patient (no. 32) elementary visual hallucinations were the first and often the only ictal symptom for most of the seizures. These were stereotyped for each patient over the years except for patient no. 32 who initially had a complex visual hallucination 'like a head of a person in the left eye' but 13 years later this was 'like fuzzy vision in the bottom of my right eye with black dots travelling along my right eye'.

Shapes, colours, numbers, size and movement (Fig. 9.2): All but two patients described multi-coloured visual hallucinations that were rarely monochromatic or dichromatic. Bright red, yellow, blue and green appear to predominate. Case 32 described 'black dots' and case 38 had a light 'like a flash of a camera switching on and off in my left eye'. Shapes were circular, spots, circles, balls or concentric rings in all but three patients who described 'bright multicoloured small squares' in the temporal hemifield, (case 35) 'multicoloured triangles and squares inside a football' (case 36), and 'blobs of fireworks'(case 37). In three other patients additional coloured square, triangular and rectangular shapes in each were experienced together with the circular patterns that predominated. Individual elements of the visual hallucinations were usually multiple (tens or hundreds), rarely single or two to four. Their size varied from 'spots' to rarely the size of a coin or slightly bigger. Their location at onset was usually unilateral appearing in the periphery of a temporal hemifield and less frequently centrally. Horizontal movements towards the other side occurred in one third of the patients, mainly those with unilateral visual hallucinations. In other patients these were flashing, spinning or rotating.

Duration. The majority of elementary visual hallucinations lasted for 5 to 30 s, rarely 1 min in all patients. They could last longer, up to 3 min, mainly prior to secondary generalization in five patients. The longest reported duration was 20 min in a patient (no. 24) who usually had brief hallucinations. Later, the experience of case 27 was similar, as detailed in his presentation (Chapter 9) with visual seizures lasting for half an hour.

The components of visual hallucinations increased in numbers, size or both for most of the patients, with progress of seizure particularly prior to other, non-visual ictal epileptic symptoms.

Frequency. Frequency varied from many per day to weekly or more rarely monthly.

Other occipital seizure symptoms with ictal elementary visual hallucinations

The elementary visual hallucinations usually started and persisted during the visual seizures, mostly without other symptoms. However, other ictal symptoms of occipital lobe origin could also occur.

Illusions of eye movement. Two patients had eye movement illusions. Patient no. 26 felt that his right sided hallucination 'draws my right eye and my head to the right' without apparent movement and case no. 31 had 'tension in the eyes. Feels similar to when you look up into your eyebrows as hard as you can. This involuntary movement of the eyes causes the pain described above. The motion to the left seems out of your control. It can be resisted but adds to nausea and general pain'.

Eyelid fluttering or repetitive eyelid-closure. Eyelid fluttering or repetitive eyelid-closure was a consistent symptom following visual hallucinations prior to GTCS in two patients (30 and 31). Additionally, eyelid fluttering, which on video-EEG looked like an exaggerated normal eyelid tremor, consistently occurred during clusters of occipital spikes in patient 35. It was not associated with impairment of consciousness or any other seizure symptoms. It would have been entirely dismissed as a normal variant without video-EEG confirmation. A similar situation was apparent on video-EEG recordings of another two patients (nos. 36 and 37) during IPS elicited occipital discharges.

Tonic deviation of the eyes. In four patients (nos. 25, 27, 33 and 34) tonic deviation of the eyes and often the head could follow elementary visual hallucinations often prior to hemiconvulsions or secondary GTCS.

Blindness and hemianopia. Five patients (nos. 24, 26, 28, 35 and 36) had rare episodic blindness lasting 1–3 min. Blindness was mainly independent of visual hallucinations. Patient no. 24 had three episodes of complete blindness immediately after diving into the sea: 'Everything went suddenly black, I could not see and I had to ask other swimmers to show me the direction to the beach'. The blindness cleared in 1 or 2 min and was followed by right-sided headache and vomiting. Only once he had had an episode of blindness preceded by visual hallucinations. Patient no. 26 had infrequent episodes of sudden blindness for 1–2 min without warning or impairment of consciousness. For patient no. 28, on 2–3 occasions, his vision went black, he felt himself spinning around and 'coloured big balls' appeared to cover his body. More interesting is patient 36 who is awakened from sleep either with her habitual elementary visual hallucinations progressing to GTCS or less often by 'white' blindness, 'all is white, I can see nothing', also progressing within seconds to GTCS. Patient no. 35 at age 7 years became blind for 15 min after an unusual sudden and brief episode of loss of consciousness, 'slumped down, was floppy, lips blue'.

Hemianopia, ictal or post-ictal, is difficult to assess, but was experienced by four patients. Patient no. 27 occasionally had his habitual visual hallucinations lasting longer, becoming bigger and probably associated with left hemianopia. Patient no. 31 consistently experienced post-ictal hemianopia, 'after this (elementary visual hallucinations) the area in which they have been is blind. You can hardly see. This lasts for between 1 and 5 min'. Similar is the situation with patient no. 36, immediately after her habitual visual seizures she 'could see only from one eye for 5–10 s'.

Complex visual hallucinations. Three patients (nos. 26, 32 and 35) experienced complex visual hallucinations. Cases 26 and 35 in the progress of their elementary visual hallucinations saw 'large objects, probably people, which I cannot identify' (case 26) or 'small faces of people' superimposed on the colours (case 35). Visual seizures of case 32 started at age 12 years with 'a fuzzy vision in the left eye that looked like the head of a person' but after 13 years she developed elementary visual hallucinations first appearing in the right side.

Level of consciousness. Consciousness was well preserved in all patients during the period of elementary visual hallucinations even if long (cases 24, 33 and 35). Some patients were well aware of symptoms that would progress to GTCS, taking precautions and informing relatives (cases 30, 32 and 38) of the impending GTCS. Consciousness is impaired in the state between visual hallucinations and hemiconvulsions or GTCS.

Temporal lobe symptoms. Complex partial seizures of temporal lobe semeiology were conspicuously absent. None of the patients had at seizure progress or any other stage, temporal lobe symptoms such as automatisms, epigastric aura or experiential phenomena. One patients (case 32) experienced 'fear' prior to nocturnal GTCS.

Hemiconvulsions and generalized tonic–clonic seizures. Hemiconvulsions (five patients) and GTCS (10 patients) were extremely rare in comparison with the eminently high frequency of visual seizures (Table 13.4). Three patients (cases 26, 28 and 35) despite numerous visual seizures never had hemiconvulsions or GTCS. Nine patients had one to a maximum of 12 hemiconvulsions or GTCS in the course of their disease. However, four patients had relatively frequent convulsions of more than 1–2 per year.

Progress of visual seizures to other non-visual manifestations. Visual seizures rarely progressed to other ictal non-visual manifestations. The pattern of progression was usually stereotypical for each patient but varied amongst patients. Progression to other ictal symptoms was usually heralded by a prolongation of the duration of the elementary visual hallucinations with their components increasing in numbers, size or both. The commonest pattern of progression is to ipsilateral eyes – head deviation and hemiconvulsions usually followed by GTCS or directly to GTCS (Table 13.4). The pattern of visual hallucinations progressing to unresponsiveness with eyelid fluttering and GTCS occurred in two patients.

Seizures without visual hallucinations. Visual seizures were by far the commonest and most frequent type of seizures in all patients except for case 39 who had a singular visual fit with secondary GTCS provoked by video-games. In 10 patients (Table 13.4) all seizures were visual alone or followed by other epileptic manifestations. In addition to visual seizures, six other patients also had other type of seizures.

Patient no. 24 had seizures of blindness and probably two motor partial seizures. Case 26 had seizures of blindness or loss of consciousness without convulsions. Case 35 had febrile convulsions and seizures of inconspicuous eyelid flutter, mild absences and a prolonged episode of blindness preceded by loss of consciousness and atonia. Cases 36 and 39 had Rolandic seizures with centrotemporal spikes. Finally, case 37 had generalized as well as occipital seizures of photosensitive epilepsy.

Precipitating factors

There were no obvious precipitating factors in 13 patients (24–34). One patient said that they were precipitated by exercise and heat, one by stress, one by hunger, one by darkness, and one by looking at bright non-flickering lights. The majority of visual seizures in these patients appeared to be spontaneous. However, in the other five patients (35–39) seizures were mainly and consistently photically induced by television, flickering lights, video-games and discotheques, alone or in combination. Only one patient (no. 39) who suffered from Rolandic seizures had a single photically-induced visual seizure with elementary visual hallucinations of a concentric multi-coloured ring followed by a GTCS.

Circadian distribution

Visual seizures were diurnal only (seven patients), diurnal mainly on awakening (three patients), diurnal and nocturnal (five patients) and nocturnal only (one patient). Three patients, despite mainly diurnal visual seizures, had only nocturnal secondary GTCS. These patients would awake with visual hallucinations or blindness before GTCS.

post-ictal symptoms of visual seizures

Headache and other migraine-like features. This refers to post-ictal symptoms after visual seizures alone and not to post-convulsions headache and vomiting. Nine patients had no post-ictal headache. Seven patients had moderate (two patients) to severe headache (five patients) which was mainly bilateral, rarely unilateral, pounding or throbbing and often associated with nausea and vomiting (four patients), photophobia and phonophobia (no. 30).

The headache would start immediately after the end of visual hallucinations or usually within 3–15 min after and would last for half an hour to 3 h, and exceptionally to half a day (no. 31). The longer the duration of visual seizures, the longer and more severe the headache was. However, even simple, elementary visual hallucinations of less than 1 min duration could be followed by severe headache in most of these patients.

Migraine symptoms

None of the patients had any other type of visual hallucinations other than their habitual visual seizures. None had the typical migraine visual aura described by Russell and Olesen[693] which 'starts with a flickering, uncoloured, unilateral zigzag line in the centre of the visual field and affects the central vision. It gradually progresses, over minutes, towards the periphery of one hemifield and often leaves

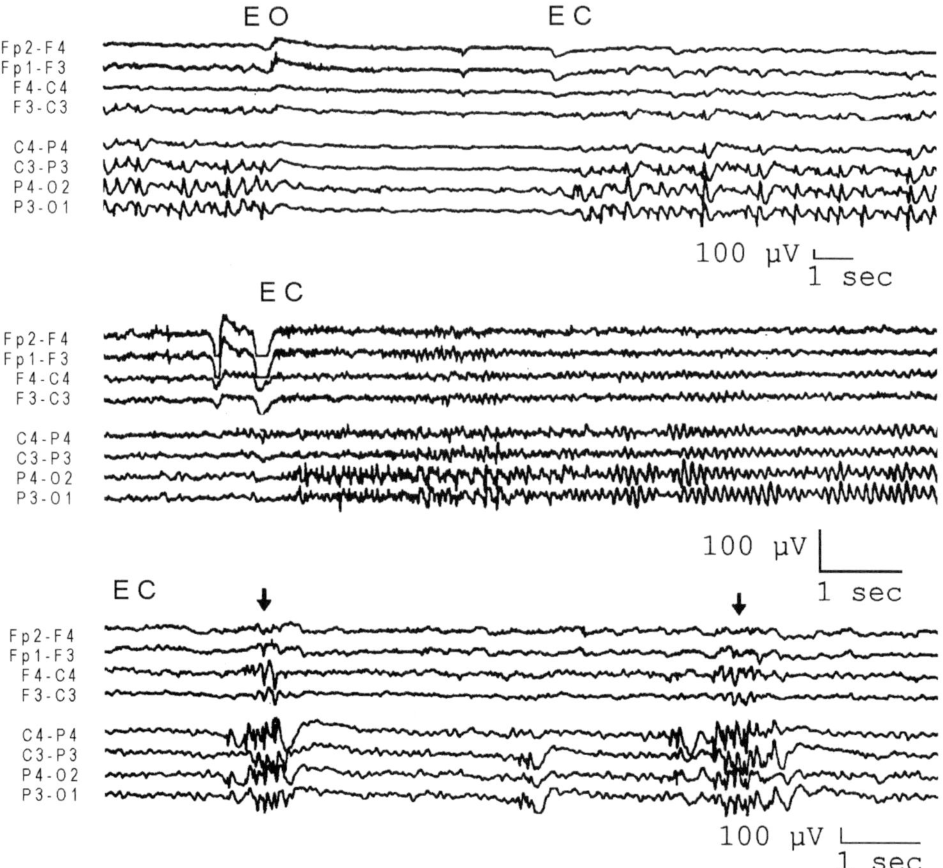

Fig. 13.1. This is from a video-EEG recording of three patients with definite idiopathic visual seizures, demonstrating the marked differences of the occipital spikes between them.
Upper: This is from case 26 which is also illustrated in more detail in Figs. 9.3 and 10.2. Occipital spikes (more accurately sharp and slow waves) occur as soon and as long as the eyes are closed because of their activation by the elimination of fixation and central vision.
Middle: This is from case 29, also illustrated in detail in Fig. 9.4.
Fast occipital spikes (ictal-like activity) appear immediately after eye-closure. This does not continue for the rest of the period when eyes are closed and disappears when eye-closure is performed in darkness. Though the patient was not clinically photosensitive, IPS also evoked occipital spikes irrespective of whether the eyes were opened or closed.
Bottom: This is from case 35 with mainly photically induced visual seizures, also illustrated in Fig. 12.3. Spontaneous clusters of occipital spikes occur when the eyes are closed, often associated with eyelid fluttering (arrows). These clusters of occipital spikes are not influenced by fixation-off. On the contrary, IPS elicits occipital spikes.

a scotoma'.[693] Four patients had frequent headaches which were never associated with visual hallucinations.

Electroencephalographic findings (Table 13.4, Figs. 13.1 and 13.2)

Non-clinically photosensitive patients. Six of 11 patients (nos. 24–34) with spontaneous seizures only,

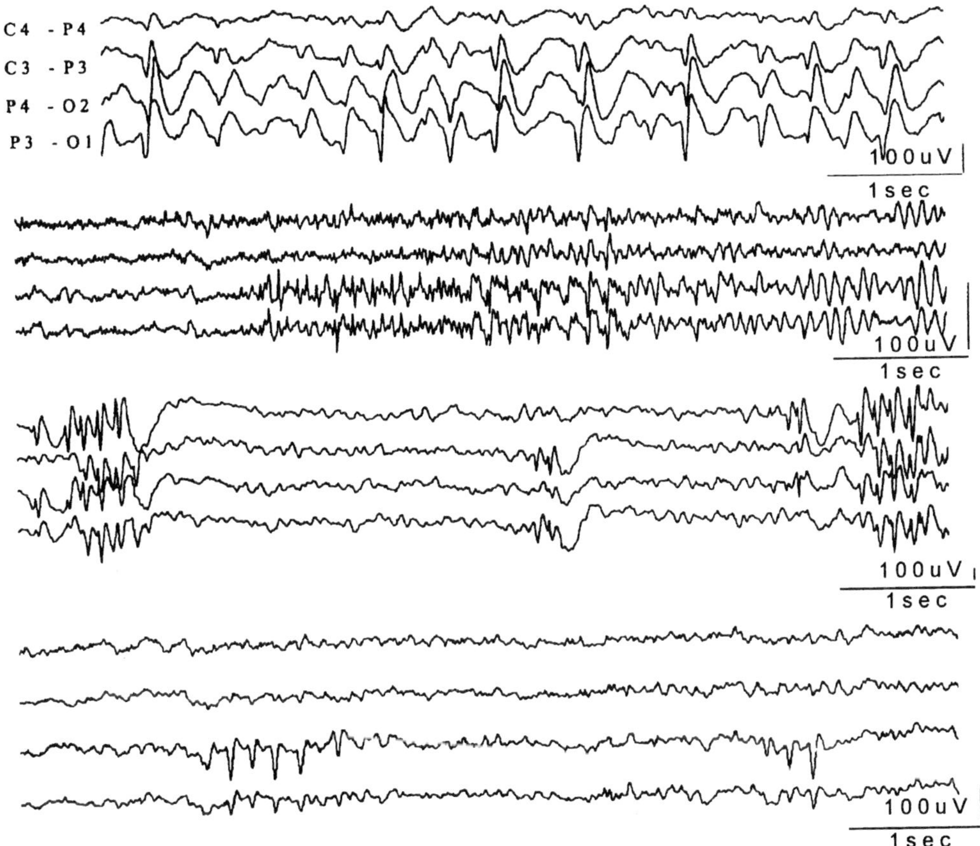

Fig. 13.2. Magnification of the occipital derivations of spontaneous EEG of four patients with visual seizures. From top to bottom are cases 26, 29, 35 and 36 consecutively. Note their marked differences.
Upper: Case 26. Occipital paroxysms occur as long as the eyes are closed, also demonstrating FOS.
Upper Middle: Case 29. Fast occipital spiking after eye-closure. Contrary to the reactivity in case 26, this type of EEG was related to occipital photosensitivity and occipital spikes were inhibited in darkness.
Lower Middle: Case 35. Spontaneous occipital spikes of case 35 who was clinically photosensitive.
Bottom: Case 36 with spontaneous and photocally induced seizures.

had abnormal EEG (Table 13.4). Three had occipital paroxysms with eyes-closed, also demonstrating fixation-off sensitivity (Figs. 13.1 and 13.2). One had brief runs of fast occipital spikes immediately after closing her eyes and photically induced occipital spikes time-locked to the flash stimulus (Figs. 13.1 and 13.2). Two had brief bursts of abortive generalized discharges of small spikes and slow waves of higher amplitude in the anterior regions and one of them additionally had occipital spikes induced by IPS. In the other five patients EEG, including sleep EEG, were consistently normal (Table 13.4).

Photosensitive patients. EEG findings were heterogeneous in five patients who had photically induced, with or without spontaneous, occipital seizures (nos. 35–39, Table 13.4). Case 35 had spontaneous clusters of occipital spikes often associated with eyelid tremor and fluttering, occasional generalized discharges of 3–4 Hz spike and slow wave and IPS evoked occipital spikes. Case 36 had centrotemporal and spontaneous occipital spikes as well as photoparoxysmal responses with posterior small spikes associated with eyelid fluttering. Case 37 had occasional spontaneous occipital spikes and IPS elicited generalized discharges or posterior spikes. Case 38 had consistently normal EEG except once on a sleep deprived EEG where IPS performed on awakening provoked brief generalized discharges of spike and slow waves after eye closure. Case 39 had centrotemporal spikes only.

Family history of migraine and epilepsy

Ten patients had no family history of migraine or epilepsy (Table 13.4) and there was no other family member of any patient having the same type of seizures. Six patients had a family history of migraine alone (one) and of epilepsy (five). The mother of patient no. 24 had two episodes of migraine with visual aura in her late 30s. A paternal sister of patient 28 has 'epilepsy' from the age of 16 years and his mother has migraine with visual aura of the zigzag lines and shimmering lights lasting for approximately 20 min before the headache. Patient 29 has a maternal half-brother with GTCS on awakening and his father also has idiopathic generalized epilepsy. Another brother suffers from common migraine, her mother had 'migraine' as a teenager and there is no relevant medical history for her remaining two brothers and four maternal half-brothers. Patient 30 has two older paternal and two maternal half-brothers. One of the paternal half-brothers has a history of 'flashing lights' in his late teens and the other had severe headaches and he passed out on a few occasions in his late teens. The father of patient 34 has severe migraine and there is a paternal grandfather with idiopathic generalized epilepsy. Patient no. 35 has a strong family history of febrile convulsions. Her maternal grandmother had migraine. Her mother had two episodes of migraine with aura in her late thirties.

Thus, from six patients having a family history of migraine, post-ictal headache occurred in three (cases 24, 29 and 30). There was no evidence of post-ictal headache in the other three despite the family history of migraine. Furthermore, four other patients had post-ictal headache with no evidence of a family history of migraine.

Diagnosis, treatment and outcome

More than half of the patients were initially misdiagnosed, sometimes for years (cases 27–30) as cases of migraine with aura, acephalgic migraine and basilar migraine, and some were unsuccessfully treated with anti-migraine medication. This diagnosis prevailed even after onset of convulsive seizures which were considered a consequence of the migraine attack or a coincidence of migraine and epilepsy (case 30). Treatment with anti-epileptic medication was delayed for years (Table 13.1) and never started before the onset of more traditionally accepted seizure symptoms such as convulsions. Even then, treatment was postponed after the first convulsive episode despite numerous and often daily visual seizures.

Details of response to treatment and prognosis are shown in Table 13.3.

Non-photosensitive patients. Six of these 11 patients were treated with carbamazepine alone and seizures stopped entirely (four patients) with occasional breakthrough of mild, brief visual seizures that were also stopped with dose adjustment (two patients). Sodium valproate, as the initial treatment for two (cases 29 and 31) was not effective and seizures stopped only when carbamazepine was added. In particular, case 29 started treatment with sodium valproate at age 14 but continued having 1–2 visual and secondary GTCS yearly. All seizures stopped at age 18 with carbamazepine add-on. She had only two secondary GTCS at age 20 years, 3 months after voluntarily stopping medication. Sodium valproate was discontinued at age 22 and she remains free of any seizures with carbamazepine alone. Case 31 despite treatment with sodium valproate from age 16 continued having visual seizures and one nocturnal secondary GTCS every year. Carbamazepine was added only 4 months ago with no further seizures. Case 32 had no minor or major seizures on treatment with carbamazepine from age 13 years. After withdrawal of medication at age 15, she started having infrequent and brief visual seizures without secondary GTCS until aged 25 when she had three visual seizures with secondary GTCS. Treatment with carbamazepine restarted 2 months ago.

Case 24 started treatment at age 11 years with phenobarbitone 90 mg daily. Seizures continued until this was changed 6 months later to cyclohexyl-2-methylamino-propranol-phenylethyl-barbiturate 150 mg daily. Since then he had only three brief visual seizures, a secondary GTCS at age 16 and a single prolonged visual seizure at age 23 years. He remained free of any seizures for 7 years after drug withdrawal. Case 33 used to have approximately four secondary GTCS every year until the age of 31 years when these stopped with a combination of phenytoin and primidone. It is not known what therapeutic attempts were made prior to this age. However, he continued having 4–5 visual seizures per year until aged 54 when he had another secondary GTCS 10 months after medication was withdrawn.

Photosensitive patients. The five photosensitive patients are difficult to assess for results of treatment as seizures also depend on exposure to photic stimuli. In case 35 sodium valproate may have had some beneficial effect as visual seizures provoked by television were reduced to one per year. Case 36 initially had, at age 10 years, six nocturnal Rolandic seizures with secondary GTCS and visual seizures provoked by television. Carbamazepine was not effective as she also developed spontaneous nocturnal GTCS preceded by elementary visual hallucinations or white blindness. Sodium valproate has been added lately. Case 37 with photically induced visual seizures, GTCS, myoclonic jerks and eyelid fluttering had only partial improvement with sodium valproate. She continues having seizures despite the addition of lamotrigine. Case 38 continued having television induced visual seizures and 3–4 nocturnal visual seizures with secondary GTCS every year despite treatment with phenytoin and later sodium valproate for 4 years. All seizures stopped when carbamazepine was added to sodium valproate at age 15 years and he remained free of seizures in the next 15 months of follow-up. Case 39 had 15 nocturnal Rolandic seizures from age 9 to 14 years when he also had a single video-game induced visual seizure with secondary GTCS. Treatment of carbamazepine was withdrawn at age 15 years. He remains well with no seizures in the next 5 years of follow-up.

In conclusion this study illustrates the following:

(a) LBOS with occipital paroxysms is a rare occurrence. Three patients in 25 years.
(b) LBOS contain rather a heterogeneous group of patients with uncertain prognosis. Some of them may suffer from symptomatic occipital epilepsy.
(c) Treatment with carbamazepine may be needed by all patients.

A comparison between Panayiotopoulos syndrome (early onset benign childhood occipital seizures) and childhood epilepsy with occipital paroxysms of Gastaut (late onset benign childhood occipital seizures)

It should be obvious from the extensive presentations in this book that the clinical manifestations of the syndrome I described (EBOS) are entirely different from those of Gastaut (LBOS). Age at onset, seizure frequency, seizure symptoms and duration, circadian distribution and prognosis are all entirely different. As a further step in the differentiation of Panayiotopoulos from Gastaut type childhood occipital seizures, I asked for statistical advice. In order to avoid any bias of selection, the 39 patients of Tables 13.1 and 13.3 were grouped according to whether their first ever reported afebrile seizure was longer or shorter than 6 min. All children with prolonged first seizure had EBOS and all children with short first seizures had LBOS. The cumulative results of comparing the characteristics of the first seizure between the two groups and their statistical values are provided in Table 13.5, and these are self-evident. All except sex are significantly different between EBOS and LBOS.

Table 13.5. Comparison between EBOS and LBOS on the basis of the first afebrile seizure

	EBOS (no. 23)	LBOS (no. 16)		
First seizure			Statistical evaluation	
	Number of patients	Number of patients	Chi^2 statistic	*P*-value
Ictal symptoms				
Visual hallucinations	0	13	28.03	< 0.001
Deviation of the eyes	19	1	22.02	< 0.001
Vomiting	18	0	23.25	< 0.001
Other non-occipital symptoms	12	2	7.73	0.005
Convulsions	13	3	5.56	0.018
Post-ictal headache	1	4	*	0.014*
Duration of seizure				
More than 6 min	23	0		
Circadian distribution				
Nocturnal only	20	3	18.14	< 0.001
Age at onset	Years	Years		
Mean ± SD	5 ± 2.1	10.2 ± 2.3	7.30**	< 0.001**
Median	5	10.5		
Range	2–12	5–14		
	No. of patients	No. of patients		
Sex-ratio M/F	11/12	9/7	0.27	0.61
Interictal EEG	22	7	13.32	< 0.001
Occipital paroxysms/spikes	2	7	4.80	0.028
Abnormal photic response	1	5	5.25	0.022
Normal				
Total seizures per life				
Mean ± SD	4 ± 4	79	z = 5.33***	< 0.001***
Median	2	29		
Range	1–15	17–100		
Age at last seizure	Years	Years		
Mean ± SD	7.0 ± 4.5	18.4 ± 10.5		
Median	6	15.5		
Range	2–25	9–54		
Age at last follow-up				
Mean ± SD	13.3 ± 6.7	20.7 ± 10.5		
Median	14	17		
Range	6–29	9–55		

*Fisher's exact test; **Unpaired t-test; ***Mann-Whitney test.

Appendix 1: Questionnaire

Visual Symptoms

Please describe your visual symptoms in detail. This is sometimes difficult. It may help if you could give examples of how they may look (like a balloon, the sun, lines, square patterns) and draw them. Children are good at drawing their symptoms.
How do they start, where in your vision and for how long ?
Please also give colour if any, shape, movement, background, number and time
How do they progress?
Do they become more intense, bigger, changing shape and position? How long do they last?
At what age did they start?
How frequent are they?
Do they occur at any particular time of the day?
Is there anything that precipitates/causes them (lights, disco, lack of food or of sleep, stress, others)?
How did they progress over the years? Do you still have them? When was the last time?

Other symptoms preceding or following the visual symptoms

Do you ever become confused, slow, lose consciousness? If yes, at what stage and for how long? Are these preceding or following the visual symptoms or are they independent?
Did you ever have any convulsions? If yes, at what stage and for how long? Are these preceding or following the visual symptoms or are they independent?
How frequently do you lose consciousness or have convulsions?
When was the last time?

Your vision, headache, vomiting, other complaints during or after the visual symptoms

How is your vision during or after the visual symptoms?
Did you ever become blind? If yes, please describe in detail.
Headache: Do you get headaches during or after the visual symptoms?
If yes, please describe when the headache starts, where it is, how strong, of what quality and for how long.
Do you ever have nausea, vomiting or other symptoms during or after the visual symptoms?
Please give details as above.

Personal history

Do you have any other diseases?
Any previous serious or related illnesses?

Family history

Are there any other members of your family having migraine and what type, epilepsy and what type, visual symptoms?
Please give details.

Treatment

Did you ever receive any treatment for your visual symptoms?
What?
When was this started and finished?
What was the effect of the treatment on your symptoms?
Are you still on treatment and what?

Tests and diagnosis

Did you visit any doctor/hospital for your visual symptoms? When? Please give names and addresses.
Did you have an EEG, Brain scan, Others? Results?

What do you know about your visual symptoms?

Anything relevant that you may wish to add?

Please draw your visual symptoms (using colours if needed)

You may need to use more sheets, please do so where necessary.

Part IV
Occipital epilepsies versus migraine with aura, acephalgic and basilar migraine

Benign Childhood Partial Seizures and Related Epileptic Syndromes. C P Panayiotopoulos
©1999 John Libbey & Company Ltd., pp. 281–302.

Chapter 14

Differentiating occipital epilepsies from migraine with aura, acephalgic migraine and basilar migraine

Some surprise may be felt that migraine is given a place in the borderland of epilepsy, but the position is justified by many relations and among them by the fact that the two maladies are sometimes mistaken and more often their distinction is difficult. *Gowers (1907)*[354]

Introduction and clarifications

In this chapter I will attempt to differentiate occipital epilepsies from migraine with aura, basilar and acephalgic migraine *with which they are often mistaken though their distinction should not be difficult today* (to paraphrase the above extract from Gowers).

My thesis and conclusions based on a 25 years, study can be summarized as follows:

The quality and the chronological sequence of ictal and post-ictal events of occipital seizures are markedly different from migraine. Visual seizures and migraine aura may imitate each other but their true identity cannot easily escape clinical scrutiny.

The concept of migralepsy and its synonymous intercalated seizures or of a migraine–epilepsy sequence needs revaluation based on accurate diagnosis. In most instances it is seizures imitating migraine. Benign visual childhood occipital seizures but also other forms of epilepsies are often misdiagnosed for basilar migraine. The erroneous concept of basilar migraine with EEG occipital paroxysms is an example of this.

Seizures may be triggered from a migrainous event or caused by a migraine stroke but this is rare. There should be no doubt that cerebral infarcts due to severe migraine can be responsible for symptomatic seizures. Also, there should be no reason why epileptic seizures, so vulnerable to extrinsic and intrinsic precipitating factors, could not also be susceptible to cortical changes introduced by migraine. Thus a migrainous attack may also be able to trigger epileptic seizures in susceptible individuals. However, both these cases are rare. In my opinion, the commonest reason for their association is coincidence of two of the commoner neurological disorders and an erroneous interpretation of epileptic seizures as migraine and less often vice versa.

The emerging and more realistic concept is of occipital seizures triggering migrainous headache which needs consideration and exploration.

More importantly, patients with daily visual seizures that may progress to convulsions merit a precise diagnosis and appropriate treatment probably with carbamazepine. Most of these patients with visual seizures are misdiagnosed as migraine with aura, basilar migraine, acephalgic migraine or migralepsy simply because physicians are not properly informed of differential diagnostic criteria. As a result, diagnosis, appropriate investigations and treatment may be delayed for years. There are numerous published reports of such a misdiagnosis.

Migraine and epilepsy are the commonest neurological disorders. Prevalence of migraine is probably around 6 per cent for men and three times more than this for women. Epilepsy is around 0.5 per cent equally affecting men and women. If there was a relation between them, this would be obvious in our everyday neurological practice. It would not be revealed only through obscure and complicated cases with bizarre symptomatology. It would be simple and common. It is not. The problem is that occipital seizures are not appropriately differentiated from migraine and therefore, they are often erroneously diagnosed as migraine.

A typical case of late onset idiopathic occipital seizures misdiagnosed as migraine with aura, acephalgic migraine, basilar migraine and migralepsy

A 10-year-old boy started having frequent attacks of visual hallucinations at age 7 years. These brief visual hallucinations could come at any time of the day and consisted of many small balls of various brilliant colours, mainly blue, yellow and red appearing in the right temporal hemifield. Within seconds they would multiply, obscuring the vision in the place of their appearance. The whole episode would last seconds to no more than half a minute. There was no impairment of consciousness. The mother, who has migraine without aura, consulted her neurologist who diagnosed that her child had acephalgic migraine and reassured the parents. These attacks continued on a daily basis. Treatment with pizotifen was ineffective. Attacks of the same quality would last longer, for 1 min, often followed by diffuse headache of moderate intensity. A routine alert EEG showed some posterior 'sharpish' components and an MRI was normal. The diagnosis was modified to migraine with aura. Treatment with propranolol was again ineffective. The boy at age 9 years also had occasional episodes of complete blindness which started and ended suddenly or were preceded by his habitual visual hallucinations and lasted for 3–5 min. There was no impairment of consciousness but strong headache could follow for 1–2 h. A new EEG during sleep showed frequent occipital spikes. The diagnosis was modified to basilar migraine, also confirmed by another paediatric neurologist. The view of a third neurologist that these were occipital seizures was denied by an authority on the basis that '*there was no ictal EEG data to prove that he had accelerated epileptic discharges during the visual hallucinations and interictal EEG does not prove that the visual symptoms are associated with a true ictal transformation (which is the only way to convincingly differentiate migraine aura from epilepsy).' (see page 295, expert assessor's view).* Treatment remained the same. Two months later the boy, after awakening, had his habitual visual hallucinations with the small balls lasting longer, becoming bigger and starting to move horizontally to the left side. He called his mother who witnessed him becoming unresponsive, eyes moving slowly to one side, eyelids opening and closing and followed within 4 min by generalized convulsions with tongue biting and incontinence of urine. He was admitted to a paediatric neurology clinic. New MRI was normal. EEG showed post-ictal slow waves, more on the left. The diagnosis was now modified to migralepsy, i.e. seizures occurring in the course of a migraine attack. Treatment with carbamazepine prescribed to avoid recurrence of seizures dramatically stopped all types of episodic events that this boy had. Attempts to reduce carbamazepine resulted in break-through of attacks of visual hallucinations. The correct diagnosis was late onset idiopathic occipital epilepsy.

Why these are occipital seizures? There was not one single symptom shown in this boy that could possibly justify migraine with aura, acephalgic or basilar migraine. Migralepsy was the result of this misdiagnosis made on the assumption that visual hallucinations, blindness and headache cannot be anything else but migraine. The daily seizures, their brief duration for seconds to a minute, their multi-coloured and spherical patterns in the lateral side of a hemifield, have no similarities with any type of migraine. The secondary generalized convulsion was an unavoidable event that was also preceded by chronological and topographic augmentation of the visual hallucinations, progressing to other seizure occipital symptoms such as deviation of the eyes and eyelid closure.

Is there any relation between migraine and epilepsy?

Migraine and epilepsy are two different groups of disorders with recurrent and paroxysmal, usually brief and abrupt, manifestations of disturbed brain function. They have different pathophysiology and different clinical presentation.

Pathophysiology: Migraine aura symptoms are due to vasomotor disturbances or the spreading depression of Leao[124,800] whereas epileptic seizures result from abnormal hypersynchronous electrical discharges in the brain. Welch, 1997[800] reviewed the prevailing hypotheses regarding the pathogenesis of migraine and concluded: 'Models of aura mechanisms include transient cerebral ischaemia and spreading depression. Models of headache involve trigeminovascular and brainstem mechanisms. The ability to trigger an attack may depend on a threshold of brain excitability. Mitochondrial disorder, magnesium deficiency, and abnormality of presynaptic calcium channels may be responsible for neuronal hyperexcitability between attacks. It remains to be determined whether cortical or brainstem centres generate the attack'.

The clinical symptomatology of migraine, with the cardinal feature of headache, is also quite different from that of epilepsy, in which convulsions and impairment of consciousness are the main manifestations. The differences between visual migraine aura and visual occipital seizures are detailed on many occasions in this book.

Relationships between migraine and epilepsy: The question of a possible relationship between migraine and epilepsy[31,33,34,39,44,66,68,73,108,263,394,419,490,509,519,529,569,590,591,663,712,718] has arisen mainly from rare cases of migraine associated with, followed by, or interposed with epileptic attacks, or by the more frequent situation of concurrent and independent migraine attacks and epileptic seizures occurring in the same subject. A possible link between the two diseases has been the subject of numerous studies on genetic, EEG, epidemiological and statistical correlations; but most of these results and views are still in conflict.[31,33,34,39,44,66,68,73,108,263,394,419,490,509,519,529,569,590,591,663,712,718] At present, it does not seem possible to formulate definite conclusions regarding a relationship between these two groups of disorders that would be generally accepted, though comorbidity has recently been postulated.[590,591,727]

The debate, as detailed by Sacks,[697] goes back to the times of Pelops, who described the sensory symptoms preceding epileptic convulsions (the aura = pnevmatiki avra = spiritual vapour), and Aretaeus, who described similar symptoms inaugurating certain migraine attacks. According to Lennox and Lennox:[478] 'Aretaeus was the first to describe the hybrid seizure, first a hallucination of colours': 'If it be near the accession of the paroxysm, there are before the sight circular flashes of purple or black colours, or all mixed together, so as to exhibit the appearance of the rainbow expanded in the heavens.'[47]

This debate on the relations of migraine and epilepsy revived scientifically with the theses by Gowers[354] and Liveing[493] at the end of the last century and by Lennox and Lennox[478] in the late 1960's who stated that: 'Of the various lands that border the state of epilepsy, migraine is the most like it and the most important. (In fact, we believe migraine is an autonomic epilepsy)'[478] (see also migralepsy, page 288–291).

Statistical and epidemiological arguments in favour of or against a relationship between migraine and epilepsy are beyond the purposes of this book. As a clinician I am interested in their differential diagnosis which has been neglected. I have previously detailed the clinical and electroencephalographic difficulties that are sometimes encountered when trying to make a definite diagnosis of migraine or epilepsy in certain cases.[602] In this book I will mainly concentrate on the differentiation between occipital seizures versus migraine with aura, acephalgic and basilar migraine.

Though migraine and its variants are well described in all relevant books, and excellent reviews exist,

I felt that some aspects of migraine should be included in this book. Appendix 1 is the presently recognized classification of migraine by the International Headache Society. Migraine with visual aura is also detailed. Furthermore, in view of the existing and continuing confusion regarding the erroneous concept of 'basilar migraine causing seizures and occipital paroxysms' I have attempted a detailed review of basilar migraine in Chapter 16.

Elementary visual hallucinations of occipital seizures versus visual aura of migraine

Visual aura of migraine: *'I was startled by a singular shadowy appearance at the outside corner of the field of vision of the left eye. It gradually advanced into the field of view and then appeared to be a pattern in straight-lined angular forms, very much in general aspects like the drawing of a fortification, with salient and re-entering angles, bastions, and ravelins with some suspicion of faint lines of colour between the dark lines.'* *Sir J.F.W. Herschel (1866)*[387]

Visual seizure: *'They commenced with the appearance of several small spheres, white in the centre with an intermediate zone of blue and outside this a ring of red, immediately to the left of the point at which the patient gazed; from here they moved either at a uniform rate or in jerks to the left and downwards...In all attacks the eyes deviated towards the left and the head turned in the same direction as soon as the visual spectra appeared.'* *G. Holmes (1927)*[396]

Introduction

Elementary visual hallucinations, blindness or both, with or without headache, are more likely to be diagnosed as migraine with aura, basilar migraine or acephalgic migraine,[602,611,618,625] despite well documented evidence that they share fundamental symptoms often with the same sequence of events as occipital seizures.[313,352,396,513,648,694,700,746,811] In a previous study[611] comparing morphology and colours of elementary visual hallucinations between the two diseases, the conclusion was that visual seizures are predominantly coloured and circular as opposed to the mainly achromatic, black and white, linear patterns of migraine aura.[611] However, it was postulated that this 'simple criterion' may not be applicable in all cases and there are many more differentiating features, as shown in Table 14.1. It has been detailed, and purposely overemphasized in this book, that the morphology and the chronological sequence of visual symptoms in migraine are entirely different from those of visual occipital seizures. Ictal elementary visual hallucinations, ictal blindness, and ictal and post-ictal headache unequivocally associated with occipital seizures have been detailed in previous chapters. In this section emphasis is placed on the elementary hallucinations and other visual symptoms associated with migraine and their differentiation from occipital seizures.

Terminology

In reviewing the medical records of patients with visual seizures or migraine aura I was impressed that the description of visual hallucinations were often abbreviated in terms such as fortification spectrum, teichopsia, scintillating scotoma, phosphenes, and their variations. Their meaning did not always represent the actual descriptions. This has been emphasized by Plant[657] in a detailed and well documented historical review of the origin of the term fortification spectra in migraine. The migrainous elementary visual hallucinations are called fortifications because of their similarities to the bastioned, star patterned, pentagonal fortifications, not because of the castellated appearances of battlements.[387] A bastion is a projecting part of a fortification, consisting of an earthwork in the form of an irregular pentagon, having its base in the main line or at an angle to the fortification.

Spectrum is used by Gowers[353] 'to mean apparition and not a coloured band of light'.

According to Airy, 1870:[19] The name 'Teichopsia' (teichos = town wall, opsis = vision) to represent the bastioned form of transient hemiopsia which I have been describing, is not without a reminiscence of some words of Tennyson:

> *as yonder walls*
> *Rose slowly to a music slowly breathed,*
> *A cloud that gathered shape* Airy (1870)[19]

Table 14.1. Differential diagnosis of basilar migraine, migraine with aura and occipital epilepsy

	BM	MA	OS
Visual hallucinations			
Mainly coloured circular patterns	+	++	++++
Mainly achromatic or black and white linear patterns	+++	++++	+
Moving from one side to the opposite side of the visual field			+++++
Expanding from the centre to the periphery of a visual hemifield	++	++++	++
Duration of a few seconds to a minute			+++++
Duration of about 15–20 min	++	++++	+
Daily in frequency			+++++
No more than one per month	++	++	+++
Evolving to blindness	++++	+	+++
Evolving to tonic deviation of eyes or other convulsive features			+++++
Evolving to impairment of consciousness without convulsions	+++	+	++++
Evolving to impairment of consciousness with convulsions	+		++++
Associated with headache	++	++++	++
Blindness and hemianopia			
Sudden without any other preceding or following symptoms*	+++		+++
Other neurological symptoms			
Brainstem symptoms (bilateral hypoasthesia and weakness, vertigo, diplopia, dizziness)	++++		
post-ictal ataxia	+		+
Vomiting			
Occurring together with visual hallucinations/blindness	++	++	+++
Occurring together with deviation of the eyes			+++++
Occurring together with impairment of consciousness	+	+	++++
post-ictal or postcritical vomiting	+++	++++	+
Headache			
Severe, throbbing, unilateral	+	++++	+
Severe, throbbing, bilateral and posterior	++++	+	++
Occurring before or at the onset of visual hallucinations	++	+++	+
Occurring during the neurological symptoms	+++	+++	+
post-ictal or postcritical severe headache	++++	++++	++
Interictal EEG			
Normal	++++	++++	++
Non-specific paroxysmal abnormalities	++++	++++	++
Occipital spikes, occipital paroxysms	+	+	++++
Photoparoxysmal responses	+	+	+++++
Ictal EEG			
Normal	++++	++++	++
Slow occipital activity	++++	++++	+
Fast spikes or fast paroxysmal occipital activity			+++++
post-ictal EEG			
Persistent occipital slow activity for hours or days	++++	++	+
Structural brain imaging			
Abnormal	+	+	++++
Ictal SPECT			
Hypoperfusion	++++	++++	
Hyperperfusion			++++
Ictal Intracranial Doppler			
Increased blood flow			++++
Decreased blood flow	++++	++++	

*If blindness or hemianopia is followed by other symptoms, the same rules as for visual hallucinations apply
+ = exceptional, ++ = rare, +++ = frequent, ++++ = as a rule, +++++ = exclusive.

Scintillating (scintilla = spark) scotoma (skotos = darkness) is also used because of the sparking appearance of the visual hallucinations of migraine (brilliant flashes of light in the periphery of dark areas in the visual fields).

Photopsias (phos = light, opsis = vision) are unformed flashes of light and sparks.

Phosphenes are subjective sensations of light due to non-luminous stimulation of the retina. The term is also used to denote visual percepts following electrical stimulation of the visual cortex, in which case they are usually coloured spots or circles.[709]

Elementary visual hallucinations, negative visual phenomena and other symptoms in migraine with aura and acephalgic migraine

Brief description

The elementary visual hallucinations of migraine with aura and acephalgic migraine are similar. The visual aura of migraine with aura and acephalgic migraine starts with predominantly flickering achromatic or black and white, linear and zigzag patterns in the centre of the visual field, gradually expanding over minutes towards the periphery of one hemifield, and often leaving a scotoma.[693] Most typically, an arc of scintillating lights appears near the point of fixation and may form a herring-bone-like pattern that expands to encompass an increasing portion of a visual hemifield.[727] It migrates across the visual field with a scintillating edge of zigzag or flashing lights which are often black and white; occasionally, coloured dots appear at the end of the white stripe but these are not predominant. Simple flashes, specks, or hallucinations of geometric forms (points, stars, lines, curves, circles, sparks, flashes, or flames) may occur and may be single or in hundreds.[727] Positive visual hallucinations may be accompanied by scotomata which are negative phenomena consisting of a blanking or graying out of vision.[727] Post-aura hemianopia is common. Less typical features of migraine visual aura and coloured patterns have been described[581,719] but clustering of other symptoms as above betray their migraine nature. Migraine complex visual hallucinations and illusions are well described in all relevant textbooks.

The visual hallucinations of migraine rarely exhibit daily frequency, cannot last for seconds, do not move en block to the contralateral side and do not progress to motor symptoms such as eye and head deviation, eyelid repetitive closures or fluttering which often characterize visual occipital seizures. It is exceptional to march to non visual epileptic seizures.[263,529,766]

Migraine headache follows, usually after a few minutes, but may precede the visual aura. Headache is mainly unilateral and throbbing, of moderate to marked severity, aggravated by head movement or physical activity and often lasts for more than 5 h to 1–3 days. Anorexia, nausea and vomiting, photophobia and phonophobia are often concurrent with the headache.

Historical and literature review

The quality and the chronological changes associated with migraine visual aura are well illustrated in all relevant textbooks and have been well studied from ancient times (see for review and illustrations 'Migraine' by Sacks[697] and for children 'migraine in childhood' by Hockaday[393]). More recent reports and studies, some of which are prospective, reach similar conclusions.[113,133,375,422,532,581,611,666,692,693,719] The most recent comprehensive prospective study is by Russell and Olesen, 1996[693] entitled 'A nosographic analysis of the migraine aura in a general population'. I quote: 'The study presented here is the first detailed nosographic analysis of migraine aura, diagnosed using the criteria of the International Headache Society, in a sufficiently large sample for statistical analysis. Of 4000 people, 163 had migraine with aura. Sixty-two had attacks of migraine aura with headache as well as migraine aura without headache, and seven had exclusively migraine aura without headache. Visual symptoms were most frequent (99 per cent), followed by sensory (31 per cent), aphasic (18 per cent) and motor (6 per cent) symptoms. Those with several types of aura symptoms had visual aura in virtually every attack, while sensory, motor and aphasic aura were present only in a small number of their attacks. The typical visual aura starts as a flickering, uncoloured, zig-zag line in the centre of the visual field and affects the central vision. It gradually progresses towards the periphery of one hemifield and often leaves a scotoma. The typical sensory aura is unilateral, starts in the hand, progresses towards the arm and then affects the face and tongue. The typical motor aura is half-sided and affects the hand and arm. The visual, sensory and aphasic auras rarely lasted 1 h, while the motor aura did in 67 per cent (six out of nine). Four people had exclusively acute onset visual aura. The duration of the aura and the characteristics of the ensuing headache were typical for migraine with aura, suggesting that acute onset aura is a real phenomenon. Headache followed the aura in 93 per cent, headache and aura occurred simultaneously in 4 per cent and aura followed headache in 3 per cent. The characteristic spread of each symptom and the sequence of different symptoms suggest that cortical spreading depression is the mechanism underlying the migraine aura. Our results do not suggest that alterations of the diagnostic criteria of the International Headache Society are needed. The intra-individual variation of aura symptoms shown in this study indicates that a simplification of the International Classification of Diseases, Neurological Adaptation is appropriate.'[693]

Details of the visual aura are as follows:[693] 'Seven people had exclusively visual aura without headache. Five people had acute onset visual aura, of these three had exclusively visual aura and headache and one had exclusively visual aura without headache. A fifth person had gradually progressing sensory and motor auras after the sudden onset of visual aura. The acute onset visual aura had a sudden onset in four people and developed during 1 min in the fifth person. It was flickering in three of the five people, and was unilateral in one person and bilateral in four people. Of the 49 people with bilateral visual aura, 21 had unilateral headache and 28 had bilateral headache. The typical visual aura starts as a flickering, uncoloured, unilateral zig-zag line in the centre of the visual field, it gradually progresses towards the periphery, often leaving a scotoma. The gradual progression lasted <30 min and the total duration of visual auras was 60 min. Only few had prolonged visual aura. Those who had visual aura exclusively tended to have shorter mean gradual progression and duration of their aura than those with visual aura in association with sensory, motor or aphasic aura.' In evaluating the significance of their results the authors commented:[693] 'The aura symptoms in the present study developed in a way which indicates a gradual spread in the great majority of people. Except for five people who only had acute onset aura, the other 158 people had gradually developed aura compatible with a contiguous spread of symptoms. This was also the case if more than one aura symptom occurred. We conclude from our nosographic analysis that cortical spreading depression of Leao remains the most likely explanation for the migraine aura. Although spreading depression most likely triggers the migraine aura, it is not always a sufficient trigger for the headache, since nearly half of the migraineurs also experienced migraine aura without headache. The severity of the migraine aura is variable, and sometimes it may be too weak to precipitate a headache. This is indirectly supported by the observation that migraine aura tended to be of longer duration if it was followed by headache ...The criterion of gradual development of aura symptoms over >4 min is essential, and caution is necessary in diagnosing migraine with acute onset aura. The gradual development of visual and sensory auras usually lasted <30 min, while the development of motor aura often lasted > 1 h. The latter may be caused by memory bias, because of the long duration of motor symptoms. We could not set suitable rules for defining gradual development of aphasic aura and therefore only recorded the duration of this symptom. The duration of visual, sensory and aphasic aura were usually < 30 min, confirming the validity of this criterion of the International Headache Society. However, motor aura can last for several hours ...We suggest that future editions of the International Classification of Diseases, Neurological Adaptation limits the subdivision of migraine with aura to comprise visual migraine, multiple types of aura, migraine aura without headache, basilar migraine and familial hemiplegic migraine.'

That colours may be seen in migraine aura is well described even by Aretaeus, 'flashes of purple or black colours before the sight ... so as to exhibit the appearance of a rainbow',[47] and Airy, 'gorgeous chromatic edgings'.[19] Also, spots, circles and beads with or without colours may also be experienced during the migraine visual aura.[179,375,719] However, colours and circular patterns in migraine are usually not dominant.[387,611]

Hemianopia and scotomas are well known visual defects of mainly migraine with aura and acephalgic migraine usually occurring during or after the characteristic visual aura described above. Monocular blindness is a common symptom of ophthalmic migraine while binocural blindness is the commonest manifestation of basilar migraine, as is detailed in Chapter 15.

Visual symptoms of basilar migraine

Basilar migraine is characterized by transient and fully reversible visual aura and symptoms of brain-stem dysfunction such as dizziness, vertigo and tinnitus, ataxia, bilateral weakness and dysaesthesia, diplopia, dysarthria and decreased hearing.[106,108,392,470,741,747] These symptoms develop gradually over 4 min and last for less than 30 min to 1 h. Visual symptoms are mainly bilateral visual impairment,[741] 'dimming of vision or blindness',[106] 'bilateral visual impairment in temporal and nasal visual fields of both eyes, transient amaurosis, diffuse reduction of vision (blurred vision, foggy vision, "everything gray"), tunnel vision, inferior hemianopia'[741], 'scotomata, transient bilateral blindness or blurred vision',[741] 'tunnel vision, total amblyopia, and bilateral positive and negative hallucinations, including teichopsia.'[392] Elementary visual hallucinations may occur and are also bilateral, described as 'teichopsia',[106,392] 'flashes or blobs of light',[108] or 'positive phenomena (flickering, flashes, teichopsia, coloured figures, dysmorphopsia)'.[741] In only one of the reported cases are 'colourful displays' mentioned.[747] Headache that follows is usually posterior, severe and bilateral. The attacks of basilar migraine are usually infrequent and over the years there is a tendency for them to cease or to be replaced by common varieties of migraine with or without aura.[106]

Basilar migraine is reviewed in Chapter 15.

Visual seizures of occipital epilepsies

The elementary visual hallucinations of occipital seizures have been detailed purposely and repeatedly in previous chapters. Briefly, they are mainly coloured, with circular patterns, have the same onset regarding localization and progress, they are often brief for seconds, develop fast and their individual components may multiply or move together to the contralateral side. They are mainly frequent, often daily, and sometimes progress to other occipital seizure symptoms such as eye and head deviation,[551,648,751] illusions of eye movement,[399] eyelid repetitive closures or fluttering[700,811] and convulsions. Blindness that lasts longer and may occur *ab initio* is not uncommon. post-ictal headache is frequent and often indistinguishable from migraine.

In view of the relative lack of relevant reports and the significance of a well designed study I have recently prospectively evaluated elementary visual hallucinations, blindness and headache in idiopathic occipital epilepsy[618] and this has been presented in detail in Chapter 13.

Migralepsy and intercalated seizures

Definition

Migralepsy is an old term deriving from migra(ine) and (epi)lepsy to 'refer to patients with classic migraine that subsequently evolved to an epilepstic seizure'[529] or more accurately to 'a seizure that may be a composite of symptoms encountered in epilepsy and migraine'.[478] Intercalated seizures denote epileptic seizures occurring between the migrainous aura and the headache phase of migraine.[525,765,766] There are no more than 30 case reports on this association and these are either occipital seizures imitating migraine or because of their complicated clinical and EEG interictal or ictal features make diagnosis extremely difficult and the conclusions may be vulnerable. It should be remembered that occipital seizures, documented with ictal recordings may present with the most uncharacteristic manifestations for epileptic seizures (see Chapters 7 and 12B).

A typical case

Over the years I was unsuccessful in finding a typical and convincing case of this situation though I have tried hard with the help of many colleagues. Whenever such a case was brought to my attention it was visual seizures, idiopathic or symptomatic which imitated migraine with aura, acephalgic and basilar migraine, alone or in combination.

Literature review, conclusions and criticism of migralepsy and intercalated seizures

Migralepsy is an old term attributed by Lennox and Lennox[478] to D. Davidson. I quote from Lennox and Lennox (pp. 450–451):[478] 'a given seizure may be a composite of symptoms encountered in epilepsy and migraine'. Such cases are more common in children than in adults. In our experience, the migraine-like symptoms appear first – the characteristics of ophthalmic migraine with perhaps nausea and vomiting, followed by symptoms characteristic of epilepsy, impairment or loss of consciousness and involuntary muscle movement. Dr Douglas Davidson calls such hybrid phenomena 'migralepsy'. I also think it important to reproduce in this section illustrative cases published by Lennox and Lennox as such examples of migralepsy. I am of the opinion that these were occipital seizures.

Case 1. Seizures a composite of epilepsy and migraine – Both a genetic and an organic background. From Lennox and Lennox.[478] pp. 451–452.

> A slender young woman of 21 was referred because of seizures which had been diagnosed as either hysteria or epilepsy. The mother and a paternal aunt have each fainted once. A maternal aunt had chronic epilepsy and a maternal cousin had seizures as a youth. The father is rigid and dominating; the mother has treated her harshly and at present suffers from involutional melancholia. Ever since she can remember, the patient has been subject to mild hemicrania on one side or the other, with slight nausea but without visual disturbance. These headaches occurred at least once a week and were only partially relieved by 10 or 15 grains of aspirin. At the age of 4 or 5, during an infection of measles, she was unconscious for 12 h. When 16, she began to have attacks described as follows: Her field of vision, more particularly the right, would be filled with yellow whirling stars, 'like driving through a snow storm.' She would then feel herself growing smaller and more distant, thoughts would be jumbled, 'like going under ether,' and she would lose consciousness. The left side of her face would twitch and the abdominal muscles would stiffen and jerk. There was cyanosis and once urinary incontinence. Unconsciousness lasted for from 20 min to 2 h, and was followed by confusion of thought and speech, sleepiness, and a short-lived bilateral headache. On several occasions there was the visual disturbance without subsequent seizure. The home situation was unhappy. The initial attack and one or two others followed emotional disturbance. During 2 years at college she was seizure-free.
>
> A characteristic attack, which occurred while she was in the hospital, was followed by a complete but transient left homonymous hemianopsia. Roentgen films disclosed multiple deposits of calcium in the right occipital pole. Dr. Sosman suggested these were either angiomas or perivascular calcification as a sequel of cerebral atrophy.
>
> The patient was placed on phenobarbital medication, 32 mg daily. There was no seizure during the following 18 months, but on two occasions a visual disturbance was followed by severe hemicrania with nausea and vomiting. An injection of ergonovine completely relieved an attack of hemicrania, so that she was given ergotamine tartrate and also amniotin for the migraine, and in the months which have elapsed she has been practically free of attacks of any kind.
>
> **In summary,** a patient with a family history of epilepsy, with exposure to emotional stress and with lime deposits in the occiput, has a migraine like visual aura followed by convulsion, and on one occasion a transient homonymous hemianopsia. With phenobarbital medication, migraine seemed to replace the convulsions. The addition of ergotamine gave freedom from attacks.

Case 3. Visual hallucinations of coloured lights or of persons, followed by migraine headache or by convulsions – Gross abnormality of EEG – Problem of driver's license. From Lennox and Lennox,[478] p. 453.

Hector Oi, was 12 years old when first seen. His paternal aunt had headaches, details not known. When 18 months old the child had a febrile convulsion. From infancy he has had attacks in which his temperature would rise to 103 ^{0}F and be accompanied by vomiting. Pain, when this could be described, was centred in the right eye. The frequency has decreased from an attack every 2 or 3 weeks to one every several months. Since about the age of 4, there has been a hallucination, a flash of red and blue round lights, principally in the right eye. This may occur frequently, as often as once a week. A headache may follow. On four occasions in the past 2 years the display of lights has been followed by the appearance of a crowd of people rushing towards him like a stampeding herd. Before they reached him he would lose consciousness and have a generalized convulsion. One such attack occurred at the onset of virus pneumonia.

In the 6 years that have intervened since the first visit, several of his EEGs have contained spike-wave discharges. For this reason Paradione, 1.2 *Gm.*, was added to his *0.065 Gm. of* phenobarbital. He has had numerous auras of colored lights, sometimes followed by headache and on a few occasions by a convulsion. Flashes might follow exposure to bright sun or snow. At last report he has been without seizures for 3 years and without medicine for two.

In the light of the invariable ophthalmic aura and in spite of an abnormal EEG, license to drive an automobile was recommended. He later entered the army.

It is interesting that in an old report of ours (1978)[629] we were emphasizing that 'Headache, often prolonged, is frequently associated with occipital seizures. Three of six patients suffered from unilateral headache which ended with vomiting. This, in the absence of any impairment of consciousness, may cause diagnostic difficulties with migraine. Lennox and Lennox[478] in reporting similar cases are of the opinion that these represent onset of migraine, progressing to an epileptic seizure that is migralepsy 'with emphasis on lepsy'. We believe that migraine and epilepsy do not co-exist in these cases. In particular, we were and still are of the opinion that case 1 from the three presented migralepsy patients by Lennox and Lennox[478] is an example of symptomatic (calcifications in the right occipital pole) visual seizures, 'migraine-like visual aura followed by convulsions and occasionally left hemianopia'.[478] Also, case 3 is most likely idiopathic occipital epilepsy with frequent elementary visual hallucinations occasionally progressing to complex visual hallucinations and secondary GTCS. Prognosis would be good.

A widely cited paper on the relation of migraine and epilepsy is by Basser.[68] Two cases 'where the same or similar aura leads sometimes to migraine and sometimes to epilepsy' are relevant to this chapter. One of these patients (case 3 in his report)[68] was a child with typical absence seizures as indicated by his EEG with 'high voltage spike and wave complexes' and brief clinical events of 'twitching of the eyelids'. There was also a complex paroxysmal symptomatology before the child 'sees a bright shining blue spot', which leads either to headache and vomiting (interpreted as migraine) or to a 'grand mal seizure'. This boy most likely had the rare form of idiopathic generalized epilepsy that may be associated with visual hallucinations (see Chapter 10). The other patient, a 37-year-old woman (case 4 in his report) had epileptic seizures in childhood preceded by 'large blobs of coloured light' and developed in adult life recurrent headaches which follow visual disturbances of 'lines and strakes of light that are white' not accompanied by epileptic fits.[68] This woman most likely had in childhood occipital seizures with secondary GTCS (it could be LBOS) and later developed migraine with aura.

There should be no reason why epileptic seizures, so vulnerable to extrinsic and intrinsic precipitating factors, could not also be susceptible to cortical changes introduced by migraine. However, this is surprisingly so extremely rare that only a few case reports are published despite the fact that migraine and epilepsy are amongst the commoner brain diseases. Most of the reported cases of 'migralepsy' are complicated cases that do not allow a meaningful and unequivocal migraine–epilepsy sequence, or they are genuine occipital seizures imitating migraine aura. None of the 1360 patients with epileptic seizures in my studies and none of my 63 patients with occipital seizures had any evidence of seizures developing from migraine aura though this was often the initial erroneous diagnosis.[611,625] Conversely, post-ictal headache and other migraine-like symptoms were common in these patients which make an epilepsy–migraine sequence[602,618] a more realistic proposition (see Chapter 13).

Marks and Ehrenberg, 1993[529] studied the relationship between migraine and epilepsy in 395 adult seizure patients. Seventy-nine patients (20 per cent) also had a migraine syndrome, and 13 of these patients (3 per cent) experienced seizures during or immediately following a migraine aura. From these 13 patients, one had a glioma in remission and two patients had cerebral infarcts attributed to migrainous ischaemia (MRI of the other patients are not reported). Five patients had complex partial seizures, three epilepsia partialis continua and EEG periodic lateralized epileptiform discharges, four had 'primary' generalized epilepsy and one partial motor seizures. Three of the 13 patients were diagnosed as having basilar migraine. Case 1, detailed in another report,[263] illustrates the diagnostic uncertainties involved as Ehrenberg admits.[263] This was a 26-year-old woman who had onset of focal febrile seizures at 16 months of age. Later in her life she had multiform epileptic seizures and she underwent a left anterior temporal lobectomy. Three months later she had 'spells of quadriparesis, random limb myoclonus and marked fading of voice with preserved consciousness' which were interpreted as basilar migraine. They could occur as frequently as 4 per day, they could last for up to 10 min and could sometimes be associated with nausea and pain behind the eye. They occasionally progressed to generalized convulsions. EEG during these 'spells' showed rhythmic spiky 3.5 Hz activity, highly and exclusively localized in the right posterior temporal electrode. On other occasions, the ictal EEG showed localized delta activity with spikes in the left posterior temporal electrode. Milder episodes could be associated with unchanged EEG activity. In this example, the brief duration of symptoms, their occurrence on average four times daily and the highly localized ictal paroxysmal activity would favour a diagnosis of epileptic seizures rather than basilar migraine. I could be wrong but certainly this cannot be considered a case of an incontrovertible basilar migraine–epileptic seizure progression. Furthermore, the EEG features during migraine attacks in this report[529] are also strikingly unusual. I am not aware of any report of EEG during basilar migraine attacks showing the abrupt onset and termination of the highly localized and brief discharges of these patients.

Manzoni *et al.*[525] and Terzano *et al.*[765,766] coined the term intercalated seizures to denote epileptic seizures occurring between the migrainous aura and the headache phase of migraine. They found that of 450 patients with migraine, 16 (3.6 per cent) also had seizures. For four of these 16 patients the two conditions appeared to be coincidental. In another five patients 'the two types of attacks were quite distinct but often an epileptic seizure was followed by a migraine attack and vice versa'. The remaining seven patients had intercalated seizures. All had a family history of migraine and two also had relatives with epilepsy. They all had visual seizures consisting of 'highly stylized contours of plain figures, or single or multicoloured spots that often rotated. They lasted for 1–2 min and came out of a scintillating scotoma slowly developing in the visual field and evolving into unilateral or bilateral hemianopia. The change of visual perception from negative to positive corresponded with the beginning of the epileptic seizure which was later followed by migraine headache. The visual epileptic symptoms were considered different from the migraine aura by the patients themselves. Seizures remitted before the age of 20 years in six of the seven patients. Migraine continued but the attacks became less frequent and responded to antimigraine treatment.' All seven patients had occipital paroxysms attenuated with eyes open and four exhibited marked photosensitivity. These patients must be exceptional in the combination of occipital paroxysms (fixation-off sensitivity) and photosensitivity in four of them. It is also interesting that none of the nine patients of the first two groups had occipital spikes or occipital seizures which were present in all patients with intercalated seizures.

De Romanis *et al.*[213,215] greatly contributed with their long follow-up studies and ictal EEG in the understanding of these conditions. Most of their patients had brief ictal visual hallucinations of 'coloured dots or discs', interictal EEG occipital paroxysms and ictal seizure EEG documenting that they had occipital epilepsy and not migraine with aura. Some of the ictal EEG of these patients are unique, such as that of their Fig. 2 with right rapid occipital spikes during left sided bright spots, 'phosphenes', followed by relative flattening of the EEG during the following phase of blindness.[213]

Basilar migraine and epilepsy

The commonly cited occurrence of basilar migraine with occipital paroxysms and seizures is probably an erroneous association. These are patients suffering from occipital, mainly idiopathic, epilepsy. The definition of basilar migraine and the associated visual and other brainstem symptoms are detailed in Chapter 16.

Basilar migraine could not escape the controversy regarding the relations of migraine with epilepsy. On the contary, because basilar migraine is often associated with impairment of consciousness and blindness[33,34,37,76,82,84,107,108,146,212,215,525,529,731,765,766,768] the relation with epilepsy appeared, erroneously in my opinion, stronger.

Bickertaff[108] mastered the differential diagnosis between basilar migraine and epilepsy and concluded that they are different disorders. However, he also accepted the 'less common' possibility that a migrainous ischaemia may precipitate seizures in 'a potentially epileptogenic brain' and one of his patients had, a few months after onset of basilar migraine, a 'full scale epileptic attack without any of the premonitory symptoms of his migraine and his EEG on this occasion was abnormal'.[108] Similar cases of occasional patients with basilar migraine also suffering from epileptic seizures have also been reported by others.[741,747]

In addition, there are also case reports of patients with intractable seizures and a plethora of ictal symptoms that have been diagnosed as basilar migraine and epilepsy. The complexities of such cases as that of Marks and Ehrenberg[529] have been discussed above earlier in this chapter (migralepsy).

Of the reported cases of basilar migraine with 'epilepsy', most suffered from occipital lobe seizures either spontaneously[33,82,84,146,212,213,215,731,765] or photically induced.[84,392,525,747,765] I would suggest that most of these patients had occipital seizures imitating migraine or their seizures were situation related.

Slatter's[731] case is widely cited as a combination of basilar migraine and seizures.[731] He described a boy of 8 years with episodes of bilateral 'bright multi-coloured wavy lines' followed by frontal headaches, often by vomiting and sometimes by fainting. EEG showed 4–5 Hz activity in the left posterior quadrant. A diagnosis of basilar migraine was made. A year later he had an episode of status epilepticus with a left occipital sharp and slow wave focus. Slatter[731] suggested that this was an example of focal brain damage caused by migraine though both the initial and subsequent symptoms could best be attributed to left occipital lobe epilepsy, possibly symptomatic.

Further interest and controversy regarding basilar migraine and occipital seizures started in 1978 with a report by Camfield *et al.*[146] of basilar migraine, seizures and severe EEG abnormalities. Their view detailed in Chapter 11 is that these patients had basilar migraine which caused seizures and EEG occipital paroxysms through migrainous ischaemic lesions. This was questioned by Panayiotopoulos[599] and later by Gastaut,[304,313] Beaumanoir and Grandjean (1987)[82] and Lerman and Kivity.[484] However, it should be emphasized that these four patients and mainly patients 2 and 3 of Camfield *et al.*[146] had a number of 'atypical' features with little resemblance to the conventional occipital seizures of Gastaut. These patients from the age of 7 to 11 years started having mainly prolonged episodes of visual hallucinations often followed by blindness, vomiting and headache. The duration of the visual hallucinations and blindness was more than 10–15 min and sometimes lasted for hours. In a patient, blindness was preceded by severe dizziness and persistent vomiting lasting from 1 to 2 h to as much as several days. All patients also had infrequent focal or generalized convulsive seizures in the course of these events or independently. The prognosis was excellent in all and that should also count against symptomatic occipital epilepsy caused by ischaemic lesions. Therefore, these patients had unusual clinical manifestations but certainly their seizures with their excellent prognosis could not be attributed to ischaemic lesions.

Beaumanoir and Grandjean[82] found three patients with 'migraine only' and five that had 'migraine and seizures' amongst 41 patients selected because of EEG occipital paroxysms which disappeared with age. 'Migrainous attacks were always characteristic of either classical or basilar migraine'. These eight patients had strange and prolonged episodes described as 'a feeling of general discomfort, perspiration, and blurred vision lasting 5 h', 'right visual field scotoma followed by diffuse headache and marked photophobia, for about 10 h', 'violent posterior headaches associated with abdominal discomfort, vomiting, vertigo, and perhaps also diplopia that lasted for a couple of hours', 'dazzling flashing lights followed by blindness, agitation, vomiting, vertigo, bilateral paraesthesia of the hands and diffuse headache mainly posterior', 'dazzling lights evolving to a red spot, hemianopia and blindness, paraesthesia of both hands with reduced awareness fluctuating for some hours after the headache stopped' and 'altitudinal hemianopia followed by diffuse headache lasting 5–24 h and associated with marked photophobia, abdominal discomfort and intermittent vomiting or a marked confusional state with agitation and ataxia'.

De Romanis *et al.*[212,213,215] reported patients with occipital paroxysms and a wide variety of ictal and post-ictal symptoms, also describing ictal EEG and long-term evolution. Most of the patients suffered from childhood occipital seizures. This may also be the case for their 14 patients reported as 'migraine and epilepsy with infantile onset and EEG findings of occipital spike-wave complexes'.[213] The ictal EEG of one of these patients clearly illustrates that the visual hallucinations, positive and negative, were epileptic. The seizure started with bilateral bright spots and EEG unilateral occipital spikes followed by amaurosis with simultaneous flattening of the EEG. post-ictally there was 'migraine accompanied by nausea, vomiting and photophobia, lasting for about 8 h'. A left homonymous hemianopsia, which disappeared after 24 h, was detected by visual field examination.

De Romanis[212] also reported seven children with 'basilar migraine with EEG findings of occipital spike-wave complexes'. 'Migraine headache was heralded in most of the patients by unilateral or bilateral visual distortions represented by circles, triangles or coloured bands lasting for seconds to minutes. Throbbing headache was localized in the occipital region or was diffuse and lasted from 5 to 12 h. Eight to 12 h of sleep or drowsiness followed'. Neurological symptoms such as ataxia, nystagmus and dysarthria alone or in combination occurred in all patients, probably during the long headache phase of the attacks.[215] Ictal EEG of all patients 'showed diffuse high voltage delta activity associated with spikes and sharp waves or diffuse delta activity which could be recorded from 1 to 7 days'. The sample of an ictal EEG provided in this report is dominated mainly by spikes and clusters of rapid spikes superimposed on slow waves.

Considering that early and late onset BCOS (Chapters 8 and 9) manifest with polymorphous ictal manifestations combining visual hallucinations, blindness, autonomic disturbances with headache and vomiting which are sometimes very prolonged, it is likely that these cases of Camfield *et al.*,[146] Beaumanoir and Grandjean[82] and De Romanis *et al.*[212,213,215] suffer from a form of occipital seizures imitating basilar migraine. This view is confirmed when ictal EEG recordings are available.[212,213,215]

I should re-emphasize that the above personal view does not mean that I do not accept the possibility of occipital seizures triggered or spontaneously occurring in patients with basilar migraine, but this would be exceptional. This may be the case for three patients with basilar migraine of Beaumanoir[76] who was able to record EEG during 'positive symptoms of coloured hallucinations' 20–40 min after the onset of the migraine and while vision had not completely recovered. During this brief period 'low amplitude, fast activity, similar to that recorded during epileptic visual seizures' was recorded.[76]

Basilar migraine and photosensitive occipital seizures

Occipital seizures induced by flickering lights[51,52,236,278,284,369–371,535,561,677] may also be another source of misdiagnosis as they frequently imitate migraine with aura and basilar migraine (see Chapter 12B). Seizures are induced by television, video-games and intermittent photic stimulation. They begin with elementary visual hallucinations which are multi-coloured and circular, often followed or associated with blindness, eyelid fluttering, tonic deviation of the eyes, epigastric discomfort, vomiting, and headache with either normal or impaired responsiveness. They may terminate with generalized convulsions.[51,236,278,284,369–371,535,561,677] Duration varies from seconds to 2–5 min but may be as long as up to 2 h.

That these symptoms, even the very prolonged and unusual ones, are ictal has been unequivocally documented with simultaneous EEG recordings by Guerrini *et al.*[370] post-ictal headache occurs in one third of the patients and may be pulsating, associated with vomiting and last up to several hours.[370] Prognosis is uncertain: Some children may have only 1–2 seizures but others may not remit. Interictal EEG shows spontaneous and photically induced occipital spikes. Centrotemporal spikes may co-exist. Ictal EEG discharges are localized to the occipital regions during the visual symptoms, and may eventually spread slowly over the temporal regions with the appearance of autonomic symptoms. These cases 'because of the clustering of visual aura, vegetative symptoms, and cephalic pain, had frequently been misdiagnosed as having migraine before adjunctive clinical and EEG evidence of epilepsy was obtained.'[370]

A well cited case of basilar migraine is case 12 of Swanson and Vick[747] despite the fact that an attack recorded with EEG during IPS was epileptic as attested by an ictal discharge of bilateral repetitive occipital spikes initially at 4 Hz, gradually increasing in amplitude for about 40 s and slowing to 1 Hz for a few seconds before disappearing completely. The discharge remained localized to the occipital areas throughout this episode. During the attack the patient became unconscious and several hours later developed generalized throbbing headache and truncal ataxia.

Another case reported as basilar migraine by Hockaday[392] was a 6-year-old child with attacks of blindness, loss of consciousness and 'convulsive movements' triggered by watching television. The interictal EEG was normal but it was rightly concluded that 'this diagnosis can not be established in the absence of either a recurrent pattern of attack or a background of unequivocal migraine and that further EEG studies may show photosensitivity'. An adolescent patient reported by Jacome[413] had photoparoxysmal discharges.

Table 14.1 indicates the main differences between basilar migraine, migraine with aura and occipital seizures.

Is there an association between basilar migraine and occipital epilepsy?

The association of basilar migraine with spontaneous or photically induced occipital lobe seizures is probably due to difficulties in differentiation between basilar migraine and occipital epilepsy. In a very small number of patients seizures may be triggered by the migrainous events but more often it is occipital seizures that initiate migraine-like symptoms.

Why are patients with occipital seizures are so often misdiagnosed as migraine with aura, acephalgic migraine or basilar migraine?

Most of my patients with occipital seizures and visual hallucinations were misdiagnosed as migraine with aura, acephalgic migraine and basilar migraine. The main reason is that the differential diagnosis of elementary visual hallucinations between the two diseases has only recently been addressed in comparative studies.[602,611,618,625] That some cases of idiopathic occipital epilepsy may cause significant difficulties in their differential diagnosis from migraine aura and particularly basilar migraine is apparent in the relevant literature[146,212] and has been debated recently.[635,720] However, the major reason for misdiagnosis is that visual hallucinations are frequently not analysed in their details, but are abbreviated in terms such as teichopsia, scintillating scotoma or fortification spectra which may misrepresent the true descriptions of the patients, as such terms are frequently unquestionably equated with migraine. This is because physicians are not properly informed of differential diagnostic criteria. In this respect it is alarming that expert assessors are reluctant to accept that the differential diagnosis between migraine aura and visual seizures is primarily based on clinical criteria. A recent systematic prospective and qualitative study of mine[618] on the characteristics of elementary visual hallucinations, blindness and headache (see Chapter 13) met with the following criticism of an expert assessor of a major neurology journal:

'The author presents subjective clinical experiences of 11 patients with idiopathic occipital

epilepsy with elementary visual hallucinations. Although he states in the abstract that 'Most of the patients are misdiagnosed as migraine...or migralepsy' he presents no ictal EEG data for any of the studied patients to prove that they had accelerated epileptic discharges during the visual hallucinations. In fact, four of the patients had normal (interictal) EEGs and this included patient 5, one of those who experienced episodes of blindness. The author asserts that 'The elementary visual hallucinations detailed cannot be anything else but visual seizures'. However, he offers no convincing data from his cases to support this: 1) The response to carbamazepine cannot be used as proof that these were not migraine episodes since it is possible that migraine could respond to this drug. 2) The progression of the symptoms to involve non-visual territories and even convulsions does not rule out migraine-triggered seizures. The interictal EEG appearance of epileptiform activity in some of these patients does not prove that the visual symptoms are associated with a true ictal tranformation (which is the only way to convincingly differentiate migraine aura from epilepsy).'

Comments of an expert assessor (April 1998)

Yet the clinical evidence offered is of clustering of symptoms as detailed in this book (Tables 14.1 and 13.5), the response to treatment is one aspect of this; ictal recordings in similar cases confirm their epileptic nature and surface EEG in 30 per cent of symptomatic occipital seizures may not show any appreciable changes. According to this assessor, all these patients suffer from migraine unless ictal recordings prove it otherwise. This is the problem.

Investigative procedures in the differentiation between occipital seizures and migraine

The differential diagnosis between occipital seizures and migraine can be adequately addressed on clinical grounds as detailed above. This is often more than sufficient for a confident diagnosis. Investigative procedures may be useful to confirm diagnosis in difficult cases or when clinical confidence is lacking. These are briefly described below.

Electroencephalography

Interictal and ictal EEG in occipital seizures

Ictal and interictal EEG findings in occipital seizures have been detailed in Chapter 10. Ictal surface EEG unequivocally confirms the epileptic nature of paroxysmal clinical events and provides information regarding localization and seizure spreading in the majority of the cases. However, it is also known that ictal surface EEG may not show any changes and this should not be considered against such a diagnosis if all other well balanced clinical and investigative criteria are satisfied.

Inter-critical EEG in migraine

The EEG is of doubtful significance in the diagnosis of migraine and may be a source of error if it is not interpreted in a well described clinical setting. The EEG of migraine patients may show increased slow, mainly posterior, episodic generalized theta activity occasionally intermixed with sharp components, an overexaggerated response to hyperventilation and to IPS. None of these abnormalities is specific for any type of migraine.[1,360a] Briefly, the EEG is not useful in migraine diagnosis and this is also the conclusion of The Quality Standards Subcommittee of the American Academy of Neurology on this matter: EEG does not improve diagnostic accuracy, does not identify headache subtypes, and cannot any longer be used as a reliable method for structural causes of headache.[1,360a]

Critical EEG in migraine

Critical EEG during an attack of migraine with aura may be normal, show some excess of localized or diffuse slow waves, or some depression of background activity.[703] The most definite abnormalities of unilateral or bilateral delta activity are recorded during attacks of hemiplegic migraine and basilar migraine. Details of EEG during attacks of basilar migraine are given in Chapter 15. Briefly, the EEG during attacks of basilar migraine is usually dominated by symmetrical high amplitude slow waves which are more abundant in the posterior regions and persist for days or a week after remission,[62,84,297,469,470, 543,548,640,643,741,747]or less commonly excessive generalized beta activity.[640,736] In a patient with '3–10 days life-threatening coma', the critical EEG showed suppression burst pattern and frontal intermittent rhythmic delta activity.[293]

Brain imaging, transcranial Doppler and brain SPECT[293,415,463,472,543,714,829]

Brain CT scan and brain MRI are normal or manifest minor non-specific abnormalities in patients with migraine with aura and basilar migraine[415] except in those few who develop cerebral infarcts. Brain imaging is also normal in idiopathic occipital epilepsy but often reveal structural occipital lesions, major or minor, in symptomatic occipital epilepsy.

Transcranial Doppler sonography shows decreased blood flow velocity during migraine aura[462,463] and increased blood flow velocity in occipital seizures.[804]

Similarly, single photon emission computed tomography (SPECT) of the brain shows hypoperfusion during migraine aura[714,737,774]and hyperprefusion in the ictal phase of occipital seizures.[70]

Clinical migraine–epilepsy syndromes

It is apparent from the relevant descriptions, examples and literature reviews detailed in this book that my thesis is that migraine–epilepsy syndromes do not exist. There are three situations where migraine and epileptic seizures may occur in the same person but these do not constitute syndromes:

(a) Coincidence, because of the high prevalence of migraine and epilesy, is expected.

(b) Severe migraine causing ischaemic and structural lesions, which is rare, may, like cerebrovascular disease, cause epileptic seizures.

(c) Seizures precipitated by migraine, which is also rare. In this setting I include the rare occasion of an epileptic seizure precipitated by migrainous changes in the brain. I also include seizures triggered by photic or other stimuli in a patient with migraine. These are isolated seizures that occur in a particular situation as for example in patients with migraine when they had their only seizure ever under aggressive photic stimulation mainly in an EEG department.[677] A similar situation may arise in normal people who do not have migraine and these are cited in the relavant sections of this book.

The reverse, that is epileptic seizures, mainly occipital seizures, causing post-ictal headache which may be indistinguishable from migraine, is common.[618]

However, this view is not shared by other, distinguished colleagues, who also have their own views and experience and these are briefly presented here. According to Andermann and Andermann,[33,37] 'there are a number of situations where migraine and epilepsy coexist or may be causally related'. They have proposed the following 'clinical migraine–epilepsy syndromes'.

(1) Epileptic seizures induced by a classical migraine aura

These are patients having migraine with aura who may have a seizure during the aura and this may then be followed by the headache phase. They refer to 'intercalated' seizures.[525,765,766] This may be the rare situation that I detailed earlier in this chapter (page 288).

(2) Epilepsy with seizures no longer triggered by migrainous aura

According to the Andermann and Andermann[33,37] 'in some of these patients seizures, particularly temporal lobe attacks, may eventually occur spontaneously, no longer triggered by a migrainous aura'. I am not aware of any such documented association.

(3) Epilepsy due to gross cerebral lesions caused by migraine

People who have a stroke related to their migraine may then develop seizures in turn related to their vascular lesion. This is well accepted and understood but also rare. It cannot constitute a separate syndrome as symptoms depend on localization of infarcts and the majority of these patients with migraine-induced infarcts may not suffer seizures. In this sense, patients with cerbrovascular disease who have seizures should also constitute a separate syndrome, which cannot be accepted as correct.

(4) a. Benign occipital epilepsy of childhood and the spectrum of the occipital epilepsies; b. Benign Rolandic epilepsy

According to Andermann and Andermann[33,37] 'there is an increased prevalence of migraine in children with benign partial epilepsies of childhood, Rolandic or occipital, and in their first-degree relatives'. This is by no means proven and most of these cases, particularly the occipital ones face the problem of correct diagnosis as detailed in other chapters.

In view of the relevance that this hypothesized syndrome has to benign partial childhood epilepsies, the readers may be interested in further details.

Andermann *et al.*[37,41,43] consider benign childhood epilepsy with centrotemporal spikes to be 'a migraine-related disease' but this view is entirely hypothetical and cannot be substantiated by the limited literature on the subject with some reports in favour[120,339] but others against such an association.[337,705] There are two reports from the last ten years that Andermann refers to: the first is by Bladin,[120] and the other by Giovanardi Rossi with associates.[337] Bladin's[120] is a clinical uncontrolled study. He found that of 30 patients with Rolandic seizures and centrotemporal spikes, 20 had 'recurrent sick headaches'. Two had classical migraine and seven children also had speech maturational problems. Headaches usually continued after the remission of seizures. A family history of migraine was obtained from 21 families. The study of Giovanardi Rossi *et al.*[337] was a designed controlled study according to well defined criteria of recurrent headaches and migraine. They found that the prevalence of recurrent headaches and migraine was not statistically different between 43 patients with Rolandic seizures and 129 control subjects. Recurrent headaches occurred in 34.9 per cent of the Rolandic group versus 28.6 per cent in the control, migraine 13.9 per cent versus 13.2 per cent and a family history of migraine 44.3 per cent versus 45 per cent.[337]

Andermann[36,37] credits the findings of Bladin[120] in support of his theory and dismisses the report of Giovanardi Rossi *et al.*[337] as follows: 'All these figures are very high, but could be explained if one believes that a predisposition to vascular headache is present in at least half the general population'. Furthermore, the recent reference (1997[36]) to the paper by Ferrie *et al.*[277] may also indicate bias by misquotation: 'Ferrie *et al.* recognized the occurrence of migraine in only 3 per cent of families of children with occipital epilepsy and this figure is considerable less than what is found in the population at large'. However, in Ferrie *et al.*[277] there is not even a word regarding migraine, there was no such a figure and this was not an epidemiological study.

Giroud and colleagues,1989[339] in a control study found that 'epilepsy with Rolandic paroxysms and migraine have a non-fortuitous association'. The incidence of migraine was studied in four groups of patients: patients with centrotemporal epilepsy, patients with absence epilepsy, patients with partial epilepsy, and non-epileptic patients with a history of cranial trauma. Migraines were present in 62 per cent of the patients with centrotemporal epilepsy, 34 per cent of the patients with absence epilepsy, 8 per cent of the patients with partial epilepsy and 6 per cent of the patients with cranial trauma. According to the authors[339] these results suggest that the association of centrotemporal epilepsy and migraine is non-fortuitous as well as, to a lesser degree, absence epilepsy and migraine. They also discussed the role of serotonin in the association of epilepsy–migraine.

On anecdotal experience, I did not find that children with Rolandic or benign occipital seizures have a higher incidence of migraine. Conversely, also on anecdotal experience, Andermann states that 'Other observers as C. Barlow, G. Waters (personal communication) and myself have confirmed the impression of Bladin[120] that a relationship exists between benign Rolandic epilepsy and migraine'.[37] I am not aware of any such reported controlled studies of the above authors or of Andermann. These are probably clinical impressions which are respected, but so are ours.

These matters cannot be solved without prospective, well controlled epidemiological studies of children with functional, age-related spikes of any location. Until then, I would follow the view that we do not know.

(5) Malignant migraine related to mitochondrial encephalomyopathy

This according to the Andermanns[33,37] is a syndrome of 'Migraine associated with a malignant form of mitochondrial disease affecting the cerebral blood vessels or MELAS syndrome. Migraine attacks, usually common migraine, often follow partial complex seizures and occasionally may precede them'.

I have discussed this in a previous (Chapter 7). Over many years Andermann and his associates[35,40,257] presented the same, approximately 10, patients, to support this syndrome. Most of them have not been confirmed as having MELAS. Also, these patients cannot be characteristic of MELAS where occipital seizures are relatively rare (14 per cent as opposed to 50 per cent of motor partial seizures) despite the predominant occipital involvement of the pathological process. These are seriously ill patients. They have headaches (why should these be migraine?), they have epileptic seizures (these are symptomatic, mainly partial seizures unrelated to headaches and migraine, not bearing any similarity to idiopathic occipital seizures) and they have stroke-like brain manifestations which may also be fatal. Why should this be a syndrome of migraine and occipital epilepsy? It cannot possibly be. Otherwise, we would have numerous and more convincing syndromes of MELAS such as stroke-like episodes with headaches and without headaches, with seizures and without seizures, with myopathy and without myopathy, with dementia and without dementia, with ataxia and without ataxia and so forth. This view of the Andermanns[33,37] can only serve as an exercise, a way of thinking but it is not documented.

(6) Alternating hemiplegia of childhood

According to the Andermanns,[33,37] 'Alternating hemiplegia of infancy has long been suspected to be migraine-related, but the evidence for this has never been conclusive. On the other hand, in our experience, mothers of these children invariably have common migraine'. I am not aware of any report documenting this experience of the Andermanns.[33,37]

(7) Ictal headaches

These also constitute another 'migraine–epilepsy' syndrome according to these authors.[33,37] There should be no doubt that headache may be an ictal event as reviewed in this book. However, why should this ictal headache, often orbital or like an uncomfortable non-specific pain, constitute a migraine–epilepsy syndrome? In this sense we should have hundreds of seizure epilepsy syndromes which also cannot be correct.

Finally, probably less important, there are no characteristic clinical pictures or entities in the proposed migraine–epilepsy syndromes. A syndrome is 'a distinct group of symptoms or signs which, associated together, form a characteristic clinical picture or entirety'.[183]

Migraine–epilepsy? Epilepsy–migraine? or A problem in their differential diagnosis?

It may be appropriate to quote here my conclusions of 1987 that I still support:[602] 'There are many cases, particularly for children, where a distinction between migraine and epilepsy is difficult if not impossible to make. Regarding the relationship between them, the prevailing view that an epileptic seizure might be triggered by a migrainous attack in a susceptible subject cannot be easily ruled out (migraine–epilepsy syndrome). However, the reverse (epilepsy–migraine syndrome) is most likely; that is, an epileptic discharge might trigger a vascular sequence of events in an individual susceptible to migraine, particularly since migraine is a neurovascular reaction in which many chemical transmitter agents appear to be involved.

Finally, a causal relationship between migraine and a secondary 'autonomous' epilepsy should not be accepted without much reservation. There is no evidence that clinical and EEG manifestations of epilepsy deteriorate progressively as would be expected from the frequent 'epileptogenic' insults of migrainous attacks to the brain, recurring sometimes throughout life. It is possible that the link suggested between migraine and epilepsy may reflect the differential diagnostic difficulties between the two diseases.

In conclusion I maintain that: (a) migraine and epilepsy are two entirely different disorders although some symptoms are common to both; (b) most of the cases presented as a migraine–epilepsy syndrome reflect problems in differential diagnosis or are pure coincidence; (c) there is no evidence that migraine, secondarily, causes epilepsy, as this would be expected to result in multiple epileptic foci and a bad prognosis; and (d) there is a strong possibility that epileptic discharges may trigger migrainous phenomena, particularly in children, and the term 'childhood epilepsy with migrainous phenomena and occipital paroxysms' to describe this disorder is proposed.'[602]

Conclusion

Elementary visual hallucinations of idiopathic occipital epilepsy are often associated with blindness and post-ictal headache. The quality and the chronological sequence of ictal elementary visual hallucinations is markedly different from thoses of the visual aura of migraine. Appropriate diagnosis of occipital seizures is of paramount importance regarding investigations and management. The concept of migralepsy or of a migraine–epilepsy sequence needs re-evaluation based on accurate diagnosis. The emerging concept of occipital seizures triggering migrainous headache, which is realistic and better documented, needs consideration and exploration. More importantly, patients with daily visual seizures that may progress to convulsions merit a precise diagnosis and appropriate treatment, probably with carbamazepine. Visual seizures and migraine aura may imitate each other but their true identity cannot easily escape clinical scrutiny. Appendix 1. (page 300) is reproduced from Cephalalgia.[169]

Appendix 1
Classification and diagnostic criteria for migraine with aura and basilar migraine proposed by 'Headache Classification Committee of the International Headache Society'[169]

1.2 Migraine with aura

Previously used terms: Classic migraine, classical migraine, ophthalmic, hemiparesthetic, hemiparetic, or aphasic migraine, migraine accompagnee, complicated migraine.

Description: Idiopathic, recurring disorder manifesting with attacks of neurological symptoms unequivocally localizable to cerebral cortex or brain stem, usually gradually developing over 5–20 min and usually lasting less than 60 min.

Headache, nausea and/or photophobia usually follow neurological aura symptoms directly or after a free interval of less than an hour. The headache usually lasts 4–72 h, but may be completely absent (1.2.5).

Diagnostic criteria:

A. At least two attacks fulfilling B.

B. At least three of the following four characteristics:

1. One or more fully reversible aura symptoms indicating focal cerebral cortical and/or brain stem dysfunction.
2. At least one aura symptom develops gradually over more than 4 min, or two or more symptoms occur in succession.
3. No aura symptom lasts more than 60 min. If more than one aura symptom is present, accepted duration is proportionally increased.
4. Headache follows aura with a free interval of less than 60 min. (It may also begin before or simultaneously with the aura.)

C. At least one of the following:

1. History, physical and neurological examinations do not suggest one of the disorders listed in groups 5–11.

   (Headache associated with head trauma, vascular disorders, non-vascular intercranial disorder, substances or their withdrawal, non-cephalic infection, metabolic disorder, disorder of cranium, neck, eyes, ears, nose, sinuses, teeth, mouth or other facial or cranial structures.)
2. History and/or physical and/or neurological examinations do suggest such disorder, but it is ruled out by appropriate investigations.
3. Such disorder is present, but migraine attacks do not occur for the first time in close temporal relation to the disorder.

Comment: Before or simultaneously with onset of aura symptoms, regional cerebral flow is decreased corresponding to the clinically affected area and often including an even wider area. Blood flow reduction usually starts posteriorly and spreads anteriorly. It is above or at the ischaemic threshold, but not infrequently below. After one to several hours, gradual transition into hyperemia is not related to headache, which usually begins during ischaemia, and may disappear during hyperemia. Cortical arteriolar vasospasm and/or spreading depression of Leao have been implied. Relationship to the headache phase and mechanisms of the headache phase are uncertain (see comment to 1.1).* The

* *The mechanisms of the attack of migraine without aura are as yet poorly understood. Regional cerebral blood flow remains normal or is perhaps slightly increased during an attack. Changes in blood composition and platelet function initiated endogenously or by environmental influences may play a triggering role. The pathophysiological process of the attack is presumed to occur in the brain, which via the trigemino-vascular and other systems interacts with intra- and extracranial vasculature and perivascular spaces.*

cerebral blood flow changes are not fully studied in the subforms, but for several (1.2.1, 1.2.2, 1.2.3, and 1.2.5) there seems to be only quantitative differences. Systematic studies have demonstrated that most patients with visual auras occasionally have symptoms in the extremities. Conversely patients with symptoms in the extremities virtually always also suffer visual aura symptoms. A distinction between ophthalmic migraine and hemiparesthetic/hemiparetic migraine is therefore probably artificial and is not recognized in this classification.

1.2.1 Migraine with typical aura

Previously used terms: Ophthalmic, hemiparetic, hemiparesthetic, hemiparetic, hemiplegic, or aphasic migraine, migraine accompagnee.

Description: Migraine with an aura consisting of homonymous visual disturbances, hemisensory symptoms, hemiparesis or dysphasia or combinations thereof. Gradual development, duration under 1 h and complete reversibility characterize the aura which is associated with headache.

Diagnostic criteria:

A. Fulfils criteria for 1.2 including all four criteria under B.

B. One or more aura symptoms of the following types:

1. Homonymous visual disturbance
2. Unilateral paresthesias and/or numbness
3. Unilateral weakness
4. Aphasia or unclassifiable speech difficulty.

***Comment*:** This is the commonest form of migraine with aura,

1.2.4 Basilar migraine

***Previously used terms*:** Basilar artery migraine, Bickerstaff's migraine, syncopal migraine.

***Description*:** Migraine with aura symptoms clearly originating from the brain stem or from both occipital lobes.

Diagnostic criteria

A. Fulfils criteria for 1.2 (migraine with aura).*

B. Two or more aura symptoms of the following types:

Visual symptoms in both the temporal and nasal fields of both eyes

Dysarthria, vertigo, tinnitus, decreased hearing, double vision, ataxia, bilateral

Paresthesias, bilateral pareses, decreased level of consciousness.

***Comment*:** Many of the symptoms listed under diagnostic criteria are subject to misinterpretation as they may occur with anxiety and hyperventilation.

Originally the term basilar artery migraine was used, but since spasm of the basilar artery may not be a mechanism of the attacks, the term basilar migraine should be preferred. Many cases have basilar attacks intermingled with attacks with typical aura. Basilar attacks are mostly seen in young adults.

1.2.5 Migraine aura without headache

Previously used terms: Migraine equivalents, acephalgic migraine.

***Description*:** Migrainous aura unaccompanied by headache.

Diagnostic criteria:

A. Fulfils criteria for 1.2 (migraine with aura).*

B. No headache.

***Comment*:** It is common for migraine with aura that headache is occasionally absent. As patients get older (*see footnote on p. 300), headache may disappear completely even if auras continue. It is less common to have always suffered exclusively from migraine aura without headache. When the onset occurs after the age of forty and for other reasons, the distinction between this entity and the thromboembolic transient ischaemic attacks may be difficult and require extensive investigations. Acute onset aura without headache is not sufficiently validated.

1.2.6 Migraine with acute onset aura

Description: Migraine with aura developing fully in less than 5 min.

Diagnostic criteria:

A. Fulfils criteria for 1.2 (migraine with aura).*

B. Neurological symptoms develop within 4 min.

C. Headache lasts for 4 to 72 h (untreated or unsuccessfully treated).

D. Headache has at least two of the following characteristics:

1. Unilateral location
2. Pulsating quality
3. Moderate or severe intensity (inhibits or prohibits daily activities)
4. Aggravation by walking stairs or similar routine physical activity.

E. During headache at least one of the following:

1. Nausea and/or vomiting
2. Photophobia and phonophobia.

F. Thromboembolic TIA and other intracranial lesion ruled out by appropriate investigations.

***Comment*:** Inaccurate history is the most common explanation of acute onset aura. Acute onset should be confirmed by repeated close questioning and preferably by prospective observation. Presence of a typical headache phase is required and the diagnosis is supported by previous migraine attacks of other type or a strong family history. Extensive investigations are usually necessary to rule out thromboembolic TIA.

Benign Childhood Partial Seizures and Related Epileptic Syndromes. C P Panayiotopoulos
©1999 John Libbey & Company Ltd., pp. 303–308.

Chapter 15

Basilar migraine: a review

Definition

Basilar migraine is characterized by transient and fully reversible aura symptoms indicating focal dysfunction of the brain stem, the occipital lobes or both, followed by headache.[106,108,392,470,741,747] Common neurological symptoms of aura include visual phenomena, mainly bilateral blurring or blindness, dizziness, vertigo and tinnitus, ataxia, bilateral weakness and dysaesthesia, diplopia, dysarthria and decreased hearing. Aura symptoms develop gradually over 4 min and last for less than 30 min to 1 h. Impairment or loss of consciousness without convulsions may occur in one quarter of patients between the aura and the headache phase. Impairment of consciousness is usually mild and brief, lasting 1 to 10 min, but in rare circumstances it may be profound and last for days. Headache usually follows but may also precede or occur simultaneously with the aura symptoms. The headache is bilateral, severe, often throbbing, mainly occipital and often combined with photo and phonophobia, nausea and vomiting. The headache phase may be prolonged for 2–6 h or longer. Frequency of the attacks varies from 1 to 2 per week, more often one or less per month, to 2–3 per life. Precipitating factors include emotions, stress, menstruation, weather changes, head injury, alcohol and food, contraceptive drugs, smoking and physical strain.

Prognosis varies from only a few age-related attacks to persistent attacks for years, often associated with other types of migraine with or without aura. Rarely cerebral infarcts may occur during a basilar migraine attack. Basilar migraine is more frequent amongst children and especially adolescents than older people. Two thirds of sufferers are women.

Basilar migraine is usually not associated with other neurological diseases but may be linked with familial hemiplegic migraine, familial episodic ataxia type 2 and CADASIL.

Visual symptoms in basilar migraine. Following a review of basilar migraine it is apparent that, with a few exceptions,[106,470,741] visual symptoms are not described in detail: 'dimming of vision or blindness',[106] 'bilateral visual impairment in temporal and nasal visual fields of both eyes, transient amaurosis, diffuse reduction of vision (blurred vision, foggy vision, "everything gray"), tunnel vision, inferior hemianopia',[741] 'scotomata, transient bilateral blindness or blurred vision'[741] and 'tunnel vision, total amblyopia, and bilateral positive and negative hallucinations, including teichopsia'[392] predominate. Elementary visual hallucinations are usually bilateral and are described as 'teichopsia',[106,392] 'flashes or blobs of light'[108] or 'positive phenomena (flickering, flashes, teichopsia, coloured figures, dysmorphopsia)'.[741] In only one of the reported cases are 'colourful displays' mentioned.[747] Bilateral visual impairment is common to as many as 86 per cent of the patients.[741] The attacks of basilar migraine are usually infrequent and over the years there is a tendency for them to cease or to be replaced by common varieties of migraine with or without aura.[106]

A typical case of basilar migraine

Probably the best example is case 1 of Bickerstaff:[106] 'A 13-year-old girl had had four menstrual periods, and three days after the end of each had had an attack in which she experienced vivid flashes of light throughout the whole visual field in both eyes. These flashes were sufficiently intense to obscure her vision completely. At the same time she had tingling in both hands and both feet, and her speech became so slurred as to be barely intelligible. She then became ataxic on attempting to walk. These symptoms lasted 15 min and then subsided, and were followed by severe throbbing occipital headache and vomiting. After vomiting, she felt better, and would sleep for several hours and awaken free from headache.

Her father and an aunt had severe migraine.

Electroencephalograms were normal, and treatment with properazine during the postmenstrual week has relieved her of these symptoms for six months.

Introduction

The original description of 'basilar artery migraine' by Edwin Bickerstaff is a classic and recommended reading.[106–108] The condition was later re-named 'basilar migraine' because the 'spasm of the basilar artery may not be the mechanism of the attacks' and it was classified as 'migraine with aura symptoms clearly originating from the brain stem or from both occipital lobes'.[169]

Basilar migraine has been the subject of many studies,[106–108,148,266,346,392,413,415,470,548,640,741,747] and more than 50 case reports.[30,50,59,100,103,137,151,172,231,248,265,281,293,297,298,336,411,412,416,463,469,472,473,530,543,643,653,656,714,717,724,734,742,743,769,828,829] The label is often applied to a patient with reversible brain stem symptoms when neuroradiological and cerebrospinal fluid examinations are normal, and it is likely that not all reported cases are basilar migraine. The possible overlap or precipitation of epileptic seizures by basilar migraine was, in the original descriptions [107,108] and continues to be, the subject of debate.[33,34,37,76,82,84,146,212,213,215,263,525,599,602,611,625,734,765,766] More recently, considerable interest has been attracted in the possible association of basilar migraine with hemiplegic migraine[374,764] and the occurrence of episodes typical of basilar migraine in patients with familial episodic ataxia type 2[62] or with cerebral autosomal dominant arteriopathy with subcortical infarcts and leucoencephalopathy (CADASIL).[157–159,233,669,696,803]

The purpose of this chapter is to review basilar migraine and explore its relation with occipital lobe epilepsy, familial episodic ataxia type 2, familial hemiplegic migraine and CADASIL.

Clinical aspects[106–108,148,156,336,346,392,416,470,548,741,747]

Basilar migraine mainly occurs in young women and children, frequently in the context of a family history of other forms of migraine.[106,470,741] Age at onset is from 4 months[392] to 62 years [741] and in more than 70 per cent it starts in the first or second decade of life. Two thirds of patients are women. Basilar migraine clinically manifests with bilateral visual symptoms associated with vertigo, ataxia, tinnitus, bilateral weakness and peripheral dysaesthesias, and sometimes other brain stem and occipital lobe symptoms. This is followed by severe, throbbing, posterior bilateral headache.

The aura symptoms of basilar migraine

The sequence of events and the clinical manifestations are well described by Bickerstaff:[108] 'The features of this syndrome have been that in an attack the patients first develop visual phenomena which differ a little from those of common migraine in that they consist either of dimming or loss of vision in the whole of both visual fields or, if there are positive phenomena, they are more often flashes or blobs of light, than the typical fortification spectra, and again affect the whole of both visual fields, often being of an intensity sufficient to blot out vision. This stage is rapidly followed by vertigo, unsteadiness of gait, occasionally tinnitus, by a speech disturbance which is undoubtedly dysarthria and not dysphasia, and by tingling in the periphery of the hands and feet on both sides, and sometimes around both sides of the mouth. These symptoms last 10–30 min and are followed by severe headache which is usually occipital.'[108]

According to Bickertaff [107,108] the aura symptoms last from two to a maximum of 45 min, usually 10–30 min, and then subside rapidly. Complete loss of vision disappears more gradually, over 5 min, through a period of greying vision. Sturzenegger and Meienberg (1985)[741] found that aura lasts for 5–60 min in 75 per cent of the patients but they also may be as short as 3 min and as long as 60 h. In children, the duration of the attacks, including the headache phase, is from minutes to many hours; the majority last less than 3–4 h.[470]

Visual aura

These are described in the definition. Although bilateral visual impairment is common, amounting to 86 per cent of the patients in one study,[741] neither every patient nor every basilar migraine attack has visual symptoms. In some reports, seven of 49 adult patients[741] and 16 of 30 children[470] did not have visual symptoms. In another study of basilar migraine in 28 children,[392] visual symptoms occurred in 14 and were described as 'tunnel vision, total amblyopia, and bilateral positive and negative hallucinations, including teichopsia.' Patients with basilar migraine may independently have episodes of migraine with aura as detailed in the relevant chapters.

Neurological symptoms (other than visual)

In basilar migraine, Bickerstaff[106] described 'vertigo, ataxia of gait, dysarthria, and occasionally tinnitus – not necessarily in this order and the ataxia was not necessarily associated with vertigo. Sensory manifestations consisted of tingling or numbness in the periphery of both hands and both feet, and sometimes around both lips and on both sides of the tongue'.

According to Sturzenegger and Meienberg (1985)[741] the commonest symptoms of aura are vertigo (63 per cent), gait ataxia (63 per cent), bilateral paraesthesia (61 per cent), bilateral weakness (57 per cent) and dysarthria (57 per cent).

In children, vertigo and staggering gait are the commonest neurological symptoms,[392,470] while cranial (mainly oculo-motor) nerve impairment occurs in severe cases.[392] Bilateral pyramidal symptoms and dysaesthesia are less frequent.

Headache, nausea and vomiting[107,108,470,741]

Headache follows the visual and neurological symptoms but in 10–30 per cent it may precede or coincide with the aura. The headache is usually severe, bilateral, posterior and pulsating. It is often associated with nausea or vomiting, photophobia and phonophobia. It lasts for 2–6 h (80 per cent)[741] but may be shorter or last for days.[107,108,392,470,741] The headache may also be bifrontal or bitemporal and less severe.

Episodic neurological symptoms may also occur without headache and can also be independent of aura.[470] Some patients never have migraine headaches.[470]

Impairment of consciousness

A quarter of patients have impairment or loss of consciousness without convulsions, usually between the aura and the headache, although impairment of consciousness may precede the other symptoms.[106,107] In one study[741] disorders of consciousness, mainly syncope, confusion and prolonged amnesia, occurred in 77 per cent of the patients. Impairment of consciousness is usually brief, lasting from 1 to 10 min, 'with features distinguished from epilepsy', as described by Bickerstaff:[107] 'The loss of consciousness is described as curiously slow in onset – never abrupt, and never causing the patient to fall or to be injured. A dreamlike state sometimes precedes impairment of consciousness. The degree of impairment of consciousness was never profound but the patients were never unrousable; on vigorous stimulation they could be aroused to co-operate but they returned to unconsciousness when the stimulation ceased.'[107]

Hockaday[392] found impairment of consciousness in 13 of 28 children with basilar migraine. This included loss of consciousness, feeling of faintness, atonic drop attacks, and profound sleep from which the patient could not be fully roused, but excluded postural syncope occurring only in the later headache phase of the attack.[392] Alteration of consciousness, observed in six of 30 children, was brief and without convulsions in one study[470] but in other studies[137,156] 12 children had loss of consciousness lasting from 1 h to one or more days.

Frequency of the basilar migraine attacks

The attacks of basilar migraine are usually infrequent and over the years there is a tendency for them to cease or to be replaced by common varieties of migraine with or without aura.[106] Women may have catamenial symptoms. Sturzenegger and Meienberg[741] found that the frequency of attacks varied considerably from patient to patient. Twenty eight of 49 patients had fewer than one attack per month and four had only one attack during an observation period of 6 months to 5 years. In patients with isolated basilar migraine, 11 of 20 had three attacks a year or less, whereas in patients who also had other migraine attacks, seven of 11 had two or more of any type of migraine per month.

In children, attack frequency also varies, with some experiencing as many as three per week and others only one to two attacks during an observation period of up to 3 years.[470]

Precipitating factors

The relationship to menstruation was described in Bickerstaff's original report.[106] Sturzenegger and Meienberg[741]studied precipitating factors in detail for 49 patients. In 35 patients these included emotion (25), stress (18), menstruation (12 of 32 females), weather changes (nine), head injury (seven), food (five), contraceptive drugs (four), smoking (two) and physical strain (two). In four patients basilar migraine attacks were initiated by head injury.[741]

Other type of attacks

Forty per cent of patients have isolated basilar migraine attacks, the remainder also experience other types of migraine.[741]

Unusual cases of basilar migraine with severe and prolonged impairment of consciousness, cerebral infarction or global amnesia

There are a few case reports of prolonged impairment of consciousness and coma[281,293,548] as well as cerebral infarction[100,148] attributed to basilar migraine.

Electroencephalography

The EEG between attacks is usually reported as normal, occasionally with borderline or non-specific abnormalities such as bursts of theta waves.[106–108,293,413,470,548,640,741,747] In four studies[106,413,470,741] from 137 children and adults with basilar migraine who had routine or 24-h ambulatory cassette EEG, 115 (84 per cent) were normal and 17 (12.4 per cent) were borderline or with non-specific paroxysmal theta activity. Five patients (3.6 per cent) had abnormal EEG sharp activity during photic stimulation (one patient), paroxysmal activity in the posterior regions (one patient), paroxysmal 'epileptogenic' activity (two patients) and generalized spikes (one patient).

The following EEG abnormalities have also been reported: Posterior rhythmic delta activity in close temporal proximity to the attacks of basilar migraine, later resolving in two children,[469,470] predominantly localized or generalized mainly paroxysmal slow wave activity in nine adults,[741] diffuse slow wave activity of higher amplitude posteriorly in eight children predominantly unilateral in five,[137,156] high amplitude monomorphic slow posterior activity in nine children and adolescents, often asymmetrical and often attenuating when eyes were open[84] and prominent posterior slowing in one woman.[297] Beaumanoir and Jekiel[84] differentiated the monomorphic and reactive slow EEG activity associated with basilar migraine attacks from the polymorphic/monomorphic, non-reactive ictal EEG abnormalities of migraine with visual aura.

The EEG during attacks of basilar migraine is usually dominated by symmetrical high amplitude slow waves which are more abundant in the posterior regions and persist for days or a week after remission.[84,297,469,470,543,548, 640,643,731,747] Parain *et al.*[640] had different findings. They described eight patients with excessive generalized beta activity during the basilar migraine attacks. The EEG returned to normal within 1–3 days after the clinical symptoms subsided. Jacome[413] found no EEG abnormalities during the 'symptomatic period' in seven patients although in one adolescent photoparoxysmal discharges were present. In a patient with '3–10 days life-threatening coma', the ictal EEG showed burst-suppression pattern and frontal intermittent rhythmic delta activity.[293]

Ictal EEG of a patient and his sister with basilar migraine-like attacks of familial episodic ataxia type 2 showed paroxysmal high amplitude, slow and sharp wave activity.[62]

Brain imaging, transcranial Doppler and brain SPECT[293,415,463,472,543,714,829]

Brain CT scan and brain MRI are normal or manifest minor non-specific abnormalities in patients with basilar migraine[415] except in those who develop cerebral infarcts. Brain MRI of 18 patients with 'non-epileptiform' basilar migraine was normal.[415] In a few subjects, mild enlargement of the cortical sulci and white matter MRI T2-weighted increased signal intensity were present.[415]

La Spina *et al.*[463] performed transcranial Doppler ultrasonography, EEG and single photon emission computed tomography (SPECT) in a case of basilar migraine during the different phases of the attack. In the aura phase, the patient had bilateral blindness and ataxia. Doppler ultrasonography demonstrated reduced mean flow velocity of blood within the posterior cerebral arteries, EEG showed slow activity confined to the posterior regions, and SPECT an area of hypoperfusion in the right parietal and occipital regions. During the headache phase, when neurological examination was normal, transcranial Doppler showed an increase in the mean flow velocity of both posterior cerebral arteries and the EEG revealed an occipital increase in slow activity. When the pain subsided, the EEG showed a progressive reduction of slow waves and transcranial Doppler became normal. After a week, SPECT and cranial MRI were normal. After a month, a follow-up EEG was also normal.

Seto *et al.*[714] reported a case of basilar migraine in a 33-year-old woman who had normal MRI and cerebral angiography. A Tc–99m HMPAO brain SPECT when she was unconscious showed a significant decrease of regional cerebral blood flow in the right temporal and occipital lobes and right cerebellar hemisphere. SPECT during a symptom-free phase was normal.

Basilar migraine, familial hemiplegic migraine, familial episodic ataxia type 2, and CADASIL

There is renewed interest in basilar migraine because affected members of three autosomal dominant diseases linked to chromosome 19 may also have basilar migraine symptoms. These are episodic familial hemiplegic migraine, episodic ataxia type 2, and CADASIL.

Familial hemiplegic migraine (FHM) is a rare autosomal dominant type of migraine with aura. A gene for FHM has been assigned to chromosome 19p13 for 50 per cent of the families tested and FHM shown to be a Ca^{2+} channelopathy allelic to episodic ataxia type 2.[13,264,373,424,425,427,587,588] Onset of FHM is at a mean age of 10 years. Attacks of migrainous headache are associated with photophobia, phonophobia, nausea and vomiting following or preceding hemiparesis, and other aura symptoms such as dysarthria or aphasia, unilateral numbness or visual hallucinations. Hemiparesis lasts for more than an hour, sometimes for weeks, may alternate from side to side and occasionally weakness may be bilateral. Visual hallucinations consist of 'blurred vision, dark spots, flashing lights, zigzag lines, tunnel or double vision'.[373] Less frequently, ataxia, confusion, dizziness, blindness and loss of consciousness may occur during the attacks. Progressive cerebellar ataxia may occur in some patients usually in the 5th decade of life. Familial hemiplegic migraine linked to chromosome 19 and familial hemiplegic migraine unlinked to chromosome 19 do not differ in clinical features.[764] However, an association with cerebellar ataxia has only been described in chromosome 19-linked families.

Several of the clinical features of FHM frequently show similarities with those of basilar migraine which made some authors suggest that FHM may be a form of basilar migraine,[402,791] and it has recently been proposed that FHM and basilar migraine are genetically linked[374] though this is controversial.[534]

Haan *et al.* (1995)[374] studied aura symptoms in 83 patients from six unrelated families suffering from familial hemiplegic migraine. Fifty-five of the patients reported symptoms meeting the criteria of basilar migraine. Conversely, in a control group of 33 patients suffering from migraine with aura and 33 patients suffering from migraine without aura, only nine patients complained of vertigo and only one patient had diplopia during one attack. None of these control patients fulfilled the criteria for basilar migraine. The authors suggested that 'familial hemiplegic migraine and basilar migraine may share certain pathophysiologic mechanisms, which may consist of a (genetically determined) disturbance of basilar artery blood flow'.

Episodic ataxia and interictal nystagmus (EA–2), allelic with FHM, is an autosomal dominant Ca^{2+} channelopathy linked to chromosome 19p13.[62,587,779] Attacks of ataxia lasting for hours are usually triggered by emotional upset and physical exertion. Acetazolamide is usually highly effective. Baloh *et al.* (1997)[62] described the clinical and oculographic findings in four families with episodic ataxia and interictal nystagmus (EA–2) linked to chromosome 19p. Episodes varied from pure ataxia to combinations of symptoms suggesting involvement of the cerebellum, brainstem and cortex. These may consist of a combination of vertigo, ataxia, visual loss, bilateral weakness and numbness. In addition, one half of the patients reported headaches meeting the criteria for migraine and seven patients had attacks which could be classified as basilar migraine. The age at onset varies from 3 to 45 years of age with the majority starting before the second decade of life. About one-half of the affected individuals had migraine headaches and several had episodes typical of basilar migraine.

CADASIL is the abbreviated term for Cerebral Autosomal Dominant Arteriopathy with Subcortical Infarcts and Leucoencephalopathy which is invariably linked to chromosome 19p13. It does not appear to be allelic with FHM and A–2.[138,157,159,199,233,405,426,511,696,803] The onset of the disease is usually in the fourth decade and it is characterized by recurrent subcortical infarcts and stepwise progressive neurological deficits leading to dementia, severe disability and early death. MRI abnormalities are found in individual members of the families with CADASIL before the development of clinical symptoms. Many patients of families with CADASIL suffer from migraine with or without aura and basilar migraine attacks prior to the onset of the strokes.[62,778,789] FHM and CADASIL have been described in the same family.[405]

Basilar migraine and occipital seizures (spontaneous, photically induced or both)

It is apparent from this review of basilar migraine that the symptoms of this disorder/syndrome are markedly different from occipital seizures, which substantiates my view that "the commonly cited occurrence of basilar migraine with occipital paroxysms and seizures is an erroneous association'. This has been detailed in Chapter 14, 292–294.

Part V

Other benign childhood partial seizures with the exceptional severe syndromes of mainly linguistic and neuropsychological deficits, seizures or both

Benign Childhood Partial Seizures and Related Epileptic Syndromes. C P Panayiotopoulos
©1999 John Libbey & Company Ltd., pp. 311–335.

Chapter 16

Other phenotypic variants of benign childhood partial seizure susceptibility syndrome

Though Rolandic seizures and Panayiotopoulos syndrome appear to be the main clinical representatives of benign childhood partial seizures, other clinical phenotypes also exist. This is expected as functional sharp and slow wave foci, the EEG marker of the benign childhood seizure susceptibility syndrome, may also occur in other than the centrotemporal and occipital locations either alone or together. It is also possible that the clinical expression of these spike foci is influenced not only by location but also by age at seizure onset, as may be the case with late onset occipital seizures. This is also expected as the result of the level of maturation of the seizure-generating structures alone or together with those at other locations where the ictal discharge may be able to spread. The most likely clinical phenotypes, other than Rolandic and occipital, are described in this chapter.

Benign partial epilepsy with affective symptoms ('benign psychomotor epilepsy')

This is a very interesting variation of benign childhood partial seizures described mainly by Dalla Bernardina and colleagues[189,191] who also acknowledged similar cases reported by Plouin, Lerique and Dulac, 1980[661] and Dulac with Arthuis 1980.[253] In their first report on 'affective symptoms during attacks of epilepsy in children', Dalla Bernardina, Bureau, Dravet, Dulac, Tassinari and Roger, 1980[189] reported 'an electroclinical study of 20 children (16 girls and four boys) having 'epileptic attacks with affective symptoms of a terrifying type'. These were often interpreted (6/20) initially as nocturnal terrors or acute anxiety attacks. Eight patients (40 per cent) had a family history of epilepsy. The age at onset was between 2 and 10 years. The attacks occurred several times during the 24 h period, both day and night, but were controlled rapidly and permanently (four children over 15 years of age have had no further attacks 4 years after discontinuing treatment), and neurological and intellectual development was normal. This benign progression was correlated with a homogeneous ictal and interictal electroclinical picture enabling an early favourable prognosis to be made. They discussed the classification of this type of epilepsy and its analogy to epilepsy with centrotemporal spikes.

The following description of this syndorme is based on an excellent publication by Dalla Bernardina, Colamaria, Chiamenti, Capovilla, Trevisan and Tassinari, 1992[191] detailing their long clinico-EEG experience.

They reported 26 otherwise normal children who experienced frequent seizures with affective symptoms; interictal EEG had fronto-temporal or parieto-temporal sharp waves and the prognosis was excellent. All patients had normal neurological and intellectual state with normal brain CT scan.

Ictal clinical manifestations

The predominant seizure symptom is sudden fright or terror. 'This terror was expressed by the child starting to scream, to yell or to call his mother (12 cases); he clung to her or to anyone nearby (14 cases) or went to a corner of the room hiding his face in his hands (three cases). This terrorized expression was sometimes associated with either chewing or swallowing movements (six cases), distressed laughter (four cases), arrest of speech with glottal noises, moans and salivation (six cases) or some kind of autonomic manifestations such as pallor, sweating or abdominal pain, that the child expressed by bringing his hands on to his abdomen and saying "It hurts me, it hurts me" (seven cases). These phenomena were associated with changes in awareness (loss of contact) that did not amount to complete unconsciousness.'

The seizures were brief, of a mean duration between 1 and 2 min and maximum 10 min. There were no post-ictal deficits other than drowsiness and fatigue.

Half of the children had frequent, several times a day, seizures from onset and these could occur with the same semeiology while awake or asleep.

Other seizures

Four children had brief and infrequent nocturnal orofacial clonic seizures in the same period as they suffered affective attacks. Tonic, clonic, tonic–clonic or atonic fits never occurred either during the active seizure period or later during the long follow-up.

Behavioural and cognitive problems during the active seizure period

At the time of frequent seizures, some children had major behavioural problems which in three cases were also associated with cognitive impairment.

Age and sex

Of the 26 patients 14 were girls. Age at onset of afebrile seizures ranged from 2 to 9 years, 'unevenly distributed with two peaks: the first between 2 and 5 years and the second between 6 and 9 years'.

Age at last examination was 7–17 years, mean 12 years.

Febrile convulsions and family history

Five children (19 per cent) had brief febrile convulsions which were generalized (three patients) or unilateral (two patients) without post-ictal defects.

Familial antecedents of epilepsy were present in 38.3 per cent of cases.

Electroencephalography

Interictal EEG

Fronto-temporal or parieto-temporal spikes, morphologically similar to the centrotemporal spikes, occurred in 19 (73 per cent) of the patients. These spikes were unilateral or bilateral, were activated by sleep and had a great tendency to appear and disappear throughout the course of the disease. In 57.6 per cent the only paroxysmal abnormalities, at least during the first months of evolution, were characterized by rhythmic sharp waves in the fronto-temporal or in the parieto-temporal areas of one hemisphere.

Brief bursts of generalized discharges of spike wave, alone or in association with one of the two types of the above focal abnormalities, occurred in 57.6 per cent of the patients. These could appear during drowsiness but never increased in frequency during slow sleep.

The background activity of awake and sleep EEG was entirely normal, even during the periods of frequent seizures.

Four of the seven patients who did not have interictal sharp waves had a relatively bad prognosis.

Ictal EEG

In 19 cases one or several seizures were recorded during waking, sleep or both.

In 15 patients the ictal discharges were clearly localized in fronto-temporal, centrotemporal or parietal areas. In the other four cases, the discharges were more diffuse without recognisable localized onset. Polygraphic records showed that the attacks were associated with various movements but never of a tonic or clonic type. For the same child, the ictal pattern was relatively stereotyped irrespective of whether the seizure occurred while awake or during sleep.

Treatment and evolution

Three patients with infrequent seizures were not treated. In all but two of the other 23 children, monotherapy with carbamazepine or phenobarbitone was effective even if delayed for 6 to 18 months. In two cases, infrequent attacks persisted for some months or years despite treatment but ultimately disappeared.

Nine cases, aged more than 13 years and off treatment for 1 or more years, did not have any further seizures.

Though at the time of frequent seizures, some children had major behavioural problems, associated in three cases with intellectual retardation, final output was excellent in all. In their last examination patients were normal without any intellectual or physical deficits. Also they did not have significant social or school difficulties.

Clinico-EEG symptoms of patients with less favourable prognosis

Dalla Bernardina *et al.*[191] provided a long follow-up of 21 patients with 'benign partial epilepsy with affective symptoms'. Sixteen subjects, aged between 15 and 28 years, were off medication and seizure free. Five patients, two were girls, aged over 18 years suffered from more or less frequent seizures despite treatment. Of these five patients one had a brain tumour, four did not have fronto-temporal or parieto-temporal spikes, and one with typical right centrotemporal spikes also had a focus of slow waves in the contralateral parietal region and brief bursts of generalized photoconvulsive discharges of spike-wave. Also, four patients had seizures 'characterized at onset by more or less important and variable "subjective" symptoms described at the end of the attacks', in one case the seizures were characterized by a significant post-ictal unilateral deficit for several minutes and 'in another case the seizures were characterized by an additional rotatory component'. Furthermore, ictal discharges in three cases were characterized at onset by a brief focal 'flattening' of the EEG activity.

Based on these observations of five cases that did not have a favourable prognosis, Dalla Bernardina *et al.*[191] concluded that the diagnosis of 'benign partial epilepsy with affective symptoms' is possible when there are no other but affective ictal symptoms, i.e. interictal abnormalities like centrotemporal spikes are present in the absence of slow wave abnormalities and of any polymorphism of the ictal discharge.

Differential diagnosis and misdiagnosis

This syndrome may be misdiagnosed as non-epileptic fear attacks, pavor nocturnus or a behavioural disorder. This is particularly the case for children with affective seizures who also have behavioural and cognitive symptoms and a normal EEG.

According to Dalla Bernardina *et al.*[191] the following features make the diagnosis relatively easy:

(a) In the majority of the cases frequent seizures occurring both during waking and while asleep are stereotyped. The nocturnal seizures usually appear on falling asleep, whereas pavor nocturnus mainly occurs during slow sleep.

(b) The manifestations of affective seizures are different from that of pavor nocturnus.

(c) The high frequency of the attacks makes ictal recordings possible, thus providing incontrovertible diagnostic evidence.

Relation with the benign childhood partial seizure susceptibility syndrome

The excellent prognosis of these patients makes 'benign partial epilepsy with affective symptoms' a benign syndrome of childhood and most likely a rare phenotypic expression of the benign childhood partial seizure susceptibility syndrome because of the age-related onset and active seizure duration, frequent personal history of febrile convulsions and familial epileptic antecedents, occurrence of other seizure types of nocturnal orofacial clonic seizures, and the morphology of focal paroxysmal abnormalities and their activation by sleep.

Dalla Bernardina *et al.*[191] stated that 'From the nosological point of view it is possible to discuss whether this epilepsy does or does not represent a separate form of idiopathic partial epilepsy. In fact, the predominance of fear over other ictal manifestations probably has not in itself an independent predictive value which is greater than that of any other ictal symptom occurring in a similar clinical context. From the practical point of view we consider that the homogeneous electroclinical pattern described above may lead the clinician to the proper diagnosis and therefore permits an early favourable prognosis to be set.' They considered that 'benign partial epilepsy with affective symptoms' does not constitute an independent form of idiopathic partial epilepsy but probably only a relatively rare variant of Rolandic seizures.[191]

Personal experience

I have not seen any definite case of the clinical and EEG features of benign partial epilepsy with affective symptoms. This may indicate that this is very rare or that these children are not referred to an epileptologist because of misdiagnosis. The closest example of this syndrome I came across is of a child that we have reported as 'an aggressive seizure and behavioural disorder following trivial head injury.'[641] Parents often attribute their child's seizures to a trivial head injury. It is our practice to disregard this association. This is the first child in whom such a relation was evident. It could not be coincidental that an aggressive seizure and behavioural disorder erupted within hours of an injury and remitted within months. We speculated that the centrotemporal spikes found in an EEG performed at a stage of clinical remission explained his susceptibility to a trivial head injury with a response similar to that of the benign childhood epilepsy with affective symptoms.[641]

> Case 16.1 This boy, born in July 1989, was well with normal development until the age of 6 years. At 8 p.m. one evening while on his bicycle in his home, he collided with another child, fell off his bicycle and hit his head on the marble floor. There was no laceration or loss of consciousness, but he cried for several minutes. He went to bed normally but on awakening looked unwell and 10 min later had a partial seizure. He walked away from his mother 'as if he did not know where he was going', his lips became blue, he salivated and was incontinent. During the next 12 h he had a further four partial seizures with one progressing to secondary generalization. On admission to a paediatric hospital he received intravenous diazepam and oral carbamazepine was initiated at 10 mg/kg daily. His neurological state, skull x-ray, EEG and CT brain scan were normal. Comprehensive haematological, biochemical and viral investigations including examination of his CSF were normal.
>
> His behaviour changed dramatically, his parents described him as 'intolerable', and there was severe impairment of concentration and learning ability. Four days later he started to have numerous, brief (up to 1 min), nocturnal and diurnal seizures consisting of frightened laughter, impairment of consciousness, rhythmic tremor of the lips and occasionally incontinence of urine. We have reviewed these seizures which were captured by the parents with a camcorder.
>
> Video-EEG of one of the seizures was described as showing 'fixation of gaze and automatisms accompa-

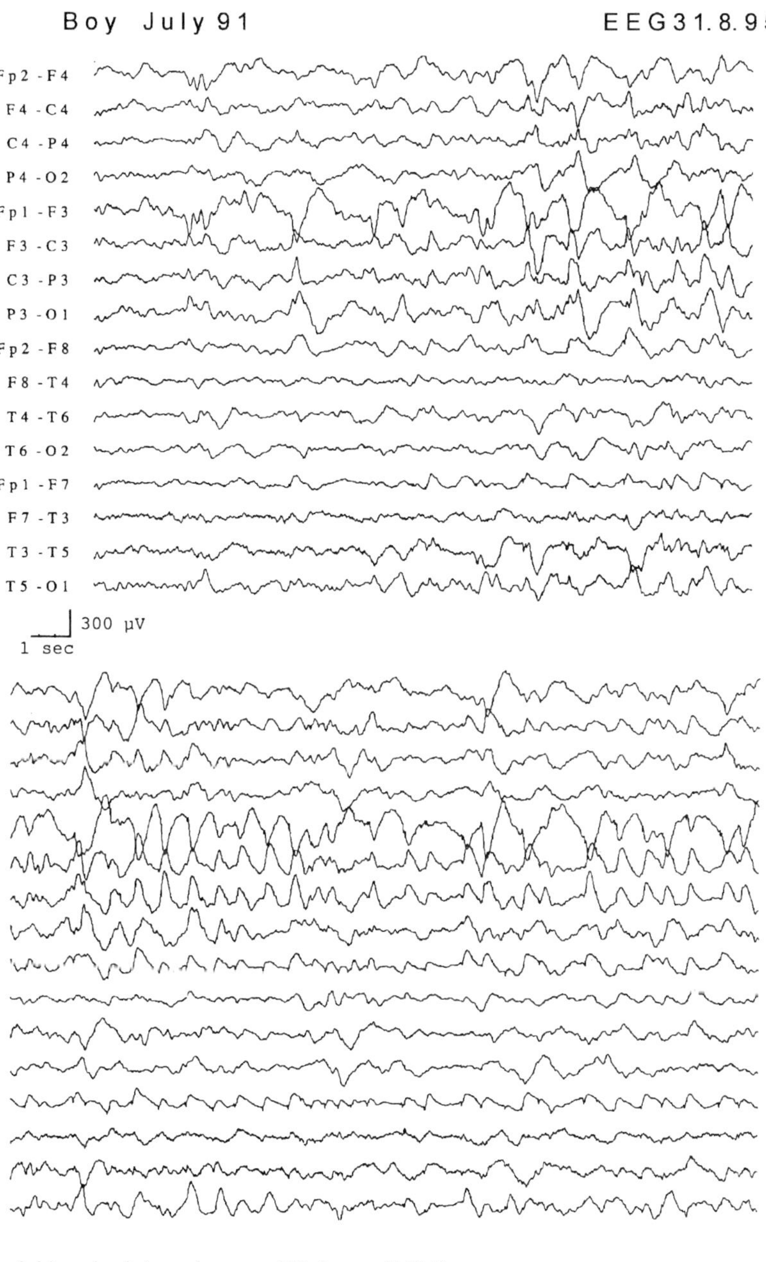

Fig. 16.1. From all-night video-EEG of a boy born July 1991 (case 16.1), 4 months after onset of symptoms (August 1995).
During sleep, there were three electrical seizures of repetitive spikes and spike-slow waves in the left frontal electrode lasting for 2–3 min. There were no detectable clinical events.
Upper: Onset with small spikes in Fp1–F3.
Lower: 45 s later, spikes and high amplitude slow waves at 2 Hz in the left fronto-central electrodes.

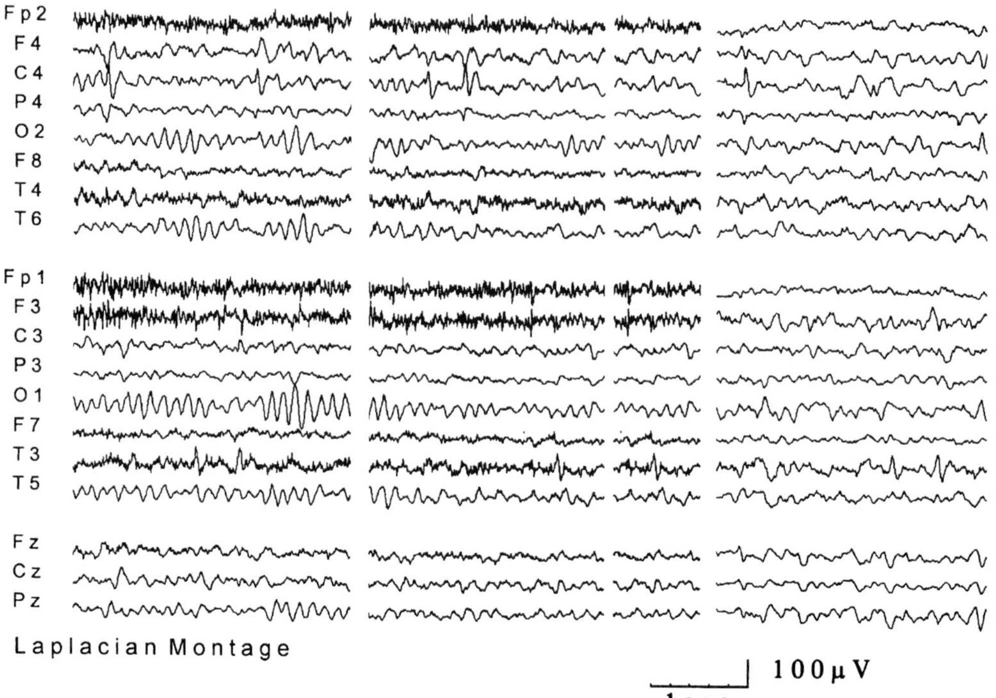

Fig. 16.2. All-night video-EEG recording of the same patient (case 16.1), one year (July 1996) after the first EEG of Fig. 16.1. The child was asymptomatic at this stage.
There are right central (C4) and left mid-temporal (T3) spikes. No frontal spikes or slow waves were seen.

nied by diffuse slow waves at 2 Hz. The background had an alpha rhythm at 7–8 Hz and bilateral runs of delta with left anterior emphasis'. High resolution MRI was performed twice and was normal.

Neither his seizures nor his behaviour changed when carbamazepine was substituted with sodium valproate. However, 2 months later seizures stopped when ox-carbazepine was added to sodium valproate. At this stage, an all-night video-EEG showed three electrical seizures of repetitive spikes and spike-slow waves in the left frontal electrode lasting for 2–3 min (Fig. 16.1). There were no detectable clinical events. In addition there were long runs of high amplitude delta waves in the left anterior quadrant.

His abnormal behaviour started to improve 1 month after cessation of seizures and he was normal 4 months later. On review, 1 year after injury, he has had no further seizures and his behaviour and school progress are normal. EEG recorded during all-night natural sleep was well organized with frequent medium amplitude sharp and slow waves localized around the right central electrode and less frequently in the left midtemporal electrode (Fig. 16.2).

Benign partial epilepsy with extreme somatosensory evoked potentials and Benign childhood epilepsy with parietal spikes

Introduction

Extreme somatosensory evoked potentials (ESEP) is an interesting EEG situation which was first described, extensively studied and well documented by De Marco[201–205] *et al.*[206–208,563,759,760] in Italy. ESEP are giant spikes (Figs. 16.3, 16.4, 16.5 and 16.6) evoked by somatosensory stimuli applied to

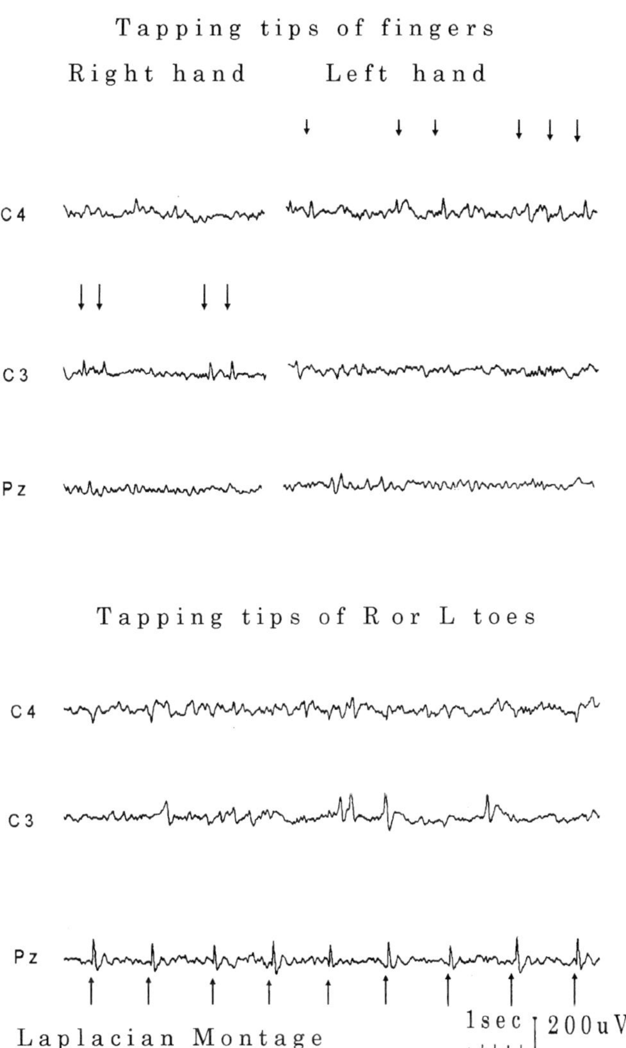

Fig. 16.3. Giant somatosensory evoked spikes on stimulating right or left tips of fingers or toes. Their EEG location is stimulus-site dependent.

the feet, fingers or both in 1–3 per cent of children.[208,290] They are called ESEP because they are exaggerated mid- or long-latency somatosensory evoked potential.[563,760]

ESEP-like centrotemporal and 'benign' spikes in other locations mostly occur in children with no evidence of seizures (more than 70 per cent). One fifth of them (19–24 per cent) have mainly partial seizures at the time of ESEP discovery and only a few (around 15 per cent) later also develop fits (see Table 16.1).

Tassinari and De Marco[759] proposed that ESEP are associated with a clinical phenotype which they called 'Benign partial epilepsy with extreme somatosensory evoked potentials',[759] a term that De Marco[205] used synonymously with 'Benign childhood epilepsy with parietal spikes'. This may not be correct as ESEP can be elicited in children with centrotemporal spikes only and, conversely, children with spontaneous parietal spikes may not have ESEP. There is evidence that both of these two EEG conditions may be associated with benign childhood partial seizures in the broad framework of a maturation-related seizure susceptibility syndrome.

Electroencephalographic aspects

ESEP and their methods of activation and study were detailed in Chapter 5. The prevalence of ESEP in two of the largest studies is given in Table 16.1.

De Marco and Tassinari, 1981[208] detailed the results of the evaluation of 15,000 children referred for an EEG mainly because of behavioural, speech and educational problems. There was a 49/51 male/female ratio. All 15,000 were tested mainly with tapping of the heel. One hundred and fifty five children (1 per cent) of whom 105 were boys had ESEP. Age at the first EEG recording of ESEP varied from 1 to 13 years with a peak at 4–8 years (91 per cent of the cases). ESEP was often the only EEG abnormality, spontaneous spikes appearing at a later age stage, usually between 1and 4 years after the first EEG with ESEP, initially during sleep and subsequently also while awake. The morphology and topography of the spontaneous focal abnormalities and the ESEP were strikingly similar according to these authors.[208]

Table 16.1. Prevalence of ESEP and seizures in two large studies

Authors	Children tested (no.)	Patients with ESEP (no.)	Patients with ESEP and non-febrile seizures
De Marco and Tassinari[208]	15,000	155 (1%)*	46 (29.7%)***
Fonseca and Tedrus[290]	6,500	186 (2.9%)**	44 (23.7%)****

*In half of the patients no hand stimulus was applied.
**All patients had hand and foot stimulation.
***These include 30 (19.4 per cent) patients who already had seizures at the time of the ESEP discovery and 16 (15.2 per cent) patients who developed seizures after a long, for years, follow-up of 105 children with ESEP who initially did not have fits.
****Only patients who had non-febrile seizures at the time of ESEP are included. Patients with no seizures did not have a follow-up.

The second largest, after the De Marco *et al.*[201–208,563,759,760] study, is that of Fonseca, Tedrus *et al.*[290–292] from Brazil. They tested 6500 children aged 2–15 years and found that 186 (2.9 per cent) had ESEP but only 44 (23.7 per cent) of them had non-febrile seizures.

Clinical correlates of ESEP

In both the study of De Marco and Tassinari[208] and Fonseca and Tedrus[290] all 21,500 children tested mainly had an EEG because of behavioural or cognitive problems. We do not know the prevalence of ESEP in a normal population of children. Of the 155 of De Marco and Tassinari[208] 30 children already had seizures at the time of the discovery of ESEP. Of the remaining 125 children without seizures, 105 children were followed up. Sixteen of them developed seizures which is the basis of these authors' concept of 'benign partial epilepsy with extreme somatosensory evoked potentials' detailed below.

In this respect the report of Fonseca and Tedrus is of significance.[290,291] They showed that 2.9 per cent of the 6500 tested children had ESEP, there was a high prevalence of febrile convulsions (20.4 per cent), and children with ESEP and seizures (23.7 per cent) had various epileptic syndromes including Rolandic seizures, benign partial seizures with affective symptoms, benign childhood occipital seizures, symptomatic and 'cryptogenic epilepsies'.[290] The term 'cryptogenic epilepsies' for 22 of these patients is probably unfortunate as all these children were of normal development, normal background EEG and were often of good prognosis. Most likely they had benign childhood parietal seizures. In detail, of 186 children with ESEP in the study of Fonseca and Tedrus[290] 44 (23.7 per cent)

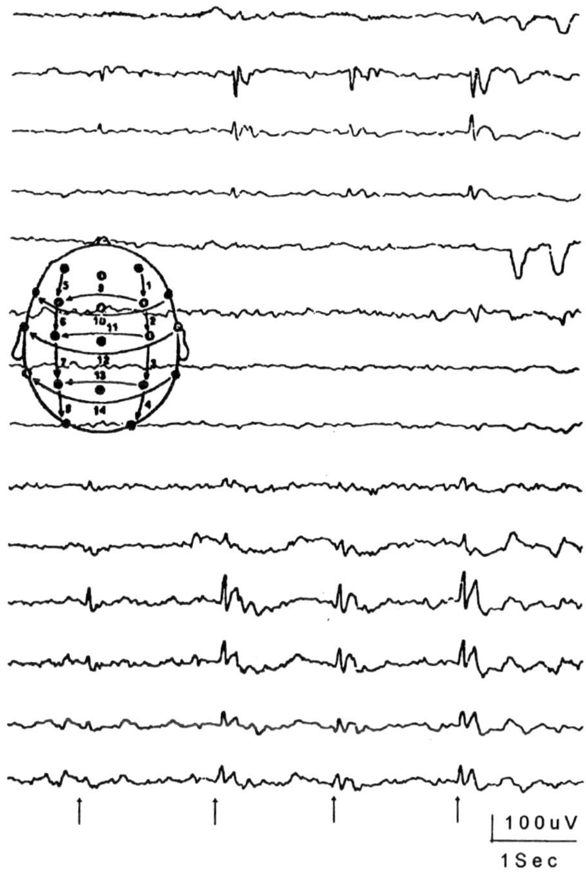

Fig. 16.4. Giant somatosensory evoked central spikes of a child aged 9 years who had at age eight and a half years a single nocturnal seizure. He was found vomiting with loss of consciousness and generalized stiffness which lasted for 5 min. Spontaneous right central spikes were also recorded. This child is also presented on page 334 (case 1 of Table 16.2).

had non-febrile seizures and 31 (16.7 per cent) had febrile convulsions only. The remaining 111 (59.7 per cent) patients without seizures had the requested EEG because of minor behavioural and scholastic problems. Of the 44 children with non-febrile seizures 21 were boys, and seven also had a previous history of febrile convulsions. These 44 patients were classified as having Rolandic seizures (12 patients with typical clinical seizures and EEG centrotemporal spikes), benign partial epilepsy with affective symptoms (one case), partial symptomatic epilepsy (four), childhood absence epilepsy (three), idiopathic generalized epilepsy (two) and cryptogenic epilepsy (22). The authors elaborated that the last group of 22 patients is classified as cryptogenic because 'they could not be included in the two forms of idiopathic benign partial epilepsy of the ILAE' despite normal neurological state and no evidence of recognisable cerebral lesion. In these 22 cases eight children had nocturnal generalized convulsions, six had versive partial fits and four had unilateral convulsions. The remaining four patients had partial complex, visual, tonic–clonic and atonic seizures each. The resting EEG was normal in three, parietal spike wave foci were recorded in 15, parietal with temporal, central or occipital foci were seen in another three and occipital spikes alone occurred in one patient. The background EEG was normal in all but one. Of 11 patients with parietal spikes, seven were seizure free for more than 1 year.

Despite the above reservations regarding the existence of a separate syndrome with ESEP, I believe that the work of De Marco *et al.*[205,208,759] cannot be omitted from a book concerned with further comparative studies between the various phenotypes of benign childhood partial seizures. The following is based on their work.[205,208,759]

Clinico-EEG evolution of 16 children with ESEP who later developed seizures

It is important to remember that the description of benign partial epilepsy with extreme somatosensory evoked potentials as portrayed by De Marco alone[205] or with Tassinari[759] is based on 16 children who developed seizures long after the discovery of ESEP in their first EEG. These 16 patients constituted 15 per cent of 105 children with a similar EEG manifestation of ESEP who were selected out of 155 patients because initially they did not have seizures. However, 30 of 155 patients with ESEP already had had fits prior to the EEG discovery of ESEP but we do not have any information about them. The other relevant point to remember is that the preferred site of stimulation of these authors[201–208,563,759,760] for ESEP was the foot. This should be less sensitive than the hand to elicit ESEP in children with centrotemporal spikes and Rolandic seizures, who have the lower Rolandic regions (face and hand) as the most hyperexitable cortical areas. Yet 155 (1 per cent) of the 15,000 tested children had ESEP but only 16 (15 per cent) of 105 developed fits.

The evolution of these 16 children followed five stages:

The first period, between 2.5 to 5.5 years of age, was characterized by the discovery of ESEP evoked by tapping of one or both feet or, less frequently, other parts of the body. EEG was otherwise normal.

The second period was signified by the appearance of spontaneous focal sharp slow-wave EEG abnormalities only during slow sleep.

The third period was characterized by the appearance of spontaneous spikes, also in awake EEG. These were parietal, central or posterior midline (Pz) spikes mainly in the side of the ESEP. The morphology and topography of the spontaneous focal spikes were strikingly similar to the ESEP. The time interval between the first discovery of ESEP to the development of spontaneous spikes varied from 9 months to 4 years with a mean of 21 months.

The fourth period was marked by electroclinical seizures which occurred 5 months to 2 years (mean approximately 1 year) after the appearance of spontaneous focal spikes.

In the fifth period, first seizures and then spikes, evoked and spontaneous, disappeared with clinical and EEG normalization before the age of 13–14 years.

Sex and age at onset of seizures

Of the 16 children, 12 (75 per cent) were boys. This male preponderance was also found in the total number of 155 children with ESEP where 105 (68 per cent) were boys.[208] However, this male prevalence was not confirmed in another study of 44 children with ESEP and seizures, where 21 were boys.[290]

The mean age at onset of seizures was 6 years (range 4.5–8 years).

Neurological and psychological state

Though the first EEG of these children was mainly performed for 'mild behavioural disturbances or poor scholastic performance' they had normal neurological state, normal brain scan and normal psychomotor development.[759] The IQ, assessed by a standard group of tests, showed normal values throughout the electroclinical evolution, 'suggesting that the seizures did not lead to psychological impairment'.[759]

Febrile convulsions

Seven (43.8 per cent) of the 16 patients had febrile convulsions.[208] Furthermore, 17 (28.3 per cent) of 60 children with ESEP without non-febrile seizures at first EEG examination had a previous history of febrile convulsions.[563] For comparison, 38 (20.4 per cent) of 186 children with ESEP studied by Fonseca and Tedrus[290] had febrile convulsions alone (16.7 per cent) or febrile and non-febrile seizures (3.8 per cent).

Seizure manifestations

According to the clinical description, most seizures in each of 16 patients were of the same type and consisted of usually brief and infrequent partial motor seizures with head and body version (12 subjects).[208] Two patients had generalized tonic–clonic seizures without apparent focal onset, while in another patient seizures were mainly of the tonic type. The last patient had somatosensory seizures with slight, if any, impairment of consciousness. They were brief and consisted of version of the head to the right, and hyperextension of the right arm, followed by a few jerks.

Seizures were usually rare, occurring two to six times a year. However, two patients had repeated seizures 'amounting to partial motor status epilepticus lasting several hours'. One of these two patients had as many as 200–800 daily for 15 days with slight impairment of consciousness only during the ictus. An illustrated[208] ictal EEG showed abrupt generalized flattening with disappearance of the pre-existing background rhythmic activity for 10–15 s. This was followed by a short period of slow theta and delta waves disturbed by artefacts. Interictal EEG had spikes in the left parietal and central regions and ESEP could be evoked by tapping the sole of the right foot. Despite clinical and interictal focal features, ictal EEG showed no focal onset. Seizures in this patient were controlled only temporarily by various treatments and finally stopped with corticotropin (ACTH) therapy. However, a second partial motor status was not responsive to ACTH and anti-epileptic drugs. Seizures eventually diminished and then stopped spontaneously after several days.

Circadian distribution

Seizures were diurnal in all but two children who also had nocturnal fits.

Treatment and evolution

The effectiveness of anti-epileptic drugs, mainly barbiturates, phenytoin, or carbamazepine, was difficult to evaluate. The seizures usually persisted for about 1 year and then subsided. Seizures remitted before the age of 9 years and did not relapse during a long follow-up period of an average of 8 years. Interictal focal spikes and ESEP usually persisted for 1–3 years or more after remission of seizures.

Benign partial epilepsy with extreme somatosensory evoked potentials and benign childhood parietal seizures: relation with the benign childhood partial seizure susceptibility syndrome

De Marco *et al.*[205,208,759] proposed that benign partial epilepsy with extreme somatosensory evoked potentials differs from Rolandic seizures because of the following:

(a) Seizures in patients with ESEP are predominantly diurnal and do not usually affect the facial muscles; their active span is brief, for 1 year.
(b) The active span of seizures is brief, for 1 year.
(c) There is a male preponderance.
(d) The EEG spikes are mostly parietal and parasagittal.
(e) ESEP were observed in only one of 100 patients with centrotemporal spikes examined by De Marco, 1980.[202]

However, only the arguments regarding seizure manifestations and EEG localization may be of some relevant value. In Rolandic seizures, there is a male preponderance, active seizure life span may be

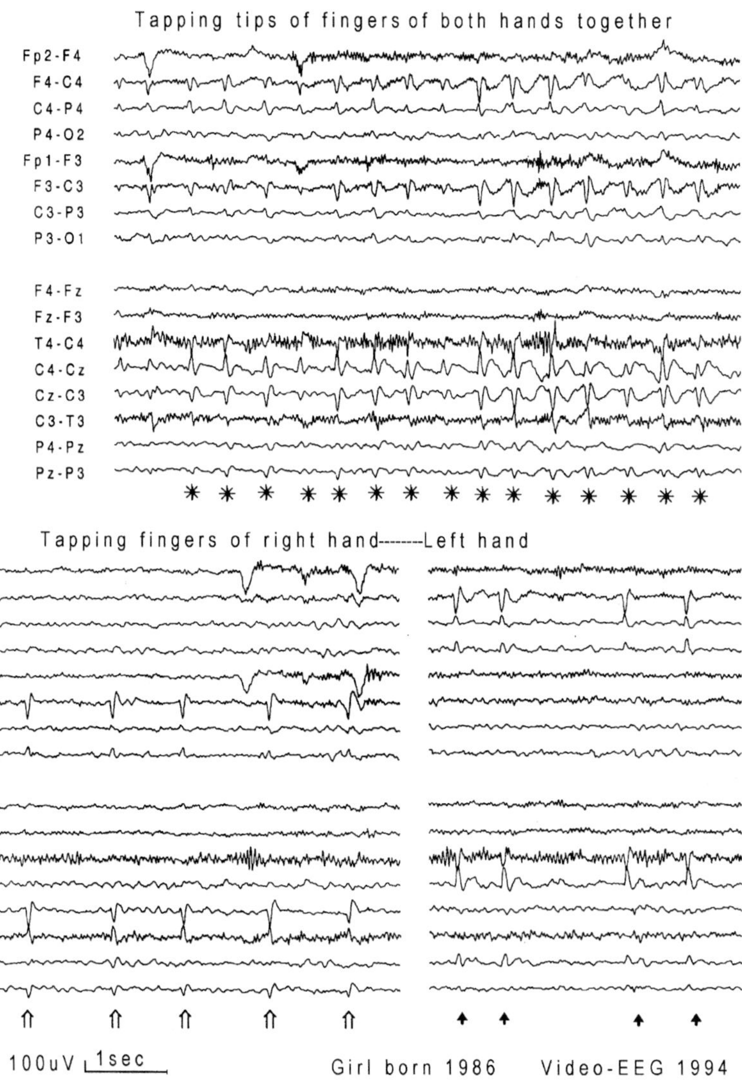

Fig. 16.5. From video-EEG recording of patient 16.2. Stars and arrows indicate timing of stimulus.

very brief, with children having only a single fit, and 10–20 per cent may also have ESEP (see Chapters 4 and 5).

My view is that these normal children with 'benign partial epilepsy with extreme somatosensory evoked potentials' are typical examples of the benign childhood partial seizure susceptibility syndrome because of:

(a) The frequent febrile convulsions;

(b) The male preponderance;

(c) The EEG sharp and slow waves being morphologically similar to the centrotemporal spikes with a life span limited to childhood;

(d) The age-related partial seizures which often remit before the disappearance of EEG spikes;

(e) The co-existence of ESEP with other functional spikes in other locations, or the frequent demonstrations of ESEP in children without seizures;

(f) The fact that children with ESEP may manifest with fits typical of Rolandic or benign childhood partial seizures from other locations, as shown by Fonseca and Tedrus.[290]

However, the clinical manifestations of seizures in children with 'benign partial epilepsy with ESEP' are frequently different from the Rolandic seizures probably because the main epileptogenic focus may be of a different localisation. In this respect another report of Fonseca and Tedrus, 1995[291] is interesting. They studied 164 children with idiopathic seizures and EEG spikes restricted to the centrotemporal (111 patients) or to the parietal regions (the other 53). Those with parietal spikes were of younger age and with onset of seizures usually before age 6 years, and had fewer oropharyngo-laryngeal or facial motor seizures (17 per cent as opposed to 44 per cent of those with centrotemporal spikes) and more frequent ESEP (40 per cent as opposed to 4 per cent of those with CTS). The authors concluded that their findings suggested that in neurologically normal children with epilepsy, the group with parietal spikes differs from those with CTS in age, age at onset, type of seizures and EEG reactivity to percussion of hands and feet.[291]

Episodic headache and dizziness in children with spontaneous and evoked centrotemporal somatosensory spikes

I detail in this section three normal children who we investigated for a similar clinical history of episodic headache and dizziness.[7] None had seizures of any type. However, their EEG showed remarkable similarities with bilateral centrotemporal spikes and giant somatosensory evoked potentials. Two of them also had brief generalized discharges.

Briefly, these three children, two boys aged 10 and 11 and one girl aged 8 years , had identical clinical presentation of recurrent bilateral headache accompanied by dizziness, nausea and/or vomiting. All had normal neurological and intellectual state. Two had normal MRI and the other had normal CT brain scan. The age at onset of headaches was 7, 10 and 7.5 years respectively. In all cases the EEG and/or video-EEG showed spontaneous bilateral centrotemporal spikes, independently right and left. They were more abundant during slow sleep. In all cases giant somatosensory evoked spikes were elicited by contralateral stimulation of the fingers. In two cases (aged 11, 8), brief (3–6 s) generalized discharges of spike/polyspike-slow waves (3–5 Hz) without clinical manifestations were seen mainly during hyperventilation. On the basis of these three children, we previously suggested that recurrent headache, dizziness and nausea may be part of the benign childhood seizure susceptibility syndrome which may also appear without overt epileptic seizures.[7]

I present these children in order to show that this EEG condition may be associated with other non-seizure symptoms though I cannot totally exclude the possibility of coincidence. These three children were selected out of probably hundreds of children with centrotemporal spikes referred for clinical or EEG evaluation over a 25 year period.

I should also emphasize that I do not consider their symptoms as migraine. Their headaches, difficult to describe by children, are not similar to those suffering from genuine migraine. I make this differentiation because some authors, mainly Andermann and Andermann,[37,41] consider benign childhood epilepsy with centrotemporal spikes a 'migraine-related' disease, a view which is hypothetical and cannot be substantiated by the limited literature on the subject (see Chapter 14), p. 297.

Case 16.2. I saw this clever and communicative normal girl, born in Sept. 1986, at age 8 (March 1994) because of 'headaches' over the previous two to three months. The headache, which she was unable to describe well, was not strong and I was uncertain whether she experienced pain or pressure. It was localized around and above the eyes, lasted for approximately 15–20 min and subsided. It occurred at any time in the day, even when she was playing. She complained that 'there is something wrong with my head', and she resumed activity as normal in about 15 min.

It is also interesting that before the onset of the 'headaches' she was complaining of abdominal pains. There is no relevant family history other than a maternal sister who suffers from common headaches.

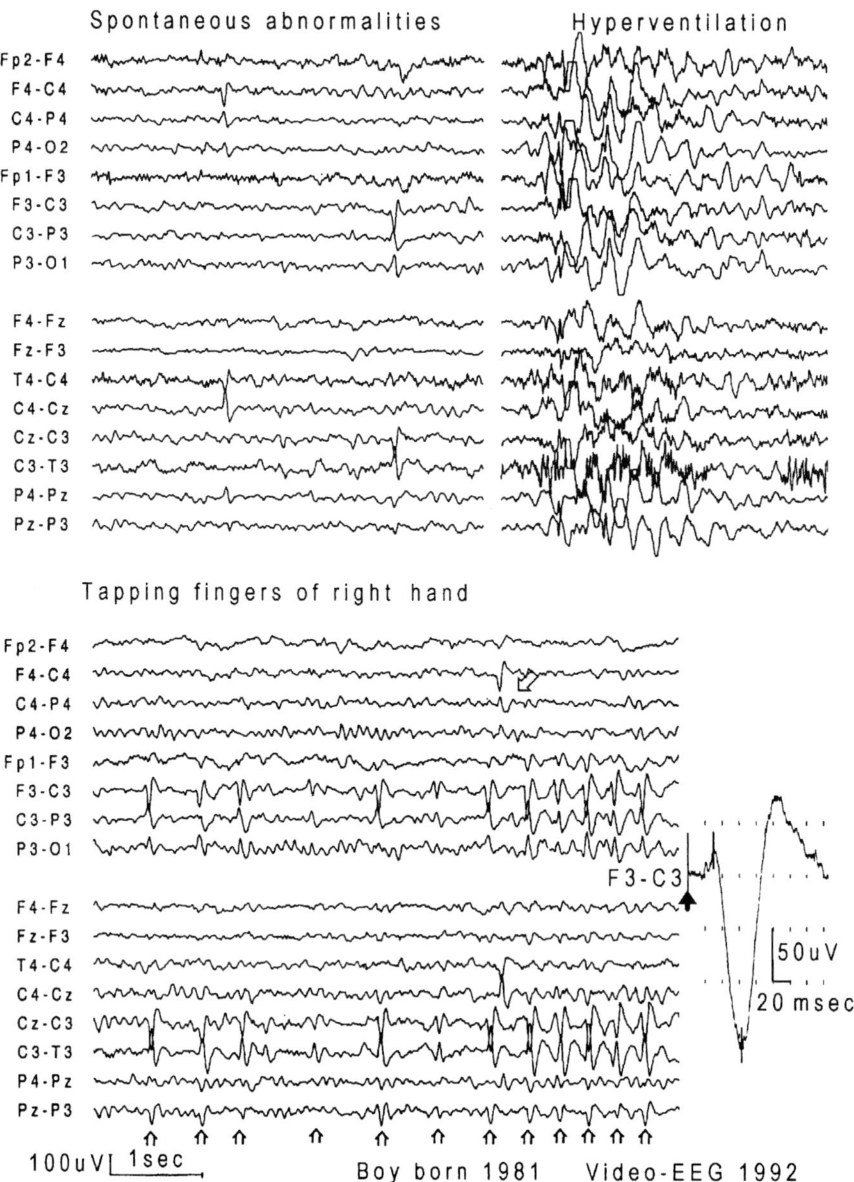

Fig. 16.6. From video-EEG recording of patient 16.3.

Neurological examination and MRI are entirely normal.

Video-EEG (Fig. 16.5) showed normal background with the following abnormalities:

(a) spontaneously central spikes, independently occurring on the right or left;

(b) somatosensory elicited high amplitude central spikes which are contralateral to the side of stimulation – simultaneous stimulation of the fingers of the hands by herself elicits simultaneous bilateral central spikes;

(c) brief, mainly anterior, bursts of polyspikes;

(d) high amplitude discharges of slow waves, 3–5 Hz, with interspersed occasional small spikes or small polyspikes. The discharges vary in duration from 3 to 6 s and they are mainly precipitated by overbreathing. There were no clinical symptoms during these discharges, verified by uninterrupted breath counting.

Somatosensory evoked spikes, using a trigger hammer connected to the evoked response machine, were bilaterally identical. The peak of the main negative wave was at 53 ms, preceded by a positive wave with onset at 28 ms and followed by a positive wave at 92 ms. The amplitude varied from 50 to 110 μV.

Symptoms improved over the following year and EEG performed elsewhere showed mainly centrotemporal spikes that were less frequent. She received no medication.

Case 16.3. This normal boy, born November 1981, was referred to me at age 11 years because of bi-temporal 'headaches' associated with dizziness and a tendency to vomit. The characteristics of the pain are not very well defined. He says that it is rather like something sharp going through his head. It lasts for the whole day, with some intervals of relaxation for approximately 5–10 min. This is also associated with dizziness, as if being in a boat. Tendency to vomit, without vomiting, follows in approximately 10–15 min after the onset of headache.

There is rivalry with his brother and his symptoms got much worse after a fight with him.

Neurological examination was entirely normal. All except EEG investigations, including CT brain scan and MRI and evaluation of his hearing, were normal.

The opinion of a child psychiatrist was that the child was under stress. 'They moved last year into an area which is rather isolated for him, his father has been overworking, his mother is over protective and he himself is a hypersensitive, introverted person with a high sense of responsibility. He is one of the best students in his class.'

Video-EEG (Fig. 16.6) showed the following abnormalities:

(a) A frequent firing focus of high amplitude sharp and slow waves mainly around the left central electrode, with some occasional localization shifting to the posterior regions. A similar but independent focus is seen on the right, which shows some localization shifting forwards. Sleep increases the frequency of the firing of the above foci.

(b) Somatosensory stimuli, mainly by tapping the right thumb, elicits a left sided central sharp and slow wave at a peak latency of about 58 ms.

(c) There are medium high amplitude spikes with occasional double spikes and slow waves, which appear usually bilateral or grossly asymmetrical in the parasaggital montage. They are of higher amplitude around the frontal electrodes.

(d) Bilateral high amplitude discharges of spikes, small spikes and occasionally multiple spikes at 3–5 Hz. They do not last more than 3 s. They are not associated with clinical manifestations. Breath counting is normal during them. There was no quantitative increase of these discharges during sleep.

Somatosensory evoked potential recordings from the central electrode were of the same latency bilaterally, with N20 at around 18 ms and P23 at 20 ms. The latest possible component was a positive one at 39 ms.

We were able to evoke the left sided spike by stimulating the right thumb. The spike appeared with a peak latency at around 58 to 60 ms.

Case 16.4: This 10-year-old boy started having recurrent bilateral headaches accompanied by dizziness, nausea and occasionally vomiting at age 7. They lasted for 10–15 min and were followed by sleepiness.

His development, intelligence and neurologic examination were normal. Brain CT scan was normal.

The family had no history of seizures or headache.

EEG showed spontaneous centrotemporal spikes, independently right and left which were more abundant during slow sleep. Evoked giant centrotemporal spikes were elicited by contralateral tapping of the fingertips. Simultaneous tapping of both hands evoked synchronous giant bilateral somatosensory spikes.

Benign childhood partial seizures with midline spikes

There is a conspicuous lack of prospective studies on children with midline spikes (Fz, Cz, Pz) who are also likely to be associated with benign childhood partial seizures.[603,605,622] Midline spikes occur

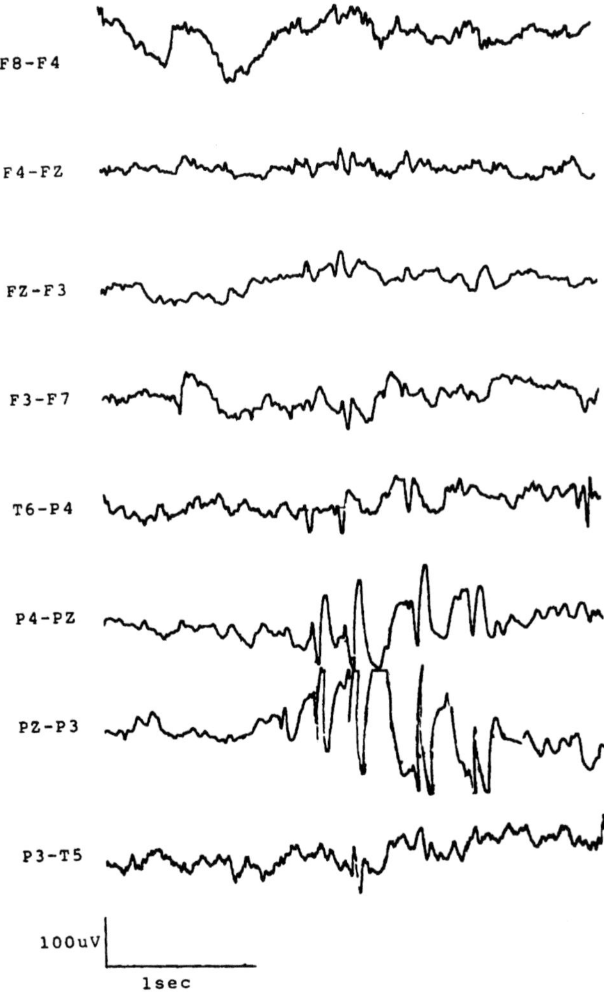

Fig. 16.7. Giant midline spikes in Pz electrode of a 5-year-old girl, patient no. 16.5 (page 327).

in 0.3 per cent[283] to 3 per cent[449] of children's EEG, and are often activated by sleep and correlate with a high prevalence of heterogeneous seizures,[211,262,449,564,664] from 70 per cent[211] to 91 per cent.[262,664] Though complex partial and generalized tonic–clonic seizures are the commonest, other types such as absences, myoclonic jerks and atonic seizures are well described[29,58,211,262,283,449,564,664] and there may be a high incidence of febrile convulsions.[449] However, these studies are retrospective, mainly from the EEG archives, and most include patients with structural lesions and often adults.

My impression is that midline spikes are not infrequent in children with benign childhood partial seizures, often together with spikes in other locations such as centrotemporal spikes (see Fig. 5.5 in Chapter 5) which are most likely to attract the attention of electroencephalographers because of their established value in the diagnosis of Rolandic seizures. Under these circumstances midline spikes are likely to be missed or under-reported, particularly in EEG recordings where relevant montages using midline electrodes are underutilized. This view is anecdotal and needs verification. However, from my prospective study of the 94 children with benign childhood partial seizures and EEG foci at various locations that I have previously detailed,[603,605,622] two children (2.1 per cent) had exclusively midline spikes (Pz), which were morphologically similar to centrotemporal spikes (Fig. 16.7). Both these two children also had ictal vomiting during their seizures[622] and their prognosis was excellent. I have recently reported them[622] with another seven children in a paper on 'extra-occipital benign childhood partial seizures with ictal vomiting and excellent prognosis' because their 'existence in the borderland between Rolandic and occipital seizures is consistent with a unified benign childhood partial seizure susceptibility syndrome'.[622] As these two children firmly document, a benign clinico-EEG course with midline spikes is described below. Considering the high prevalence of benign childhood partial seizures amongst children, benign childhood partial seizures with midline spikes may not be that unusual. EEG midline spikes with other functional spikes in childhood certainly occur more frequently than reported.

In case 16.5, seizures were nocturnal, also featuring symptoms common in Rolandic (oropharyngolaryngeal movements, speech arrest) and early onset benign childhood occipital seizures (ictal vomiting). Conversely, she also had hemiconvulsions of the leg which, unusual in Rolandic and EBOS seizures, can be explained from the EEG spike localization (Pz).

Case 16.5. (case 3 of Panayiotopoulos, 1999)[622] is a 13-year-old clever and normal girl who had at age four, within 3 months, two nocturnal seizures with left-sided clonic convulsions associated with oropharyngolaryngeal movements, vomiting, hypersalivation and speech arrest. The left sided hemiconvulsions were very brief, 3–5 jerks, and on the first occasion they involved face, arm and leg but on the second seizure were restricted to the leg, 'her left leg jerked once or twice'. She was unable to speak but could understand and on recovery she asked 'why could I not speak?'. Consciousness was intact. The seizures lasted for 10 min. She was treated with cyclohexyl-2-methylamino-propranol-phenylethyl barbiturate for 3 years with no further seizures. Two EEG at ages 4 and 5 showed high amplitude singular or clusters of spikes localized in the posterior mid-line (Pz) electrode (Fig. 16.7). All subsequent annual EEG were normal and no further seizures had occurred up to the last follow-up at age 13 years.

The second case had nocturnal seizures indistinguishable from those of Panayiotopoulos syndrome. Conversely, these were frequent, weekly, which has never so far been observed in Panayiotopoulos syndrome. Also he had Todd's hemiparalysis which is also unusual in EBOS.

Case 16.6 (case 4 of Panayiotopoulos, 1999)[622] is a 19-year-old normal boy who developed at age 5 years frequent, sometimes weekly, nocturnal seizures manifested with deviation of the eyes to the left associated with vomiting and followed by left sided hemiconvulsions for 3–5 min. They all occurred within the first half an hour of sleep and were followed by mild post-ictal left hemiparesis for 10–20 min. Seizure control was achieved with phenobarbitone at age 6 years. A similar nocturnal seizure occurred at age 10 years upon gradual discontinuation of treatment. He was again treated with cyclohexyl-2-methylamino-propranol-phenylethyl barbiturate for five years with no further seizures. Treatment was withdrawn at age 15. His first EEG available to me at age 10 years, showed high amplitude midline spikes mainly in the Pz electrode. All subsequent annual EEG showed an excess of slow waves with no spikes. He was an excellent pupil at school and no further seizures had occurred up to the last follow-up at age 19 years.

Literature review of midline spikes

Ehle *et al.*, 1981[262] studied the clinical correlates of midline spikes in 21 children. These were compared with 63 age-matched children (group 1) and 24 children with centrotemporal spikes (group 2). Midline spikes correlated well with a history of seizures (91 per cent vs. 73 per cent in group 1 and 76 per cent in group 2) and neurologic abnormality (38 per cent vs. 29 per cent in group 1 and 22 per cent in group 2). No patient had progressive neurologic disease or brain tumour. The authors assumed that there are two different mechanisms in the genesis of midline spikes. These either represent generalized epileptiform abnormalities in most or they may be analogous to centrotemporal spikes in a few.

Fischer and Clancy, 1987[283] reported the clinico-EEG manifestations of 21 neonates and children younger than 13 years with midline spikes. They represented 0.3 per cent of all 7051 consecutive

EEG. EEG was requested because of single or recurrent seizures (17/21), attention deficit disorder (2/21), psychomotor retardation (1/21) and headache (1/21). Clinical seizure types were diverse and included simple partial (5/17), complex partial (2/17), generalized tonic–clonic (4/17), mixed (2/17), and neonatal (4/17). The majority (13/21) of patients had an identifiable aetiology for their disorder; CT scans verified mass lesions in two patients. Midline epileptogenic foci were present during wakefulness in 14 of 17 older children and restricted to sleep in the others. Midline foci were exquisitely confined to Fz, Cz, and Pz in six of 17 older children. In five other children, midline foci spread preferentially to the adjacent central-parietal regions and closely resembled the appearance of benign Rolandic foci in the longitudinal EEG montages. This according to the authors is 'a potentially serious cause of EEG misinterpretation in view of the high incidence of neuropathology in this patient group'.[283]

Konishi and colleagues, 1988[449] studied the clinico-EEG manifestations of 45 children with midline spikes. The incidence of midline spikes was 3 per cent in children's EEG. Boys and girls were equally affected. Cz was the most frequent localization (31 patients), followed by Pz (11) and Fz (only three). Midline spikes were the only epileptiform EEG abnormality in 22 patients while the other 23 had additional focal spikes or generalized spike-wave discharges. Age at first discovery of midline spikes ranged from one month to 12 years, with a mean at 5 years. Thirty two of the 45 patients (71 per cent) had clinical seizures; 16 with febrile and 16 with non-febrile epileptic fits. Of the remaining 13 patients without a history of seizures, the EEG was requested because of post-meningitis in four, developmental delay in four, migraine in one and for miscellaneous reasons in four. The authors concluded that midline spikes might not have a strong correlation with clinical seizures. Ten patients had a family history of epilepsy and/or febrile convulsions. In the patients with seizures, generalized tonic–clonic seizures were the most frequent type (18 primary GTCS and 10 partial with secondary GTCS). Symptoms of partial seizures were variable (focal motor in five, Jacksonian march in one, aversive in one, autonomic in two and automatism in five), 'which might be related to the other lesions such as temporal and/or frontal lobes'. Seizure control was mostly good except for two patients with brain damage. Other neurological symptoms were not progressive.

Pourmand *et al.* 1984[664] found that of 32 patients with Cz and Pz spikes, two-thirds were neurologically impaired and 91 per cent had heterogeneous epileptic seizures.

Nelson *et al.*, 1983[564] compared the clinical features of 40 patients with midline spikes with those of age- and sex-matched controls. Seizure incidence was significantly greater in the study group than in the controls (85 per cent vs. 45 per cent). Tonic–clonic seizures were the most frequent type. Eighteen patients from the study group had additional focal or generalized epileptiform abnormalities. This subgroup had a significantly greater incidence of seizures than patients with only midline spikes (100 per cent vs. 73 per cent). Midline spikes were more common in children and markedly activated by sleep.

de Paola *et al.*, 1990[211] reported the clinical and EEG characteristics of 13 patients (80 per cent were children) with midline, parasaggital spikes, or both, which were facilitated by sleep in 73 per cent. Neurologic examination was normal in the majority of the patients. Seizures occurred in 70 per cent and these were GTCS (60 per cent), complex partial and partial with secondary generalization.

Amit and Crumrine, 1993[29] reported eight patients, aged 5 weeks to 17 years, who had ictal midline discharges during seizures which were heterogeneous, such as complex partial, simple sensory and myoclonic. The ictal EEG showed spike and spike and slow wave complexes, rhythmic theta, background attenuation, and paroxysmal fast activity. Based on reports from animal experiments and on a variety of types of clinical seizures and their ictal EEG correlates, the authors concluded that the midline scalp EEG discharges do not represent the anatomical focus of origin of the seizures. They probably reflect secondary extension and summation of a remote source of epileptogenic activity.

Bagdorf and Lee, 1993[58] retrospectively examined clinical and EEG features in 57 patients of all ages with midline spikes as the only epileptiform activity in their EEG. They represented approximately

0.2 per cent of all patients. The majority of them (86 per cent) occurred in children from neonate to younger than 16 years. Midline spikes were activated by sleep in children but not adults. Forty eight (84 per cent) of the 57 patients had seizures that varied from absences (3.5 per cent), atonic (12.2 per cent), GTCS (14 per cent), myoclonic (10.5 per cent), tonic (1.8 per cent) to the most common of all, complex partial seizures (50.1 per cent). Five patients had more than one type of seizures. This series included eight adult patients with severe brain disease such as metastasis, cerebral atrophy or coma from cardiac arrest. Of 29 patients who were followed for 6 months to 9 years, only 15 (52 per cent) achieved good seizure control, which was determined as less than one seizure per 6 months. The authors concluded that 'epilepsy with midline spikes is not necessarily benign and that future studies with larger patient groups may be necessary to identify factors that influence prognosis'. I should add that future studies should aim at more homogeneous groups of patients regarding age and underlying diseases. Based on my experience and the literature review, I have no doubt in my mind of the existence of benign childhood seizures with midline spikes as the sole EEG manifestation of this age-related seizure susceptibility syndrome. However, midline spikes are also most likely to occur together with spike foci in other locations. Their clinical representative has to be defined.

Benign childhood frontal seizures

Beaumanoir and Nahory,1983[85] were the first to describe 'benign frontal partial epilepsy' of 11 patients. These represented 8.9 per cent of patients with functional EEG spike and benign partial childhood seizures. These were well selected on strict inclusion criteria, mainly on the basis of at least two partial seizures, EEG focal or multifocal functional spikes in the frontal regions (Fp2, Fp1, F3, F4 and Fz), normal EEG background, normal neurological examination and at least 5 years free of seizures.

Clinical findings

Two children had some learning difficulties and one had behavioural problems. Three had a family history of epilepsy.

The diurnal seizures were infrequent and polymorphic. The commonest description was of an absence-like seizure associated with autonomic disturbances or motor, tonic or atonic, symptoms. In particularly the following ictal symptoms were observed: impairment of consciousness (10 cases), tonic deviation of the head (six), head and body (six), of the mouth (two), smile (one), drop (amyotonic) of one arm (three), drop of the head (two), unilateral myoclonic jerks of an arm during the hypnagogic phase of sleep (one), redness of the face (nine), urine incontinence (two), sweating (one), lacrimation (one) and headache (one). Four patients also had post-ictal headache. In four cases typical absence seizures were described by observers.

The nocturnal seizures were frequent, usually described as GTCS or prolonged clonic seizures. However, in three cases, observed from the beginning, these were adversive seizures with secondary GTCS. In these three cases the diurnal seizures never progressed to secondary GTCS.

The frequency of the seizures was variable. Two patients had only two seizures. All but one patient were treated with anti-epileptic drugs for at least 2 years.

One patient had typical absence seizures which started at age 4 years with generalized 3 Hz spike and waves. The first frontal spike appeared 5 months prior to the first partial seizure at age 7 years. Another child had febrile convulsions at age 1 year with normal EEG.

Age at onset of seizures was 4–8 years and the last seizure occurred between 6 to 11 years. However, two patients had GTCS and another two partial seizures a long time after the disappearance of the EEG focus and drug withdrawal. In the two patients with GTCS these were precipitated by head injury in one and after excessive alcohol consumption with sleep deprivation in the other. The two patients with partial seizures were under stress at the time. In one of them, the EEG one week later showed only generalized discharges of spike and wave. This patient also had another GTCS at age 21 years.

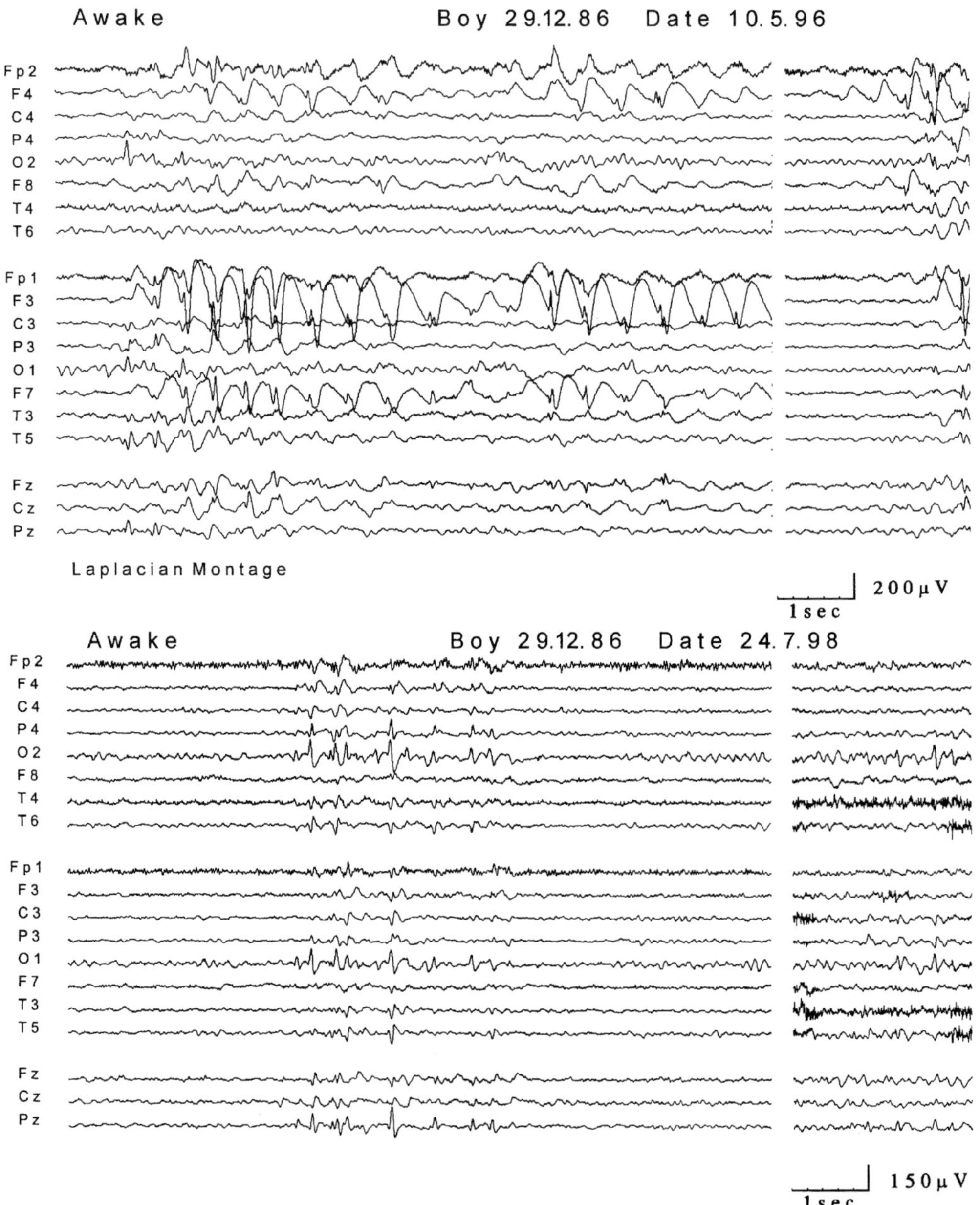

Fig. 16.8a. From video-EEG recordings of patient 16.7 recorded at onset of seizures (upper, May 1996) and two years later when he was free of seizures (lower, July 1998). Also compare with the multiple spike foci that he had in the video EEG of December 1997 (Fig. 16.8b).

EEG findings

The EEG focus was consistently recorded in the same location in successive EEG in only three cases. It was not associated with spikes localized in other brain regions. However, 3 Hz generalized spike and slow wave discharges occurred in six patients and one of them also had clinical manifestations

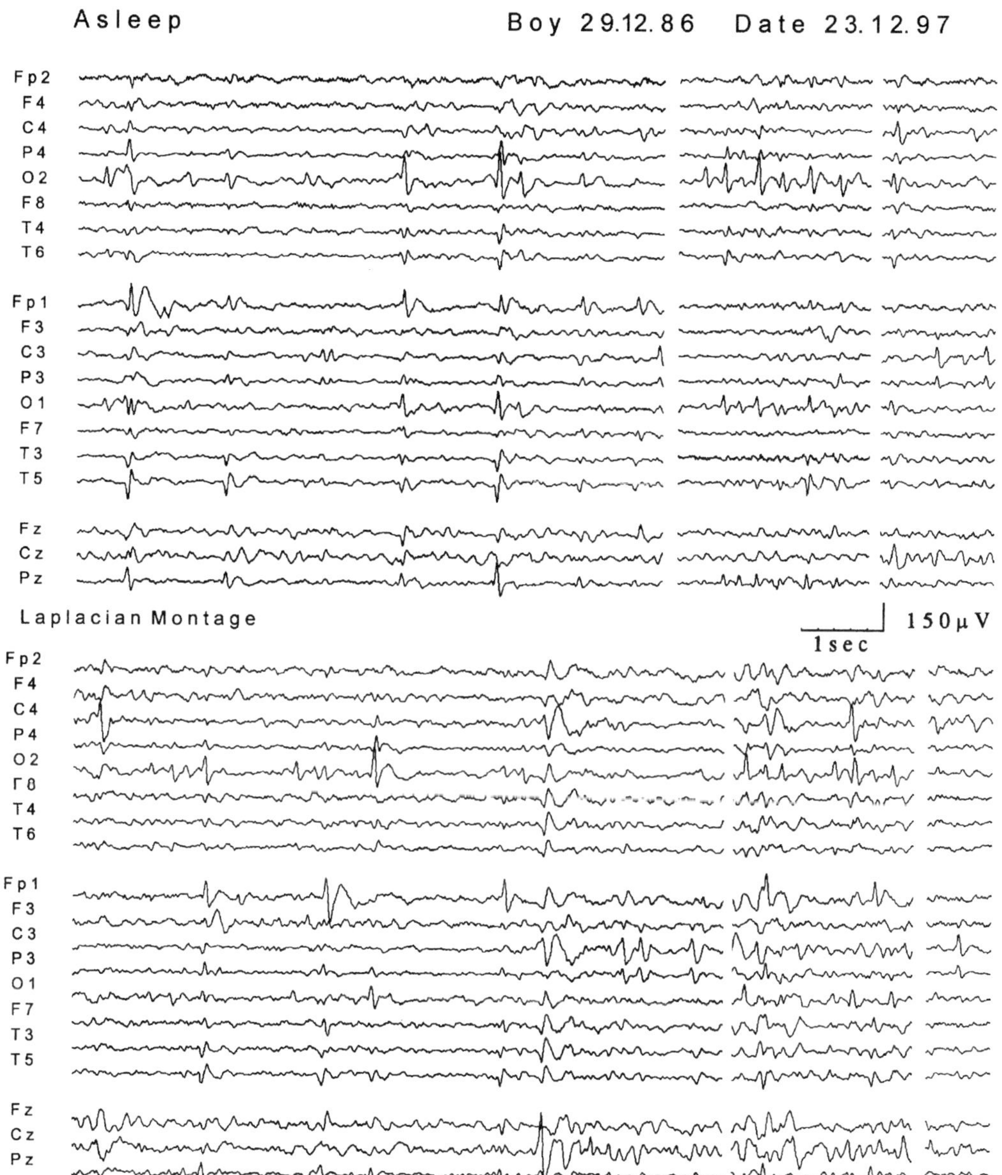

Fig. 16.8b. From video-EEG recordings of patient 16.7 recorded in December 1997. High amplitude sharp and slow waves are seen in nearly all brain locations.
Compare with Fig. 16.8a at onset of seizures (upper, May 1996) and two years later (lower, July 1998).

of absence. Sleep EEG showed good organization with exacerbation of the focal spikes and a tendency to spread to the contralateral frontal regions, to the whole ipsilateral hemisphere or diffusely over both hemispheres.

It is not certain when the frontal EEG spike disappears.

Ictal EEG was recorded in four cases and it appeared that the discharge starts from one and spreads to both frontal poles irrespective of lateralization and other interictal EEG findings.

Comment

There should be no doubt that functional frontal spikes exist. These may occur in normal children or associated with seizures which have a good prognosis. However, functional frontal spikes are much less frequent than in any other location and they do not appear to have a particular age-related preference, occurring in children of any age between 1 and 12 years. In my limited experience with these frontal spikes, their EEG features are not as typical as of other locations. Also, after a seizure, there are also marked frontal slow waves or long runs of spikes and slow wave which are not morphologically similar to those of other benign childhood partial epilepsies. Thanks to Beaumanoir and Nahory,1983[85] we know that these benign childhood frontal seizures exist and they are of good prognosis. Fifteen years after their report, we know no more.

These two cases of mine may add some thoughts to those who would like to make a contribution to this significant topic.

> Case 16.7. This boy of normal physical and intellectual state, born in Dec. 1986, had three febrile convulsions as a baby. At age 9 years he had within a month three partial seizures with secondary GTCS while awake and while asleep. One was witnessed from the beginning. He had a fixed gaze, lying still in bed, and gradually convulsions started, with the left side of the face first, then the limbs of the same side. Though medication with carbamazepine was advised, the parents were reluctant to initiate treatment or even give him a very small dose. He had approximately another 12 seizures which were either left hemiconvulsions or secondary GTCS. An unusual seizure occurred while he was writing: 'His gaze became fixed but he continued his work without knowing what he was doing. I asked him what he could see, he told me and returned back to normal'. The last seizure occurred six months from onset when carbamazepine at appropriate dose started. Since then he has been well, happy, co-operative and a good student. Last follow-up was 2 years from last seizure.
>
> Two high resolution MRI were normal. However, alert and sleep video-EEG were dramatically abnormal (Figs. 16.8a and 16.8b). The first EEG at age 9 years showed long, nearly continuous, runs of high amplitude, 2–3 Hz, slow waves in the anterior regions, more persistently on the left. Small spikes were intermixed with the slow waves. Also, on a few occasions there were some simultaneous small occipital spikes. One year later the abnormalities consisted mainly of high amplitude, more than 600 μV, runs of spike and slow wave complexes mainly localized around the left frontal electrode but also starting from the right. Occasional occipital spikes also occurred. Based on my principle that a highly epileptogenic EEG of a normal child should raise the possibility of benign childhood partial seizures, I reluctantly discussed this with his parents, although the frontal spike and wave complexes were not morphologically similar to the functional spikes of children and the EEG continued having runs of anterior delta waves. Confirmation of my diagnosis came from his EEG at age 11 years which showed functional spikes in every possible location of the brain. The last EEG at age 12 years is improving, showing only clusters of occipital spikes.

The next is one of the two patients with frontal spikes that I reported amongst 94 children with benign childhood partial seizures case 5 of table 16.2.[603,622]

> Case 16.8. This 14-year-old boy had at age 5 years, within 2 weeks, two nocturnal seizures witnessed from onset. These consisted of simultaneous tonic deviation of the eyes to the right with vomiting for 10 min. He could understand but was unable to speak. He started medication with carbamazepine 200 mg daily with one further similar nocturnal seizure that lasted for 20 min one year later. No further seizures occurred and in the last follow-up at age 14 years he was well with normal EEG and no medication. His first EEG 2 days after the second seizure, at age 5 years, showed high amplitude bursts of slow wave mainly bi-frontally. However, six months later the EEG had severe abnormalities consisting of frequent, nearly continuous runs of high amplitude sharp and slow wave complexes in the bi-frontal or mainly left side (similar to Fig. 16.8a). These were consistently recorded in the next two years until normalization at age 9 years.

Extra-occipital benign childhood partial seizures with ictal vomiting and excellent prognosis

This section aims to describe the prevalence, clinical and electroencephalographic manifestations, and the prognosis of benign childhood partial seizures with ictal vomiting in other than occipital localizations. The purpose is not to present another syndrome but at show that benign childhood partial seizures may manifest with ictal symptoms of another phenotype but at different interictal EEG localization or with normal EEG. By virtue of an excellent prognosis, they classify within the age-related seizure susceptibility syndrome, which includes centrotemporal and occipital seizures, its main representatives.

Despite some differences of clinical and EEG manifestations from early onset benign childhood occipital seizures (EBOS), childhood seizures with ictal vomiting and extra-occipital EEG foci are of equally excellent prognosis as EBOS. Their existence in the borderland between centrotemporal and occipital seizures offers a further argument in favour of a unified benign childhood partial seizure susceptibility syndrome. Their recognition is important for prognostic and therapeutic reasons.

Of the 24 children with ictal vomiting I reported in 1988,[603] 12 had Panayiotopoulos syndrome and three had symptomatic epilepsy. The remaining nine children with extra-occipital EEG foci (six) or normal EEG were followed clinically and with EEG for a median of 9 years after their first seizure, and they have only recently been reported.[622] All but one child had nocturnal seizures which manifested with ictal vomiting, eye deviation and unilateral clonic convulsions with or without impairment of consciousness. The median onset of seizures was 5 years and seizure life span was brief with four children having a single fit, four 2–3 and only one child many seizures prior to the initiation of medication. Prognosis was excellent with no seizures and good development in the long follow-up period. All nine patients were of normal neurological state and development with normal brain scan.

Prevalence

These nine children with ictal vomiting constitute 9.1 per cent of 99 patients with benign childhood partial seizures (94 of them had EEG spike foci) or 2.2 per cent of 418 patients with onset of seizures before the age of 13 years.

Sex, age and other chronological data

These are shown in Table 16.2. There are eight boys and one girl with a median onset of seizures at 5 years (range 2–11), a median age at last seizure of 6 years (4–11) and a median age at last follow-up of 14 years (6–23).

Neurological, mental state and development

By inclusion criteria all patients were of normal neurological, mental state and development. All patients attended main stream schools and most of them were good students. Patient 2 was mildly hyperkinetic with low grade school records. Patient 4 was considered to be badly behaved by his parents.

Family history

There was no other member of the family with similar seizures. Patient 6 had a strong family history of febrile convulsions.

Clinical data

All patients had seizures which were characterized by ictal vomiting either from the onset or during the ictus (Table 16.2). All seizures in all but one patient occurred during sleep. Only one patient had frequent seizures before onset of treatment. All others had a single to a maximum of three fits during the long follow-up period.

Table 16.2. Chronological, ictal and EEG data

Case	Age (years) of			Seizures			
No./Sex	Last FU	Onset	Last seizure	Number	Sleep/ awake	Free (years)	Ictal symptoms
1M	14	8.5	8.5	1	Sleep	5.5	V-LOC-Stiffness
2M	16	5.5	6	2	Sleep	10	LHC-V-LOC-Flaccid-IU
3F	13	4	4.5	2	Sleep	8.5	LHC-OPLS-V-Salivation-Speech arrest
4M	19	5	10	50	Sleep	9	ED-V-LOC-LHC, post-ictal HP
5M	14	5	7	3	Sleep	7	ED-V-Speech arrest
6M	6	3.5	3.5	1	Sleep	2.5	V-ED-LOC-GCStatus
7M	6	2	4	3	Sleep	2	ED-V-LOC-RHC, post-ictal HP
8M	23	6	6	1	Awake	17	Dizzinesss-Speech arrest-V-P-GTCS
9M	15	11	11	1	Sleep	4	V-LOC-RHC
Mean	14	5.6	6.7	7.1		7.3	
SD	5.5	2.7	2.6	16.1		4.6	
Median	14	5.3	6.4	2		7.1	
Maximum	23	11	11	50		17	
Minimum	6	2	4	1		2	

FU = Follow-up; V = Vomiting; LOC = Loss of consciousness; LHC or RHC = Left (L) or right (R) sided clonic convulsions; IU = Incontinence of urine; ED = Deviation of the eyes; P = Pallor; GSStatus = Generalized convulsive status epilepticus; OPLS = oropharyngolaryngeal symptoms; HP = Hemiparesis; GSSES = Giant somatosensory evoked spikes; SD = Standard deviation.

Description of seizures

Case 1 had at age eight and a half years a single nocturnal seizure. He was found vomiting with loss of consciousness and generalized stiffness which lasted for 5 min.

Case 2 had at age five and a half years a nocturnal seizure with clonic convulsions of the left arm and concurrent vomiting for 30 min. He subsequently became flaccid with loss of consciousness and incontinence of urine. A second, shorter and milder, episode occurred again during sleep, one year later.

Case 3 with midline spikes is detailed on page 327 (case 16.5).

Case 4 with midline spikes is detailed on page 327 (case 16.6).

Case 5 with frontal spikes is detailed on page 332 (case 16.8).

Case 6, with a strong family history of febrile convulsions, had three febrile convulsions at age 2–3 years and started treatment with phenobarbitone. At age three and a half and 3 days after sudden withdrawal of phenobarbitone, he had a nocturnal seizure with vomiting, deviation of the eyes and unresponsiveness followed within 5 min by generalized convulsive status epilepticus.

Case 7 had at age 2 years a nocturnal seizure with eyes deviated to the right, vomiting and loss of consciousness followed within 5 min by prolonged right hemiconvulsions and post-ictal hemiparesis. A similar but milder episode with the same sequence of events and brief hemiconvulsions occurred 2 months later. Despite treatment with phenobarbitone he had another seizure at age 4 which was witnessed from the beginning. He sat up in his bed, his eyes opened and immediately deviated to the right. Within seconds he started vomiting and became unresponsive for 5 min before going to sleep again without convulsions.

Case 8 had at age 6 years a diurnal seizure that started with dizziness, inability to speak and vomiting. He was pale. Consciousness was not impaired. This lasted for approximately 5 min, ending with generalized convulsions.

Case 9 had at age 11 years a single nocturnal seizure with vomiting and unresponsiveness which lasted for half an hour before ending with hemiconvulsions.

Electroencephalography

All patients had 1–3 EEG in the first year after their first seizure and annual EEG in the next 3–7 years. The EEG spike foci were seen only once and in their first EEG (cases 3 and 4) or persisted for 1–2 years (cases 1 and 2). Cases 1 and 2 had right central spikes and giant somatosensory spikes (Fig. 16.4). Cases 3 and 4 had midline (Pz) spikes (Fig. 16.7). Case 5 had no spikes in the first EEG but all subsequent EEG from age 6–8 years consistently showed a high amplitude spike and slow wave focus in the left frontal electrode, before complete normalization at age 9. All spike foci in all patients were of high amplitude and morphologically similar to the centrotemporal or occipital paroxysms of benign childhood partial seizures (Figs. 16.4 and 16.7).

Case 6 had a normal EEG at age 2 years but another EEG one year later showed a brief photoparoxysmal response of generalized spike and slow wave which was not seen in subsequent EEG. Cases 7, 8 and 9 had consistently normal EEG.

Treatment and prognosis

Cases 1 and 7 did not receive any treatment. Cases 2, 5 and 8 were treated with carbamazepine and cases 3, 4, 6 and 7 with phenobarbitone or cyclohexyl-2-methylamino-propranol-phenylethyl barbiturate for 2–6 years. All patients did well with no further seizures and good development during the follow-up period of a median of 9 years (range 3–17) from their first seizure (Table 16.2).

Irrespective of pathogenetic mechanisms, it is important to recognize that ictal vomiting is unequivocally associated with benign childhood partial seizures.[150,192,270,277,367,370,443,517,615,793,826]

'That these nine children with partial seizures and ictal vomiting have an entirely benign condition is well documented with the long follow-up. Most of them had a total 1–3 mainly nocturnal fits in early childhood and all developed well with no further seizures. In this respect they classify amongst the benign childhood partial seizures.'

These nine children signify with their symptoms and EEG findings that the unified concept of benign childhood partial epilepsies is justified. They all have ictal vomiting which is a cardinal symptom of Panayiotopoulos syndrome, yet none of them had occipital spikes in their EEG. Conversely, five of them had central, giant somatosensory, frontal or midline spikes of benign childhood partial seizures which do not manifest with ictal vomiting. Furthermore, some of these patients also have, concurrently with ictal vomiting, symptoms such as hemiclonic seizures, oropharyngolaryngeal movements, aphemia and hypersalivation which characterize other than occipital benign childhood partial seizures.

Thus, these nine children, constituting approximately 10 per cent of benign childhood partial seizures, present with ictal symptoms and EEG findings sharing features of Rolandic seizures, EBOS and other phenotypic variations of the benign childhood seizure susceptibility syndrome. Irrespective of their categorization, they present with sound clinico-EEG manifestations which are unlikely to occur in other than benign epilepsies and in this respect are important to recognize for prognostic purposes. Most of them may not even need treatment.[622]

Benign Childhood Partial Seizures and Related Epileptic Syndromes. C P Panayiotopoulos
©1999 John Libbey & Company Ltd., pp. 337–360.

Chapter 17

Severe syndromes of mainly linguistic and neuropsychological deficits, seizures or both and marked EEG abnormalities from the Rolandic and neighbouring regions

Landau–Kleffner syndrome or Acquired epileptic aphasia

Introduction

Landau–Kleffner syndrome or acquired epileptic aphasia is a severe, partly reversible, age-related childhood clinical syndrome with mainly linguistic decline and neuropsychological abnormalities as the cardinal clinical symptoms.[46,75,105,112,122,139,174,187,226,250,252,268,318,320,349,358,366,390,403,467,468,489,524,526,528,544,545,547,558,577,583,592,639,671,678,690,715,733,739,745,820a,785,836] It is a functional disorder of childhood manifested with acquired verbal auditory agnosia and other predominantly linguistic deficits which often occur together with other cognitive and neuropsychological-behavioural abnormalities. Clinically, seizures may also occur in three-quarters of the patients but these are usually infrequent and of good prognosis. EEG is characterized by mainly posterior temporal foci of sharp and slow waves which are often multifocal and bisynchronous, markedly facilitated by slow sleep (Figs. 17.1 and 17.2a). Continuous spikes and waves during slow sleep may occur but this is not a prerequisite for diagnosis. Structural brain imaging is often normal but functional brain imaging demonstrates abnormalities mainly in the left temporal lobe. Seizures and EEG abnormalities remit by mid-teen with concomitant improvement of linguistic and behavioural impairment but often with permanent sequelae. Landau–Kleffner syndrome is probably the result of an epileptogenic functional lesion in the speech cortex during a critical period of child development, and should be differentiated from symptomatic cases (see pathology, page 346).[733]

Though this, predominantly linguistic, disturbance is often associated with functional EEG sharp and slow wave foci activated by sleep, the diagnosis of Landau–Kleffner syndrome is clinical, irrespective of EEG and other seizure features. Conversely, the diagnosis of a similarly age-related condition of 'epilepsy with continuous spikes and waves during slow sleep (ECSWS)', detailed in a subsequent section, is based on EEG criteria irrespective of clinical manifestations. Landau–Kleffner syndrome by definition cannot exist without linguistic manifestations while ECSWS cannot be diagnosed without EEG continuous spikes and wave during sleep. It is a matter of selection criteria.

I found 248 publications in the Medline retrieval system on all aspects of Landau–Kleffner syndrome during the last 32 years. This chapter is based on the most significant of these publications and excellent reviews on the Landau–Kleffner syndrome mainly by Beaumanoir (1992),[75] Deonna and Roulet (1995),[221] Dugas *et al.* (1995)[251] and Smith (1997).[733]

Synonyms

Landau–Kleffner-syndrome[251]
Acquired epileptic aphasia[177]
Acquired aphasia with convulsive disorder in children[468]

Abbreviations

CSWS = Continuous spikes and waves during slow sleep
ECSWS = Epilepsy with continuous spikes and waves during slow sleep
ESESS = Electrical status epilepticus during slow sleep

Definition

According to the Commission on Classification and Terminology of the International League Against Epilepsy,1989[177] 'acquired epileptic aphasia (Landau–Kleffner syndrome) is a childhood disorder in which an acquired aphasia, multifocal spike, and spike and wave discharges are associated. Epileptic seizures and behavioural and psychomotor disturbances occur in two-thirds of the patients. There is verbal auditory agnosia and rapid reduction of spontaneous speech. The seizures, usually GTCS or partial motor, are rare, and remit before the age of 15 years, as do the EEG abnormalities.'[177]

Nomenclature

The proposed name by Landau and Kleffner[468] was 'acquired aphasia with convulsive disorder in children' and 'acquired epileptic aphasia' is the official term used by the Commission on Classification and Terminology of the International League Against Epilepsy,1989.[177] However, one quarter of children with Landau–Kleffner syndrome do not have convulsive disorders and acquired auditory verbal agnosia, not aphasia, is the prominent deficit. Therefore, 'acquired verbal auditory agnosia with EEG paroxysms' would probably be more accurate. However, the terminology of Landau–Kleffner syndrome is now well established and this is followed in this book until an aetiological cause is found.

The eponym Landau–Kleffner syndrome was first proposed in 1977 by M. Dugas (cited by Dugas *et al.*).[251] Landau,1992[467] in an editorial 'Landau–Kleffner syndrome. An eponymic badge of ignorance' emphasized that little progress has been made in the understanding of this syndrome and he wished that future advances would allow an aetiological terminology. I quote from Landau, 1992:[467]

> From the personal perspective of attaining three score and seven and the condition of Status Eponymicus, I can find no basis for ego gratification.... Here is a condition of variable and really unpredictable prognosis, of unknown cause, and for which we have no convincing evidence of empirically effective therapy. Every major neurologic centre sees one to several cases a year. Surely the time is ripe to call for a tightly organized interinstitutional and, if possible, international study. The primary questions to be tackled concern (1) aetiology, (2) pathological physiology, (3) rational therapy (based on knowledge of aetiology), and (4) empirical therapy (not quite so rational) ... Elementary genetic linkage analyses could be assayed in a large number of patients already on the books who are long-term survivors. There is also complete absence of epidemiologic data of every sort in regard to geography, infectious disease, toxins, nutrition, or environmental exposures.
>
> The first step must be a collective agreement about the clinical diagnostic criteria. At the outset, I submit

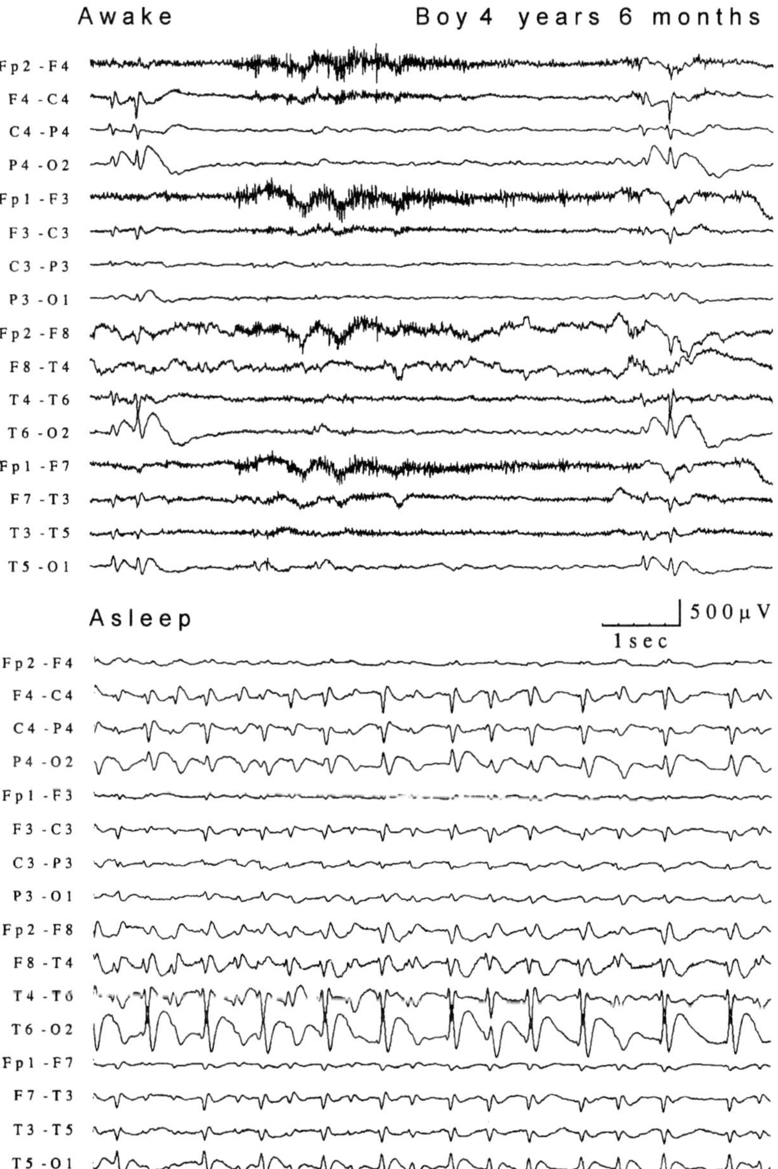

Fig. 17.1. This 4 years and 6 months old boy was referred for an EEG because of suspected absences. This EEGs with mainly right sided posterior temporal sharp and slow wave complexes while awake (upper) and continuous bisynchronous sharp and slow waves at 1–4 Hz during sleep, prompted a proper evaluation for Landau–Kleffner syndrome which was clinically confirmed (see Chapter 2 regarding the contribution of EEG to clinical diagnosis.

that these criteria should be very narrow. Borderline variants of the condition surely occur, but one believes that they should be excluded from the first effort research protocol in order to maximize the significance of correlative studies. All participants must agree to enlist available patients into agreed-upon diagnostic studies, both old-fashioned and newfangled, as intelligence may occur. Randomization and, if possible, double-blind therapeutic studies are essential ...

Just as Schilder's disease has become a more intellectually gratifying illness called adrenoleukodystrophy, Frank Kleffner and I hope that an organized research effort may spare the next generation of paediatric neurologists from the useless chore of recalling our names.[467] [See also his recent views in reference [467a]].

Historical aspects

In 1957 Landau and Kleffner[468] reported six children with a syndrome of 'acquired aphasia with a convulsive disorder'. Aphasia developed over days to months and then persisted from two weeks to several years. The associated seizures included GTCS, absences, and myoclonic seizures which were easily controlled with medication and had a relatively good prognosis. EEG showed paroxysmal epileptiform abnormality that was usually bilateral, and most prominent over the temporal lobes. They felt that although the relationship was not perfect, the severity of the paroxysmal disturbance on EEG did correspond to the severity of language disturbance. They hypothesized that 'persistent convulsive discharge in brain tissue largely concerned with linguistic communication results in the functional ablation of these areas for normal linguistic behaviour'. Their thesis was supported by the fact that these children did not have clouded consciousness like patients in non-convulsive status epilepticus and had good performance on nonverbal intelligence tests.[468] This original report by Landau and Kleffner[468] has been recently reproduced in *Neurology* (November 1998) as a landmark article, together with a commentary by Landau.[467a]

In England this syndrome is best known through the report of Worster–Drought.[820a]

Prevalence

This is another rare condition with a prevalence of around 0.2 per cent amongst children with epileptic seizures.[454] Despite the interest that Landau–Kleffner syndrome is generating through its clinico-EEG features for epileptologists, psychologists, neurophysiologists, paediatric neurologists and neurosurgeons, there are no more than 300 reported cases and not all of them have Landau–Kleffner syndrome.[467a,544]

According to Landau 1992[467] 'every major neurologic centre sees one to several cases a year'. Dugas *et al.*, 1982[252] see one new patient per year in a specialized clinic.

Age at onset and sex

Age at onset is mainly before 6 years, after age-appropriate speech has been acquired. Exceptionally, Landau–Kleffner syndrome may start after 8 years to as late as 10–13. Boys are twice as likely to suffer from it as girls.

Family history and personal antecedents

A family history of epilepsy is found in approximately 12 per cent of those with Landau–Kleffner syndrome and seizures. This is reduced to 5 per cent in Landau–Kleffner syndrome without seizures. Three per cent of the patients have encephalopathy.

Probably the only familial incidence of Landau–Kleffner syndrome is of two brothers[524] and a brother with his sister.[558]

Acquired epileptic aphasia and other predominantly linguistic deficits

Though the language disturbance is described as an acquired aphasia, the main deficit is verbal auditory agnosia[671,672] occurring in an initially normal child who achieved developmental milestones at appropriate ages and has already acquired age-appropriate speech. Whether an earlier onset of the same pathological process can prevent language development is debatable, but this by definition is not Landau–Kleffner syndrome.

The first symptom is usually verbal auditory agnosia. The parents notice a gradual inability of the child to respond to their calls despite raising their voices. Verbal auditory agnosia may later progress to non-linguistic sound agnosia such as the telephone ringing. Children with Landau–Kleffner syndrome become incapable of attributing a semantic value to acoustic signals, thus making them appear as hypoacousic or autistic children. It is because of this that the diagnosis is often delayed, mistaken for acquired deafness or mutism. Many of these children have an audiogram which is normal. The onset may be subacute, progressive or step-wise (stuttering), and gradually worsens until it affects other linguistic functions with impairment of expressive speech, paraphasias, stereotypes, perseverations and phonological errors. Probably all types of aphasia can occur. The children express themselves in a telegraphic style or in very simple sentences and in some cases may develop 'fluent aphasia' or jargon'. Finally, the child may become entirely mute, also failing to respond to even nonverbal sounds. One of the most puzzling features of Landau–Kleffner syndrome is the fluctuating course of the linguistic disturbances, characterized by remissions and exacerbations.[639]

In most cases, Landau–Kleffner syndrome starts before the children have learned reading and writing. Older children who have acquired these skills can lose them.

Psychomotor disturbances

Cognitive and behavioural problems occur in more than three quarters of patients with Landau–Kleffner syndrome. Behavioural disorders such as hyperactivity and attention deficits are common and, rarely, there is progression to severe disinhibition and psychosis.

The severity of the linguistic, behavioural and cognitive problems can vary over time in the same child and between children. Long-term follow-up studies have shown that Landau–Kleffner syndrome is not always associated with intellectual deterioration.

The language deficit may be undermined because of other behavioural or cognitive problems.

Seizures

Seizures occur in three-quarters of children with Landau–Kleffner syndrome. In one third of them these are single or isolated status epilepticus occurring mainly around 5–10 years. Seizures are often nocturnal, infrequent, respond well to treatment and remit before the age of 13–15 years. Onset is between 4–6 years, only 20 per cent of patients continue having seizures after the age of 10 years and in only three cases have these persisted after the age of 15.[80] Frequency and severity of seizures are not determined by severity of EEG abnormalities or severity of linguistic and behavioural problems.

Seizure symptoms and seizure type are not well described. They may be heterogeneous. Generalized tonic–clonic seizures (GTCS) and partial motor seizures are emphasized by the Commission.[177] However, atypical absences, atonic seizures with head drop, minor automatisms and secondary GTCS are reported.. Complex partial seizures of temporal lobe origin are very rare and tonic seizures are probably incompatible with Landau–Kleffner syndrome.

Morrell, 1995[544] in a neurosurgical series of patients with Landau–Kleffner syndrome and EEG continuous spikes and waves during slow sleep (CSWS) found with video-EEG that 'many patients have seizures that are subtle and often missed by the family. These may be minor motor manifestations such as isolated clonic deviation of the eyes, sometimes associated with blinking or occasionally only subjective behavioural manifestations such as "roaring in my eyes", sounds like a lion, accompanied by covering both ears with the hands. Such phenomena have been found to be correlated with electrographic seizure discharges. Descriptions such as those in [double] quotation marks above were obtained when the seizures began and before the onset of aphasia, or rarely after recovery as they are remembered, but the gesture of suddenly covering the ears with a terrified expression is something done by even those children who are already mute.'

A seizure of a child of Dr C. Ferrie with Landau–Kleffner syndrome was video-EEG recorded in our department and is presented in Figs. 17.2a and 17.2b.

Case 17.1. This boy, born March 1989, had a video-EEG prior to brain PET scan in February 1997. He

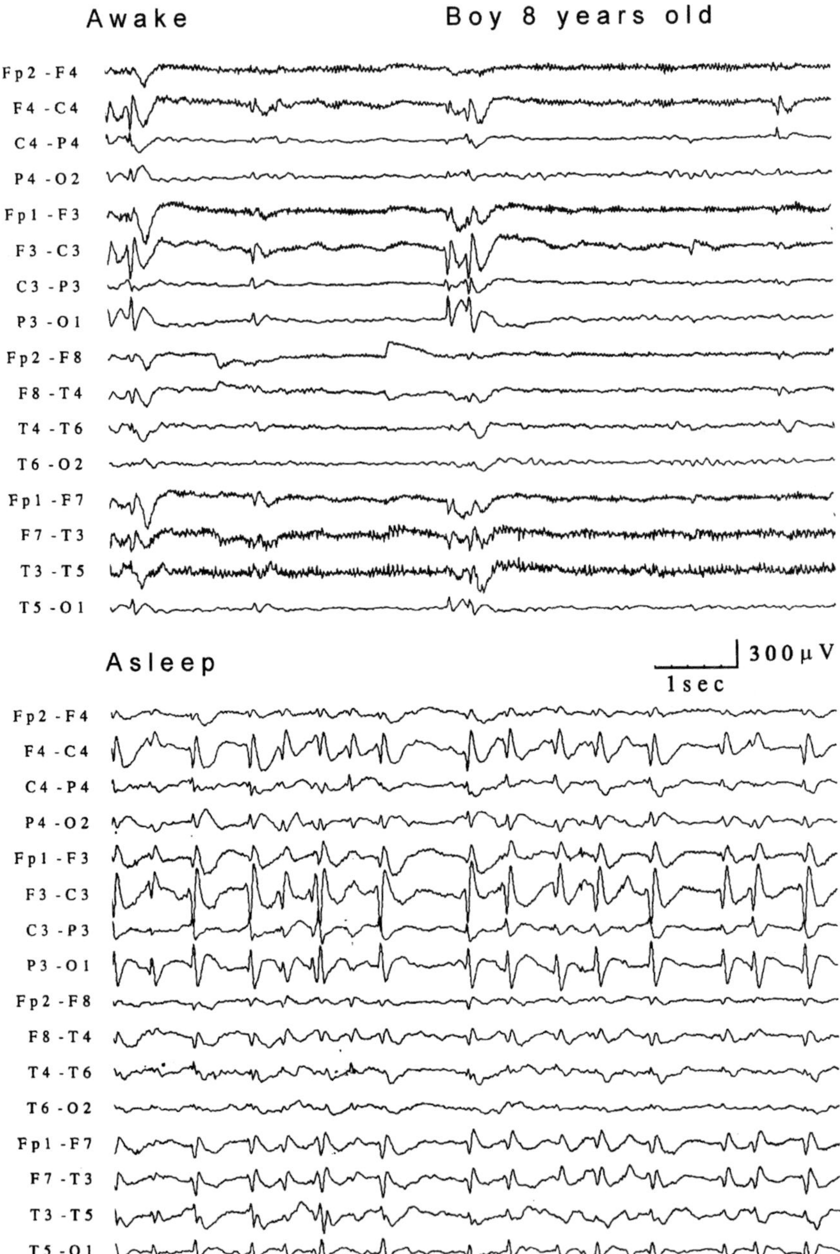

Fig. 17.2a. This is the interictal EEG of case 17.1 (see text) with Landau–Kleffner syndrome and a hemiconvulsive seizure recorded with video-EEG which is illustrated in Fig. 17.2b.

has Landau–Kleffner syndrome and 'occasional complex partial seizures with prominent motor components affecting the left side of his body with frequent atypical absences'. During the alert state there were abundant (one every 1–4 s) sharp and slow wave complexes mainly localized in the left centroparietal region. They showed maximal electronegativity around the C3, P3, T3 electrodes and maximal electro-

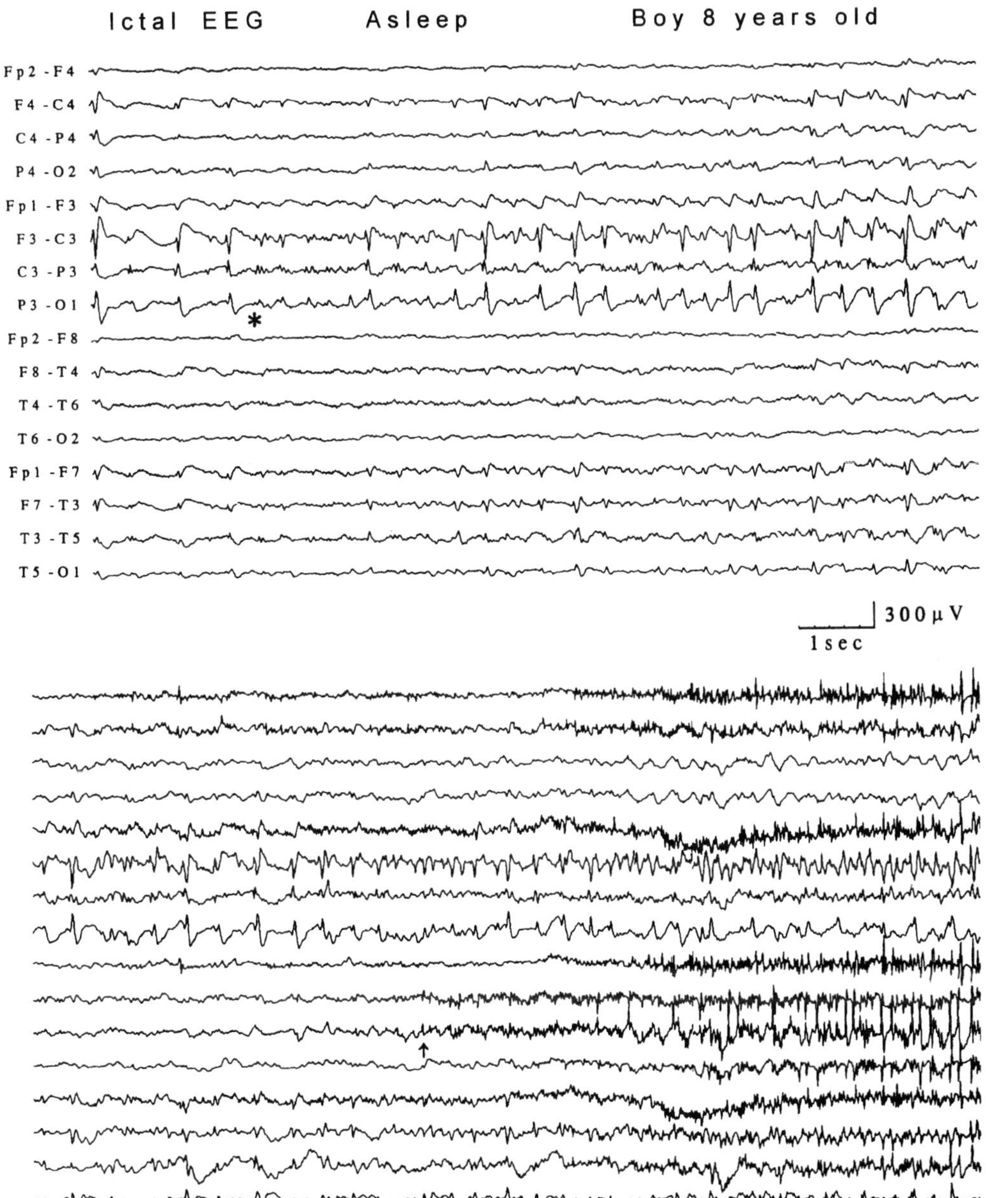

Fig. 17.2b. Ictal EEG of case 17.1 with Landau–Kleffner syndrome and a hemiconvulsive seizure recorded with video-EEG. Note the relative cessation of the sleep abnormalities prior to seizure and the onset of localized fast spike activity (asterisk). The clinical symptoms of the seizure start at arrow (see text).

positivity over the frontal areas. They were frequently displayed bisynchronously over both hemispheres with higher voltage on the left. There were also some single discharges of spike-wave independently over the right central and/or centrotemporal regions. In addition there was a consistent poverty of the alpha rhythm over the left parieto-occipital regions, while this was relatively well preserved on the right.

During sleep, simultaneously with the drop-out of the alpha rhythm on the right, the record started showing continuous bisynchronous centrotemporal spikes with higher voltage on the left with a repetitition rate at 1–1.5 per s (Fig. 17.2a).

A motor partial seizure was recorded during sleep which lasted for 2.5 min (Fig. 17.2b). The electrical status during sleep reduced and focal activity of fast rhythms at 20–25 Hz over the left central regions started intermixed with repetitive left spikes (asterisk) in the same location, mainly C3–P3. This focal fast activity increased in amplitude and became slower at 7–10 Hz intermixed with less frequent C3–P3 spikes.

The clinical seizure started at arrow (Fig. 17.2b) with a tonic spasm of the right facial muscles, swallowing and eye opening. Afterwards, the partial clonic phase started from the face, involving, within 5 s, the right eyelid. The fluttering of the right eyelid became gradually very fast, associated with tonic deviation of the head to the right. Ten seconds later there was involvement of the right arm, at the begining with tonic extension and afterwards (9 s) with clonic movements. One min later the video recording stopped due to technical problems. The seizure ended 1 min later. The EEG recording continued for 40 s after the onset of the clonic phase. It showed high voltage continuous fast-spike activity at 10–15 Hz intermixed with a few slower waves. It was localized over the left central regions, spreading to the temporal areas. The EEG activities over the right hemisphere are very difficult to differentiate from the muscle artefacts.

Post-ictally the record showed electrical status (continuous bisynchronous centrotemporal spikes). The child was drowsy, having his eyes opened or closed. He opened his eyes spontaneously 1 min after the end of the seizure.

Electroencephalography

The EEG of Landau–Kleffner syndrome, though not specific, is usually characterized by multiple foci of high amplitude sharp-slow waves with a preferential posterior temporal localization and marked slow wave sleep activation when bisynchronous discharges predominate (Figs. 17.1 and 17.2a)[75,112,174,221,250,349,390,544,547,671,739,745] The main activating EEG focus is probably in the intrasylvian region of the dominant hemisphere.

Awake EEG

The awake EEG shows relatively well preserved physiological rhythms with frequent clusters of high amplitude spikes or more likely sharp and slow wave foci which are variable in time and location (Figs. 17.1 and 17.2a). The posterior-temporal region is their preferred location, probably in more than two-thirds of the patients. Parieto-occipital regions are their second preference. Anterior and mid-temporal foci are rarer. Commonly, there are multiple foci which occur either constantly, or during certain active periods of the disease. They are often bilateral, bi-synchronous with no clear cut hemispheric preponderance but unilateral, also predominantly temporal, foci may occur in 15 per cent. Hyperventilation and photic stimulation do not appear to influence these EEG foci. Awake EEG may be normal in less than 10 per cent of the cases, even at a stage where sleep may activate very abnormal spike-and-wave complexes.

The age of appearance of these EEG abnormalities depends on the time of the first EEG which is abnormal in more than 90 per cent of the cases. This is usually performed because of clinical symptoms, between 3 and 9 years of age, with a peak at 3 to 5. EEG normalizes after the age of 15 years.

Sleep EEG

Sleep, immediately after onset, activates the EEG spike-wave foci which tend to become bi-synchronous and diffuse (Figs. 17.1 and 17.2a). This may be continuous but it is usually interrupted by normal sleep patterns.

The spread of the spikes and waves during slow sleep stages may be identical[390] or similar[112,528] to that of continuous spikes and waves during slow sleep. In Genton *et al.* 1990,[320] the case of a 3-year-old girl with Landau–Kleffner syndrome, the facilitation of spike waves was dramatically increased during REM sleep. A substantial number of patients with Landau–Kleffner syndrome show CSWS at a certain stage of the disease which may persist for a long time.

Spike localization in Landau–Kleffner syndrome

Morrell, 1995,[544] in one of his last papers before his tragic and untimely death, detailed the results of his team's extraordinary research in patients with Landau–Kleffner syndrome. This is a highly recommended reading that cannot be surpassed. These are some extracts:

With the use of the methohexital suppression test, intracarotid amobarbital, and EEG dipole mapping, Morrell,1995[544] showed that 'despite the apparent bilaterality and widespread distribution of the disturbance EEG pattern of these patients with Landau–Kleffner syndrome, the actual source of the epileptiform abnormalities in both hemispheres was dependent on the discharge emanating from the left. In other words, this bilateral and hypersynchronous EEG epileptiform activity is generated by a primary epileptogenic focus which is unilateral and exquisitely localized. In fact, there is a very consistent and striking organization of a spike dipole with the temporal site being positive to the negativity at the suprasylvian derivation. This distribution of electrical charge is most easily interpreted as reflecting a tangentially oriented dipole with an origin on the superior surface of the superior temporal gyrus.'

Furthermore, Morrell states:[544] 'Tangential dipoles are particularly well delineated by magnetic source imaging. Signals detected in magnetic recording are those of transmembrane synaptic currents oriented in a plane tangential to the surface of the skull. The method is particularly appropriate for the detection of potential generators in the depths of sulci such as the Sylvian fissure. A 37-channel planar gradiometer was used. EEG and magnetoencephalographic (MEG) data were simultaneously collected with EEG discharges serving as a time marker for MEG. The dipole fit derived from magnetic source data superimposed upon a previously obtained MRI. Evoked potentials to peripheral shocks and to pure tone stimuli were also recorded and were displayed on the MRI together with the spontaneous spike potentials. A series of sequential coronal sections beginning anteriorly and extending posteriorly revealed the distribution of the magnetic dipoles of each recorded spike.'

With this method Morrell and collaborators[544] found that the primary focus is typically larger and more widely distributed on the planum temporale than is the secondary site. 'There was a strikingly consistent localization of these generators on the dorsal surface of the superior temporal gyrus. It is important to remember that these well-localized discharges are responsible for the extraordinarily widespread abnormalities and there was a close proximity of the sites of the auditory evoked potentials elicited by pure tones to the epileptogenic areas'. A similar localization was documented by Paetau, 1994[592] in a patient with Landau–Kleffner syndrome.

In another Landau–Kleffner patient of Morrell and collaborators,[544] the entire dipole, including its orientation, was displayed on the MR image. 'In the sagittal reconstruction, the dipolar orientation was perpendicular to the Sylvian fissure and was angled so that the suprasylvian projection is anterior to that of the infrasylvian one. This distribution was comparable with the dipolar organization derived from electrical mapping of extracellular current flow.'

Morrell goes even further:[544] 'The magnetoencephalograph provides a striking demonstration of the intrasylvian location of these discharging sources, despite their apparent widespread distribution as viewed in the standard EEG. Magnetic source imaging revealed the origin of the abnormality to be on the dorsal surface of the superior temporal gyrus, essentially in the auditory association cortex, with the spike dipole being oriented tangentially to the scalp surface. This localization and the unilaterality of its origin was confirmed by electrocorticographic recording from within the Sylvian fissure. At times the epileptogenic region was confined within the Sylvian fissure near Heschl's gyrus.'

The highly specific, consistent and unilateral localization of the epileptogenic process indicated in the above studies was also confirmed with electrocorticography. There was an 'extraordinarily localized and very high voltage discharge recorded from an electrode on the superior surface of the superior temporal gyrus'. Interestingly, an adventitious noise in the operating theatre resulted in prompt but temporary suppression of this discharge and this acoustical suppression could then be reproduced intentionally time after time. The interaction of acoustic input with the epileptiform potentials suggested that the latter were generated in neocortical tissue normally engaged in acoustic processing.'

Finally, Morrell and collaborators[544] were able to demonstrate that transaction of the intrasylvian source and the secondary activated tissue surrounding it resulted in disappearance of the widespread discharge in the operated hemisphere and also in the opposite contralateral cortex. Furthermore, Morrell and collaborators[544] observed that in 11 of 14 Landau–Kleffner syndrome patients their neurosurgical procedure as above resulted in cessation of seizures, normalization of the EEG and gradual recovery of speech.[544,545]

Audiogram and auditory evoked potentials

Tonal audiogram[672] is normal in Landau–Kleffner syndrome. There is nothing wrong with the hearing. The defect is cortical. However, auditory evoked responses may be abnormal.[408a]

Brain imaging

Structural neuroimaging with computed tomography (CT) and magnetic resonance imaging (MRI) is normal. The findings of functional neuroimaging are of interest.

da Silva and colleagues, 1997[187] evaluated 17 children (aged 2.4 to 10.6 years) with Landau–Kleffner syndrome using positron emission tomography (PET) with 2-deoxy-2-[18F]fluoro-D-glucose (FDG). Patients were awake for the uptake period of FDG, and the EEG was monitored. On visual analysis of the PET images, patients showed metabolic abnormalities in the temporal lobes. Fifteen patients showed bilateral temporal hypometabolism, and comparison of these patients with a neurologically normal age-matched control group (n = 8) demonstrated significantly reduced glucose metabolism bilaterally in the middle temporal gyrus ($P < 0.02$). The remaining two children had focal hypermetabolism in the left temporal cortex, one of whom also showed right temporal cortex hypometabolism. Other cortical regions could display hypometabolism but these regions were not consistently abnormal in all patients. The authors concluded that 'The finding of temporal lobe abnormalities in all Landau–Kleffner syndrome patients suggests that temporal lobe structures are important in the pathophysiology of this syndrome, whereas the presence of additional cortical abnormalities in many patients indicates that extensive brain functional disturbances are common.'[187]

De Volder *et al.* 1994[216a] studied regional brain glucose utilization with PET and FDG in a case of Landau–Kleffner syndrome associated with a left sylvian arachnoid cyst. CT and MRI had failed to disclose any mass effect of the cyst on surrounding brain structures. Sequential metabolic measurements showed a comparable pronounced hypometabolism in cortical regions around the cyst, involving speech areas, and suggested mild but chronic compression of the developing brain. After placement of a cyst-peritoneal shunt system, significant metabolic improvement occurred in all cortical regions, especially the inferior frontal gyrus and the perisylvian area, with predominant residual deficit in the left superior temporal gyrus. These findings were concomitant with a pronounced improvement in word fluency and slower progress in verbal auditory comprehension.

Guerreiro and colleagues, 1996[366] reported that all five Landau–Kleffner syndrome children tested with SPECT had abnormal perfusion in the left temporal lobe.

Pathology

The pathology of Landau–Kleffner syndrome is well reviewed by Smith:[733] 'The pathological findings associated with Landau–Kleffner syndrome in the literature are similar to those seen in other partial epilepsies; such as encephalitis, vasculitis, subpial gliosis, cysticercosis, and neuronal migration disorders. The biopsy material taken from the temporal pole, at a distance from the primary epileptic site, in one surgical series of 14 patients with Landau–Kleffner syndrome revealed a variety of pathological abnormalities in 13.'[733]

Evolution and prognosis

Seizures and EEG abnormalities are age-dependent and remit by the age of 15 years though 10 to 20 per cent of the reported cases continue having infrequent partial motor seizures or GTCS. Language and other neuropsychological disturbances gradually improve at the same age as the disappearance of EEG epileptiform activity, but although some 10–20 per cent may achieve complete normalization all others are left with permanent sequelae which may be very severe. There is a general consensus that early onset of Landau–Kleffner syndrome is related to the worsened prognosis regarding language recovery. Outcome does not depend on frequency and type of seizures. Only half of patients with Landau–Kleffner syndrome may be able to live a relatively normal social and professional life.[75]

Treatment

Medical treatment

Seizures in Landau–Kleffner syndrome are infrequent, often age-limited and easily controlled with anti-epileptic drugs. Therefore seizures are not a problem. The pharmaceutical attempt is to reduce the epileptiform EEG discharges on the assumption that these are responsible for the linguistic, behavioural and other neuropsychological abnormalities of children with Landau–Kleffner syndrome. All traditional anti-epileptic drugs, including sleep modifying drugs such as amitriptyline and amphetamine, have been tried with disappointing results. However, some children responded rather well to high doses of corticosteroid therapy, either with ACTH or prednisone.

The consensus is to first treat Landau–Kleffner syndrome with sodium valproate, ethosuximide and clonazepam or clobazam, alone or in combination. If this fails, which is most likely, ACTH or prednisone should be the treatment of choice, especially in new and younger patients who may respond better, need shorter steroid treatment and are at a higher risk for significant residual neuropsychological sequelae. There is an empirical view that the results depend on early treatment with high initial doses of steroids. A proposed strategy is to use prednisone 3–5 mg/kg daily or ACTH 80 IU/day for at least 3 months. Continuation of treatment after this period depends on response and side effects. Some children with a good response may relapse and this may necessitate long, probably for years, continuation of treatment. Steroids are usually used together with valproate or benzodiazepines and these may continue after steroid withdrawal.

The effect of treatment should be monitored with appropriate neuropsychological evaluation and serial awake and sleep EEG.

Neurosurgical treatment

Morrell *et al.*,1995[544,545] reported their results on the treatment of Landau–Kleffner syndrome with subpial intracortical transection. Utilizing this new surgical technique, designed to eliminate the capacity of cortical tissue to generate seizures while preserving the normal cortical physiological function, they treated 14 children with aphasia, seizures and a severely abnormal EEG by multiple subpial transection of the epileptogenic cortex. Seven of the 14 patients (50 per cent) recovered age-appropriate speech, attended regular classes in school and no longer required speech therapy. Four of the 14 (29 per cent) showed marked improvement, speaking and understanding verbal with instruction with regard to speech therapy. Thus, 11 of the 14 (79 per cent), none of whom had used language to communicate for at least 2 years, were able to speak – a rate of sustained improvement considered unusual in this disorder. This study documented the value of a treatment modality not previously used in Landau–Kleffner syndrome. Success depends on selection of cases having severe epileptogenic abnormality that can be demonstrated to be unilateral in origin despite a bilateral electrographic manifestation.

Sawhney and colleagues, 1995[706] had three mute patients with Landau–Kleffner syndrome who showed substantial recovery of speech after multiple subpial transection.

Epilepsy with continuous spikes and waves during slow sleep (ECSWS) or Epilepsy with electrical status epilepticus during slow sleep (ESESS)

Introduction

Epilepsy with continuous spikes and waves during slow sleep (ECSWS) or epilepsy with electrical status epilepticus during slow sleep (ESESS) is a partly reversible, age-related childhood syndrome characterized by the triad of (a) EEG continuous spikes and waves during slow sleep, (b) seizures, and (c) neuropsychological decline.[79,80,144,197,209,210,318,461,527,539,540,578,589,644,733,755–757] Continuous spikes and waves during slow sleep are a prerequisite for the diagnosis of epilepsy with CSWS which follows three stages of evolution. The first stage manifests with mainly infrequent nocturnal motor partial seizures, often hemiclonic status epilepticus and EEG with focal and bi-synchronous generalized discharges. In the second stage, EEG show continuous spikes and waves during slow sleep, seizures become worse and polymorphous with frequent atypical absences and atonic but never tonic fits, while neuropsychological decline and behavioural abnormalities are severe. In the third stage, seizures improve and finally remit entirely followed by gradual normalization of EEG and improvement of the neuropsychological state, which rarely may reach average normal but more frequently patients are left with significant deficits.

Definition

The Commission on Classification and Terminology of the International League Against Epilepsy,1989[177] named this condition 'epilepsy with continuous spikes and waves during slow sleep' (ECSWS) to the dismay of Tassinary[755] who insists in his first proposition that this is 'epilepsy with electrical status epilepticus during slow sleep (ESESS).'

The Commission[177] classified ECSWS amongst the epilepsies and syndromes undetermined as to whether they are focal or generalized and it is defined as follows: 'Epilepsy with CSWS results from the association of various seizure types, partial or generalized, occurring during sleep, and atypical absences when awake. Tonic seizures do not occur. The characteristic EEG pattern consists of continuous diffuse spike-waves during slow wave sleep, which is noted after onset of seizures. Duration varies from months to years. Despite the usually benign evolution of seizures, prognosis is guarded because of the appearance of neuropsychological disorders.'[177]

Synonyms

Subclinical 'electical status epilepticus' induced by sleep in children.[644]
Electrical status epilepticus during sleep (ESES)[755,757]

Historical aspects

Patry, Lyagoubi and Tassinari, 1971[644] were the first to report subclinical 'electical status epilepticus' induced by sleep in four boys and two girls, aged 7–12 years. The clinical situation was heterogeneous. Five patients had epileptic seizures, five were mentrally retarded, two failed to acquire language and one was mute. Seizures were described as atonic, generalized tonic–clonic, convulsive, clonic and atypical absences. Because the degree of mental retardation was related to the age of onset of the seizures, the authors speculated that this syndrome represented a form of encephalopathy secondary to a focal or multifocal brain lesion. They attributed the EEG paroxysmal activity during sleep to an activating synchronizing system of slow sleep.

Tassinari prefers[755] the term 'electrical status epilepticus during sleep'. However, according to Bureau,

1995[144] this name was criticized in the workshop held in Marseille (July,1983) because (a) it was difficult to accept that continuous spikes and waves during sleep can be considered as a status without detectable simultaneous clinical signs, and (b) continuous spikes and waves during sleep can occur in non-epileptic children. Therefore, the term 'continuous spikes and waves during sleep' (CSWS) was preferred by the Commission,[177] also accepting this as a separate epileptic syndrome.

Prevalence

This must be a very rare condition of no more than 0.4 per cent amongst children with seizures. Morikawa *et al.*[539,540] reported 31 cases with ECSWS from 12,854 patients with childhood epilepsies that they had examined in the past 10 years. Kramer and colleagues,1998,[454] in a cohort of 440 consecutive paediatric patients with at least two seizures, found that ECSWS and Landau–Kleffner syndrome were extremely rare (0.2 per cent each) as compared to Rolandic seizures (8 per cent) or benign childhood occipital seizures (2 per cent). Despite their interest in this condition only 31 cases were found by the physicians in the famous Centre St-Paul, Marseille between 1968 and 1992.[144]

Genetics

A family history of epilepsy is quite uncommon (approxiamtely 10 per cent). There are no genetic studies regarding sleep EEG in siblings and other relatives. It should be reminded that both clinical and EEG features are age-dependent, disappearing later in life.

Neurological state and personal antecedents

More than one third of patients with ECSWS have abnormal neurological and neuroradiological signs such as unilateral or diffuse cortical atrophy, porencephaly and developmental brain malformations. Pre- or perinatal illness, neonatal convulsions, congenital hemiparesis or tetraparesis, psychomotor or language retardation are found in approxiamtely half of the cases. These cannot be included in the idiopathic form of the benign childhood partial seizures described in this book.

Age at onset and sex

This syndrome is age-dependent, occurring only in children. Onset of seizures is between 1 and 10 years, with a peak at 4–5 years. The age at onset of CSWS is not certain but may peak at 8 years, usually starting after 1–2 years from the first seizure.

There may be a male preponderance (62 per cent, 18 of 29 cases of Tassinari *et al.*, 1992).[757]

Electroclinical features

First stage before the discovery of CSWS

Seizures prior to the development of CSWS

The first seizure is usually nocturnal in half of the cases and in 40 per cent consists of unilateral convulsions often lasting for more than half an hour, thus constituting hemiclonic status epilepticus. In the other cases the first seizure may be partial motor–clonic, generalized tonic–clonic, complex partial seizures or myoclonic absence. Motor manifestations involving the facial muscles with a mandibular contraction and loss of consciousness were described in four and hemifacial motor seizure in only one of 29 cases in a study.[757]

Neuropsychological state prior to CSWS

Of 29 patients with ECSWS, 13 had normal psychomotor development prior to CSWS, five had linguistic impairment and 11 already exhibited psychomotor retardation.[757]

Electroencephalographic findings prior to the development of CSWS

The interictal awake routine EEG after the first seizure usually, in more than two thirds of the patients, show 'more or less generalized spikes and waves, sometimes in bursts, clinically accompanied or not by impairment of consciousness with twitching of the eyelids'.[757] Also, half of the patients have focal interictal spikes or sharp-slow waves localized in the frontotemporal or centrotemporal regions associated with diffuse abnormalities. Rarely, in less than one fifth of the cases, focal or multifocal abnormalities without generalized discharges may occur.[539,540,757] These abnormalities are activated by sleep without altering their morphology. Sleep patterns and cyclic organization do not change.

Thus, for the majority of these children there would be an EEG warning of a stormy disease process with the appearance of bi-synchronous, generalized spikes or sharp and slow waves, sometimes accompanied with subtle clinical events such as impairment of consciousness, eyelid flickering or both. These do not occur in Rolandic seizures or other forms of benign childhood partial seizures. Exceptions in medicine are the rule, but there are very few, if any, in the proposed association of Rolandic seizures and ECSWS.

Second stage with CSWS

The discovery of CSWS is usually because of seizure increase and neuropsychological symptoms that prompt a sleep EEG. This is probably 1–2 years after the first seizure with a peak at 8 years and a range of 4–10 years. The duration of CSWS is also difficult to assess, ranging from one month to several months, up to 6–7 years.

Seizures during the stage of CSWS

After a variable time, up to 1–2 years, of infrequent seizures these become more frequent and complicated with other type of seizures such as typical or more frequently atypical absences, myoclonic absences, absence status, atonic or clonic fits, oro-facial and generalized tonic–clonic convulsions. It is at this stage that the CSWS EEG pattern is usually discovered and this is also associated with a neuropsychological decline.

Of 26 patients described by Tassinari, 1992[757] three had only motor seizures (myoclonic absences, GTCS or oro-facial seizures), 12 also developed typical absences 'similar to those of childhood absence epilepsy' and 12 had 'atypical absences, frequently with atonic and clonic components leading to sudden falls'.[757]

The general consensus is that tonic seizures do not occur at any stage and these are probably incompatible with the diagnosis of ECSWS.

In the course of the disease, seizures may rarely be infrequent but most likely, in over 90 per cent, these are numerous from several per week to several per day.

Neuropsychological state during the stage of CSWS

There is a dramatic, sometimes sudden but often insidious decline of the psychomotor development of these children at the time when CSWS is discovered.

The decline of the neuropsychological state and behaviour abnormalities are the most cardinal and disturbing clinical features of ECSWS. Many of these children suffer from complex and severe neuropsychological impairment, mainly of language-related functions, with mental impairment and psychiatric disturbances that may be life long, despite some improvement, after an age-related remission of seizures and CSWS.[112,539,540,757]

Tassinari and colleagues, 1992[757] distinguished two groups according to their premorbid state:

Group A:

In all 18 patients with a normal psychomotor development who attended main stream schools prior to the occurrence of CSWS there was, during CSWS, a severe decrease in IQ, ranging from 45 to 78, as measured by the Wechsler Intelligence Scale for Children. Also, all showed behavioural abnormalities with reduced attention span, hyperkinesia, aggressiveness, difficulty in contact, sometimes dysinhibition and two patients suffered psychotic states.

Two thirds (eight children) exhibited a very marked reduction of language function though five of them already had an isolated speech retardation prior to the probable onset of CSWS and in two of them there was an expressive dysphasia. In another five untested cases, severe impairment of language was noted. Therefore in 13/18 cases there was a marked reduction of language function. Furthermore, 10 also suffered very marked impairment of temporo-spatial orientation.

Group B

All 11 cases with abnormal psychomotor development prior to the occurrence of CSWS had during CSWS a worsening of mental deficiency, impairment of temporo-spatial orientation and three exhibited severe aggression.

EEG continuous spikes and waves during slow sleep

ECSWS is mainly an EEG defined condition. So what is CSWS? Let us learn from Tassinari *et al.*, 1992:[757]

> As soon as the patient falls asleep continuous bilateral and diffuse slow spike and wave (SW) appear, persisting through all the slow sleep stages. It is not a matter of an 'important' or 'almost subcontinuous' activation. Indeed, the discharges are continuous and the SW index ranges from 85 to 100 per cent. The SW index was calculated during all-night sleep EEG recordings. It is equal to the total sum of all spike-waves (min) x 100 divided by the total non-REM duration (min). However, other authors (Calvet, 1978;[145] Billard *et al.*, 1981[112]) also include diseases with a SW index higher than 50 per cent. Thus, they considerably widen the definition of CSWS, from a continuous status of SW, as in our own definition, to a considerable amount of SW during slow sleep. With this method, we have noted that the percentage of CSWS is more marked during the first cycle of sleep (95–100 per cent) than in the following cycles (80–70 per cent), but the overall percentage is equal to 85. The physiological sleep patterns (spindles, K complexes or vertex spikes) were seldom distinguishable. In some cases, focal abnormalities, with frontal predominance, can be observed during the rare short periods (seconds) of fragmented diffuse SW discharges in non-REM sleep. During REM sleep the electrical status disappears and the paroxysmal abnormalities consist of rare bursts of diffuse SW, or of focal, predominantly frontal discharges. In four patients (also three described by Dalla Bernardina *et al.,* 1978)[197] focal, fronto-central rhythmic discharges organized as a subclinical seizure were observed at the end of REM sleep.

The CSWS consists mainly of spike and wave with no polyspikes or fast episodic activity which is against this diagnosis. The intradischarge frequency is usually slow, 1.5–2 Hz, but faster rates, 3–4 Hz, can occur. CSWS is a consistent finding over the active phase of this condition.

The differentiation of non-REM and REM sleep is possible because of the preservation of EEG and polygraphic REM sleep patterns concomitant with the non-REM-related discontinuation of CSWS. The cyclic organization of sleep is grossly preserved, 80 per cent of sleep is non-REM and there are no apparent sleep disorders. On awakening, EEG abnormalities are similar to those of the wakefulness prior to sleep.

Third stage of remission

After a variable period of months to usually 2–7 years this aggressive, neuropsychological and electroencephalographic disorder starts improving and finally all patients remit regarding seizures, and EEG gradually improves to normalization. Neuropsychological problems also improve though often severe sequelae remain.

Remission of seizures

Seizures gradually become less frequent and less severe before they finally remit in all, symptomatic

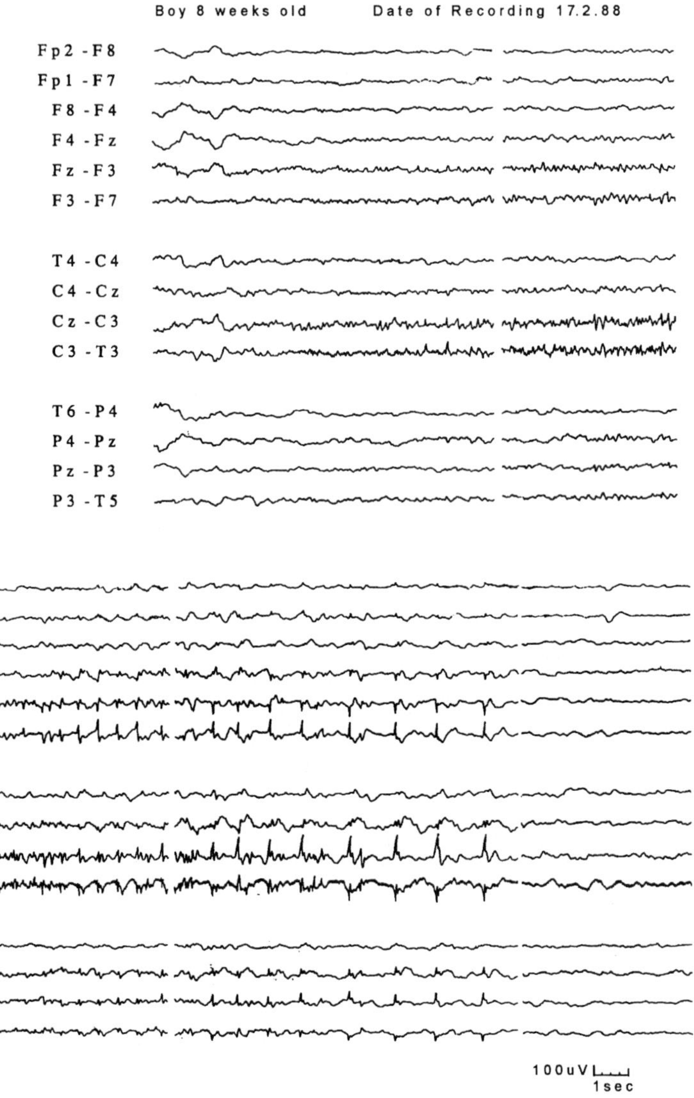

Fig. 17.3a. EEG of patient 17.2 when he was 8 weeks old. The EEG is continuous. Note the electrical discharge starting with fast rhythms and small spikes in the left central region.

or idiopathic, cases at about the age of 10–15 years. Seizure improvement may be simultaneous, precede or follow the disappearance of CSWS.

The total duration of the active seizure period varies from 4 to 17 years.

Neuropsychological status after the remission of seizures and CSWS

Though all patients show a global psychomental and behavioural improvement after the remission of CSWS and seizures, recovery is always slow and often only partial. Less than a quarter of the patients

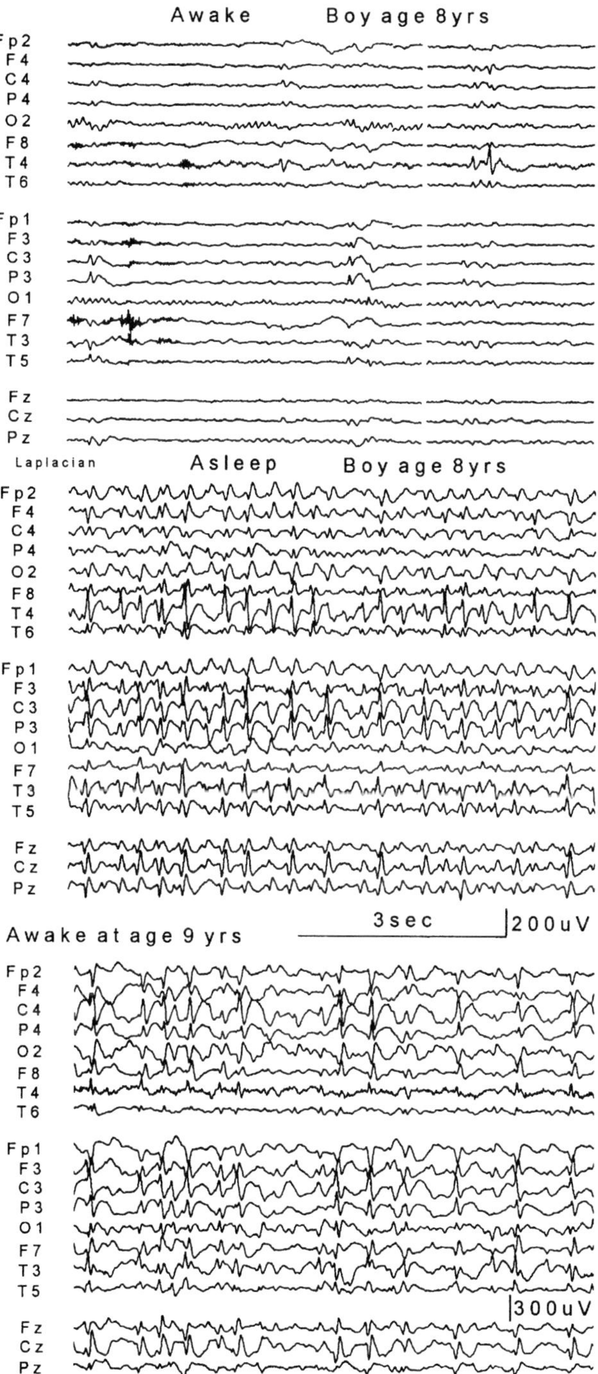

Fig. 17.3b. Longitudinal evolution of EEG of patient 17.2. His first EEG at age 2 months is shown in Fig. 17.3a. Awake EEG at age 8 years shows infrequent right and left centrotemporal spikes (upper) but during sleep there is CSWS (middle). At age 9 even awake EEG shows nearly continuous spike-wave activity (bottom).

will resume acceptable social and professional levels and these are more likely amongst those who had a normal pre-morbid neuropsychological state and a shorter CSWS life span.

In the long follow-up of Tassinari *et al.*, 1992[757] neuropsychiatric disturbances improved but the global evaluation at last follow-up showed that only 15 of 29 patients lived a normal life.

The neuropsychological and social prognosis does not depend on age of discovery of CSWS, severity of epilepsy, presence or absence of a cerebral lesion but is likely to be worse if the duration of CSWS is long.

Relative normalization of EEG

Longitudinal sleep EEG show a progressive, over approximately 3 years, improvement towards normalization after an average age of about 11 years. The discharges during sleep EEG become less frequent and more fragmented and gradually they allow the reappearance of physiological patterns. Rare focal sharp and slow wave complexes may persist, particularly in sleep EEG, long after clincal improvement.

After CSWS remission, in all cases, sleep organization is normal, sleep stages have their normal percentage and the EEG patterns are bilateral and symmetrical.

An interesting case of epilepsy with continuous spikes and waves during slow sleep

The following is a very interesting case who at age 9 years had ECSWS. Though he had three partial motor seizures at age 2 months, his development was normal without seizures and he was an excellent student until age 7 years when seizures started again, and these were followed by gradual mental deterioration and EEG development of CSWS (Figs. 17.3a and 17.3b). He had two normal MRI.

This boy is a patient of Dr G. Du Mond, Consultant in Paediatrics at St. Thomas' Hospital who allowed me to publish it here. I know about the case because of EEG follow-up in our department from age 2 months.

> Case 17.2. This boy, born 17 December 1987, had at age 8 weeks three right sided convulsions which mainly involved face and upper limbs. An EEG six days later showed during sleep 'a classical electrical seizure' in the left central regions (Fig. 17.3a). No clinical manifestations were noticed but the child was lying in mum's arms. Treatment with sodium valproate was initiated. He did not have any further seizures and his next EEG six months later (21.7.88) both while awake and during sleep was normal. A brain MRI on 11.2.88 was reported as normal. Sodium valproate was stopped ten months later in November 1988.
>
> No further seizures occurred and he developed well until the age of 7 years, when he had three seizures. 'His hands started shaking and if he is holding something he will drop it'. He is unable to speak during these and trembles. They last for 1–2 min and he does not lose consciousness during them. Two occurred on the same day and one was precipitated by a knock on the forehead. Following the attack, his right arm is stiff and this resolves after 10 min or so.' A repeat EEG in September 1994 and MRI were normal.
>
> Treatment with sodium valproate was initiated again but soon after he had approximately six seizures. These were right sided partial motor of the face and arm. A new EEG elsewhere was highly abnormal with continuous high amplitude spike, multiple spike and slow wave in all regions. I reviewed this and started to wonder whether during this EEG he was in any type of epileptic status (myoclonic, absence).
>
> In April 1995, he was admitted to our hospital because 'of increasing seizures. On discharge he had a number of further fits where he just dribbles or is subject to more extensive fits involving his right arm and becoming secondary generalized. This settled with the addition of lamotrigine.' A new EEG in April 1995 was severely abnormal (Fig. 17.3b).
>
> Subsequent to these events, the situation got out of hand. He continued to have frequent fits. Two of these lasted for approximately 25 min. It is interesting that in, April 1996, he had a seizure which was different from all others. He woke up at night unable to see. His eyes were deviated and he was shaking and hysterical. The episode lasted for about 5 min. His vision gradually returned and he fell asleep. He also continued having attacks of dribbling from the corner of his mouth and making a clicking noise. This lasted for 2–3 min and he was well afterwards.
>
> 'It was at this time in 1996 that his school work also started being affected. He used to be regularly at the

top of his class and this was no longer happening. He has difficulty in concentration, sometimes falls asleep at school and he is often too tired to complete his home work.'

In October 1996, he was referred to a Specialized Paediatric Neurology Clinic. Since then things have got even worse, though some response to steroids was noticed. In particular, in a recent medical report dated July 1997 it was noted that 'he has made a remarkable improvement following his course of steroids, he has apparently been doing very well at school and gained some very creditable marks in the end of term examination'.

Autosomal dominant Rolandic epilepsy and speech dyspraxia: A new syndrome with anticipation

'Autosomal dominant Rolandic epilepsy and speech dyspraxia: a new syndrome with anticipation' appears to be a rare hereditary condition that was newly described by the Australian team of Scheffer *et al*,.1995.[708] They extensively studied a family of nine affected individuals over three generations with nocturnal orofaciobrachial partial seizures, secondary generalized partial seizures, and centrotemporal epileptiform discharges, associated with oral and speech dyspraxia and cognitive impairment. The authors assessed that 'The speech disorder was prominent, but differed from that of Landau–Kleffner syndrome and of epilepsy with continuous spike and wave during slow-wave sleep' and that 'The electroclinical features of this new syndrome of autosomal dominant Rolandic epilepsy resemble those of benign Rolandic epilepsy, a common inherited epilepsy of childhood. This family shows clinical anticipation of the seizure disorder, the oral and speech dyspraxia, and cognitive dysfunction, suggesting that the genetic mechanism could be expansion of an unstable triplet repeat. Molecular studies on this syndrome, where the inheritance pattern is clear, could also be relevant to identifying a gene for benign Rolandic epilepsy where anticipation does not occur and the mode of inheritance is uncertain.'

However, the clinical presentation of these patients with permanent neurologic deficit, sometimes preceding the seizures, can hardly be considered as 'resembling benign Rolandic epilepsy' or 'epitomize the archetypal benign Rolandic epileptic attack'[708] which the authors believe.

Let us take for example their first patient, the proband:

> 'This 5-year-old boy presented with a 2-month history of ataxia, inability to combine two words, drooling, incontinence, and irritability, and was in nonconvulsive status epilepticus (NCSE). Birth history was unremarkable. Global developmental delay had been recognized at 21 months when he spoke only a single word. Nocturnal seizures began at 2.5 years and were diagnosed at 3.5 years when he had a 30-min right-sided facio-brachial seizure. Sodium valproate was commenced with improvement in his speech. Partial seizures increased at 4.5 years and were characterized by nocturnal right-sided facial and upper limb twitching and drooling, and sometimes secondary generalization. He sometimes staggered to his parents' bedroom during a seizure, leaning to the right. He had difficulty speaking and he stuttered. Further episodes of NCSE occurred at 6 and 7 years.
>
> On examination, oral coordination was poor with abnormal fluency, accuracy, and rate of speech. Speech was slow and effortful, and at times unintelligible. Some functional oral tasks were poorly performed including managing solid foods, blowing out candles on his birthday cake and sucking through a straw. Receptive and expressive language skills on formal assessment were below expectation based on his Verbal Intelligence Quotient (VIQ) of 79.
>
> EEG studies performed between 3 years 10 months and 6.5 years showed frequent bilaterally independent centrotemporal epdeptiform activity. Discharges had the morphology of a sharp wave followed by a prominent slow wave and the field of a horizontal dipole. His EEG during NCSE showed continuous epdeptiform activity consisting predominantly of discharges localized to the right centrotemporal region with occasional left centrotemporal discharges, both awake and asleep.'

Patients of previous generations were not so severely affected but they also had neurological deficits mainly of oral and speech dyspraxia without evidence of dysarthria.

This is an extraordinarily rare family that was meticulously investigated by one of the most competent teams in the world, who by the time of publication may already have progressed to the identification of the relevant gene in this family. However, this has little relevance to millions of normal children with Rolandic seizures all over the world.

Atypical benign partial epilepsy of childhood

Atypical benign partial epilepsy of childhood is a term coined by Aicardi and Chevrie, 1982[16] for a rare condition that they initially described in seven children with normal neurological and intellectual state and a final good output. The term 'benign' was not because of possible similarities with Rolandic seizures but in order to distinguish them from the severe epileptic syndromes of childhood and mainly the Lennox–Gastaut syndrome 'for which it is regularly mistaken because of the repeated falls, absences, and diffuse slow spike-wave activity when drowsiness or sleep records are obtained'. These seven children had 'partial motor seizures ocurring on falling asleep or on awakening, reminiscent of those seen in benign partial epilepsy of childhood, absences clinically similar to those of petit mal epilepsy, brief atonic or myoclonic seizures responsible for repeated falls; and generalized tonic–clonic seizures mostly nocturnal'. EEG showed a striking contrast between waking state which usually displayed focal central spikes, and sleep with an almost continuous, diffuse, slow spike-wave activity. Age at onset was in early childhood and 'although the electroclinical features suggested the diagnosis of Lennox–Gastaut syndrome or myoclonic epilepsy, the seizures remitted spontaneously in the five oldest patients and may well do so in the two youngest ones'.[304]

The following description of atypical benign partial epilepsy of childhood is based on a recent review of Aicardi[15] with his accumulated experience of 12 cases[17] and on a few more cases in the literature.[224,240,431,585,831]

Clinical manifestations

The onset is between 2 and 6 years of age in children with normal development and neurological examination. At the active seizure periods there is some degree of mental slowing or behavioural disturbance which is often subtle and disappears during seizure-free periods. All patients have at least two different seizure types: atonic attacks and nocturnal partial Rolandic-like seizures.

Atonic seizures are the most characteristic of all and occur in clusters lasting for one to several weeks, usually separated by free intervals of several weeks or months. They may involve the whole axial musculature and/or both lower limbs with multiple daily falls which can produce severe injuries. On other occasions, they may be localized, manifested with brief 1–2 s sudden head drop or hand focal atonia demonstrated by having the patient maintain his arms extended. Brief focal atonia in seven patients of Oguni and colleagues 1992[585] was observed as a transient dropping of one arm, lasting from 100 to 150 ms when patients were asked to keep both arms outstretched in front of the body. The brief focal atonia of the arm occasionally would progress to atonic seizures or atonic absence seizures.

Atonic attacks are associated with the slow-wave component of spike-wave complexes, and the location of the EEG discharges corresponds to that of the atonic episodes.[431,585]

Nocturnal partial seizures similar to Rolandic seizures are often infrequent and the initial seizure type.

Other type of seizures. Some patients may additionally have generalized tonic–clonic seizures, brief absences and occasionally jerks. Focal sensory-motor fits are exceptional.

In some patients, absence seizures may be more prominent as in the two twin sisters reported by Yoshimura *et al.*, 1993.[831] These two girls had diurnal atypical absences and nocturnal partial seizures.

Deonna *et al.*1986[224] reported six other cases that closely resembled those of Aicardi and Chevrie[16], although the focal clinical and EEG features were not as striking as in their cases.

Doose and Baier 1989[240] called this condition of atypical benign partial epilepsy of childhood 'pseudo-Lennox syndrome'. They reported that repeated minor seizures may combine to a series or status resembling the Lennox–Gastaut syndrome and maintained that overt and subclinical status epilepticus may in some cases lead to transient or persisting deterioration of the psychomental state or to severe dementia or Landau–Kleffner syndrome.

Electroencephalographic manifestations

Sleep EEG are similar or identical to the continuous spikes and waves during slow sleep (CSWS). This occurs mainly during the active period of atonic seizures and may disappear in between. The awake EEG shows centrotemporal spikes, often with considerable contralateral and generalized spread. Generalized 3-Hz spike-waves are frequent with or without clinical absences.

Oguni and colleagues, 1992[585] studied unilateral, brief, 100–150 ms, focal atonia in their seven patients with polygraphic video-EEG. The dropping of the arm corresponded exactly with a single sharp and slow wave complex arising from the contralateral centro-temporo-parietal region. The brief focal atonia of the arm occasionally would progress to atonic seizures or atonic absence seizures, when the localized epileptic discharge evolved into generalized discharges. In one patient they found that the intensity of brief focal atonia was proportional to the amplitude of the contralateral epileptic discharges and concluded that 'the apparently interictal single sharp and slow wave complex in the Rolandic region may inhibit contralateral motor control, thus producing brief focal atonia that corresponds with the spike amplitude'.[585]

Yoshimura *et al.*[831] 1993 reported that, in their two twin girls, atypical absences showed in EEG bursts in the bilateral parietal and temporal regions during the waking state and almost continuous diffuse spike-waves during sleep. Seizures were controlled with phenytoin.

Kanazawa and Kawai, 1990[431] reported two cases of discontinuous status epilepticus characterized by repetitive asymmetrical atonic episodes associated with diffuse but asymmetrical spike waves. Both patients also had partial seizures and interictal Rolandic discharges. Dynamic EEG topography was performed to investigate the location or propagation of each ictal discharge overlying the scalp during status, and showed immediate bilateral spread of discharges originating from a primary epileptogenic focus in a Rolandic area.

Treatment

Anti-epileptic drugs were probably ineffective against the seizures and did not modify the EEG paroxysms. ACTH or steroids were tried unsuccesfully in a few cases. Deonna *et al.* 1986[224] reported that the therapeutic benefit of the various drugs tried was difficult to assess, but the behaviour was often perturbed by medication. In the two cases of Yoshimura *et al.*[831] seizures were controlled with phenytoin.

Prognosis

The course of 15 patients studied and reviewed by Aicardi[15] has been self-limited with apparently complete remission, maintained for up to 12 years, in the 11 children who have been followed after 9 years of age. None of them had any gross cognitive or behavioural sequelae though no detailed psychological study has been performed. All attended main stream schools.

Differential diagnosis from Lennox–Gastaut syndrome

As already stated, Aicardi and Chevrie, 1982[16] used the term 'benign' for this atypical benign partial epilepsy of childhood in order to distinguish it mainly from the Lennox–Gastaut syndrome 'for which it is regularly mistaken'. According to Aicardi:[15] 'The good outcome of atypical benign partial epilepsy of childhood is in sharp contrast with that of the Lennox–Gastaut syndome and certainly justifies their differentiation in order to avoid errors in prognosis and escalation of treatment. In atypical benign partial epilepsy of childhood as opposed to the Lennox–Gastaut syndrome there is no evidence of lasting mental or behavioural deterioration even after some months of evolution, there are no tonic fits, central spikes occur frequently and the relatively good awake EEG is in marked contrast with the sleep deterioration compatible with CSWS'.[15]

Carbamazepine induced 'atypical benign partial seizures of childhood' in children with Rolandic seizures

Caraballo *et al.*[149] described clinical features similar to the atypical benign partial epilepsy of childhood induced by carbamazepine. Though none of the cases described by Aicardi[15] could be attributed to carbamazepine, this possibility should be raised in children with Rolandic seizures and dramatic deterioration after treatment with this drug.

The following is an interesting relevant case that I saw when she was aged 6 years.

> Case 17.3. This 12-year-old girl of normal neurological, intellectual and developmental state started having frequent, brief, diurnal minor seizures at age 4 years. These were described as inconspicuous clonic movements of the right upper lip which lasted for seconds and occurred daily for 1–2 months. However, at age 5 she had on the same night two typical Rolandic seizures of 'excessive salivation, deviation of the mouth to one side, eyes looked vague and was unable to speak'. A post-ictal EEG, next day, was markedly abnormal. There were: (a) Nearly continuous, bi-synchonous, high amplitude (up to 400 μV) spike and slow wave complexes at a fluctuating 1–2 Hz frequency. They were more abundant in the bitemporal regions, left more than right. (b) Long runs of rhythmic delta activity, 2–4 Hz, in the left temporal and parietal regions. The alpha rhythm was well formed on the right, but was missing or of small amplitude on the left. An attempt to treat her with carbamazepine resulted immediately in an increased number of right sided hemifacial seizures and a brief, absence-like episode. Sodium valproate was added 2 weeks later but after 3 days she had a nocturnal generalized tonic–clonic seizure. Serum drug levels of both drugs were at low therapeutic target (carbamazepine at 6 mg/l and sodium valproate 46 mg/l). Subsequently, she developed longer hemifacial convulsions and also brief atonic attacks of head drop forwards or backwards. Sodium valproate was increased, carbamazepine was withdrawn and the situation came under control, but 4 months later diurnal hemifacial seizures recurred and within 5 months she had seven nocturnal right facial seizures, spreading to the right arm, and secondary GTCS. Her development, intellect, language and school performance were not affected.
>
> Figure 17.4 is her all-night video-EEG while on monotherapy with sodium valproate (drug levels were adequate at 406 μmol/l). The awake EEG showed frequent multifocal sharp or spike and slow waves mainly on the left but sleep EEG was characterized by continuous spikes and waves during slow sleep with bisynchronous spikes and waves predominating in the left hemisphere and of higher amplitude in the left posterior temporal electrode.
>
> Having not appreciated the previous deteriorating effect of carbamazepine on her, I erroneously attempted to re-introduce this drug add-on with the existing medication of sodium valproate. The result was catastrophic. Within days, at carbamazepine 300 mg daily, she suffered nearly continuous, brief atonic attacks of head and arm drop (probably atonic status epilepticus) and also absences. Fortunately, all stopped upon withdrawal of carbamazepine and introduction of phenytoin. The remainder of her story is provided to me by her paediatric neurologist (Dr H. Skouteli), to whom I am grateful, who followed her over many years. Her last ever brief hemifacial seizure was at age 6 years. Also her EEG gradually started improving, showing only some infrequent sharp-slow waves in the left posterior temporal electrode until complete normalization at age 8 years. Sodium valproate was discontinued at age 9 and phenytoin at age 11 years. In her last evaluation 'she is off medication for 1 year and has had no more seizures. She is a charming young lady, doing reasonably well at school with no learning disability but rather mediocre personal performance. Normal neurological state. Normal awake and sleep EEG'.

Commentary: What is this case? Certainly, she has all the clinico-EEG features of the atypical benign partial epilepsy of childhood: diurnal hemifacial and nocturnal Rolandic, atonic seizures and absences in clusters, and EEG with continuous spikes and waves during slow sleep. Also, there should be no doubt that carbamazepine had a serious aggrevating effect as the atonic seizures and absences occurred only and soon after she was exposed to this drug, which were abolished completely upon withdrawal of carbamazepine and initiation of phenytoin. However, even without carbamazepine, she was not a typical case of a child with Rolandic seizures, as indicated by her first EEG in an untreated stage, and the subsequent EEG with continuous spikes and waves during slow sleep without carbamazepine. Bureau[144] never saw CSWS in 70 children with Rolandic seizures and this is probably the general consensus. It is important to know for practical reasons if cases with carbamazepine-induced atonic

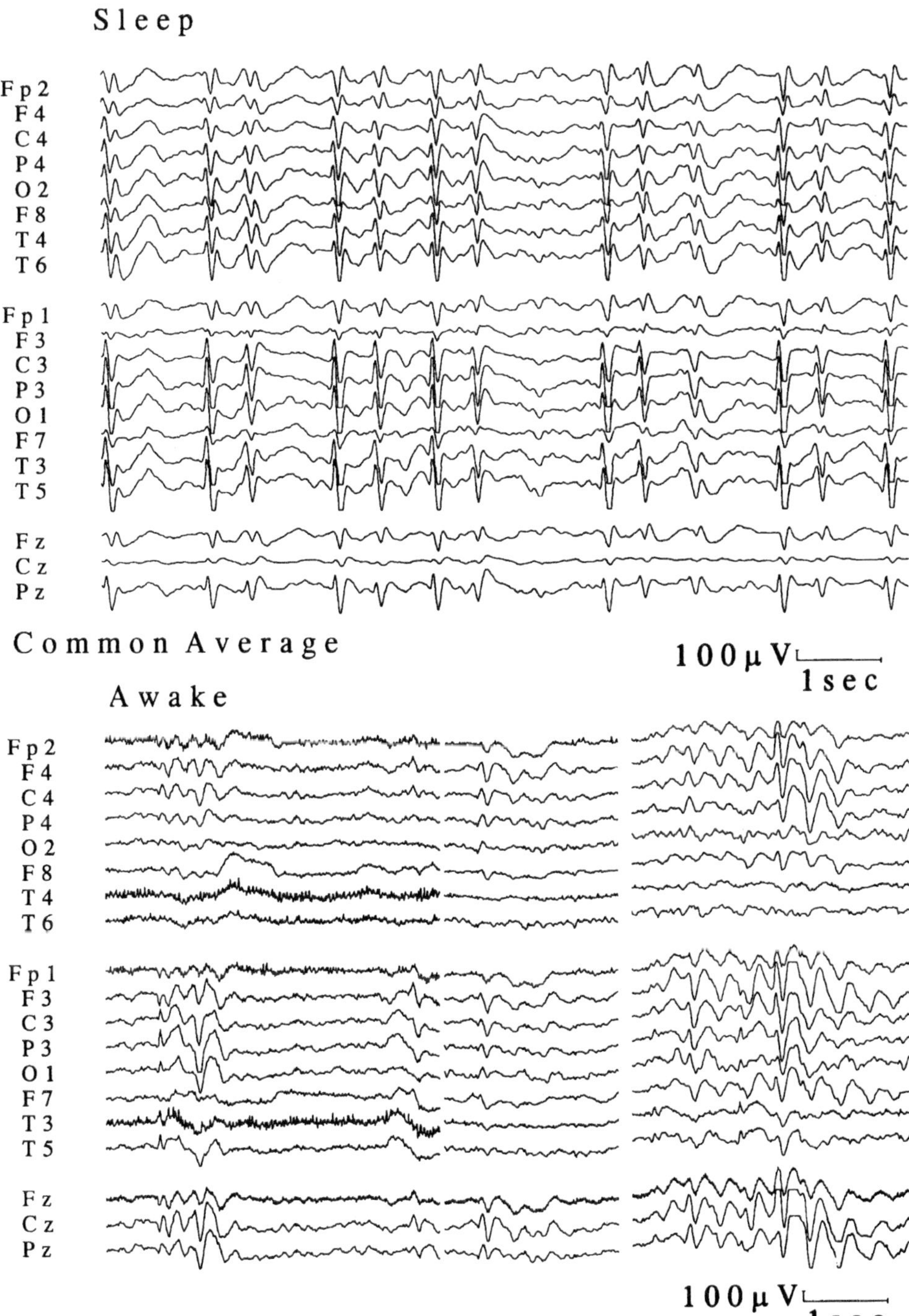

Fig. 17.4. Awake and all-night sleep video-EEG of patient 17.3 at age 5 years when she was only on sodium valproate.

and absence seizures refer to typical cases of Rolandic seizures or if they are all atypical, as for this patient. Another important point is that she never had any learning, behavioural or linguistic problems despite continuous spikes and waves during slow sleep. This is significant because there are doubts whether, in atypical benign partial epilepsy of childhood, the deterioration of EEG during sleep reaches the state of continuous spikes and waves during slow sleep[144] and exists without intellectual deterioration. This girl had continuous spikes and waves during slow sleep documented with all-night video-EEG and she never exhibited any intellectual or other abnormalities that were clinically detectable by an experienced paediatric neurologist. Furthermore, phenytoin proved the beneficial therapeutic drug for her condition, signifying the contribution of the old anti-epileptic drugs in the modern management of epilepsy.

Symptomatic cases of atypical benign partial epilepsy of childhood

Aicardi[15] has emphasized that the above described clinico-EEG features of atypical benign partial epilepsy of childhood can occur in children with brain neurological deficits. He described six patients with hemiparesis and variable degrees of mental retardation who had 'a type of epilepsy reminiscent of atypical benign partial epilepsy, e.g. with diffusion of the EEG abnormalities and atonic seizures'.[15] In these patients, atonic seizures of very brief duration (usually less than 1 s) affected either the axial muscles (neck, trunk and lower limbs), with consequent falls or head nods, or the upper limbs, resulting in 'negative myoclonus'. During the active periods, the EEG displayed continuous spike-wave activity in slow sleep and occasionally in the awake state. The paroxysmal activity often predominated over the side of the brain lesion but was always diffuse. The attacks were grouped in episodes of nonconvulsive status epilepticus lasting usually several days. Despite the presence of a lesion, the seizures eventually remitted in three patients followed up for 3 years or more.[15]

Benign Childhood Partial Seizures and Related Epileptic Syndromes. C P Panayiotopoulos
©1999 John Libbey & Company Ltd., pp. 361–363.

Chapter 18

Epilogue and conclusions

From the detailed analysis of historical, clinical, epidemiological, EEG and other relevant aspects of benign childhood partial seizures it is apparent that these are a group of syndromes of probably one functional disorder of maturation as they share common clinical and EEG characteristics that are age-dependent and reversible. Seizures are infrequent, usually nocturnal and remit within 1–3 years from onset. Brief or prolonged seizures, even status epilepticus, may be the only clinical event in the patient's lifetime. Ictal hypersalivation, vomiting, headache, pallor or sweating and behavioural changes, unusual in other epileptic syndromes, are frequent and may occasionally appear in isolation. Children with the clinical and EEG characteristics of one may evolve into or simultaneously develop features of another form of benign childhood partial seizures. Febrile convulsions are common. Neurological examination and intellect are normal, but some children may experience mild and reversible neuropsychological problems at the active stage of the disorder. Brain imaging is normal. EEG abnormalities are severe and disproportionate to seizure infrequency. Epileptogenic EEG foci, irrespective of their location, manifest with abundant, high amplitude sharp-slow wave complexes, mainly in clusters. They are often bilateral, independent or synchronous, frequently combined with foci from other cortical areas or brief generalized discharges, and are exaggerated in stages I–IV of sleep. A normal awake EEG is exceptional and should provoke a sleep EEG study. Other precipitating factors include somatosensory stimuli for the centrotemporal, parietal or midline spikes and elimination of central vision and fixation for the occipital spikes. Photosensitivity may occur though intermittent photic stimulation usually has an inhibitory effect initially in some children with occipital paroxysms which becomes excitatory at a later stage. Similar EEG features, also resolving with age, are frequently found in 2–4 per cent of normal children aged 2–13 years, and children having an EEG for reasons other than seizures.

There is no reason to maintain that all these syndromes differ from each other merely because an 'epileptogenic' focus is a little anterior or posterior, lateral or medial to the centrogyral regions. A unified concept of benign childhood partial seizures is also suggested by the frequency of more than one type of benign childhood partial seizures and EEG foci in more than one location in an affected child, siblings or both.

It is likely that all these conditions are linked together due to a common, genetically determined, mild and reversible, functional derangement of the brain cortical maturational process which I propose to call 'childhood seizure susceptibility syndrome'.

Electroencephalographic manifestations of childhood seizure susceptibility syndrome

In more than 90 per cent of affected children, this condition is often clinically silent, manifested only by EEG sharp and slow waves with an age-related localization. These EEG sharp and slow wave foci are mainly occipital in younger children with a peak age at 4–5 years in their first appearance and mainly centrogyral in older children with a peak age at 7–9 years. Their attrition rate varies from one to many years before their final disappearance usually before the age of 13 to a maximum of 16 years. Centrotemporal (62 per cent) are approximately 2.5 times more common than occipital (25 per cent). Spike foci in other locations are less prevalent (13 per cent). Centrotemporal, occipital and spikes in other locations may co-exist or appear in the same child at different locations in longitudinal EEG. One spike may synchronize with another in the same contralateral region or with other spikes in different locations. Bilateral synchrony of occipital spikes is probably due to the activating effect of elimination of central vision and fixation.

The EEG spike foci are mainly facilitated by slow wave sleep. Other means of precipitation, depending on localization, are somatosensory stimuli, elimination of central vision and fixation, and less often photic stimulation.

Seizures of childhood seizure susceptibility syndrome

Less than 10 per cent of affected children with the EEG markers of childhood seizure susceptibility syndrome may have seizures. These are often infrequent age- and localization-related idiopathic seizures. Seizures are localization related because clinical and EEG manifestations arise from a cortical locus. They are age related because they occur only in children at a certain age of their development. They are idiopathic because physical, mental and laboratory examinations other than EEG are normal.

Benign childhood partial seizures are common, comprising about one quarter of all epilepsies with onset between 2 and 13 years of age. With their good prognosis, they exemplify the importance of the syndromic classification of epilepsies and mandate a precise diagnosis which is usually easy on clinical and EEG grounds.

Rolandic seizures are the commonest, followed in prevalence by Panayiotopoulos syndrome. However, there are also other clinical variants of benign childhood partial seizures with EEG spikes in other cortical regions, such as parietal, frontal or midline spikes. Furthermore, clinical manifestations may be different despite EEG spikes in the same location, probably as a result of other interfering factors such as age. An example of this may be the rare form of late onset benign childhood occipital seizures.

Rolandic seizures are the clinical representative of centrotemporal spikes and Panayiotopoulos syndrome is the clinical representative of occipital spikes. Like their EEG counterparts, Rolandic seizures have a peak age at onset of 7–9 years and are 2.5 more frequent than early onset benign childhood occipital seizures which have an earlier peak age at onset of 5 years. Rolandic seizures may appear later in a child with Panayiotopoulos syndrome. Seizures with symptoms from other locations may also occur. Irrespective of location, seizures are mainly nocturnal, one third of children may have only one seizure and prognosis is excellent with no more than 2 per cent later developing infrequent GTCS.

Neuropsychological and linguistic symptoms in childhood seizure susceptibility syndrome

It is possible that a few of these children, with or without seizures, may also have usually minor and fully reversible neuropsychological symptoms. These are rarely clinically overt, requiring special neuropsychological testing for their detection. Finally, there may be a very small, less than 2 per cent, number of patients for whom this derangement of the brain maturation process may be derailed, resulting in a more aggressive condition of seizures, neuropsychological manifestations and EEG abnormalities of various combinations and various degree of severity, such as in atypical benign partial epilepsy of childhood, Landau–Kleffner syndrome or epilepsy with continuous spike and slow waves during sleep. The reason for the derailment of such a benign condition is not known but may be related to location or other intrinsic and external superimposed factors.

Pathophysiology of childhood seizure susceptibility syndrome

The pathophysiology of benign childhood seizure susceptibility is unknown. It is a cortical hyperexcitability possibly due to a mild and reversible derangement of the brain maturation process. This may be genetically determined though external factors interfering with the maturation of certain cortical areas are also possible.

The various EEG and seizure manifestations often follow an age (maturation)-related localization and prevalence. Thus, benign childhood seizure susceptibility is expressed from the occipital cortex of younger children while the centrogyral and neighbouring cortex is involved at a later age. Therefore, the clinico-EEG differences between the various forms of benign childhood partial seizures are localization dependent which in turn are age related. Irrespective of localization, the pathophysiological process should be the same. In this sense, it is not the functional spikes that migrate. It is rather that the pathophysiological process may follow an age-related cortical, regional, sequence of localization.

Treatment of childhood seizure susceptibility syndrome

Children with EEG foci only do not need treatment. There is no consensus on whether to treat those who develop seizures with anti-epileptic drugs. Most authors recommend 1–2 or a few more years of treatment, mainly with carbamazepine, after a second documented seizure, but treatment may not be needed. Prevention of prolonged seizures with diazepam is necessary. Epileptogenesis secondary to kindling has been feared by some authors; but the benign course of benign childhood partial seizures is reassuring.

Present and future directions regarding childhood seizure susceptibility syndrome

It is probably not realized by the medical community that childhood seizure susceptibility syndrome is one of the most common paediatric conditions, affecting 2–4 per cent of all children (based on EEG data) and approximately 25 per cent of children with seizures. It is also probably not realized that it is harmful to equate these benign seizures indiscriminately with 'epilepsy'. Their prognosis is better than that for febrile convulsions.

With such a high prevalence and significance regarding prognosis and treatment strategies, childhood seizure susceptibility syndrome should be well understood and well known by those who care for the medical welfare of children such as paediatricians, paediatric neurologists, electroencephalographers and allied specialities. In this sense, it is the responsibility of the editors of general paediatric and specialized medical journals to campaign for childhood seizure susceptibility syndrome and make this knowledge widely available.

Despite the significant progress detailed in this book, we still do not know many important aspects of childhood seizure susceptibility syndrome regarding genetics and other contributing external or internal factors, epidemiology (other than seizure clinical manifestations), interactions with a co-existing brain lesion or with other genetic seizure background, pathophysiology, neurophysiology, neuropsychology and learning.

I have tried to present in this book a thorough, honest and direct account of what I know about the clinical, EEG and other manifestations of childhood seizure susceptibility syndrome. I based this on the published reports of eminent colleagues, known and unknown, and my long-term clinical and EEG research. I hope that this effort will increase awareness and attract wider interest in this common condition which affects millions of children all over the world. Childhood seizure susceptibility syndrome is not simply Rolandic seizures or centrotemporal spikes which, although initiating studies and contributing to our understanding, are by no means the end or the whole of the story.

'Though much is taken, much abides'

References

1. A.A.N. (1995): Practice parameter: the electroencephalogram in the evaluation of headache (summary statement). Report of the Quality Standards Subcommittee of the American Academy of Neurology. *Neurology* **45,** 1411–1413.
2. Aarts, J.H., Binnie, C.D., Smit, A.M. & Wilkins, A.J. (1984): Selective cognitive impairment during focal and generalized epileptiform EEG activity. *Brain* **107,** 293–308.
3. Abad-Alegria, F., Ramis, M. & Pedrol, J.C. (1980): Benign epilepsy in childhood. *Act. Luso-Espan. Neurol. Psiqu. Cienc. Af.* **8,** 11–20.
4. Abe, K., Oda, N., Araki, R. & Igata, M. (1989): Macropsia, micropsia, and episodic illusions in Japanese adolescents. *J. Amer. Acad. Child & Adolescent Psychiatry* **28,** 493–496.
5. Acharya, J.N., Satischandra, P., Asha, T. & Shankar, S.K. (1993): Lafora's disease in south India: a clinical, electrophysiologic, and pathologic study. *Epilepsia* **34,** 476–487.
6. Acharya, J.N., Satishchandra, P. & Shankar, S.K. (1995): Familial progressive myoclonus epilepsy: clinical and electrophysiologic observations. *Epilepsia* **36,** 429–434.
7. Agathonikou, A., Koutroumanidis, M. & Panayiotopoulos, C.P. (1996): Episodic headache and dizziness in children with spontaneous and evoked giant centrotemporal spikes without overt seizures. *Epilepsia* **37 Suppl 4,** S90.
8. Agathonikou, A., Koutroumanidis, M. & Panayiotopoulos, C.P. (1997): Fixation-off-sensitive epilepsy with absences and absence status: video-EEG documentation. *Neurology* **48,** 231–234.
9. Agathonikou, A. & Panayiotopoulos, C.P. (1996): Benign Partial Epilepsy with Centro-Temporal Spikes and Idiopathic Generalised Seizures. *Epilepsia* **37 Suppl 4,** S86.
10. Agathonikou, A., Panayiotopoulos, C.P., Koutroumanidis, M. & Rowlinson, A. (1997): Idiopathic regional occipital epilepsy imitating migraine. *J. Epilepsy* **10,** 287–290.
11. Aguglia, U., Zappia, M. & Quattrone, A. (1987): Carbamazepine-induced nonepileptic myoclonus in a child with benign epilepsy. *Epilepsia* **28,** 515–518.
12. Ahmed Sharoqi, I., Parker, A. & Agathonikou, A. (1997): Early onset benign childhood occipital seizures (Panayiotopoulos' syndrome). *Epilepsia* **38 Suppl 3,** 223.
13. Ahmed, M.A., Reid, E., Cooke, A., Arngrimsson, R., Tolmie, J.L. & Stephenson, J.B. (1996): Familial hemiplegic migraine in the west of Scotland: a clinical and genetic study of seven families. *J. Neurol. Neurosurg. Psychiatry* **61,** 616–620.
14. Aicardi, J. (1979): Benign epilepsy of childhood with Rolandic spikes. *Brain Dev.* **1,** 71–73.
15. Aicardi, J. (1994): *Epilepsy in Children*. New York: Raven Press.
16. Aicardi, J. & Chevrie, J.J. (1982): Atypical benign partial epilepsy of childhood. *Dev. Med. Child Neurol.* **24,** 281–292.
17. Aicardi, J. & Gomes, A.L. (1992): Clinical and electroencephalographic symptomatology of the 'genuine' Lennox–Gastaut syndrome and its differentiation from other forms of epilepsy of early childhood. In: *Benign localized and generalized epilepsies of early childhood,* eds. R. Degen & F.E. Dreifuss, pp. 185–193. Amsterdam: Elsevier.
18. Aicardi, J. & Newton, R. (1987): Clinical findings in children with occipital spike wave complexes suppressed by eye opening. In: *Migraine and epilepsy,* eds. F. Andermann & E. Lugaresi, pp. 111–124. Boston MA: Butterworths.
19. Airy, H. (1870): On a distinct form of transient hemiopsia. *Philos. Trans. R. Soc. Lond.* **160,** 247–270.

20. Akutsu, T., Sakai, F., Hata, T., Iizuka, T. & Tazaki, Y. (1992): Neurological and neuroimaging studies of eclampsia. *Rinsho Shinkeigaku* **32,** 701–707.
21. Aldrich, M.S., Vanderzant, C.W., Alessi, A.G., Abou-Khalil, B. & Sackellares, J.C. (1989): Ictal cortical blindness with permanent visual loss. *Epilepsia* **30,** 116–120.
22. Ambrosetto, G., Antonini, L. & Tassinari, C.A. (1992): Occipital lobe seizures related to clinically asymptomatic celiac disease in adulthood. *Epilepsia* **33,** 476–481.
23. Ambrosetto, G., Dalla Bernardina, B., Beghini, G., Gobbi, G. & Ambrosetto, P. (1977): Benign epilepsy in childhood with Rolandic and/or mid-temporal paroxysmal EEG discharges: study of the intercritical and critical activity during sleep. *Riv. Neurol.* **47,** 243–251.
24. Ambrosetto, G., Giovanardi Rossi, P. & Tassinari, C.A. (1987): Predictive factors of seizure frequency and duration of antiepileptic treatment in Rolandic epilepsy: a retrospective study. *Brain Dev.* **9,** 300–304.
25. Ambrosetto, G. & Gobbi, G. (1975): Benign epilepsy of childhood with Rolandic spikes, or a lesion? EEG during a seizure. *Epilepsia* **16,** 793–796.
26. Ambrosetto, G. & Tassinari, C.A. (1990): Antiepileptic drug treatment of benign childhood epilepsy with Rolandic spikes: is it necessary? *Epilepsia* **31,** 802–805.
27. Ambrosetto, G., Tinuper, P. & Baruzzi, A. (1985): Relapse of benign partial epilepsy of children in adulthood: report of a case. *J. Neurol. Neurosurg. Psychiatry* **48,** 90.
28. Amit, R. (1987): Benign focal epilepsy of childhood: individual and intrafamilial multifocality of spikes. *Clin. Electroencephalogr.* **18,** 169–172.
29. Amit, R. & Crumrine, P.K. (1993): Ictal midline epileptiform discharges. *Clin. Electroencephalogr.* **24,** 67–69.
30. Amit, R., Shapira, Y., Flusser, H. & Aker, M. (1986): Basilar migraine manifesting as transient global amnesia in a 9-year-old child. *Headache* **26,** 17–18.
31. Andermann, E. & Andermann, F. (1987): Migraine–epilepsy relationships: Epidemiological and genetic studies. In: *Migraine and epilepsy,* eds. F. Andermann & E. Lugaresi, pp. 281–291. Boston, MA: Butterworths.
32. Andermann, E.D. (1972): Focal epilepsy and related disorders: genetic, metabolic, and prognostic studies. Ph.D. Thesis, McGill University.
33. Andermann, F. (1987): Clinical features of migraine–epilepsy syndromes. In: *Migraine and epilepsy,* eds. F. Andermann & E. Lugaresi, pp. 3–30. Boston, MA: Butterworths.
34. Andermann, F. (1987): Migraine and epilepsy: An overview. In: *Migraine and epilepsy,* eds. F. Andermann & E. Lugaresi, pp. 405–422. Boston, MA: Butterworths.
35. Andermann, F. (1993): Occipital epileptic abnormalities im mitochondrial disorders–preferential involvement, illustrations of clinical patterns, current progress in neurobiology and a hypothesis. In: *Occipital seizures and epilepsies in children,* eds. F. Andermann, A. Beaumanoir, L. Mira, J. Roger & C.A. Tassinari, pp. 111–118. London: John Libbey & Company Ltd.
36. Andermann, F. (1997): The benign occipital epilepsies of childhood: How many syndromes? In: *Annual Course Handbook. December 1997,* pp. B1-B13. Boston, MA: American Epilepsy Society.
37. Andermann, F. & Andermann, E. (1992): Migraine and epilepsy, with special reference to the benign epilepsies of childhood. *Epilepsy Research – Supplement* **6,** 207–214.
38. Andermann, F., Beaumanoir, A., Mira, E., Roger, J. & Tassinari, C.A. (1993): *Occipital seizures and epilepsies in children.* London: John Libbey & Company Ltd.
39. Andermann, F. & Lugaresi. E. (1987): *Migraine and Epilepsy.* Boston, MA: Butterworths.
40. Andermann, F., Lugaresi, E., Dvorkin, G.S. & Montagna, P. (1986): Malignant migraine: the syndrome of prolonged classical migraine, epilepsia partialis continua, and repeated strokes; a clinically characteristic disorder probably due to mitochondrial encephalopathy. *Functional Neurology* **1,** 481–486.
41. Andermann, F. & Oguni, H. (1990): Do epileptic foci in children migrate? The pros. *Electroencephalogr. Clin. Neurophysiol.* **76,** 96–99.
42. Andermann, F., Salanova, V., Olivier, A. & Rasmussen, T. (1993): Occipital lobe epilepsy in children – electroclinical manifestations, surgical implications and treatment. In: *Occipital seizures and epilepsies in children,* eds. F. Andermann, A. Beaumanoir, L. Mira, J. Roger & C.A. Tassinari, pp. 213–220. London: John Libbey & Company Ltd.
43. Andermann, F. & Zifkin, B. (1998): The benign occipital epilepsies of childhood: an overview of the idiopathic syndromes and of the relationship to migraine. *Epilepsia* **39 Suppl 4,** S9-S23.
44. Anonymous (1969): Migraine and epilepsy. *Lancet* **2,** 527–528.
45. Anyamwu, E., Harding, G.F., Jeavons, P.M. & Edson, A. (1995): 'Telephillic syndrome' in pattern and photosensitive epilepsy: report of three cases. *East African Med. J.* **72,** 402–405.

46. Appleton, R.E. (1995): The Landau–Kleffner syndrome. *Arch. Dis. Child.* **72,** 386–387.

47. Aretaeus (1856): *The extant Works of Aretaeus the Cappadocian* (Francis Adams' translation: printed for the Sydenham Society). London: Wertheimer & Co.

48. Arts, W.F., Tjiam, A.T. & Tillema-The, P. (1984): Benign midtemporal epilepsy in childhood. *Nederlands Tijdschrift voor Geneeskunde* **128,** 1704–1708.

49. Arzimanoglou, A. & Evrard, P. (1997): Clinical and pathological findings in Sturge–Weber syndrome and other congenital neurological diseases with epilepsy and calcifications. In: *Epilepsy and other neurological disorders in coeliac disease,* eds. G. Gobbi, F. Andermann, S. Naccarato & G. Banchin, pp. 161–170. London: John Libbey & Company Ltd.

50. Asencio Marchante, J.J., Heras Perez, J.A. & Juan-Togores Veguero, J.M. (1985): Basilar migraine and 5-allyl-beta-oxypropylmalonylurea. *Medic. Clin.* **85,** 431.

51. Aso, K., Watanabe, K., Negoro, T., Furune, A., Takahashi, I., Yamamoto, N. & Nomura, K. (1988): Photosensitive partial seizure: The origin of abnormal discharges. *J. Epilepsy* **1,** 87–93.

52. Aso, K., Watanabe, K., Negoro, T., Takaesu, E., Furune, A., Takahashi, I., Yamamoto, N. & Nomura, K. (1987): Visual seizures in children. *Epilepsy Research* **1,** 246–253.

53. Autret, A. (1995): Sleep and intra-ictal epileptic electroencephalographic activities. *Neurophysiol. Clin.* **25,** 263–282.

54. Autret, A., Lucas, B., Hommet, C., Corcia, P. & De Toffol, B. (1997): Sleep and the epilepsies. *J. Neurol.* **244,** S10–7.

55. Avanzini, G. (1993): Structures and functions of the occipital lobe. In: *Occipital seizures and epilepsies in children,* eds. F. Andermann, A. Beaumanoir, J. Roger & C.A. Tassinari pp. 31–41. London: John Libbey & Company Ltd.

56. Ayala, G. (1929): Status epilepticus amauroticus. *Boll. Accad. Med. Roma* **55,** 288–290.

57. Babb, T.L., Halgren, E., Wilson, C., Engel, J. & Crandall, P. (1981): Neuronal firing patterns during the spread of an occipital lobe seizure to the temporal lobes in man. *Electroencephalogr. Clin. Neurophysiol.* **51,** 104–107.

58. Bagdorf, R. & Lee, S.I. (1993): Midline spikes: is it another benign EEG pattern of childhood? *Epilepsia* **34,** 271–274.

59. Bahemuka, M. (1981): Basilar artery migraine in a child: excellent response to propranolol. *East African Med. J.* **58,** 75–79.

60. Bakshi, R., Bates, V.E., Mechtler, L.L., Kinkel, P.R. & Kinkel, W.R. (1998): Occipital lobe seizures as the major clinical manifestation of reversible posterior leukoencephalopathy syndrome: magnetic resonance imaging findings. *Epilepsia* **39,** 295–299.

61. Baldy-Moulinier, M. (1992): Sleep organization in benign childhood partial epilepsies. *Epilepsy Research – Supplement* **6,** 121–124.

62. Baloh, R.W., Yue, Q., Furman, J.M. & Nelson, S.F. (1997): Familial episodic ataxia: clinical heterogeneity in four families linked to chromosome 19p. *Ann.Neurol.* **41,** 8–16.

63. Bancaud, J. (1969): Les crises epileptiques d'origine occipitale (etude stereo-electroencephalographique). *Rev. Oto-Neuro-Ophtalmologie* **41,** 299–311.

64. Bancaud, J. (1987): Clinical symptomatology of epileptic seizures of temporal origin. *Rev. Neurol.* **143,** 392–400.

65. Bancaud, J., Colomb, J. & Dell, M.B. (1958): Les pointes rolandiques: un symptome EEG propre a l'enfant. *Rev. Neurol.* **99,** 206–209.

66. Barolin, G.S. (1965): Relations between migraine and epilepsy. *Munch. Medizin. Wochenschrift* **107,**1843–1847.

67. Barry, E., Sussman, N.M., Bosley, T.M. & Harner, R.N. (1985): Ictal blindness and status epilepticus amauroticus. *Epilepsia* **26,** 577–584.

68. Basser, L.S. (1969): The relation of migraine and epilepsy. *Brain* **92,** 285–300.

69. Battistella, P.A., Mattesi, P., Casara, G.L., Carollo, C., Condini, A., Allegri, F & Rigon, F. (1987): Bilateral cerebral occipital calcifications and migraine-like headache. *Cephalalgia* **7,** 125–129.

70. Bauer, J., Schuler, P., Feistel, H., Hilz, M.J. & Stefan, H. (1991): Blindness as an ictal phenomenon: investigations with EEG and SPECT in two patients suffering from epilepsy. *J. Neurol.* **238,** 44–46.

71. Baumgartner, C., Doppelbauer, A., Lischka, A., Graf, M., Lindinger, G., Olbrich, A., Novak, K., Aull, S., Serles, W., Lurger, S. & Deecke, L. (1995): Benign focal epilepsy of childhood – a combined neuroelectric and neuromagnetic study. In: *Biomagnetism: fundamental research and clinical applications,* eds. C. Baumgartner, L. Deecke, G. Stroink & S.J. Williamson, pp. 39–42. Amsterdam: Elsevier Science. IOS Press.

72. Baumgartner, C., Graf, M., Doppelbauer, A., Serles, W., Lindinger, G., Olbrich, A. Bacher, J., Pataraia, E., Almer, G. & Lischka, A. (1996): The functional organization of the interictal spike complex in benign Rolandic epilepsy. *Epilepsia* **37,** 1164–1174.

73. Bazil, C.W. (1994): Migraine and epilepsy. *Neurologic Clinics* **12,** 115–128.

74. Beaumanoir, A. (1983): Infantile epilepsy with occipital focus and good prognosis. *Eur. Neurol.* **22,** 43–52.

75. Beaumanoir, A. (1992): The Landau–Kleffner syndrome. In: *Epileptic syndromes in infancy, childhood and adolescence,* eds. J. Roger, M. Bureau, C. Dravet, F.E. Dreifuss, A. Perret & P. Wolf, pp. 231–243. London: John Libbey & Company Ltd.

76. Beaumanoir, A. (1993): An EEG contribution to the study of migraine and of the association between migraine and epilepsy in childhood. In: *Occipital seizures and epilepsy in children,* eds. F. Andermann, A. Beaumanoir, L. Mira, J. Roger & C.A. Tassinari, pp. 101–110. London: John Libbey & Company Ltd.

77. Beaumanoir, A. (1993): Semiology of occipital seizures in infants and children. In: *Occipital seizures and epilepsies in children,* eds. F. Andermann, A. Beaumanoir, L. Mira, J. Roger & C.A. Tassinari, pp. 71–86. London: John Libbey & Company Ltd.

78. Beaumanoir, A., Ballis, T., Varfis, G. & Ansari, K. (1974): Benign epilepsy of childhood with Rolandic spikes. A clinical, electroencephalographic, and telencephalographic study. *Epilepsia* **15,** 301–315.

79. Beaumanoir, A., Bureau, M., Deonna, T., Mira, L. & Tassinari, C.A. (1995) *Continuous spikes and waves during slow sleep . Electrical status epilepticus during slow sleep.* London: John Libbey & Company Ltd.

80. Beaumanoir, A., Bureau, M. & Mira, L. (1995): Identification of the syndrome. In: *Continuous spikes and waves during slow sleep. Electrical status epilepticus during slow sleep. Acquired epileptic aphasia and related conditions,* eds. A. Beaumanoir, M. Bureau, T. Deonna, L. Mira & C.A. Tassinari, pp. 243–249. London: John Libbey & Company Ltd.

81. Beaumanoir, A., Capizzi, G., Nahory, A. & Yousfi, Y. (1989): Scotogenic seizures. In: *Reflex seizures and reflex epilepsies,* eds. A. Beaumanoir, H. Gastaut & J. Roger, pp. 219–223. Geneve: Medecine & Hygiene.

82. Beaumanoir, A. & Grandjean, E. (1987): Occipital spikes, migraine and epilepsy. In: *Migraine and epilepsy,* eds. F. Andermann & E. Lugaresi, pp. 97–110. Boston, MA: Butterworths.

83. Beaumanoir, A., Inderwildi, B. & Zagury, S. (1981): Paroxysms EEG non epileptiques. *Medecine et Hygiene* **39,** 1911–1918.

84. Beaumanoir, A. & Jekiel, M. (1987): Electrographic observations during atttacks of classical migraine. In: *Migraine and epilepsy,* eds. F. Andermann & E. Lugaresi, pp. 163–180. Boston, MA: Butterworths.

85. Beaumanoir, A. & Nahory, A. (1983): Benign partial epilepsies: 11 cases of frontal partial epilepsy with favorable prognosis. *Rev. EEG Neurophysiol.* **13,** 207–211.

86. Beaumanoir, A. & Thomas, P. (1992): Benign epilepsy of childhood with occipital paroxysms. *Epilepsy Research, Supplement* **6,** 105–109.

87. Beaussart, M. (1972): Benign epilepsy of children with Rolandic (centrotemporal) paroxysmal foci. A clinical entity. Study of 221 cases. *Epilepsia* **13,** 795–911.

88. Beaussart, M. (1975): Benign epilepsy of children with Rolandic paroxysmal electroencephalographic foci. *Pediatrie* **30,** 249–263.

89. Beaussart, M. (1981): Epileptic seizures after recovery from an epilepsy with Rolandic paroxysms. *Rev. EEG Neurophysiol.* **11,** 489–492.

90. Beaussart, M. & Faou, R. (1976): Paroxysmal Rolandic epilepsy pre-study of 293 cases. *Lille Medical* **21,** 414–422.

91. Beaussart, M. & Faou, R. (1978): Evolution of epilepsy with Rolandic paroxysmal foci: a study of 324 cases. *Epilepsia* **19,** 337–342.

92. Beaussart, M., Roger, J. & Loiseau, P. (1999): The discovery of 'benign Rolandic epilepsy'. In: *Genetics of focal epilepsies,* eds. S.F. Berkovic, P. Genton, E. Hirsch & F. Picard, pp. 3–6. London: John Libbey & Company Ltd.

93. Benbadis, S.R. & Luders, H.O. (1996): Epileptic syndromes: an underutilized concept [editorial]. *Epilepsia* **37,** 1029–1034.

94. Bennett, A.H. (1884): *On epilepsy and its treatment.* London: H.K. Lewis.

95. Berg, A.T. & Shinnar, S. (1991): The risk of seizure recurrence following a first unprovoked seizure: a quantitative review. *Neurology* **41,** 965–972.

96. Berkovic, S.F. (1997): Progressive myoclonuc epilepsies. In: *Epilepsy: A comprehensive textbook,* eds. J.J. Engel & T.A. Pedley, pp. 2455–2468. Philadelphia: Lippincott-Raven Publishers.

97. Berkovic, S.F., Kennerson, M.L., Howell, R.A., Scheffer, I.E., Hwang, P.A. & Nicholson, G.A. (1994): Phenotypic expression of benign familial neonatal convulsions linked to chromosome 20. *Arch.Neurol.* **51,** 1125–1128.

98. Berkovic, S.F. & Scheffer, I.E. (1997): Epilepsies with single gene inheritance. *Brain Dev.* **19,** 13–18.

99. Bernardina, B.D. & Beghini, G. (1976): Rolandic spikes in children with and without epilepsy (20 subjects polygraphically studied during sleep). *Epilepsia* **17,** 161–167.

100. Bernsen, H.J., Van de Vlasakker, C., Verhagen, W.I. & Prick, M.J. (1990): Basilar artery migraine stroke. *Headache* **30,** 142–144.

101. Beun, A.M., Beintema, D.J., Binnie, C.D., Debets, R.M., Overweg, J. & Van Heycop ten Ham, M.W. (1984): Epileptic nystagmus. *Epilepsia* **25,** 609–614.

102. Beydoun, A., Garofalo, E.A. & Drury, I. (1992): Generalized spike-waves, multiple loci, and clinical course in children with EEG features of benign epilepsy of childhood with centrotemporal spikes. *Epilepsia* **33,** 1091–1096.

103. Bharani, A.K., Babbar, P., Jain, A.C. & Sepaha, G.C. (1985): Basilar artery migraine. *Journal of the Ass. Physicians of India* **33,** 239.

104. Bhatia, K.P., Brown, P., Gregory, R., Lennox, G.G., Manji, H., Thompson, P.D., Ellison, D.W. & Marsden, C.D. (1995): Progressive myoclonic ataxia associated with coeliac disease. The myoclonus is of cortical origin, but the pathology is in the cerebellum. *Brain* **118,** 1087–1093.

105. Bhatia, M.S., Shome, S., Chadda, R.K. & Saurabh. (1994): Landau–Kleffner syndrome in cerebral cysticercosis. *Indian Pediatrics* **31,** 584–587.

106. Bickerstaff, E.R. (1961): Basilar artery migraine. *Lancet* **i,** 15–17.

107. Bickerstaff, E.R. (1961): Impairment of consciousness in migraine. *Lancet* **ii,** 1057–1059.

108. Bickerstaff, E.R. (1962): The basilar artery and the migraine–epilepsy syndrome. *Proc. R. Soc. Med.* **55,** 167–169.

109. Bickford, R.G. & Klass, D.W. (1969): Sensory precipitation and reflex mechanisms. In: *Basic mechanisms of the epilepsies,* eds. H.H. Jasper, A.A. Ward & A. Pope, pp. 543–564. Boston, MA: Little, Brown and Co.

110. Bidzinski, J., Bacia, T. & Ruzikowski, E. (1992): The results of the surgical treatment of occipital lobe epilepsy. *Acta Neurochir. (Wien)* **114,** 128–130.

111. Biervert, C., Schroeder, B.C., Kubisch, C., Berkovic, S.F., Propping, P., Jentsch, T.J. & Steinlein, O.K. (1998): A potassium channel mutation in neonatal human epilepsy. *Science* **279,** 403–406.

112. Billard, C., Autret, A., Laffont, F., De Giovanni, E., Lucas, B., Santini, J.J., Dulac, O. & Plouin, P. (1981): Acquired aphasia in epileptic children – four cases with electrical infraclinic status epilepticus during sleep. *Rev. EEG Neurophysiol.* **11,** 457–467.

113. Bille, B. (1968): Headaches in children. In: *Handbook of clinical neurology,*eds. P.J. Vinken & G.W. Bruyn, pp. 239–246. Amsterdam: North-Holland/ Elsevier.

114. Binnie, C.D. (1993): Significance and management of transitory cognitive impairment due to subclinical EEG discharges in children. *Brain Dev.* **15,** 23–30.

115. Binnie, C.D., de Silva, M. & Hurst, A. (1992): Rolandic spikes and cognitive function. *Epilepsy Research – Supplement* **6,** 71–73.

116. Binnie, C.D., Harding, G.F., Richens, A. & Wilkins, A. (1994): Video games and epileptic seizures – a consensus statement. Video-Game Epilepsy Consensus Group. *Seizure* **3,** 245–246.

117. Binnie, C.D. & Marston, D. (1992): Cognitive correlates of interictal discharges. *Epilepsia* **33 Suppl 6,** S11–7.

118. Binnie, C.D. & Prior, P.F. (1994): Electroencephalography. *J.Neurol.Neurosurg.Psychiatry* **57,** 1308–1319.

119. Binnie, C.D. & Wilkins, A.J. (1998): Visually induced seizures not caused by flicker (intermittent light stimulation). *Adv. Neurol.* **75,** 123–138.

120. Bladin, P.F. (1987): The association of benign Rolandic epilepsy with migraine. In: *Migraine and epilepsy,*eds. F. Andermann & E. Lugaresi, pp. 145–152. Boston, MA: Butterworths.

121. Bladin, P.F. & Berkovic, S.F. (1987): Juvenile migraine and epilepsy: EEG and neuropathological findings in a fatal case. In: *Migraine and epilepsy,* eds. F. Andermann & E. Lugaresi, pp. 181–188. Boston, MA: Butterworths.

122. Blagosklonova, N.K. & Mastiukova, E.M. (1994): The seizure syndrome combined with sensorimotor aphasia and alalia (the Landau–Kleffner syndrome). *Zhurnal Nevropatologii i Psikhiatrii Imeni S - S - Korsakova* **94,** 46–51.

123. Blau, J.N. (1992): Classical migraine: symptoms between visual aura and headache onset. *Lancet* **340,** 355–356.

124. Blau, J.N. (1992): Migraine: theories of pathogenesis. *Lancet* **339,** 1202–1207.

125. Blom, S. & Brorson, L.O. (1966): Central spikes or sharp waves (Rolandic spikes) in children's EEG and their clinical significance. *Acta Paediatr. Scand.* **55,** 385–393.

126. Blom, S. & Heijbel, J. (1975): Benign epilepsy of children with centrotemporal EEG foci. Discharge rate during sleep. *Epilepsia* **16,** 133–140.

127. Blom, S. & Heijbel, J. (1982): Benign epilepsy of children with centrotemporal EEG foci: a follow-up study in adulthood of patients initially studied as children. *Epilepsia* **23,** 629–632.

128. Blom, S., Heijbel, J. & Bergfors, P.G. (1972): Benign epilepsy of children with centrotemporal EEG foci. Prevalence and follow-up study of 40 patients. *Epilepsia* **13,** 609–619.

129. Blume, W.T. (1982): *Atlas of pediatric electroencephalography*. New York: Raven.

130. Blume, W.T. (1990): Do epileptic foci in children migrate? The cons. *Electroencephalogr Clin. Neurophysiol.* **76,** 100–105.

131. Blume, W.T., Whiting, S.E. & Girvin, J.P. (1991): Epilepsy surgery in the posterior cortex. *Ann. Neurol.* **29,** 638–645.

132. Blume, W.T. & Young, G.B. (1987): Ictal pain: unilateral, cephalic, and abdominal. In: *Migraine and epilepsy,* eds. F. Andermann & E. Lugaresi, pp. 235–247. Boston, MA: Butterworths.

133. Bodensteiner, J.B. (1990): Visual symptoms in childhood migraine. *J. Child. Neurol.* **5,** 190

134. Bossu van Nieuwenhuyse, C., Pasquier, C. & Pouplard, F. (1980): Rolandic paroxysmal epilepsy. Prognostic, electric, clinical limits. Study of 28 cases. *Semaine des Hopitaux* **56,** 559–564.

135. Boulloche, J., Husson, A., Le Luyer, B. & Le Roux, P. (1990): Dysphagia, speech disorders and centrotemporal spikes-waves. *Arch. Franc. Pediatr.* **47,** 115–117.

136. Bouma, P.A., Bovenkerk, A.C., Westendorp, R.G. & Brouwer, O.F. (1997): The course of benign partial epilepsy of childhood with centrotemporal spikes: a meta-analysis. *Neurology* **48,** 430–437.

137. Bouquet, F. & Cernibori, A. (1981): Prolonged consciousness disorders in attacks of basilar artery migraine. *Riv. Neurobiol.* **27,** 671–676.

138. Bousser, M.G. & Tournier-Lasserve, E. (1994): Summary of the proceedings of the First International Workshop on CADASIL. Paris, 19–21 May, 1993. *Stroke* **25,** 704–707.

139. Boyd, S.G., Rivera-Gaxiola, M., Towell, A.D., Harkness, W. & Neville, B.G. (1996): Discrimination of speech sounds in a boy with Landau–Kleffner syndrome: an intraoperative event-related potential study. *Neuropediatrics* **27,** 211–215.

140. Bray, P.F. & Wiser, W.C. (1964): Evidence for a genetic etiology of temporal-central abnormalities in focal epilepsy. *New Engl. J. Med.* **271,** 926–933.

141. Bray, P.F. & Wiser, W.C. (1965): The relation of focal to diffuse epileptiform EEG discharges in genetic epilepsy. *Arch.Neurol.* **13,** 223–237.

142. Bray, P.F. & Wiser, W.C. (1965): Hereditary characteristics of familial temporal-central focal epilepsy. *Pediatrics* **36,** 207–221.

143. Brinciotti, M., Matricardi, M., Pelliccia, A. & Trasatti, G. (1994): Pattern sensitivity and photosensitivity in epileptic children with visually induced seizures. *Epilepsia* **35,** 842–849.

144. Bureau, M. (1995): 'Continuous spikes and waves during slow sleep' (CSWS): definition of the syndrome. In: *Continuous spikes and waves during slow sleep. Electrical status epilepticus during slow sleep. Acquired epileptic aphasia and related conditions,*eds. A. Beaumanoir, M. Bureau, T. Deonna, L. Mira & C.A. Tassinari, pp. 17–26. London: John Libbey & Company Ltd.

145. Calvet, V. (1978): Epilepsies nocturnes de l' enfant: epilepsies benignes. These Medecine, Toulouse. (Cited by Balby-Moulinier, M.[61])

146. Camfield, P.R., Metrakos, K. & Andermann, F. (1978): Basilar migraine, seizures, and severe epileptiform EEG abnormalities. *Neurology* **28,** 584–588.

147. Capizzi, G., Vigliano, P., Pengo, A.M. & Balona, M. (1993): Occipital symptomatic epilepsy: epidemiological aspects. In: *Occipital seizures and epilepsies in children,* eds. F. Andermann, A. Beaumanoir, L. Mira, J. Roger & C.A. Tassinari, pp. 183–188. London: John Libbey & Company Ltd.

148. Caplan, L.R. (1991): Migraine and vertebrobasilar ischemia. *Neurology* **41,** 55–61.

149. Caraballo, R., Fontana, E., Michelizza, B., Zullini, B., Sgro, V., Pajno-Ferrara, F. *et al.* (1989): Carbamazepina, 'assenze atipiche', 'crisi atoniche', 'crisi atoniche' e stato di PO continua del sonno. *Boll. Lega. It. Epil.* **66/67,** 379–381.

150. Caraballo, R.H., Cersosimo, R.O., Medina, C.S., Tenembaum, S. & Fejerman, N. (1997): Epilepsias parciales idiopaticas con paroxysmos occipitales. *Revist. Neurolog.* **25,** 1052–1058.

151. Castels-van Daele, M., Standaert, L., Boel, M., Smeets, E., Colaert, J. & Desmyter, J. (1981): Basilar migraine and viral meningitis. *Lancet* **1,** 1366

152. Catania, S., De Sousa, C. & Boyd, S.G. (1999): New epileptic attacks with lamotrigine in benign Rolandic epilepsy. *Electroencephalogr. Clin. Neurophysiol.* (in press).

153. Cavazzuti, G.B. (1980): Epidemiology of different types of epilepsy in school age children of Modena, Italy. *Epilepsia* **21,** 57–62.

154. Cavazzuti, G.B., Cappella, L. & Nalin, A. (1980): Longitudinal study of epileptiform EEG patterns in normal children. *Epilepsia* **21,** 43–55.

155. Cavazzuti, G.B., Rozzi, N. & Ferrari, F. (1978): Longitudinal study of 129 cases of infantile focal benign epilepsy. *Riv. Neurol.* **48,** 539–545.

156. Cernibori, A. & Bouquet, F. (1984): Loss of consciousness during basilar artery migraine attack in childhood: EEG and clinical studies. *Electroencephalogr. Clin. Neurophysiol.* **58,** 72.

157. Chabriat, H., Joutel, A., Vahedi, K., Iba-Zizen, M.T., Tournier-Lasserve, E. & Bousser, M.G. (1996): CADASIL (cerebral autosomal dominant arteriopathy with subcortical infarcts and leukoencephalopathy). *J. Mal. Vascul.* **21,** 277–282.

158. Chabriat, H., Tournier-Lasserve, E., Vahedi, K., Leys, D., Joutel, A., Nibbio, A, Escaillas, J.P., Iba-Zizen, M.T., Bracard, S., Tehindrazanarivelo, A. *et al.* (1995): Autosomal dominant migraine with MRI white-matter abnormalities mapping to the CADASIL locus. *Neurology* **45,** 1086–1091.

159. Chabriat, H., Vahedi, K., Iba-Zizen, M.T., Joutel, A., Nibbio, A., Nagy, T.G., Krebs, M.O., Julien, J., Dubois, B., Ducrocq, X. *et al.* (1995): Clinical spectrum of CADASIL: a study of 7 families. Cerebral autosomal dominant arteriopathy with subcortical infarcts and leukoencephalopathy. *Lancet* **346,** 934–939.

160. Chadwick, D. (1990): Diagnosis of epilepsy. *Lancet* **336,** 291–295.

161. Chadwick, D. (1994): Epilepsy. *J.Neurol.Neurosurg.Psychiatry* **57,** 264–277.

162. Chang, W.N., Lui, C.C. & Chang, J.M. (1996): CT and MRI findings of eclampsia and their correlation with neurologic symptoms. *Chung Hua I Hsueh Tsa Chih (Taipei)* **57,** 191–197.

163. Chinnery, P.F. & Turnbull, D.M. (1997): Clinical features, investigation, and management of patients with defects of mitochondrial DNA [editorial]. *J.Neurol.Neurosurg.Psychiatry* **63,** 559–563.

164. Critchley, M. (1949): Metamorphopsia of central origin. *Trans. Ophthalmol. Soc. U.K.* **69,** 111–121.

165. Critchley, M. (1951): Types of visual perseveration: 'palinopsia' and 'illusory visual spread'. *Brain* **74,** 267–299.

166. Critchley, M.(1986): *Butterworths Medical Dictionary*. London: Butterworth & Co. (Publishers) Ltd.

167. Cirignotta, F., Lugaresi, E. & Montagna, P. (1987): Occipital EEG acticity induced by darkness: The critical role of central vision. In: *Migraine and epilepsy,*eds. F. Andermann & E. Lugaresi, pp. 139–145. Boston, MA: Butterworths.

168. Clark, J.M., Marks, M.P., Adalsteinsson, E., Spielman, D.M., Shuster, D., Horoupian, D. & Albers, G.W. (1996): MELAS: Clinical and pathologic correlations with MRI, xenon/CT, and MR spectroscopy. *Neurology* **46,** 223–227.

169. Classification Committee of the International Headache Society (1988): Classification of headache disorders, cranial neuralgias and facial pain; and diagnostic criteria for primary headache disorders. *Cephalalgia* **8 suppl,** 1–96.

170. Clemens, B. & Majoros, E. (1987): Sleep studies in benign epilepsy of childhood with Rolandic spikes. II. Analysis of discharge frequency and its relation to sleep dynamics. *Epilepsia* **28,** 24–27.

171. Clemens, B. & Olah, R. (1987): Sleep studies in benign epilepsy of childhood with Rolandic spikes. I. Sleep pathology. *Epilepsia* **28,** 20–23.

172. Cohn, D.F., Vardi, Y., Flechter, S. & Streifler, M. (1980): Basilar artery migraine. *Schweiz. Medizin. Wochenschrift Journal Suisse de Me*, 26–28.

173. Colamaria, V., Sgro, V., Caraballo, R., Simeone, M., Zullini, E., Fontana, E., Zanetti, R., Grimau-Merino, R. & Dalla Bernardina, B. (1991): Status epilepticus in benign Rolandic epilepsy manifesting as anterior operculum syndrome. *Epilepsia* **32,** 329–334.

174. Cole, A.J., Andermann, F., Taylor, L., Olivier, A., Rasmussen, T., Robitaille, Y. & Spire, J.P. (1988): The Landau–Kleffner syndrome of acquired epileptic aphasia: unusual clinical outcome, surgical experience, and absence of encephalitis. *Neurology* **38,** 31–38.

175. Commission of Classification and Terminology of the International League Against Epilepsy (1981): Proposal for revised clinical and electroencephalographic classification of epileptic seizures. *Epilepsia* **22,** 489–501.

176. Commission on Classification and Terminology of the International League Against Epilepsy (1985): Proposal for classification of epilepsy and epileptic syndromes. *Epilepsia* **26,** 268–278.

177. Commission on Classification and Terminology of the International League Against Epilepsy (1989): Proposal for revised classification of epilepsies and epileptic syndromes. *Epilepsia* **30,** 389–399.

178. Conde-Lopez, M. & Picornell-Darder, I. (1986): Contribucion al estudio de la epilepsia benigna de la infancia con paroxismos rolandicos: a proposito de una crisis focal registrada durante el suono espontaneo diurno. *Rev. Espan. Epilepsia* **1**,25–28.

179. Congdon, P.J. & Forsythe, W.I. (1979): Migraine in childhood. A review. *Clinical Pediatrics* **18,** 353–359.

180. Cooper, G.W. & Lee, S.I. (1991): Reactive occipital epileptiform activity: is it benign? *Epilepsia* **32,** 63–68.
181. Courjon, J. & Cotte, M.R. (1959): Les decharges pseudo-rythmiques localisees chez l'enfant et leur evolution a la puberte. In: Anonymous, pp. 247–250. *22eme Congres de Pediatrie de Langue Francaise.* Montpellier: De han.
182. Courjon, J., Moene, Y., Revol, M. & Genin, P. (1968): Occipital attacks triggered by photic stimulation. *Electroencephalogr. Clin. Neurophysiol.* **25,** 587.
183. Cross, H. (1998): Significance of the EEG after the first afebrile seizure: Commentary. *Arch. Dis. Child.* **78,** 576–577.
184. Cuvellier, J.C., Vallee, L. & Nuyts, J.P. (1996): Celiac disease, cerebral calcifications and epilepsy syndrome. *Arch. Pediatrie* **3,** 1013–1019.
185. D'Alessandro, P., Piccirilli, M., Tiacci, C., Ibba, A., Maiotti, M., Sciarma, T. & Testa, A. (1990): Neuropsychological features of benign partial epilepsy in children. *It. J. Neurol. Sci.* **11,** 265–269.
186. D'Alessandro, R., Sacquegna, T., Pazzaglia, P. & Lugaresi, E. (1987): Headache after partial complex seizures. In: *Migraine and epilepsy,* eds. F. Andermann & E. Lugaresi, pp. 273–278. Boston, MA: Butterworths.
187. da Silva, E.A., Chugani, D.C., Muzik, O. & Chugani, H.T. (1997): Landau–Kleffner syndrome: metabolic abnormalities in temporal lobe are a common feature. *J. Child Neurol.* **12,** 489–495.
188. Dahl, M. & Dam, M. (1985): Sleep and epilepsy. *Ann. Clin. Research* **17,** 235–242.
189. Dalla Bernardina, B., Bureau, M., Dravet, C., Dulac, O., Tassinari, C.A., & Roger, J. (1980): Affective symptoms during attacks of epilepsy in children. *Rev. EEG Neurophysiol.* **10,** 8–18.
190. Dalla Bernardina, B., Colamaria, V., Capovilla, G. & Bondavalli, S. (1984): Sleep and benign partial epilepsies of childhood. In: *Epilepsy, sleep and sleep deprivation,* eds. R. Degen & R. Niedermeyer, pp. 119–133. Amsterdam: Elsevier.
191. Dalla Bernardina, B., Colamaria, V., Chiamenti, C., Capovilla, G., Trevisan, E. & Tassinari, C.A. (1992): Benign partial epilepsy with affective symptoms ('benign psychomotor epilepsy'). In: *Epileptic syndromes in infancy, childhood and adolescence,* eds. J. Roger, M. Bureau, C. Dravet, F.E. Dreifuss, A. Perret & P. Wolf, pp. 219–223. London: John Libbey & Company Ltd.
192. Dalla Bernardina, B., Fontana, E., Caraballo, R., Zullini, E., Darra, F. & Collamaria, V. (1993): The partial occipital epilepsies in childhood. In: *Occipital seizures and epilepsies in children,* eds. F. Andermann, A. Beaumanoir, L. Mira, J. Roger & C.A. Tassinari, pp. 173–181. London: John Libbey and Company Ltd.
193. Dalla Bernardina, B., Sgro, V., Caraballo, R., Fontana, E., Colamaria, V., Zullini, E., Simone, M. & Zanetti, R. (1991): Sleep and benign partial epilepsies of childhood: EEG and evoked potentials study. *Epilepsy Research –* **Suppl 2,** 83–96.
194. Dalla Bernardina, B., Sgro, V., Caraballo, R., Montagna, P., Colamaria, V., Zullini, E., Simeone, M. & Zanetti, R. (1991): Sleep and benign partial epilepsies of childhood. In: *Epilepsy, sleep and sleep deprivation,* eds. R. Degen & E.A. Rodin, pp. 83–96. Amsterdam: Elsevier.
195. Dalla Bernardina, B., Sgro, V., Fontana, E., Colamaria, V. & La Selva, L. (1992): Idiopathic partial epilepsies in children. In: *Epileptic syndromes in infancy, childhood and adolescence,* eds. J. Roger, M. Bureau, C. Dravet, F.E. Dreifuss, A. Perret & P. Wolf, pp. 173–188. London: John Libbey & Company Ltd.
196. Dalla Bernardina, B. & Tassinari, C.A. (1975): EEG of a nocturnal seizure in a patient with 'benign epilepsy of childhood with Rolandic spikes'. *Epilepsia* **16,** 497–501.
197. Dalla Bernardina, B., Tassinari, C.A., Dravet, C., Bureau, M., Beghini, G. & Roger, J. (1978): Benign focal epilepsy and 'electrical status epilepticus' during sleep. *Rev. EEG Neurophysiol.* **8,** 350–353.
198. Davidoff, R.A. & Johnson, L.C. (1963): Photic activation and photoconvulsive responses in a nonepileptic subject. *Neurology* **13,** 617–621.
199. Davous, P. & Bequet, D. (1995): Cadasil – a new model for subcortical dementia. *Rev. Neurol.* **151,** 634–639.
200. de Carolis, P., Tinuper, P. & Sacquegna, T. (1991): Migraine with aura and photosensitive epileptic seizures: a case report. *Cephalalgia* **11,** 151–153.
201. De Marco, P. (1971): Peculiar aspect of evoked potentials during sensory stimulation. Preliminary note. *Riv. Neurobiol.* **17,** 177–183.
202. De Marco, P. (1980): An unusual case of 'somatosensory epilepsy'. *Clin. Electroencephalogr.* **11,** 169–172.
203. De Marco, P. (1980): Evoked parietal spikes and childhood epilepsy. *Arch.Neurol.* **37,** 291–292.
204. De Marco, P. (1980): Possibilities of a temporal relationship between the morphology and frequency of parietal somato-sensory evoked spikes and the occurrence of epileptic manifestations. *Clin. Electroencephalogr.* **11,** 132–135.
205. De Marco, P. (1989): Benign infantile epilepsy with 'parietal spikes' (also called 'with extreme sensory evoked potentials'). In: *Reflex seizures and reflex epilepsies,* eds. A. Beaumanoir, H. Gastaut & R. Naquet, pp. 69–74. Geneve: Editions Medecine & Hygiene.

206. De Marco, P., Lorenzi, E. & Miotello, P. (1980): A special form of epileptic signs in childhood. *Z. Elektroenzephalogr. Elektromyogr. und Verwandte Gebiete* **11,** 107–109.

207. De Marco, P. & Negrin, P. (1973): Parietal focal spikes evoked by contralateral tactile somatotopic stimulation in four non-epileptic subjects. *Electroencephalogr. Clin. Neurophysiol.* **34,** 308–312.

208. De Marco, P. & Tassinari, C.A. (1981): Extreme somatosensory evoked potential (ESEP): an EEG sign forecasting the possible occurrence of seizures in children. *Epilepsia* **22,** 569–575.

209. De Negri, M. (1997): Electrical status epilepticus during sleep (ESES). Different clinical syndromes: towards a unifying view?. *Brain Dev.* **19,** 447–451.

210. De Negri, M., Baglietto, M.G., Battaglia, F.M., Gaggero, R., Pessagno, A. & Recanati, L. (1995): Treatment of electrical status epilepticus by short diazepam (DZP) cycles after DZP rectal bolus test. *Brain Dev.* **17,** 330–333.

211. de Paola, L., Balliana, M.O., Silvano, C.E. & de Paola, D. (1990): Irritative midline and parasaggital foci: a clinical and electroencephalographic correlation. *Arquiv. Neuro-Psiquiatria* **48,** 183–187.

212. De Romanis, F., Buzzi, M.G., Assenza, S., Brusa, L. & Cerbo, R. (1993): Basilar migraine with electroencephalographic findings of occipital spike-wave complexes: a long-term study in seven children. *Cephalalgia* **13,** 192–196.

213. De Romanis, F., Buzzi, M.G., Cerbo, R., Feliciani, M., Assenza, S. & Agnoli, A. (1991): Migraine and epilepsy with infantile onset and electroencephalographic findings of occipital spike-wave complexes. *Headache* **31,** 378–383.

214. De Romanis, F. & Feliciani, M. (1988): Occipital epilepsy: a non-benign pediatric syndrome. *Clinica Terapeutica* **124,** 25–32.

215. De Romanis, F., Feliciani, M. & Cerbo, R. (1988): Migraine and other clinical syndromes in children affected by EEG occipital spike-wave complexes. *Functional Neurology* **3,** 187–203.

216. De Romanis, F., Feliciani, M. & Ruggieri, S. (1986): Rolandic paroxysmal epilepsy: a long term study in 150 children. *It. J. Neurol. Sci.* **7,** 77–80.

216a. De Volder, A.G., Michel, C., Thauvoy, C., Willems, G. & Ferriere, G. (1994): Brain glucose utilisation in acquired childhood aphasia associated with a sylvian arachnoid cyst: recovery after shunting as demonstrated by PET. *Neurol. Neurosurg. Psychiatr.* **57,** 296–300.

217. Degen, R. & Degen, H.E. (1990): Some genetic aspects of Rolandic epilepsy: waking and sleep EEGs in siblings. *Epilepsia* **31,** 795–801.

218. Degen, R. & Degen, H.E. (1992): Contribution to the genetics of Rolandic epilepsy: waking and sleep EEGs in siblings. *Epilepsy Research* – **Suppl 6,** 49–52.

219. Degen, R., Degen, H.E. & Hans, K. (1991): A contribution to the genetics of febrile seizures: waking and sleep EEG in siblings. *Epilepsia* **32,** 515–522.

220. Delwaide, P.J., Barragan, M. & Gastaut, H. (1971): Remarks about a partial epilepsy: occipital epilepsy. *Acta Neurol. Belg.* **71,** 383–391.

221. Deonna, T. & Roulet, E. (1995): Acquired epileptic aphasia (AEA): definition of the syndrome and current problems. In: *Continuous spikes and waves during slow sleep. Electrical status epilepticus during slow sleep. Acquired epileptic aphasia and related conditions,* eds. A. Beaumanoir, M. Bureau, T. Deonna, L. Mira & C.A. Tassinari, pp. 37–45. London: John Libbey & Company Ltd.

222. Deonna, T. & Ziegler, A.L. (1994): So-called benign epilepsies in children. *Rev. Medic. Suisse Romande* **114,** 861–867.

223. Deonna, T., Ziegler, A.L. & Despland, P.A. (1984): Paroxysmal visual disturbances of epileptic origin and occipital epilepsy in children. *Neuropediatrics* **15,** 131–135.

224. Deonna, T., Ziegler, A.L. & Despland, P.A. (1986): Combined myoclonic-astatic and 'benign' focal epilepsy of childhood ('atypical benign partial epilepsy of childhood'). A separate syndrome? *Neuropediatrics* **17,** 144–151.

225. Deonna, T., Ziegler, A.L., Despland, P.A. & van Melle, G. (1986): Partial epilepsy in neurologically normal children: clinical syndromes and prognosis. *Epilepsia* **27,** 241–247.

226. Deonna, T.W. (1991): Acquired epileptiform aphasia in children (Landau–Kleffner syndrome). *J. Clin. Neurophysiol.* **8,** 288–298.

227. Deonna, T.W., Roulet, E., Fontan, D. & Marcoz, J.P. (1993): Speech and oromotor deficits of epileptic origin in benign partial epilepsy of childhood with Rolandic spikes (BPERS). Relationship to the acquired aphasia–epilepsy syndrome. *Neuropediatrics* **24,** 83–87.

228. Dermirbilek, A., Dervent, A., Cacmak, O. & Korkmaz, B. (1996): Electroclinical survey on benign epilepsy with occipital paroxysms. *Epilepsia* **37 (Suppl 4),** 95

229. Devinsky, O., Frasca, J., Pacia, S.V., Luciano, D.J., Paraiso, J. & Doyle, W. (1995): Ictus emeticus: further evidence of nondominant temporal involvement. *Neurology* **45,** 1158–1160.

230. Dhuna, A., Pascual-Leone, A. & Talwar, D. (1991): Exacerbation of partial seizures and onset of nonepileptic myoclonus with carbamazepine. *Epilepsia* **32,** 275–278.

231. Diamond, S. (1987): Basilar artery migraine. A commonly misdiagnosed disorder. *Postgr. Med.* **81,** 45–46.

232. Diaz, Y. and Diaz H. (1976): Paroxysmal epileptic headache. *Neurol.Neurocir.Psiquiatria* **17,** 85–94.

233. Dichgans, M., Mayer, M., Muller-Myhsok, B., Straube, A. & Gasser, T. (1996): Identification of a key recombinant narrows the CADASIL gene region to 8 cM and argues against allelism of CADASIL and familial hemiplegic migraine. *Genomics* **32,** 151–154.

234. Dinner, D.S. (1989): Sleep and pediatric epilepsy. *Clev.Cl. J. Med.* **56 Suppl Pt 2,** S234–9.

235. Dobrzynska, L. & Kamraj-Mazurkiewicz, K. (1978): Benign childhood epilepsy with spike activity in the area of the precentral gyrus. *Neurol. Neurochir. Polska* **12,** 561–568.

236. Donnet, A. & Bartolomei, F. (1997): Migraine with visual aura and photosensitive epileptic seizures. *Epilepsia* **38,** 1032–1034.

237. Doose, H. (1989): Symptomatology in children with focal sharp waves of genetic origin. *European J. Pediatr.* **149,** 210–215.

238. Doose, H. (1992): Pathogenesis of epilepsy in childhood and adolescence. *Monatsschrift Kinderheilkunde* **140,** 385–390.

239. Doose, H. & Baier, W.K. (1988): Theta rhythms in the EEG: a genetic trait in childhood epilepsy. *Brain Dev.* **10,** 347–354.

240. Doose, H. & Baier, W.K. (1989): Benign partial epilepsy and related conditions: multifactorial pathogenesis with hereditary impairment of brain maturation. *European J. Pediatr.* **149,** 152–158.

241. Doose, H. & Baier, W.K. (1991): A genetically determined basic mechanism in benign partial epilepsies and related non-convulsive conditions. *Epilepsy Research – Supplement* **4,** 113–118.

242. Doose, H., Baier, W.K., Ernst, J.P., Tuxhorn, I. & Volzke, E. (1988): Benign partial epilepsy – treatment with sulthiame [letter]. *Dev. Med. Child Neurol.* **30,** 683–684.

243. Doose, H., Brigger-Heuer, B. & Neubauer, B. (1997): Children with focal sharp waves: clinical and genetic aspects. *Epilepsia* **38,** 788–796.

244. Doose, H., Gerken, H., Kiefer, R. & Volzke, E. (1977): Genetic factors in childhood epilepsy with focal sharp waves. II. EEG findings in patients and siblings. *Neuropadiatrie* **8,** 10–20.

245. Doose, H., Neubauer, B. & Carlsson, G. (1996): Children with benign focal sharp waves in the EEG – developmental disorders and epilepsy. *Neuropediatrics* **27,** 227–241.

246. Doose, H. & Sitepu, B. (1983): Childhood epilepsy in a German city. *Neuropediatrics* **14,** 220–224.

247. Drabek, P. (1989): Basilar artery migraine. *Ceskoslovenska Neurol. Neurochir.* **52,** 424–428.

248. Dravet, C. (1994): Benign epilepsy with centrotemporal spikes: do we know all about it? In: *Epileptic seizures and syndromes*, ed. P. Wolf, pp. 231–240. London: John Libbey & Company Ltd.

249. Drury, I. & Beydoun, A. (1991): Benign partial epilepsy of childhood with monomorphic sharp waves in centrotemporal and other locations. *Epilepsia* **32,** 662–667.

250. Dugas, M. (1982): The Landau–Kleffner syndrome. Infantile 'acquired' aphasia, paroxysmal electroencephalographic changes and epileptic seizures. *Nouvelle Presse Medicale* **11,** 3787–3791.

251. Dugas, M., Franc, S., Gerard, C.L. & Lecendreux, M. (1995): Evolution of acquired epileptic aphasia with or without continuous spikes and waves during slow sleep. In: *Continuous spikes and waves during slow sleep. Electrical status epilepticus during slow sleep. Acquired epileptic aphasia and related conditions,* eds. A. Beaumanoir, M. Bureau, T. Deonna, L. Mira & C.A. Tassinari, pp. 47–55. London: John Libbey & Company Ltd.

252. Dugas, M., Masson, M., Le Heuzey, M.F. & Regnier, N. (1982): Childhood acquired aphasia with epilepsy (Landau–Kleffner syndrome). 12 personal cases. *Rev. Neurol.* **138,** 755–780.

253. Dulac, O. & Arthuis, M. (1980): Epilepsie psychomotrice benigne de l'enfant. *Journees parisiennes de padiatrie* 211–220.

254. Dulac, O., Chiron, C., Valenza, A., Jalin, C. & Plouin, P. (1986): Epilepsie generalisee primaire avec crises partielles. *Boll. Lega Ital. Epil.* **54/55,** 71–74.

255. Dulac, O., Cusmai, R. & de Oliveira, K. (1989): Is there a partial benign epilepsy in infancy? *Epilepsia* **30,** 798–801.

256. Duncan, J.S. and Panayiotopoulos, C.P. (1996): *Eyelid myoclonia with absences.* London: John Libbey & Company Ltd.

257. Dvorkin, G.S., Andermann, F., Carpenter, S., Melanson, D., Verret, S., Jacob, J.C., Sherwin, A., Bekhor, S., Lugaresi, E., Sackellares, C., Willoughby, J. & MacGregor, D. (1987): Classical migraine, intractable epilepsy, and multiple strokes: A syndrome related to mitochondrial encephalomyopathy. In: *Migraine and epilepsy,* eds. F. Andermann & E. Lugaresi, pp. 203–232. Boston, MA: Butterworths.

258. Eeg-Olofsson, O. (1992): Further genetic aspects in benign localized epilepsies in early childhood. *Epilepsy Research* – **Suppl 6,** 117–119.

259. Eeg-Olofsson, O., Osterland, C.K., Guttmann, R.D., Andermann, F., Prchal, J.F., Andermann, E. & Janjua, N.A. (1988): Immunological studies in focal epilepsy. *Acta Neurol. Scand.* **78,** 358–368.

260. Eeg-Olofsson, O., Petersen, I. & Selden, U. (1971): The development of the electroencephalogram in normal children from the age of 1 through 15 years. *Neuropadiatrie* **2,** 375–404.

261. Eeg-Olofsson, O., Safwenberg, J. & Wigertz, A. (1982): HLA and epilepsy: an investigation of different types of epilepsy in children and their families. *Epilepsia* **23,** 27–34.

262. Ehle, A., Co, S. & Jones, M.G. (1981): Clinical correlates of midline spikes. An analysis of 21 patients. *Arch.Neurol.* **38,** 355–357.

263. Ehrenberg, B.L. (1991): Unusual clinical manifestations of migraine and 'the borderland of epilepsy' – reexplored. *Seminars in Neurology* **11,** 118–127.

264. Elliott, M.A., Peroutka, S.J., Welch, S. & May, E.F. (1996): Familial hemiplegic migraine, nystagmus, and cerebellar atrophy. *Ann. Neurol.* **39,** 100–106.

264a. Elmslie, F.V., Rees, M., Williamson, M.P., Kerr, M., Kjeldsen, M.J., Pang, K.A., Sundqvist, A., Friis, M.L., Chadwick, D., Richens, A., Santos, M., Arzimanoglou, A., Panayiotopoulos, C.P., Curtis, D., Whitehouse, W.P. & Gardiner, R.M. (1997): Genetic mapping of major susceptibility locus for juvenile myoclonic epilepsy on chromosome 15q. *Human Molecular Genetics* **6,** 1329–1334.

265. Erdemoglu, A.K. (1996): Psychogenic basilar migraine [letter; comment]. *Neurology* **47,** 302–303.

266. Eviatar, L. (1981): Vestibular testing in basilar artery migraine. *Ann.Neurol.* **9,** 126–130.

267. Faure, J. & Loiseau, P. (1960): Une correlation clinique particuliere de pointe-ondes rolandiques sans signification focale. *Rev. Neurol.* **102,** 399–406.

268. Fayad, M.N., Choueiri, R. & Mikati, M. (1997): Landau–Kleffner syndrome: consistent response to repeated intravenous gamma-globulin doses: a case report. *Epilepsia* **38,** 489–494.

269. Fazio, C., Manfredi, M. & Piccinelli, A. (1975): Treatment of epileptic seizures with clonazepam. A reappraisal. *Arch.Neurol.* **32,** 304–307.

270. Fejerman, N. (1996): Atypical evolutions of benign partial epilepsies in children. *International Pediatrics* **11,** 351–356.

271. Fejerman, N. (1996): Atypical evolution of benign partial epilepsy in children. *Revist. Neurol.* **24,** 1415–1420.

272. Fejerman, N. (1997). New idiopathic partial epilepsies. *Epilepsia* **38 Suppl 7,** 26.

273. Fejerman, N. & Di Blasi, A.M. (1987): Status epilepticus of benign partial epilepsies in children: report of two cases. *Epilepsia* **28,** 351–355.

274. Ferraro, S.M., Daraio, M.C., Mazzola, M.E., Fiori, R., Solis, S., Aqosta, G. & Castano, J. (1997): Coexistence of two forms of benign childhood partial epilepsies. *Epilepsia* **38 Suppl 7,** 38.

275. Ferraro, S.M., Daraio, M.C., Solis, S., Menzano, E. & Castano, J. (1997): Is the ILAE classification comprehensive to pediatric epileptic patients? *Epilepsia* **38 Suppl 7,** 37.

276. Ferri, R., Musumeci, S.A., Elia, M., Del Gracco, S., Scuderi, C. & Bergonzi, P. (1994): BIT-mapped somatosensory evoked potentials in the fragile X syndrome. *Neurophysiol. Clin.* **24,** 413–426.

277. Ferrie, C.D., Beaumanoir, A., Guerrini, R., Kivity, S., Vigevano, F., Takaishi, Y, Watanabe, K., Mira, L., Capizzi, G., Costa, P., Valseriati, D., Grioni, D., Lerman, P., Ricci, S., Vigliano, P., Goumas-Kartalas, A., Hashimoto, K., Robinson, R.O. & Panayiotopoulos, C.P. (1997): Early-onset benign occipital seizure susceptibility syndrome. *Epilepsia* **38,** 285–293.

278. Ferrie, C.D., De Marco, P., Grunewald, R.A., Giannakodimos, S. & Panayiotopoulos, C.P. (1994): Video game induced seizures. *J. Neurol. Neurosurg. Psychiatry* **57,** 925–931.

279. Ferrie, C.D., Robinson, R.O., Giannakodimos, S. & Panayiotopoulos, C.P. (1994): Video-game epilepsy. *Lancet* **344,** 1710–1711.

280. Ferrie, C.D., Robinson, R.O., Knott, C. & Panayiotopoulos, C.P. (1995): Lamotrigine as an add-on drug in typical absence seizures. *Acta Neurol. Scand.* **91,** 200–202.

281. Finelli, P.F. (1978): Confusional state and basilar artery migraine. *Neurology* **28,** 1201

282. Fiol, M.E., Leppik, I.E., Mireles, R. & Maxwell, R. (1988): Ictus emeticus and the insular cortex. *Epilepsy Research* **2,** 127–131.

283. Fischer, R.A. & Clancy, R.R. (1987): Midline foci of epileptiform activity in children and neonates. *J. Child Neurol.* **2,** 224–228.

284. Fischer-Williams, M., Bickford, R.G. & Whisnant, J.R. (1964): Occipito-Parieto-Temporal Seizure Discharge with Visual Hallucinations and Aphasia. *Epilepsia* **5,** 279–292.

285. Foerster, O. & Penfield, W. (1929): The structural basis of traumatic epilepsy and results of radical operation. *Assoc. Res. Nerv. Ment. Dis.* **7,** 569–591.

286. Fois, A., Borgheresi, S. & Luti, E. (1968): Clinical correlates of focal epileptic discharges in children without seizures. A study of 110 cases. *Helv. Paediatr. Acta* **23,** 257–265.

287. Fois, A., Malandrini, F. & Tomaccini, D. (1988): Clinical findings in children with occipital paroxysmal discharges. *Epilepsia* **29,** 620–623.

288. Fois, A., Vascotto, M., Di Bartolo, R.M. & Di Marco, V. (1994): Celiac disease and epilepsy in pediatric patients. *Childs Nervous System* **10,** 450–454.

289. Fonseca, L.C. & Tedrus, G.M. (1994): Occipital paroxysms before eye closure. Clinico-electroencephalographic correlations in 24 cases. *Arq. Neuro-Psiquiatria* **52,** 510–514.

290. Fonseca, L.C. & Tedrus, G.M. (1994): Epileptic syndromes in children with somatosensory evoked spikes. *Clin. Electroencephalogr.* **25,** 54–58.

291. Fonseca, L.C. & Tedrus, G.M. (1995): Epilepsy with centrotemporal spikes and parietal spikes: comparative study. *Arq. Neuro-Psiquiatria* **53,** 208–212.

292. Fonseca, L.C., Tedrus, G.M., Bastos, A., Bosco, A. & Laloni, D.T. (1996): Reactivity of Rolandic spikes. *Clin. Electroencephalogr.* **27,** 116–120.

293. Frequin, S.T., Linssen, W.H., Pasman, J.W., Hommes, O.R. & Merx, H.L. (1991): Recurrent prolonged coma due to basilar artery migraine. A case report. *Headache* **31,** 75–81.

294. Fukusako, T., Yamamoto, K., Takase, Y., Nogaki, H. & Morimatsu, M. (1990): A case of reflex epilepsy with binasal visual field defects attack induced by family computer game. *Rinsho Shinkeigaku – Clinical Neurology* **30,** 540–543.

295. Furman, J.M., Crumrine, P.K. & Reinmuth, O.M. (1990): Epileptic nystagmus. *Ann. Neurol.* **27,** 686–688.

296. Gallet, S., Revol, M., Isnard, H. & Gilly, R. (1986): Visual seizures and benign epilepsy in children with paroxysmal occipital discharges. *Pediatrie* **41,** 383–391.

297. Ganji, S. (1986): Basilar artery migraine: EEG and evoked potential patterns during acute stage. *Headache* **26,** 220–223.

298. Ganji, S., Hellman, S., Stagg, S. & Furlow, J. (1993): Episodic coma due to acute basilar artery migraine: correlation of EEG and brainstem auditory evoked potential patterns. *Clin. Electroencephalogr.* **24,** 44–48.

299. Garofalo, E.A., Drury, I. & Goldstein, G.W. (1988): EEG abnormalities aid diagnosis of Rett syndrome. *Pediatr. Neurol.* **4,** 350–353.

300. Gastaut, H. (1950): Evidences electrographiques d'un mechanisme sous-cortical dans certaines epilepsies partielles. La signification clinique des 'secteures areo-thalamiques'. *Rev. Neurol.* **83,** 396–401.

301. Gastaut, H. (1960): Un aspect meconnu des decharges neuroniques occipitales: la crise occuloclonique ou 'nystagmus epileptique'. In: *Les grandes activites du lobe occipital,* ed. T. Alajouanine, pp. 169–185. Paris: Masson.

302. Gastaut, H. (1981): Benign epilepsy with occipital spike waves in children. *Bulletin et Memoires de l' Academie Royale de Medecine de Belgique* **136,** 540–555.

303. Gastaut, H. (1982): A new type of epilepsy: Benign partial epilepsy of childhood with occipital spike-waves. In: *Brain Dev. in Epileptology: XIIIth Epilepsy International Symposium* eds. H. Akimoto, H. Kazamatsuri, M. Seino & A. Ward, pp. 19–24. New York: Raven Press.

304. Gastaut, H. (1982): A new type of epilepsy: benign partial epilepsy of childhood with occipital spike-waves. *Clin. Electroencephalogr.* **13,** 13–22.

305. Gastaut, H. (1982): The benign epilepsy in childhood with occipital spike wave complexes. *EEG-EMG Zeitschrift fur Elektroenzephalographie Elektromyographie und Verwandte Gebiete* **13,** 3–8.

306. Gastaut, H. (1982): Benign spike-wave occipital epilepsy in children. *Rev. EEG Neurophysiol.* **12,** 179–201.

307. Gastaut, H. (1983): Classification of status epilepticus. *Adv. Neurol.* **34,** 15–35.

308. Gastaut, H. (1985): Benign epilepsy of childhood with occipital paroxysms. In: *Epilepsy syndromes in infancy, childhood and adolescence,* eds. J. Roger, C. Dravet, M. Bureau, F.E. Dreifuss & P. Wolf, pp. 159–170. London: John Libbey & Company Ltd.

309. Gastaut, H., Regis, H., Bostem, F. & Beaussart, M. (1960): Etude electroencephalographique de 35 sujets ayant presente des crises au cours d'un spectacle televise. *Rev. Neurol.* **102,** 533–534.

310. Gastaut, H., Roger, J. & Bureau, M. (1992): Benign epilepsy of childhood with occipital paroxysms. Up-date. In: *Epileptic syndromes in infancy, childhood and adolescence,* eds. J. Roger, M. Bureau, C. Dravet, F.E. Dreifuss, A. Perret & P. Wolf, pp. 201–217. London: John Libbey & Company Ltd.

311. Gastaut, H., Roger, J. & Gastaut, Y. (1948): Les formes experimentales de l'epilepsie humaine: 1. L'epilepsie induite par la stimulation lumineuse intermittente rythmee ou epilepsie photogenique. *Rev. Neurol.* **80,** 161–183.

312. Gastaut, H. & Zifkin, B.G. (1984): Ictal visual hallucinations of numerals. *Neurology* **34,** 950–953.

313. Gastaut, H. & Zifkin, B.G. (1987): Benign epilepsy of childhood with occipital spike and wave complexes. In: *Migraine and epilepsy,* eds. F. Andermann & E. Lugaresi, pp. 47–81. Boston, MA: Butterworths.

314. Gastaut, Y. (1952): Un element deroutant de la semeiologie electroencephalographique: les points prerolandiques sans signification focale. *Rev. Neurol.* **87,** 488–499.

315. Geladze, T.S., Toidze, O.S. & Lomashvili, N.D. (1983): Importance of timely diagnosis of benign childhood epilepsy with Rolandic peaks. *Zhurnal Nevropatologii i Psikhiatrii Imeni S - S - Korsakova* **83,** 1492–1496.

316. Genton, P., Borg, M., Vigliano, P., Pellissier, J.F. & Roger, J. (1989): Semi-late onset and rapidly progressive case of Lafora's disease with predominant cognitive symptoms. *Eur. Neurol.* **29,** 333–338.

317. Genton, P., Bureau, M., Dravet, C. & Roger, J. (1988): Napping sleep EEG in partial childhood epilepsy. *Neurophysiol. Clin.* **18,** 333–343.

318. Genton, P. & Guerrini, R. (1993): What differentiates Landau–Kleffner syndrome from the syndrome of continuous spikes and waves during slow sleep? *Arch.Neurol.* **50,** 1008–1009.

319. Genton, P. & Guerrini, R. (1994): Idiopathic localization-related epilepsies: the non-Rolandic types. In: *Epileptic seizures and syndromes,*ed. P. Wolf, pp. 241–256. London: John Libbey & Company Ltd.

320. Genton, P., Maton, B., Ogihara, M., Samoggia, G., Guerrini, R., Medina, M.T., Dravet, C. & Roger, J. (1992): Continuous focal spikes during REM sleep in a case of acquired aphasia (Landau–Kleffner syndrome). *Sleep* **15,** 454–460.

321. Gerken, H., Kiefer, R., Doose, H. & Volzke, E. (1977): Genetic factors in childhood epilepsy with focal sharp waves. I. Clinical data and familial morbidity for seizures. *Neuropadiatrie* **8,** 3–9.

322. Giannakodimos, S., Ferrie, C.D. & Panayiotopoulos, C.P. (1995): Qualitative and quantitative abnormalities of breath counting during brief generalized 3 Hz spike and slow wave 'subclinical' discharges. *Clin. Electroencephalogr.* **26,** 200–203.

323. Giannakodimos, S. & Panayiotopoulos, C.P. (1996): Eyelid myoclonia with absences in adults: a clinical and video-EEG study. *Epilepsia* **37,** 36–44.

324. Gibbs, E.L., Fois, A. & Gibbs, F.A. (1955): The electroencephalogram in retrolental fibroplasia. *New Engl. J. Med.* **253,** 1102–1106.

325. Gibbs, E.L. & Gibbs, F.A. (1981): Electroencephalogram in congenital anophthalmia. *EEG-EMG Zeitschrift fur Elektroencephalographie Elektromyographie und Verwandte Gebiete* **12,** 171 173.

326. Gibbs, E.L., Gillen, H.W. & Gibbs, F.A. (1954): Disappearance and migration of epileptic foci in childhood. *Am. J. Dis. Child* **88,** 596–603.

327. Gibbs, F.A., & Gibbs, E.L. (1952): *Atlas of electroencephalography*, Vol. 2. *Epilepsy,* pp. 214–290. Reading, MA: Addison-Wesley.

328. Gibbs, F.A. & Gibbs, E.L. (1960): Good prognosis of midtemporal epilepsy. *Epilepsia* **1,** 448–453.

329. Gibbs, F.A. & Gibbs, E.L. (1963): Age factor in epilepsy. A Summary and Synthesis. *New Engl. J. Med.* 1230–1236.

330. Gibbs, F.A. & Gibbs, E.L. (1964): *Atlas of electroncephalography.* Reading, MA: Addison-Wesley.

331. Gibbs FA & Gibbs EL. (1967): *Medical Electroencephalography.* Reading, MA: Addison-Wesley.

332. Gibbs, F.A. & Gibbs, E.L. (1970): Clinical correlates and prognostic significance of various types of mid-temporal spike focus. *Clin. Electroencephalogr.* **1,** 45–64.

333. Gibbs, F.A., Gibbs, E.L. & Gibbs, T.J. (1968): Relation between specific types of occipital dysrhythmia and visual defects. *Johns Hopkins Medical Journal* **122,** 343–349.

334. Gil, R., Lefevre, J.P. & Burelout, Y. (1984): Migraine, seizures and epileptic focal E.E.G. abnormalities in a young adult: a nine-year follow-up. *Headache* **24,** 23–25.

335. Gilliam, F. & Wyllie, E. (1995): Ictal amaurosis: MRI, EEG, and clinical features. *Neurology* **45,** 1619–1621.

336. Gilroy, J. & Lerman, V.J. (1982): Cardiac arrhythmia in basilar migraine. *Headache* **22,** 140.

337. Giovanardi Rossi, P., Santucci, M., Gobbi, G., D'Alessandro, R. & Sacquegna, T. (1987): Epidemiological study of migraine in epileptic patients. In: *Migraine and epilepsy,* eds. F. Andermann & E. Lugaresi, pp. 313–322. Boston, MA: Butterworths.

338. Giroud, M., Borsotti, J.P., Michiels, R., Tommasi, M. & Dumas, R. (1990): Epilepsy and bilateral occipital calcifications: 3 cases. *Rev. Neurol.* **146,** 288–292.

339. Giroud, M., Couillault, G., Arnould, S., Dauvergne, M., Dumas, R. & Nivelon, J.L. (1989): Epilepsy with Rolandic paroxysms and migraine, a non-fortuitous association. Results of a controlled study. *Pediatrie* **44,** 659–664.

340. Giroud, M., Soichot, P., Weyl, M., Dauvergne, M., Alison, M. & Dumas, R. (1986): Epilepsy with occipital spike waves. Its place among the benign epilepsies. *Ann. Pediatrie* **33,** 131–135.

341. Gobbi, G., Andermann, F., Naccarato, S., Banchini, G., Gobbi, G., Andermann, F., Naccarato. S. & Banchini, G. (eds) (1997): *Epilepsy and other neurological disorders in coeliac disease.* pp. 1–378. London: John Libbey & Company Ltd.

342. Gobbi, G., Bertani, G. & Italian Working Group on Coeliac Disease and Epilepsy (1997): Coeliac disease and epilepsy. In: *Epilepsy and other neurological disorders in coeliac disease,* eds. G. Gobbi, F. Andermann, S. Naccarato & G. Banchini, pp. 65–79. London: John Libbey & Company Ltd.

343. Gobbi, G., Bouquet, F., Greco, L., Lambertini, A., Tassinari, C.A., Ventura, A. & Zaniboni, M.G. (1992): Coeliac disease, epilepsy, and cerebral calcifications. The Italian Working Group on Coeliac Disease and Epilepsy. *Lancet* **340,** 439–443.

344. Gobbi, G. & Guerrini, R. (1997): Childhood epilepsy with occipital spikes and other benign localization-related epilepsies. In: *Epilepsy: A Comprehensive Textbook,* eds. J.J. Engel & T.A. Pedley, pp. 2315–2326. Philadelphia: Lippincott-Raven Publishers.

345. Gobbi, G., Sorrenti, G., Santucci, M., Rossi, P.G., Ambrosetto, P., Michelucci, R & Tassinari, C.A. (1988): Epilepsy with bilateral occipital calcifications: a benign onset with progressive severity. *Neurology* **38,** 913–920.

346. Golden, G.S. & French, J.H. (1975): Basilar artery migraine in young children. *Pediatrics* **56,** 722–726.

347. Goldstein, M.J., Parker, R.L. & Dewan, D.M. (1996): Status epilepticus amauroticus secondary to meningitis as a cause of postpartum cortical blindness. *Regional Anesthesia* **21,** 595–598.

348. Gonzalez de Dios, J., Moya Benavent, M., Izura Azanza, V. & Pastore Olmedo, C. (1997): Electrophysiological studies in the follow-up of children with perinatal asphyxia history. *An. Espan. Pediatria* **46,** 597–602.

349. Gordon, N. (1997): The Landau–Kleffner syndrome: increased understanding. *Brain Dev.* **19,** 311–316.

350. Gowers, W.R. (1879): Cases of cerebral tumors illustrating diagnosis and localisation. *Lancet* 363–365.

351. Gowers, W.R. (1881): Epilepsy and other chronic convulsive diseases: their causes, symptoms and treatment. London: J. & A. Churchill.

352. Gowers, W.R. (1885): *Symptoms. General characters of epileptic fits,* pp. 31–58. New York: William Wood & Co.

353. Gowers, W.R. (1904): *Subjective sensations of sight and sound; Abiotrophy and other lectures.* Philadelphia: P. Blackinston's Son & Co.

354. Gowers, W.R. (1907): *The borderland of epilepsy. Faints, vagal attacks, vertigo, migraine, sleep symptoms, and their treatment.* Philadelphia: P. Blackinston's Son & Co.

355. Gozukirmizi, E., Derewet, A., Altinel, A., Zelbinci, N. (1982): All night sleep recordings in benign childhood epilepsy. *Electroencephalogr. Clin. Neurophysiol.* **53,** 28P.

356. Graf, W.D., Chatrian, G.E., Glass, S.T. & Knauss, T.A. (1994): Video game-related seizures: a report on 10 patients and a review of the literature. *Pediatrics* **93,** 551–556.

357. Grecory, R.P., Oates, T. & Merry, R.T.C. (1993): EEG epileptiform abnormalities in candidates for aircrew training. *Electroencephalogr. Clin. Neurophysiol.* **86,** 75–77.

358. Green, J.B. (1995): Regarding 'Sounds trigger spikes in the Landau–Kleffner syndrome'. *J. Clin. Neurophysiol.* **12,** 203.

359. Gregory, D.L. & Wong, P.K. (1984): Topographical analysis of the centrotemporal discharges in benign Rolandic epilepsy of childhood. *Epilepsia* **25,** 705–711.

360. Gregory, D.L. & Wong, P.K. (1992): Clinical relevance of a dipole field in Rolandic spikes. *Epilepsia* **33,** 36–44.

360a. Gronseth, G.S. & Greenberg, M.K. (1995): The utility of the electroencephalogram in the evaluation of patients presenting with headache: a review of the literature. *Neurology* **45,** 1263–1267.

361. Gropen, T.I., Prohovnik, I., Tatemichi, T.K. & Hirano, M. (1994): Cerebral hyperemia in MELAS. *Stroke* **25,** 1873–1876.

362. Grunewald, R.A., Aliberti, V. & Panayiotopoulos, C.P. (1992): Exacerbation of typical absence seizures by progesterone. *Seizure* **1,** 137–138.

363. Grunewald, R.A., Chroni, E. & Panayiotopoulos, C.P. (1992): Delayed diagnosis of juvenile myoclonic epilepsy. *J. Neurol. Neurosurg. Psychiatry* **55,** 497–499.

364. Grunewald, R.A. & Panayiotopoulos, C.P. (1993): Juvenile myoclonic epilepsy. A review. *Arch. Neurol.* **50,** 594–598.

365. Grunewald, R.A. & Panayiotopoulos, C.P. (1996): The diagnosis of epilepsies. *J. R. Coll. Phys. Lond.* **30,** 122–127.

366. Guerreiro, M.M., Camargo, E.E., Kato, M., Menezes Netto, J.R., Silva, E.A., Scotoni, A.E., Silveira, D.C. & Guerreiro, C.A. (1996): Brain single photon emission computed tomography imaging in Landau–Kleffner syndrome. *Epilepsia* **37,** 60–67.

367. Guerrini, R., Battaglia, A., Dravet, C., Bureau, M. & Genton, P. (1993): Outcome of idiopathic childhood epilepsy with occipital paroxysms. In: *Occipital seizures and epilepsies in children,* eds. F. Andermann, A. Beaumanoir, L. Mira, J. Roger & C.A. Tassinari, pp. 165–171. London: John Libbey & Company Ltd.

368. Guerrini, R., Belmonte, A., Veggiotti, P., Mattia, D. & Bonanni, P. (1997): Delayed appearance of interictal EEG abnormalities in early onset childhood epilepsy with occipital paroxysms. *Brain Dev.* **19,** 343–346.

369. Guerrini, R., Bonanni, P., Parmeggiani, L. & Belmonte, A. (1997): Adolescent onset of idiopathic photosensitive occipital epilepsy after remission of benign Rolandic epilepsy. *Epilepsia* **38,** 777–781.

370. Guerrini, R., Dravet, C., Genton, P., Bureau, M., Bonanni, P., Ferrari, A.R. & Roger, J. (1995): Idiopathic photosensitive occipital lobe epilepsy. *Epilepsia* **36,** 883–891.

371. Guerrini, R., Ferrari, A.R., Battaglia, A., Salvadori, P. & Bonanni, P. (1994): Occipitotemporal seizures with ictus emeticus induced by intermittent photic stimulation. *Neurology* **44,** 253–259.

372. Gutierrez, A.R., Brick, J.F. & Bodensteiner, J. (1990): Dipole reversal: an ictal feature of benign partial epilepsy with centrotemporal spikes. *Epilepsia* **31,** 544–548.

373. Haan, J., Terwindt, G.M., Bos, P.L., Ophoff, R.A., Frants, R.R. & Ferrari, M.D. (1994): Familial hemiplegic migraine in The Netherlands. Dutch Migraine Genetics Research Group. *Clin. Neurol. Neurosurg.* **96,** 244–249.

374. Haan, J., Terwindt, G.M., Ophoff, R.A., Bos, P.L., Frants, R.R., Ferrari, M.D., Krommenhoek, T., Lindhout, D.L., Sandkuyl, L.A. & Van Eyk, R. (1995): Is familial hemiplegic migraine a hereditary form of basilar migraine? *Cephalalgia* **15,** 477–481.

375. Hachinski, V.C., Porchawka, J. & Steele, J.C. (1973): Visual symptoms in the migraine syndrome. *Neurology* **23,** 570–579.

376. Hagne, I., Witt-Engerstrom, I. & Hagberg, B. (1989): EEG development in Rett syndrome. A study of 30 cases. *Electroencephalogr. Clin. Neurophysiol.* **72,** 1–6.

377. Harding, G.F.A. & Jeavons, P.M. (1994): *Photosensitive epilepsy.* London: MacKeith Press.

378. Harris, C.M., Boyd, S., Chong, K., Harkness, W. & Neville, B.G. (1997): Epileptic nystagmus in infancy. *J. Neurol. Sci.* **151,** 111–114.

379. Hart, Y.M., Sander, J.W., Johnson, A.L. & Shorvon, S.D. (1990): National General Practice Study of Epilepsy: recurrence after a first seizure. *Lancet* **336,** 1271–1274.

380. Hauser, W.A., Rich, S.S., Annegers, J.F. & Anderson, V.E. (1990): Seizure recurrence after a 1st unprovoked seizure: an extended follow- up. *Neurology* **40,** 1163–1170.

381. Hauswald, M. (1987): Cortical blindness and late postpartum eclampsia. *American Journal of Emergency Medicine* **5,** 130–132.

382. Heijbel, J. (1976): Benign epilepsy of children with centrotemporal EEG foci. Clinical, genetic and neurophysiological aspects. Thesis. Umea University, Sweden.

383. Heijbel, J., Blom, S. & Bergfors, P.G. (1975): Benign epilepsy of children with centrotemporal EEG foci. A study of incidence rate in outpatient care. *Epilepsia* **16,** 657–664.

384. Heijbel, J., Blom, S. & Rasmuson, M. (1975): Benign epilepsy of childhood with centrotemporal EEG foci: a genetic study. *Epilepsia* **16,** 285–293.

385. Heijbel, J. & Bohman, M. (1975): Benign epilepsy of children with centrotemporal EEG foci: intelligence, behavior, and school adjustment. *Epilepsia* **16,** 679–687.

386. Herranz Tanarro, F.J., Saenz Lope, E. & Cristobal Sassot, S. (1984): La pointe-onde occipitale avec et sans epilepsie benigne chez l'enfant. *Rev. EEG Neurophysiol.* **14,** 1–7.

387. Herschel, J.F.W. (1866): *Familiar lectures on scientific aspects.* London: Alexander Straham.

388. Hirano, M. & DiMauro, S. (1997): Primary Mitochondrial Diseases. In: *Epilepsy. A comprehensive textbook,* eds. J.J. Engel & T.A. Pedley, pp. 2563–2570. Philadelphia: Lippincott-Raven.

389. Hirano, M. & Pavlakis, S.G. (1994): Mitochondrial myopathy, encephalopathy, lactic acidosis, and strokelike episodes (MELAS): current concepts. *J. Child Neurol.* **9,** 4–13.

390. Hirsch, E., Marescaux, C., Maquet, P., Metz-Lutz, M.N., Kiesmann, M., Salmon, E., Franck, G. & Kurtz, D. (1990): Landau–Kleffner syndrome: a clinical and EEG study of five cases. *Epilepsia* **31,** 756–767.

391. Hishikawa, Y., Yamamoto, J., Furuya, E., Yamada, Y., Miyazaki, K. & Kaneko, Z. (1967): Photosensitive epilepsy: relationships between the visual evoked responses and the epileptiform discharges induced by intermittent photic stimulation. *Electroencephalogr. Clin. Neurophysiol.* **23,** 320–334.

392. Hockaday, J.M. (1979): Basilar migraine in childhood. *Dev. Med. Child Neurol.* **21,** 455–463.

393. Hockaday, J.M. (1988): *Migraine in Childhood.* London: Butterworths.

394. Hockaday, J.M. & Newton, R.W. (1988): Migraine and Epilepsy. In: *Migraine in childhood* ed. J.M. Hockaday, pp. 88–143. London: Butterworths.

395. Hoekelman, R.A. (1991): A pediatrician's view. The first seizure – a terrifying event [editorial]. *Pediatric Annals* **20,** 9–10.

396. Holmes, G. (1927): Sabill memorial oration on focal epilepsy. *Lancet* **i,** 957–962.

397. Holmes, G.L. (1992): Rolandic epilepsy: clinical and electroencephalographic features. *Epilepsy Research – Supplement* **6,** 29–43.

398. Holmes, G.L. (1993): Benign focal epilepsies of childhood. *Epilepsia* **34 Suppl 3,** S49–61.

399. Holtzman, R.N. (1977): Sensations of ocular movement in seizures originating in occipital lobe. *Neurology* **27,** 554–556.

400. Hopkins, A., Garman, A. & Clarke, C. (1988): The first seizure in adult life. Value of clinical features, electroencephalography, and computerised tomographic scanning in prediction of seizure recurrenc. *Lancet* **1,** 721–726.

401. Horita, H. & Maekawa, K. (1993): A case of benign childhood epilepsy with centrotemporal spike diagnosed by a seizure during polysomnography and clinical and EEG follow-up. *No to Hattatsu [Brain Dev.]* **25,** 563–568.

402. Hosking, G.P., Cavanagh, N.P.C. & Wilson, J. (1978): Alternating hemiplegia: complicated migraine of infancy. *Arch. Dis. Child.* **53,** 656–659.

403. Hu, S.X., Wu, X.R., Lin, C. & Hao, S.Y. (1989): Landau–Kleffner syndrome with unilateral EEG abnormalities – two cases from Beijing, China. *Brain Dev.* **11,** 420–422.

404. Huott, A.D., Madison, D.S. & Niedermeyer, E. (1974): Occipital lobe epilepsy. A clinical and electroencephalographic study. *Eur. Neurol.* **11,** 325–339.

405. Hutchinson, M., O'Riordan, J., Javed, M., Quin, E., Macerlaine, D., Wilcox, T., Parfrey, N., Nagy, T.G. & Tournier-Lasserve, E. (1995): Familial hemiplegic migraine and autosomal dominant arteriopathy with leukoencephalopathy (CADASIL). *Ann. Neurol.* **38,** 817–824.

406. Inazuki, G. & Kaji, S. (1988): Two BECCT (benign partial epilepsy of childhood with temporo central foci) cases with carbamazepine-exacerbated seizures. *No to Hattatsu [Brain Dev.]* **20,** 320–324.

407. International Federation of Societies for Electroencephalography and Clinical Neurophysiology (1974): A glossary of terms most commonly used by clinical electroencephalographers. *Electroencephalogr. Clin. Neurophysiol.* **37,** 538–548.

408. Isler, H., Wieser, H.G. & Egli, M. (1987): Hemicrania epileptica: Synchronous ipsilateral ictal headache with migraine features. In: *Migraine and epilepsy* eds. F. Andermann & E. Lugaresi, pp, 249–263. Boston, MA: Butterworths.

408a. Isnard, J., Fuscher, C., Bastuji, H., Batinand, N. & de Villard, R. (1995). Auditory (early) and middle-latency evoked potentials in patients with CSWS and Landau–Kleffner syndrome. In: *Continuous spikes and waves during slow sleep. Electrical status epilepticus during slow sleep. Acquired epileptic aphasia and related conditions* eds. A. Beaumanoir, N. Bureau, T. Deonna, L. Mira & C.A. Tassinari, pp. 99–103. London: John Libbey & Company Ltd.

409. Italian Working Group on coeliac disease and epilepsy (1993): Coeliac disease, epilepsy and cerebral calcifications: a multicentric study. In: *Occipital seizures and epilepsies* eds. F. Andermann, A. Beaumanoir, L. Mira, J. Roger & C.A. Tassinari, pp. 189–196. London: John Libbey & Company Ltd.

410. Iwasaki, N., Hamano, K., Kawashima, K., Takeya, T., Horigome, Y. & Takita, H. (1992): A case of childhood epilepsy with occipital paroxysms (CEOP) presenting particular EEG findings. *No to Hattatsu [Brain Dev.]* **24,** 364–369.

411. Jacobson, S.L. & Redman, C.W. (1989): Basilar migraine with loss of consciousness in pregnancy. Case report. *British J. Obst. Gynaec.* **96,** 494–495.

412. Jacome, D.E. (1986): Basilar artery migraine after uncomplicated whiplash injuries. *Headache* **26,** 515–516.

413. Jacome, D.E. (1987): EEG features in basilar artery migraine. *Headache* **27,** 80–83.

414. Jacome, D.E. & FitzGerald, R. (1982): Ictus emeticus. *Neurology* **32,** 209–212.

415. Jacome, D.E. & Leborgne, J. (1990): MRI studies in basilar artery migraine. *Headache* **30,** 88–90.

416. Jacome, D.E. & Risko, M. (1986): The non-epileptiform basilar artery migraine. *Headache* **26,** 447–450.

417. Jacome, D.E. & Suarez, M. (1988): Ictus emeticus induced by photic stimulation. *Clin. Electroencephalogr.* **19,** 214–218.

418. Jaffe, S.J. & Roach, E.S. (1988): Transient cortical blindness with occipital lobe epilepsy. *J. Cl. Neuro-Ophthalm.* **8,** 221–224.

419. Jay, G.W. (1982): Epilepsy, migraine, and EEG abnormalities in children: a review and hypothesis. *Headache* **22,** 110–114.

420. Jeavons, P.M., Harding, G.F., Panayiotopoulos, C.P. & Drasdo, N. (1972): The effect of geometric patterns combined with intermittent photic stimulation in photosensitive epilepsy. *Electroencephalogr. Clin. Neurophysiol.* **33,** 221–224.

421. Jeavons, P.M. & Harding, G.F.A. (1975): *Photosensitive epilepsy*. London: W. Heinemann Medical Books.

422. Jensen, K., Tfelt-Hansen, P., Lauritzen, M. & Olesen, J. (1986): Classic migraine. A prospective recording of symptoms. *Acta Neurol. Scand.* **73,** 359–362.

423. Joseph, J.M. & Louis, S. (1995): Transient ictal cortical blindness during middle age. A case report and review of the literature. *J. Neuro-Ophthalm.* **15,** 39–42.

424. Joutel, A., Bousser, M.G., Biousse, V., Labauge, P., Chabriat, H., Nibbio, A., Maciazek, J., Meyer, B., Bach, M.A., Weissenbach, J. *et al.* (1993): A gene for familial hemiplegic migraine maps to chromosome 19. *Nature Genetics* **5,** 40–45.

425. Joutel, A., Bousser, M.G., Biousse, V., Labauge, P., Chabriat, H., Nibbio, A., Maciazek, J., Meyer, B., Bach, M.A., Weissenbach, J. *et al.* (1994): Familial hemiplegic migraine. Localization of a responsible gene on chromosome 19. *Rev. Neurol.* **150,** 340–345.

426. Joutel, A., Corpechot, C., Ducros, A., Vahedi, K., Chabriat, H., Mouton, P., Alamowitch, S., Domenga, V., Cecillion, M., Marechal, E., Maciazek, J., Vayssiere, C., Cruaud, C., Cabanis, E.A., Ruchoux, M.M., Weissenbach, J., Bach, J.F., Bousser, M.G. & Tournier-Lasserve, E. (1996): Notch3 mutations in CADASIL, a hereditary adult-onset condition causing stroke and dementia. *Nature* **383,** 707–710.

427. Joutel, A., Tournier-Lasserve, E. & Bousser, M.G. (1995): Hemiplegic migraine. *Presse Medicale* **24,** 411–414.

428. Kabiraj, M.M., al Rajeh, S., Awada, A., Abduljabbar, M., Daif, A., al Tahan, A. & al Bunyan, M. (1997): Centro-temporal benign epilepsy in Saudi children. *Seizure* **6,** 139–144.

429. Kajitani, T., Kimura, T., Sumita, M. & Kaneko, M. (1992): Relationship between benign epilepsy of children with centrotemporal EEG foci and febrile convulsions. *Brain Dev.* **14,** 230–234.

430. Kajitani, T., Ueoka, K., Nakamura, M. & Kumanomidou, Y. (1981): Febrile convulsions and Rolandic discharges. *Brain Dev.* **3,** 351–359.

431. Kanazawa, O. & Kawai, I. (1990): Status epilepticus characterized by repetitive asymmetrical atonia: two cases accompanied by partial seizures. *Epilepsia* **31,** 536–543.

432. Kaplan, P.W. & Lesser, R.P. (1989). Vertical and horizontal epileptic gaze deviation and nystagmus. *Neurology* **39,** 1391–1393.

433. Kaplan, P.W. & Tusa, R.J. (1993): Neurophysiologic and clinical correlations of epileptic nystagmus. *Neurology* **43,** 2508–2514.

434. Karbowski, K. & Donati, F. (1992): Benign localised epilepsies in childhood: historical aspects. *Epilepsy Research* – **Suppl 6,** 23–27.

435. Kasteleijn-Nolst Trenite, D.G. (1989): Photosensitivity in epilepsy. Electrophysiological and clinical correlates. *Acta Neurol. Scand.* **Suppl 125,** 3–149.

436. Kasteleijn-Nolst Trenite, D.G. (1994): Video-game epilepsy. *Lancet* **344,** 1102–1103.

437. Kasteleijn-Nolst Trenite, D.G. (1998): Reflex seizures induced by intermittent light stimulation. *Adv. Neurol.* **75,** 99–121.

438. Kellaway, P. (1980): The incidence, significance and natural history of spike foci in children. In: *Current Clinical Neurophysiology. Update on EEG and Evoked Potentials.* ed. C.E. Henry, pp. 151–175. New York: Elsevier/North Holland.

439. Kellaway, P. (1985): Sleep and epilepsy. *Epilepsia* **26 Suppl 1,** S15–30.

440. Kellaway, P., Bloxsom, A. & MacGregor, D. (1955): Occipital spike foci associated with retrolental fibroplasia and other forms of retinal loss in children. *Electroencephalogr. Clin. Neurophysiol.* **7,** 469–470.

441. Kinast, M., Lueders, H., Rothner, A.D. & Erenberg, G. (1982): Benign focal epileptiform discharges in childhood migraine (BFEDC). *Neurology* **32,** 1309–1311.

442. Kivity, S. & Lerman, P. (1989): Benign partial epilepsy of childhood with occipital discharges. In: *Adv. Epileptol. XVIIth Epilepsy International Symposium,* eds. J. Manelis, E. Bental, J.N. Loeber & F.E. Dreifuss, pp. 371–373. New York: Raven Press.

443. Kivity, S. & Lerman, P. (1992): Stormy onset with prolonged loss of consciousness in benign childhood epilepsy with occipital paroxysms. *J.Neurol.Neurosurg.Psychiatry* **55,** 45–48.

444. Kluger, G., Bohm, I., Laub, M.C. & Waldenmaier, C. (1996): Epilepsy and fragile X gene mutations. *Pediatr. Neurol.* **15,** 358–360.

445. Kohlheb, O., Szego, L. & Halasz, P. (1980): Benign epilepsy in childhood with centrotemporal focus in EEG. *Kinderarztliche Praxis* **48,** 299–304.

446. Kohrogi, T. & Mitsudome, A. (1993): MRI hippocampal volumetric measurements in benign childhood epilepsy with centrotemporal spike(s) and temporal lobe epilepsy of childhood onset. *No to Hattatsu [Brain Dev.]* **25,** 548–553.

447. Kolmel, H.W. (1985): Complex visual hallucinations in the hemianopic field. *J.Neurol.Neurosurg.Psychiatry* **48,** 29–38.

448. Kolmel, H.W. (1993): Visual illusions and hallucinations. *Baillieres Clinical Neurology* **2,** 243–264.

449. Konishi, T., Naganuma, Y., Hongou, K., Murakami, M., Yamatani, M. & Okada, T. (1988): Clinical and EEG evaluation of mid-line spikes in childhood. *No to Shinkei – Brain & Nerve* **40,** 1189–1193.

450. Kosnik, E., Paulson, G.W. & Laguna, J.F. (1976): post-ictal blindness. *Neurology* **26,** 248–250.

451. Koutroumanidis, M., Koepp, M.J., Richardson, M.P., Camfield, C., Agathonikou, A., Ried, S., Papadimitriou, A., Plant, G.D., Duncan, J.S. & Panayiotopoulos, C,P. (1988): The variants of reading epilepsy. A clinical and video-EEG study of 17 patients with reading-induced seizures. *Brain* **121,** 1409–1427.

451a. Koutroumanidis, M., Binnie, C.D., Elwes, R.D., Polkey, C.E., Speed, P., Alarcon, G., Cox, T., Barrington, S., Marsden, P., Maisey, M.N. & Panayiotopoulos, C.P. (1998): Interictal regional slow activity in temporal lobe epilepsy correlates with lateral temporal hypometabolism as imaged with 18FDG PET: neurological and metabolic implications. *J. Neurol. Neurosurg. Psychiatr.* **65,** 170–176.

452. Kowacs, P.A., Muszkat, M., De Albuquerque, M. & de Campos, C.J. (1991): Rolandic epilepsy: report of 53 cases. *Arquiv. Neuro-Psiquiatria* **49,** 155–158.

453. Kramer, R.E., Luders, H., Goldstick, L.P., Dinner, D.S., Morris, H.H., Lesser, R.P. & Wyllie, E. (1988): Ictus emeticus: an electroclinical analysis. *Neurology* **38,** 1048–1052.

454. Kramer, U., Nevo, Y., Neufeld, M.Y., Fatal, A., Leitner, Y. & Harel, S. (1998): Epidemiology of epilepsy in childhood: a cohort of 440 consecutive patients. *Pediatr. Neurol.* **18,** 46–50.

455. Kriz, M. & Gazdik, M. (1978): Epilepsy with centrotemporal (Rolandic) spikes. A peculiar seizure disorder of childhood. *Neurol. Neurochir. Polska* **12,** 413–419.

456. Kurihara, M., Kumagai, K., Ohi, S., Maekawa, K. & Suenaga, K. (1993): Clinico-polysomnographical evolutions in benign epilepsy in childhood with centrotemporal foci. *Jap. J. Psychiatry Neurol.* **47,** 327–328.

457. Kuzniecky, R., Gilliam, F., Morawetz, R., Faught, E., Palmer, C. & Black, L. (1997): Occipital lobe developmental malformations and epilepsy: clinical spectrum, treatment, and outcome. *Epilepsia* **38,** 175–181.

458. Kuzniecky, R. & Rosenblatt, B. (1987): Benign occipital epilepsy: a family study. *Epilepsia* **28,** 346–350.

459. Kuzniecky, R.I. (1998): Symptomatic occipital lobe epilepsy. *Epilepsia* **39 suppl 4,** S24–31.

460. Kuzniecky, R.I. & Jackson, G.D. (1997): Developmental disorders. In: *Epilepsy: A comprehensive textbook,* eds. J.J. Engel & T.A. Pedley, pp. 2517–2532. Philadelphia: Lippincott-Raven Publishers.

461. Kyllerman, M., Nyden, A., Praquin, N., Rasmussen, P., Wetterquist, A.K. & Hedstrom, A. (1996): Transient psychosis in a girl with epilepsy and continuous spikes and waves during slow sleep (CSWS). *European Child & Adolescent Psychiatry* **5,** 216–221.

462. La Spina, I., Calloni, M.V. & Porazzi, D. (1994): Transcranial Doppler monitoring of a migraine with aura attack from the prodromal phase to the end. *Headache* **34,** 593–596.

463. La Spina, I., Vignati, A. & Porazzi, D. (1997): Basilar artery migraine: transcranial Doppler EEG and SPECT from the aura phase to the end. *Headache* **37,** 43–47.

464. Lairy, G.C., Harrison, A. & Leger, E.M. (1964): Foyers EEG bi-occipitaux asynchrones de pointes chez l'enfant mal voyant et aveugle d'age scholaire. *Rev. Neurol.* **3,** 351–353.

465. Lance, J.W. (1976): Simple formed hallucinations confined to the area of a specific visual field defect. *Brain* **99,** 719–734.

466. Lance, J.W. & Smee, R.I. (1989): Partial seizures with visual disturbance treated by radiotherapy of cavernous hemangioma. *Ann.Neurol.* **26,** 782–785.

467. Landau, W.M. (1992): Landau–Kleffner syndrome. An eponymic badge of ignorance [editorial; comment]. *Arch.Neurol.* **49,** 353.

467a. Landau, W.M. (1998): Commentary. Syndrome of acquired aphasia with convulsive disorder in children. *Neurology* **51**, 1241.

468. Landau, W.M. & Kleffner, F.R. (1957): Syndrome of acquired aphasia with convulsive disorder in children. *Neurology* **7,** 523–530. Also reproduced in *Neurology* **51** (November 1998), Landmark Article.

469. Lapkin, M.L., French, J.H., Golden, G.S. & Rowan, A.J. (1977): The electroencephalogram in childhood basilar artery migraine. *Neurology* **27,** 580–583.

470. Lapkin, M.L. & Golden, G.S. (1978): Basilar artery migraine. A review of 30 cases. *Am. J. Dis. Child.* **132,** 278–281.

471. Laplante, P., Saint-Hilaire, J.M. & Bouvier, G. (1983): Headache as an epileptic manifestation. *Neurology* **33,** 1493–1495.

472. Laurent, B., Michel, D., Antoine, J.C. & Montagnon, D. (1984): Basilar migraine with alexia but not agraphia: arterial spasm on arteriography and the effect of naloxone. *Rev. Neurol.* **140,** 663–665.

473. LaWall, J.S. & Oommen, K.J. (1978): Single case study basilar artery migraine presenting as conversion hysteria. *J. Nerv. Ment. Dis.* **166,** 809–811.

474. Leblanc, R., Feindel, W. & Ethier, R. (1983): Epilepsy from cerebral arteriovenous malformations. *Can. J. Neurol. Sci.* **10,** 91–95.

475. Lefebre, C. & Kolmel, H.W. (1989): Palinopsia as an epileptic phenomenon. *Eur. Neurol.* **29,** 323–327.

476. Legarda, S. & Jayakar, P. (1995): Electroclinical significance of Rolandic spikes and dipoles in neurodevelopmentally normal children. *Electroencephalogr. Clin. Neurophysiol.* **95,** 257–259.

477. Legarda, S., Jayakar, P., Duchowny, M., Alvarez, L. & Resnick, T. (1994): Benign Rolandic epilepsy: high central and low central subgroups. *Epilepsia* **35,** 1125–1129.

478. Lennox, W.G. & Lennox, M.A. (1960): *Epilepsy and related disorders.* Boston, MA: Little, Brown & Co.

479. Leppert, M., Anderson, V.E., Quattlebaum, T., Stauffer, D., O'Connell, P., Nakamura, Y., Lalouel, J.M. & White, R. (1989): Benign familial neonatal convulsions linked to genetic markers on chromosome 20. *Nature* **337,** 647–648.

480. Lerman, P. (1970): Benign focal epilepsy in children. *Electroencephalogr. Clin. Neurophysiol.* **28,** 642.

481. Lerman, P. (1992): Benign partial epilepsy with centrotemporal spikes. In: *Epileptic syndromes in infancy, childhood and adolescence,* eds. J. Roger, M. Bureau, C. Dravet, F.E. Dreifuss, A. Perret & P. Wolf, pp. 189–200. London: John Libbey & Company Ltd.

482. Lerman, P. (1997): Benign childhood epilepsy with centrotemporal spikes. In: *Epilepsy: A comprehensive textbook,* eds. J.J. Engel & T.A. Pedley, pp. 2307–2314. Philadelphia: Lippincott-Raven Publishers.

483. Lerman, P. & Kivity, S. (1975): Benign focal epilepsy of childhood. A follow-up study of 100 recovered patients. *Arch.Neurol.* **32,** 261–264.

484. Lerman, P. & Kivity, S. (1991): The benign partial nonrolandic epilepsies [Review] *J. Clin. Neurophysiol.* **8,** 275–287.

485. Lerman, P. & Kivity-Ephraim, S. (1981): Focal epileptic EEG discharges in children not suffering from clinical epilepsy: etiology, clinical significance, and management. *Epilepsia* **22,** 551–558.

486. Lesser, R.P., Arroyo, S., Crone, N. & Gordon, B. (1998): Motor and sensory mapping of the frontal and occipital lobes. *Epilepsia* **39 suppl 4,** S69–80

487. Levinson, J.D., Gibbs, E.L., Stillermann, M.L. & Peristein, M.A. (1951): Electro-encephalogram in eye disorders. *Pediatrics* **7,** 422–427.

488. Lewis, T.B., Leach, R.J., Ward, K., O'Connell, P. & Ryan, S.G. (1993): Genetic heterogeneity in benign familial neonatal convulsions: identification of a new locus on chromosome 8q. *Am. J. Hum. Genet.* **53,** 670–675.

489. Li, M., Hao, X.Y., Qing, J. & Wu, X.R. (1996): Correlation between CSWS and aphasia in Landau–Kleffner syndrome: a study of three cases. *Brain Dev.* **18,** 197–200.

490. Lipton, R.B., Ottman, R., Ehrenberg, B.L. & Hauser, W.A. (1994): Comorbidity of migraine: the connection between migraine and epilepsy. *Neurology* **44,** S28–32.

491. Lischka, A. & Graf, M. (1992): Benign Rolandic epilepsy of childhood: topographic EEG analysis. *Epilepsy Research – Supplement* **6,** 53–58.

492. Liu, X. (1918): Benign focal epilepsy of childhood (BFEC). *Chung-Hua Shen Ching Ching Shen Ko Tsa Chih [Chinese J. Neurol. & Psychiatry]* **25,** 136–138.

493. Liveing, E. (1873): *On megrim, sick-headache, and some allied disorders: A contribution to the pathology of nerve-storms.* London: Churchill.

494. Lloyd-Smith, D.L. & Henderson, L.R. (1951): Epileptic patients showing susceptibility to photic stimulation alone. *Electroencephalogr. Clin. Neurophysiol.* 378–379.

495. Loiseau, J., Loiseau, P., Guyot, M., Duche, B., Dartigues, J.F. & Aublet, B. (1990): Survey of seizure disorders in the French southwest. I. Incidence of epileptic syndromes. *Epilepsia* **31,** 391–396.

496. Loiseau, P. (1993): Benign focal epilepsies of childhood. In: *The treatment of epilepsy: Principles and practices,* ed. E. Wyllie, pp. 503–512. Philadelphia: Lee & Febiger.

497. Loiseau, P. & Beaussart, M. (1969): Hereditary factors in partial epilepsy. *Epilepsia* **10,** 23–31.

498. Loiseau, P. & Beaussart, M. (1973): The seizures of benign childhood epilepsy with Rolandic paroxysmal discharges. *Epilepsia* **14,** 381–389.

499. Loiseau, P., Cohadon, F. & Mortureux, Y. (1967): A propos d'une forme singuliere d'epilepsie de l'enfant. *Rev. Neurol.* **116,** 244–248.

500. Loiseau, P. & Duche, B. (1988): Rolandic paroxysmal epilepsy or partial benign epilepsy in children. *Revue du Praticien* **38,** 1194–1196.

501. Loiseau, P. & Duche, B. (1989): Benign childhood epilepsy with centrotemporal spikes. *Clev. Clin. J. Med.* **56 Suppl Pt 1,** S17–22; discussion S40–2.

502. Loiseau, P. & Duche, B. (1992): Benign Rolandic epilepsy. *Advan. Neurol.* **57,** 411–417.

503. Loiseau, P., Duche, B. & Cohadon, S. (1992): The prognosis of benign localized epilepsy in early childhood. *Epilepsy Research* – **Suppl 6,** 75–81.

504. Loiseau, P., Duche, B., Cordova, S., Dartigues, J.F. & Cohadon, S. (1988): Prognosis of benign childhood epilepsy with centrotemporal spikes: a follow-up study of 168 patients. *Epilepsia* **29,** 229–235.

505. Loiseau, P., Duche, B. & Loiseau, J. (1991): Classification of epilepsies and epileptic syndromes in two different samples of patients. *Epilepsia* **32,** 303–309.

506. Loiseau, P. & Faure, J. (1961): Une forme particuliere d'epilepsie de la seconde enfance. *J. Med. Bourdeaux* **138,** 381–389.

507. Loiseau, P., Pestre, M., Dartigues, J.F., Commenges, D., Barberger-Gateau, C. & Cohadon, S. (1983): Long-term prognosis in two forms of childhood epilepsy: typical absence seizures and epilepsy with Rolandic (centrotemporal) EEG foci. *Ann. Neurol.* **13,** 642–648.

508. Lombroso, C.T. (1967): Sylvian seizures and midtemporal spike foci in children. *Arch.Neurol.* **17,** 52–59.

509. Lossius, R. (1995): Is there a connection between epilepsy and migraine? *Tidsskrift for Den Norske Laegeforening* **115,** 2669–2670.

510. Lu, C.S., Thompson, P.D., Quinn, N.P., Parkes, J.D. & Marsden, C.D. (1986): Ramsay Hunt syndrome and coeliac disease: a new association? *Movement Disorders* **1,** 209–219.

511. Lucas, C., Pasquier, F., Leys, D., Ruchoux, M.M. & Pruvo, J.P. (1995): Cadasil: a new familial disease responsible for cerebral infarction and dementia. *Rev. Medec.Interne* **16,** 290–292.

512. Luders, H.O., Lesser, R.P., Dinner, D.S. & Morris III, H.H. (1987): Benign focal epilepsy of childhood. In: *Epilepsy. Electroclinical syndromes.* eds. H. Luders & R.P. Lesser, pp. 303–346. Berlin, Heidelberg: Springer-Verlag.

513. Ludwig, B.I. & Marsan, C.A. (1975): Clinical ictal patterns in epileptic patients with occipital electroencephalographic foci. *Neurology* **25,** 463–471.

514. Lugaresi, E., Cirignotta, F. & Montagna, P. (1984): Occipital lobe epilepsy with scotosensitive seizures: the role of central vision. *Epilepsia* **25,** 115–120.

515. Maeda, Y., Kurokawa, T., Sakamoto, K., Kitamoto, I., Ueda, K. & Tashima, S. (1990): Electroclinical study of video-game epilepsy. *Dev. Med. Child Neurol.* **32,** 493–500.

516. Magaudda, A., Dalla Bernardina, B., De Marco, P., Sfaello, Z., Longo, M., Colamaria, V., Daniele, O., Tortorella, G., Tata, M.A., Di Perri, R. *et al.* (1993): Bilateral occipital calcification, epilepsy and coeliac disease: clinical and neuroimaging features of a new syndrome. *J.Neurol.Neurosurg.Psychiatry* **56,** 885–889.

517. Maher, J., Ronen, G.M., Ogunyemi, A.O. & Goulden, K.J. (1995): Occipital paroxysmal discharges suppressed by eye opening: variability in clinical and seizure manifestations in childhood. *Epilepsia* **36,** 52–57.

518. Malafosse, A., Leboyer, M., Dulac, O., Navelet, Y., Plouin, P., Beck, C., Laklou, H, Mouchnino, G., Grandscene, P., Vallee, L. *et al.* (1992): Confirmation of linkage of benign familial neonatal convulsions to D20S19 and D20S20. *Hum.Genet.* **89,** 54–58.

519. Mancia, D., Manzoni, G.C., Terzano, M.G., Pavesi, G., Marchini, M., & Dalla Bernardina, B. (1986): Partial seizures and migraine. *Functional Neurol.* **1,** 439–453.

520. Mandelkern, D. & Burger, A. (1992): Cortical blindness in postpartum preeclampsia progressing to eclampsia: case report. *Mount Sinai Journal of Medicine* **59,** 72–74.

521. Manford, M., Hart, Y.M., Sander, J.W. & Shorvon, S.D. (1992): National General Practice Study of Epilepsy (NGPSE): partial seizure patterns in a general population. *Neurology* **42,** 1911–1917.

522. Manganotti, P., Miniussi, C., Santorum, E., Tinazzi, M., Bonato, C., Marzi, C.A., Fiaschi, A., Dalla Bernardina, B. & Zanette, G. (1998): Influence of somatosensory input on paroxysmal activity in benign Rolandic epilepsy with 'extreme somatosensory evoked potentials'. *Brain* **121,** 647–658.

523. Manonmani, V. & Tan, C.T. (1994): Malaysian children with: 'benign epilepsy of childhood with centrotemporal spikes'. *Singapore Med. J.* **35,** 247–249.

524. Mantovani, J.F. & Landau, W.M. (1980): Acquired aphasia with convulsive disorder: course and prognosis. *Neurology* **30,** 524–529.

525. Manzoni, G.C., Terzano, M.G. & Mancia, D. (1979): Possible interference between migrainous and epileptic mechanisms in intercalated attacks. Case report. *Eur. Neurol.* **18,** 124–120.

526. Maquet, P., Hirsch, E., Dive, D., Salmon, E., Marescaux, C. & Franck, G. (1990): Cerebral glucose utilization during sleep in Landau–Kleffner syndrome: a PET study. *Epilepsia* **31,** 778–783.

527. Maquet, P., Hirsch, E., Metz-Lutz, M.N., Motte, J., Dive, D., Marescaux, C. & Franck, G. (1995): Regional cerebral glucose metabolism in children with deterioration of one or more cognitive functions and continuous spike-and-wave discharges during sleep. *Brain* **118,** 1497–1520.

528. Marescaux, C., Hirsch, E., Finck, S., Maquet, P., Schlumberger, E., Sellal, F., Metz-Lutz, M.N., Alembik, Y., Salmon, E. & Franck, G. (1990): Landau–Kleffner syndrome: a pharmacologic study of five cases. *Epilepsia* **31,** 768–777.

529. Marks, D.A. & Ehrenberg, B.L. (1993): Migraine-related seizures in adults with epilepsy, with EEG correlation. *Neurology* **43,** 2476–2483.

530. McDonald, J.V. (1990): Basilar artery migraine. Case report. *J. Neurosurg.* **72,** 289–291.

531. McLachlan, R.S. (1987): The significance of head and eye turning in seizures. *Neurology* **37,** 1617–1619.

532. Melen, O., Olson, S.F. & Hodes, B.L. (1978): Visual disturbances in migraine. *Postgrad. Med.* **64,** 139–143.

533. Menini, C. & Silva-Barrat, C. (1998): The photosensitive epilepsy of the baboon. A model of generalized reflex epilepsy. *Adv. Neurol.* **75,** 29–47.

534. Merikangas, K. (1995): Common heredity of familial hemiplegic migraine and basilar artery migraine? [comment]. *Cephalalgia* **15,** 449.

535. Michelucci, R. & Tassinari, C.A. (1993): Television-induced occipital seizures. In: *Occipital seizures and epilepsies in children,* eds. F. Andermann, A. Beaumanoir, L. Mira, J. Roger & C.A. Tassinari, pp. 141–144. London: John Libbey & Company Ltd.

536. Minami, T., Gondo, K., Yamamoto, T., Yanai, S., Tasaki, K. & Ueda, K. (1996): Magnetoencephalographic analysis of Rolandic discharges in benign childhood epilepsy. *Ann .Neurol.* **39,** 326–334.

537. Mitchell, W.G., Greenwood, R.S. & Messenheimer, J.A. (1983): Abdominal epilepsy: Cyclic vomiting as the major symptom of simple partial seizures. *Arch. Neurol.* **40,** 251–252.

538. Morikawa, T., Osawa, T., Ishihara, O. & Seino, M. (1979): A reappraisal of 'benign epilepsy of children with centrotemporal EEG foci'. *Brain Dev.* **1,** 257–265.

539. Morikawa, T., Seino, M. & Watanabe, M.D. (1995): Long-term outcome of CSWS syndrome. In: *Continuous spikes and waves during slow sleep. Electrical status epilepticus during slow sleep. Acquired epileptic aphasia and related conditions,* eds. A. Beaumanoir, M. Bureau, T. Deonna, L. Mira & C.A. Tassinari, pp. 27–36. London: John Libbey & Company Ltd.

540. Morikawa, T., Seino, M. & Yagi, K. (1992): Long-term outcome of four children with continuous spike-waves during sleep. In: *Epileptic syndromes in infancy, childhood and adolescence,* eds. J. Roger, M. Bureau, C. Dravet, F.E. Dreifuss, A. Perret & P. Wolf, pp. 257–265. London: John Libbey & Company Ltd.

541. Morikawa, T., Seino, M. & Yagi, K. (1992): Is Rolandic discharge a hallmark of benign partial epilepsy of childhood? *Epilepsy Research* – **Suppl 6,** 59–69.

542. Morikawa, T., Terauchi, N., Shigematsu, H., Tsuji, M., Fukai, M., Yagi, K. & Seino, M. (1986): Functional partial epilepsies in childhood. *Jap. J. Psychiatry Neurol.* **40,** 301–306.

543. Morimoto, Y., Nakajima, S., Nishioka, R. & Nakamura, H. (1993): Basilar artery migraine with transient MRI and EEG abnormalities. *Rinsho Shinkeigaku – Clin. Neurol.* **33,** 61–67.

544. Morrell, F. (1995): Electrophysiology of CSWS in Landau–Kleffner syndrome. In: *Continuous spikes and waves during slow sleep. Electrical status epilepticus during slow sleep. Acquired epileptic aphasia and related conditions,* eds. A. Beaumanoir, M. Bureau, T. Deonna, L. Mira & C.A. Tassinari, pp. 77–90. London: John Libbey & Company Ltd.

545. Morrell, F., Whisler, W.W., Smith, M.C., Hoeppner, T.J., de Toledo-Morrell, L., Pierre-Louis, S.J., Kanner, A.M., Buelow, J.M., Ristanovic, R., Bergen, D. *et al.* (1995): Landau–Kleffner syndrome. Treatment with subpial intracortical transection. *Brain* **118,** 1529–1546.

546. Morrell, M.J. & Druzin, M.L. (1997): Disorders of Pregnancy. In: *Epilepsy: A comprehensive textbook,* eds. J.J. Engel & T.A. Pedley, pp. 2635–2642. Philadelphia: Lippicott-Raven Publishers.

547. Mouridsen, S.E. (1995): The Landau–Kleffner Syndrome: a review. *Eur. Child & Adolescent Psychiatr.* **4,** 223–228.

548. Muellbacher, W. & Mamoli, B. (1994): Prolonged impaired consciousness in basilar artery migraine. *Headache* **34,** 282–285.

549. Mukhin, K.I., Temin, P.A. & Rykova, E.A. (1995): Rolandic epilepsy. *Z. Nevropat. Psikhiatrii Imeni S - S - Korsakova* **95,** 78–84.

550. Muller, T., Buttner, T., Kuhn, W., Heinz, A. & Przuntek, H. (1995): Palinopsia as sensory epileptic phenomenon. *Acta Neurol. Scand.* **91,** 433–436.

551. Munari, C., Bonis, A., Kochen, S., Pestre, M., Brunet, P., Bancaud, J. *et al.*(1983): Eye movement and occipital seizures in man. *Acta Neurochirurg.* **33 Suppl,** 47–52.

552. Munari, C., Tassi, L., Francione, S., Kahane, P., Malapani, C., Lo Russo, G. & Hoffmann, D. (1993): Occipital seizures with childhood onset in severe partial epilepsy: a surgical perspective. In: *Occipital seizures and epilepsies in children,* eds. F. Andermann, A. Beaumanoir, L. Mira, J. Roger & C.A. Tassinari, pp. 203–211. London: John Libbey & Company Ltd.

553. Musicco, M., Beghi, E., Solari, A. & Viani, F. (1997): Treatment of first tonic–clonic seizure does not improve the prognosis of epilepsy. First Seizure Trial Group (FIRST Group). *Neurology* **49,** 991–998.

554. Musumeci, S.A., Colognola, R.M., Ferri, R., Gigli, G.L., Petrella, M.A., Sanfilippo, S, Bergonzi, P. & Tassinari, C.A. (1988): Fragile-X syndrome: a particular epileptogenic EEG pattern. *Epilepsia* **29,** 41–47.

555. Musumeci, S.A., Elia, M., Ferri, R., Scuderi, C. & Del Gracco, S. (1994): Evoked spikes and giant somatosensory evoked potentials in a patient with fragile-X syndrome. *It. J. Neurol. Sci.* **15,** 365–368.

556. Musumeci, S.A., Ferri, R., Elia, M., Colognola, R.M., Bergonzi, P. & Tassinari, C.A. (1991): Epilepsy and fragile X syndrome: a follow-up study. *Amer. J. Med. Genet.* **38,** 511–513.

557. Nagendran, K., Prior, P.F. & Rossiter, M.A. (1990): Benign occipital epilepsy of childhood: a family study. *J. Royal Soc. Med.* **83,** 804–805.

558. Nakano, S., Okuno, T. & Mikawa, H. (1989): Landau–Kleffner syndrome. EEG topographic studies. *Brain Dev.* **11,** 43–50.

559. Nakken, K.O. (1996): Ictus emeticus. Vomiting as epileptic manifestation. *Tidsskrift for Den Norske Laegeforening* **116,** 369–371.

560. Nalin, A., Ruggerini, C., Ferrari, E., Galli, V., Ferrari, P. & Finelli, T. (1989): Clinical aspects, differential diagnosis and evolution of visual epileptic seizures in children. *Neurophysiol. Clin.* **19,** 25–36.

561. Naquet, R., Fegersten, L. & Bert, J. (1960): Seizure discharges localised to the posterior cerebral regions in man, provoked by intermittent photic stimulation. *Electroencephalogr. Clin. Neurophysiol.* **12,** 305–316.

562. Nayrac, P. & Beaussart, M. (1958): Les pointes-ondes prerolandiques: expression EEG tres particuliere. Etude electroclinique de 21 cas. *Rev. Neurol.* **99,** 201–206.

563. Negrin, P. & De Marco, P. (1977): Parietal focal spikes evoked by tactile somatotopic stimulation in sixty non-epileptic children: the nocturnal sleep and clinical and EEG evolution. *Electroencephalogr. Clin. Neurophysiol.* **43,** 312–316.

564. Nelson, K.R., Brenner, R.P. & de la Paz, D. (1983): Midline spikes. EEG and clinical features. *Arch.Neurol.* **40,** 473–476.

565. Neubauer, B.A., Kampfer, F., Fredler, B., Schwabe, G., Doose, H., & Stephani, U.(1997): Towards the mapping of a gene responsible for Rolandic epilepsy. *Epilepsia* **38 Suppl 3,** 201.

565a. Neubauer, B.A., Fiedler, B., Himmelein, B., Kampfer, F., Lassker, U., Schwabe, G., Spanier, I., Tams, D., Bretscher, C., Moldenhauer, K., Kurlemann, G., Weise, S., Tedroff, K., Eeg-Olofsson, O., Wadelius, C. & Stephani, U. (1998): Centrotemporal spikes in families with Rolandic epilepsy: linkage to chromosome 15q14. *Neurology* **51,** 1608–1612.

566. Neubauer, B.A., Moises, H.W., Lassker, U., Waltz, S., Diebold, U. & Stephani, U. (1997): Benign childhood epilepsy with centrotemporal spikes and electroencephalography trait are not linked to EBN1 and EBN2 of benign neonatal familial convulsions. *Epilepsia* **38,** 782–787.

567. Newmark, M.E. & Penry, J.K. (1980): *Genetics of Epilepsy: A Review,* pp. 1–122. New York: Raven Press.

568. Newton, R. & Aicardi, J. (1983): Clinical findings in children with occipital spike-wave complexes suppressed by eye-opening. *Neurology* **33,** 1526–1529.

569. Niedermeyer, E. (1993): Migraine-triggered epilepsy. *Clin. Electroencephalogr.* **24,** 37–43.

570. Niedermeyer, E. & Lopes da Silva, F. (1993): *Electroencephalography. Basic principles, clinical applications, and related fields,* 3rd edn. Baltimore: Williams & Wilkins.

571. Niedermeyer, E. & Naidu, S. (1989): Blocking of Rolandic spikes by hand and finger movements. In: *Reflex seizures and reflex epilepsies,* eds.A. Beaumanoir, H. Gastaut & R. Naquet, pp. 89–95. Geneve: Editions medecine & Hygiene.

572. Niedermeyer, E. & Naidu, S. (1990): Further EEG observations in children with the Rett syndrome. *Brain Dev.* **12,** 53–54.

573. Niedermeyer, E., Naidu, S.B. & Plate, C. (1997): Unusual EEG theta rhythms over central region in Rett syndrome: considerations of the underlying dysfunction. *Clin. Electroencephalogr.* **28,** 36–43.

574. Niedermeyer, E., Riggio, S. & Santiago, M. (1988): Benign occipital lobe epilepsy. *J. Epilepsy* **1,** 3–11.

575. Nielsen, C.J. (1978): Benign partial epilepsy in childhood. *Ugeskrift for Laeger* **140,** 341–343.

576. Nieto Barrera, M., Jimenez Ayllon, M. & Lopez Guerrero, D. (1978): Epilepsy with centrotemporal E.E.G. foci. *Anal. Espan. Pediatr.* **11,** 195–204.

577. Nieto Barrera, M., Lopez Alcaide, M.I., Candau Fernandez-Mensaque, R., Ruiz, P., del Portal Bermudo, L., Rufo Campos, M. & Correa Charro, A. (1997): Acquired aphasic epilepsy (Landau–Kleffner syndrome). Report of 10 cases. *An. Espan. Pediatr.* **47,** 611–617.

578. Nieto-Barrera, M., Aguilar-Quero, F., Montes, E., Candau, R. & Prieto, P. (1997): Epileptic syndromes which show continuous spike and wake complexes during slow wave sleep. *Rev. Neurologia* **25,** 1045–1051.

579. Nishiura, N. & Iwakoshi, M. (1990): A new scoring system of EEGs of benign epilepsy and centrotemporal delta activity (CTDA). *Jap. J. Psychiatry Neurol.* **44,** 362–364.

580. Nishiura, N. & Miyazaki, T. (1976): Clinico-electroencephalographical study of focal epilepsy with special reference to 'benign epilepsy of children with centrotemporal EEG foci' and its age dependency. *Fol. Psychiatr. Neurolog. Japon.* **30,** 253–261.

581. O'Connor, P.S. & Tredici, T.J. (1981): Acephalgic migraine. Fifteen years experience. *Ophthalmology* **88,** 999–1003.

582. O'Donohoe, N.V. (1985): *Epilepsies of childhood.* 2nd edn. London: Butterworths.

583. O'Tuama, L.A., Urion, D.K., Janicek, M.J., Treves, S.T., Bjornson, B. & Moriarty, J.M. (1992): Regional cerebral perfusion in Landau–Kleffner syndrome and related childhood aphasias. *J. Nuclear Medic.* **33,** 1758–1765.

584. Ochs, R., Gloor, P., Quesney, F., Ives, J. & Olivier, A. (1984): Does head-turning during a seizure have lateralizing or localizing significance? *Neurology* **34,** 884–890.

585. Oguni, H., Sato, F., Hayashi, K., Wang, P.J. & Fukuyama, Y. (1992): A study of unilateral brief focal atonia in childhood partial epilepsy. *Epilepsia* **33,** 75–83.

586. Okubo, Y., Matsuura, M., Asai, T., Asai, K., Kato, M., Kojima, T. & Toru, M. (1994): Epileptiform EEG discharges in healthy children: prevalence, emotional and behavioral correlates, and genetic influences. *Epilepsia* **35,** 832–841.

587. Ophoff, R.A., Terwindt, G.M., Vergouwe, M.N., van Eijk, R., Oefner, P.J., Hoffman, S.M., Lamerdin, J.E., Mohrenweiser, H.W., Bulman, D.E., Ferrari, M., Haan, J., Lindhout, D., van Ommen, G.J., Hofker, M.H., Ferrari, M.D. & Frants, R.R. (1996): Familial hemiplegic migraine and episodic ataxia type–2 are caused by mutations in the Ca+2 channel gene CACNL1A4. *Cell* **87,** 543–552.

588. Ophoff, R.A., van Eijk, R., Sandkuijl, L.A., Terwindt, G.M., Grubben, C.P., Haan, J., Lindhout, D., Ferrari, M.D. & Frants, R.R. (1994): Genetic heterogeneity of familial hemiplegic migraine. *Genomics* **22,** 21–26.

589. Ortega, J.J., Belda, V.J., Tripiana, J.L., Gil, M., Salas, R., Orenga, J.V., Serrano *et al.* (1996): Electrical status epilepticus during sleep. *Rev. Neurolologia* **24,** 1551–1553.

590. Ottman, R. & Lipton, R.B. (1994): Comorbidity of migraine and epilepsy. *Neurology* **44,** 2105–2110.

591. Ottman, R. & Lipton, R.B. (1996): Is the comorbidity of epilepsy and migraine due to a shared genetic susceptibility? *Neurology* **47,** 918–924.

592. Paetau, R. (1994): Sound triggers spikes in the Landau–Kleffner syndrome. *J. Clin. Neurophysiol.* **11,** 231–241.

593. Panayiotopoulos, C.P.(1972): A study of photosensitive epilepsy with particular reference to occipital spikes induced by intermittent photic stimulation. Ph.D. Thesis. Aston University in Birmingham.

594. Panayiotopoulos, C.P. (1974): Effectiveness of photic stimulation on various eye-states in photosensitive epilepsy. *J. Neurol.Sci.* **23,** 165–173.

595. Panayiotopoulos C.P. (1977): 'Eye closure' and 'eyes closed' EEG abnormalities: Discrimination and effectiveness of light and dark. *Electroencephalogr. Clin. Neurophysiol.* **43,** 523 [Abstract].

596. Panayiotopoulos, C.P. (1978): Occipital epilepsy. *Materia Med. Gr.* **30,** 557–564.

597. Panayiotopoulos, C.P. (1979): Self-induced pattern-sensitive epilepsy. *Arch.Neurol.* **36,** 48–50.

598. Panayiotopoulos, C.P. (1979): Conversion of photosensitive to scotosensitive epilepsy: report of a case. *Neurology* **29,** 1550–1554.

599. Panayiotopoulos, C.P. (1980): Basilar migraine? Seizures, and severe epileptic EEG abnormalities. *Neurology* **30,** 1122–1125.

600. Panayiotopoulos, C.P. (1981): Inhibitory effect of central vision on occipital lobe seizures. *Neurology* **31,** 1330–1333.

601. Panayiotopoulos, C.P. (1983): Inhibitory effect of central vision on occipital lobe seizures. *Neurology* **33,** 523–524.

602. Panayiotopoulos, C.P. (1987): Difficulties in differentiating migraine and epilepsy based on clinical and EEG findings. In: *Migraine and epilepsy,* eds. F. Andermann & E. Lugaresi, pp. 31–46. Boston, MA: Butterworths.

603. Panayiotopoulos, C.P. (1988): Vomiting as an ictal manifestation of epileptic seizures and syndromes. *J.Neurol.Neurosurg.Psychiatry* **51,** 1448–1451.

604. Panayiotopoulos, C.P. (1989): Fixation-off-sensitive epilepsies. In: *Reflex seizures and reflex epilepsies,* eds .A. Beaumanoir, H. Gastaut & R. Naquet, pp. 203–217. Geneva: Medecine et Hygiene.

605. Panayiotopoulos, C.P. (1989): Benign childhood epilepsy with occipital paroxysms: a 15-year prospective study. *Ann.Neurol.* **26,** 51–56.

606. Panayiotopoulos, C.P. (1989): Benign nocturnal childhood occipital epilepsy: a new syndrome with nocturnal seizures, tonic deviation of the eyes, and vomiting. *J. Child Neurol.* **4,** 43–49.

607. Panayiotopoulos, C.P. (1991): Basilar migraine. *Neurology* **41,** 1707

608. Panayiotopoulos, C.P. (1993): Benign childhood epilepsy with occipital paroxysms. In: *Occipital seizures and epilepsies in children,* eds. F. Andermann, A. Beaumanoir, L. Mira, J. Roger & C.A. Tassinari, pp. 151–164. London: John Libbey & Company Ltd.

609. Panayiotopoulos, C.P. (1993): Benign childhood partial epilepsies: benign childhood seizure susceptibility syndromes [editorial]. *J.Neurol.Neurosurg.Psychiatry* **56,** 2–5.

610. Panayiotopoulos, C.P. (1994): Juvenile myoclonic epilepsy: an underdiagnosed syndrome. In: *Epileptic seizures and syndromes,* ed. P. Wolf, pp. 221–230. London: John Libbey & Company Ltd.

611. Panayiotopoulos, C.P. (1994): Elementary visual hallucinations in migraine and epilepsy. *J. Neurol. Neurosurg. Psychiatry* **57,** 1371–1374.

612. Panayiotopoulos, C.P. (1995): Typical absences are syndrome related. In: *Typical absences and related epileptic syndromes,* eds .J.S. Duncan & C.P. Panayiotopoulos, pp. 304–310. London: Churchill Communications Europe.

613. Panayiotopoulos, C.P. (1996): The diagnosis of epilepsies: still a central problem? *Eur. J. Neurol.* **3 Suppl 3,** 3–8.

614. Panayiotopoulos, C.P. (1996): Juvenile myoclonic epilepsy. In: *Epilepsy in Children,* ed. S. Wallace, pp. 333–347. London: Chapman & Hall.

615. Panayiotopoulos, C.P. (1996): Ictus emeticus. *Neurology* **46,** 1785.

616. Panayiotopoulos, C.P. (1996): Epilepsies characterized by seizures with specific modes of precipitation (reflex epilepsies). In: *Epilepsy in Children,* ed. S. Wallace, pp. 355–375. London: Chapman & Hall.

617. Panayiotopoulos, C.P. (1997): Absence epilepsies. In: *Epilepsy: A comprehensive Textbook,* eds J.J. Engel & T.A. Pedley, pp. 2327–2346. Philadelphia: Lippincott-Raven Publishers.

618. Panayiotopoulos, C.P. (1999): Elementary visual hallucinations, blindness and headache in idiopathic occipital epilepsy: Differentiation from migraine. *J.Neurol.Neurosurg.Psychiatry* (in press).

619. Panayiotopoulos, C.P. (1998): Significance of the EEG after the first afebrile seizure. *Arch. Dis. Child.* **78,** 575–576.

620. Panayiotopoulos, C.P. (1998): Fixation-off, scotosensitive, and other visual-related epilepsies. *Adv. Neurol.* **75,** 139–157.

621. Panayiotopoulos, C.P. (1998): Benign childhood occipital seizures. *Arch. Dis. Child.* **78,** 3–4.

622. Panayiotopoulos, C.P. (1999) Extra-occipital benign childhood seizures with ictal voniting and excellent prognosis. *J.Neurol.Neurosurg.Psychiatry* **66,** 82–85.

622a. Panayiotopoulos, C.P. (1999): Early onset benign childhood occipital seizures: A syndrome to recognise. *Epilepsia* (in press).

622b. Panayiotopoulos, C.P. (1999): The benign occipital epilepsies of childhood: Diagnostic and management problems. *Epilepsia* (in press).

623. Panayiotopoulos, C.P., Agathonikou, A., Koutroumanidis, M., Giannakodimos, S., Rowlinson, S. & Carr, C.P. (1996): Eyelid myoclonia with absences: the symptoms. In: *Eyelid myoclonia with absences,* eds J.S. Duncan & C.P. Panayiotopoulos, pp. 17–26. London: John Libbey & Company Ltd.

624. Panayiotopoulos, C.P., Agathonikou, A., Sharoqi, I.A. & Parker, A.P. (1997): Vigabatrin aggravates absences and absence status. *Neurology* **49,** 1467.

625. Panayiotopoulos, C.P., Ahmed Sharoqi, I. & Agathonikou, A. (1997): Occipital seizures imitating migraine aura. *J. Royal Soc. Med.* **90,** 255–257.

626. Panayiotopoulos, C.P., Binnie, C.D. & Takahashi, T. (1994): Fixation-off-sensitive epilepsies:clinical and EEG characteristics. In: *Epileptic seizures and syndromes,* ed. P. Wolf, pp. 55–66. London: John Libbey & Company Ltd.

627. Panayiotopoulos, C.P., Chroni, E., Daskalopoulos, C., Baker, A., Rowlinson, S. & Walsh, P. (1992): Typical absence seizures in adults: clinical, EEG, video-EEG findings and diagnostic/syndromic considerations. *J.Neurol.Neurosurg.Psychiatry* **55,** 1002–1008.

628. Panayiotopoulos, C.P., Giannakodimos, S., Agathonikou, A. & Koutroumanidis, M. (1996): Eyelid myoclonia is not a manoeuvre for self-induced seizures in eyelid myoclonia with absences. In: *Eyelid myoclonia with absences,*eds. J.S. Duncan & C.P. Panayiotopoulos, pp. 93–106. London: John Libbey & Company Ltd.

629. Panayiotopoulos, C.P., Hatziconstantinou, M. & Scarpalezos, S. (1978): Clinical and EEG observations on occipital lobe epilesy. *Arch. Med. Soc. Proc.* (Greece), **4,** 254–256.

630. Panayiotopoulos, C.P. & Igoe, D.M. (1992): Cerebral insult-like partial status epilepticus in the early- onset variant of benign childhood epilepsy with occipital paroxysms. *Seizure* **1,** 99–102.

631. Panayiotopoulos, C.P., Jeavons, P.M. & Harding, G.F. (1970): Relation of occipital spikes evoked by intermittent photic stimulation to visual evoked responses in photosensitive epilepsy. *Nature* **228,** 566–567.

632. Panayiotopoulos, C.P., Jeavons, P.M. & Harding, G.F. (1972): Occipital spikes and their relation to visual responses in epilepsy, with particular reference to photosensitive epilepsy. *Electroencephalogr. Clin. Neurophysiol.* **32,** 179–190.

633. Panayiotopoulos, C.P., Koutroumanidis, M., Giannakodimos, S. & Agathonikou, A. (1997): Idiopathic generalised epilepsy in adults manifested by phantom absences, generalised tonic–clonic seizures, and frequent absence status. *J.Neurol.Neurosurg.Psychiatry* **63,** 622–627.

634. Panayiotopoulos, C.P., Obeid, T. & Tahan, A.R. (1994): Juvenile myoclonic epilepsy: a 5-year prospective study. *Epilepsia* **35,** 285–296.

635. Panayiotopoulos, C.P., Sharoqi, I.A. & Agathonikou, A. (1997): Acephalgic migraine or childhood occipital seizures? *Neurology* **49,** 1479.

636. Panayiotopoulos, C.P. & Siafacas, A. (1980): Triggering factors in occipital lobe epilepsy. *Acta Neurol. Scand.* **62 (Suppl 79),** 112.

637. Panayiotopoulos, C.P., Tahan, R. & Obeid, T. (1991): Juvenile myoclonic epilepsy: factors of error involved in the diagnosis and treatment. *Epilepsia* **32,** 672–676.

638. Paolozzi, C., Colucci, D.C & Bravaccio, F. (1970): Unusual electro-clinical aspects of a case of epileptic nystagmus. *Acta Neurol. (Napoli)* **25,** 450–456.

639. Paquier, P.F., Van Dongen, H.R. & Loonen, C.B. (1992): The Landau–Kleffner syndrome or 'acquired aphasia with convulsive disorder'. Long-term follow-up of six children and a review of the recent literature. *Arch. Neurol.* **49,** 354–359.

640. Parain, D. & Samson-Dollfus, D. (1984): Electroencephalograms in basilar artery migraine. *Electroencephalogr. Clin. Neurophysiol.* **58,** 392–399.

641. Parker, A.P., Agathonikou, A. & Panayiotopoulos, C.P. (1997): An aggressive seizure and behavioural disorder following trivial head injury. *Seizure* **6,** 499–501.

642. Parker, A.P.J., Agathonikou, A., Robinson, R.O. & Panayiotopoulos, C.P. (1998): Inappropriate use of carbamazepine in typical absences. *Dev. Med. Child Neurol.* **40,** 517–519.

643. Passier, P.E., Vredeveld, J.W. & de Krom, M.C. (1994): Basilar migraine with severe EEG abnormalities. *Headache* **34,** 56–58.

644. Patry, G., Lyagoubi, S. & Tassinari, C.A. (1971): Subclinical 'electrical status epilepticus' induced by sleep in children. A clinical and electroencephalographic study of six cases. *Arch.Neurol.* **24,** 242–252.

645. Patterson, M.C., Tomlinson, F.H. & Stuart, G.G. (1988): Palinacousis: a case report. *Neurosurgery* **22,** 1088–1090.

646. Pazzaglia, P., Sabattini, L. & Lugaresi, E. (1970): Occipital seizures precipitated by darkness. *Riv. Neurol.* **40,** 184–192.

647. Penfield, W. & Erickson, T.C. (1941): *Epilepsy and cerebral localization. A study of the mechanism, treatment and prevention of epileptic seizures.* London: Bailliere,Tindall, and Cox.

648. Penfield, W. & Jasper, H.H. (1954): *Epilepsy and the functional anatomy of the human brain.* Boston: Little, Brown & Co.

649. Penfield, W. & Kristiansen, K. (1951): *Epileptic seizure patterns.* Springfield, IL: Charles C. Thomas.

650. Penfield, W.& Perot, P. (1963): The brain's record of auditory and visual experience. *Brain* **86,** 595–696.

651. Penfield, W. & Rasmussen, T. (1957): *The cerebral cortex of man:A clinical study of localisation of function.* 4th edn. New York: The Macmillan Company.

652. Petersen, J., Nielsen, C.J. & Gulmann, N.C. (1983): Atypical EEG abnormalities in children with benign partial (Rolandic) epilepsy. *Acta Neurol. Scand.* **Suppl 94,** 57–62.

653. Peterson, J., Scruton, D. & Downie, A.W. (1977): Basilar artery migraine with transient atrial fibrillation. *B.M.J.* **2,** 1125–1126.

654. Piccirilli, M., D'Alessandro, P., Sciarma, T., Cantoni, C., Dioguardi, M.S., Giuglietti, M., Ibba, A. & Tiacci, C. (1994): Attention problems in epilepsy: possible significance of the epileptogenic focus. *Epilepsia* **35,** 1091–1096.

655. Piccirilli, M., D'Alessandro, P., Tiacci, C. & Ferroni, A. (1988): Language lateralization in children with benign partial epilepsy. *Epilepsia* **29,** 19–25.

656. Pierzchala, K., Rosciszewska, D. & Kwiecinski, J. (1992): Severe case of basilar migraine treated with flunarizine. *Neurol. Neurochir. Polska* **26,** 879–882.

657. Plant, G.T. (1986): The fortification spectra of migraine. *B.M.J. Clinical Research Ed.* **293,** 1613–1617.

658. Plant, G.T. (1996): Anatomy and physiology of the eyelids. In: *Eyelid myoclonia with absences,* eds. J.S. Duncan & C.P. Panayiotopoulos, pp. 1–11. London: John Libbey & Company Ltd.

659. Plasmati, R., Michelucci, R., Forti, A., Rubboli, G., Salvi, F., Saba, E. & Tassinari, C.A. (1992): The neurophysiological features of benign partial epilepsy with Rolandic spikes. *Epilepsy Research* – **Suppl 6,** 45–48.

660. Plazzi, G., Tinuper, P., Cerullo, A., Provini, F. & Lugaresi, E. (1994): Occipital lobe epilepsy: a chronic condition related to transient occipital lobe involvement in eclampsia. *Epilepsia* **35,** 644–647.

661. Plouin, P., Lerique, A. & Dulac, O. (1980): Etude electroclinique et evolution dans 7 observations de crises partielles complexes dominees par un comportement de terreur chez l'enfant. *Boll. Lega Ital. Epil.* **29/30,** 139–143.

662. Porro, G., Matricardi, M., Guidetti, V. & Benedetti, P. (1988): Prognosis of partial epilepsy. *Arch. Dis. Child.* **63,** 1192–1197.

663. Post, R.M. & Silberstein, S.D. (1994): Shared mechanisms in affective illness, epilepsy, and migraine. *Neurology* **44,** S37–47.

664. Pourmand, R.A., Markand, O.N. & Thomas, C. (1984): Midline spike discharges: clinical and EEG correlates. *Clin. Electroencephalogr.* **15,** 232–236.

665. Pressler, R.M., Wilson, A.G., Robinson, R.O., McCartney, D., Coleshill, S.G. & Binnie, C.D. (1999): Transitory cognitive impairment in children with benign partial epilepsy. *Electroencephalogr. Clin. Neurophysiol.* 1998 (in press) Abstract.

666. Queiroz, L.P., Rapoport, A.M., Weeks, R.E., Sheftell, F.D., Siegel, S.E. & Baskin, S.M. (1997): Characteristics of migraine visual aura. *Headache* **37,** 137–141.

667. Quirk, J.A., Fish, D.R., Smith, S.J., Sander, J.W., Shorvon, S.D. & Allen, P.J. (1995): First seizures associated with playing electronic screen games: a community-based study in Great Britain. *Ann.Neurol.* **37,** 733–737.

668. Radhakrishnan, K., Silbert, P.L. & Klass, D.W. (1995): Reading epilepsy: An appraisal of 20 patients diagnosed at the Mayo Cliinic, Rochester, Minnesota, between 1949 and 1989, and delineation of the epileptic syndrome. *Brain* **118,** 75–89.

669. Ragno, M., Tournier-Lasserve, E., Fiori, M.G., Manca, A., Patrosso, M.C., Ferlini, A, Sirocchi, G., Trojano, L., Chabriat, H. & Salvi, F. (1995): An Italian kindred with cerebral autosomal dominant arteriopathy with subcortical infarcts and leukoencephalopathy (CADASIL). *Ann. Neurol.* **38,** 231–236.

670. Ramani, V. (1998): Reading epilepsy. *Adv. Neurol.* **75,** 241–262.

671. Rapin, I. (1995): Acquired aphasia in children [editorial]. *J. Child Neurol.* **10,** 267–270.

672. Rapin, I., Mattis, S., Rowan, A.J. & Golden, G.G. (1977): Verbal auditory agnosia in children. *Dev. Med. Child Neurol.* **19,** 197–207.

673. Rees, M., Diebold, U., Parker, K., Doose, H., Gardiner, R.M. & Whitehouse, W.P. (1993): Benign childhood epilepsy with centrotemporal spikes and the focal sharp wave trait is not linked to the fragile X region. *Neuropediatrics* **24,** 211–213.

674. Ribacoba Montero, R., Salas Puig, J., Fernandez Toral, J., Fernandez Martinez, J.M. & Moral Rato, M. (1995): Fragile X syndrome and epilepsy. *Neurologia* **10,** 70–75.

675. Ricci, G. & Vizioli, R. (1966): A case of epileptic nystagmus. *Riv. Neurol.* **36,** 40–48.

676. Ricci, S., Cusmai, R., Di Capua, M., Fusco, L. & Vigevano, F. (1991): Seizures with vomiting, eye deviation and semiconvulsion: epilepsy or migraine? In: *Juvenile Headache,* eds. V. Gallai & V. Giudetti, pp. 193–196.

677. Ricci, S. & Vigevano, F. (1993): Occipital seizures provoked by intermittent light stimulation: ictal and interictal findings. *J. Clin. Neurophysiol.* **10,** 197–209.

678. Rintahaka, P.J., Chugani, H.T. & Sankar, R. (1995): Landau–Kleffner syndrome with continuous spikes and waves during slow-wave sleep. *J. Child Neurol.* **10,** 127–133.

679. Robb, S.A., Harden, A. & Boyd, S.G. (1989): Rett syndrome: an EEG study in 52 girls. *Neuropediatrics* **20,** 192–195.

680. Robert, J., Miro, O., Pedrol, E. & Cardellach, F. (1995): Palinopsia as a manifestation of migraine associated with other symptoms. *Medicina Clinica* **105,** 76–77.

681. Robertson, R., Langill, L., Wong, P.K. & Ho, H.H. (1988): Rett syndrome: EEG presentation. *Electroencephalogr. Clin. Neurophysiol.* **70,** 388–395.

682. Roger, J., Bureau, M., Genton, P. & Dravet, C. (1990): Idiopathic partial epilepsies. In: *Comprehensive epileptology,* eds. M. Dam & L. Gram, pp. 155–170. New York: Raven Press.

683. Roger, J., Dravet, C., Bureau, M., Dreifuss, F.E. & Wolf, P. (1985): Introduction. In: *Epileptic syndromes in infancy, childhood and adolescence,* eds. J. Roger, C. Dravet, M. Bureau, F.E. Dreifuss & P. Wolf, pp.vii-viii. London: John Libbey Eurotext Ltd.

684. Roger, J., Genton, P., Bureau, M. & Dravet, C. (1992): Progressive myoclonus epilepsies in childhood and adolescence. In: *Epileptic syndromes in childhood and adolescence,* eds. J. Roger, M. Bureau, C. Dravet, F.E. Dreifuss, A. Perret & P. Wolf, pp. 381–400. London: John Libbey & Company Ltd.

685. Roger, J., Pellissier, J.F., Bureau, M., Dravet, C., Revol, M. & Tinuper, P. (1983): Early diagnosis of Lafora disease. Significance of paroxysmal visual manifestations and contribution of skin biopsy. *Rev. Neurol.* **139,** 115–124.

686. Ronen, G.M., Rosales, T.O., Connolly, M., Anderson, V.E. & Leppert, M. (1993): Seizure characteristics in chromosome 20 benign familial neonatal convulsions. *Neurology* **43,** 1355–1360.

687. Rose, D. & Duron, B. (1984): Prognostic value of EEG abnormalities observed during sleep in epilepsy with Rolandic spikes. *Rev. EEG Neurophysiol.* **14,** 217–226.

688. Rosenbaum, D.H., Siegel, M. & Rowan, A.J. (1986): Contraversive seizures in occipital epilepsy: case report and review of the literature. *Neurology* **36,** 281–284.

689. Rosenberg, M.L. & Jabbari, B. (1991): Miosis and internal ophthalmoplegia as a manifestation of partial seizures. *Neurology* **41,** 737–739.

690. Rossi, P.G., Pazzaglia, P. & Frank, G. (1976): Acquired aphasia with convulsion anomalies in the developmental age: clinical neuropsychological and electroencephalographic study of a case. *Riv. Neurol.* **46,** 130–162.

691. Roulet, E., Deonna, T. & Despland, P.A. (1989): Prolonged intermittent drooling and oromotor dyspraxia in benign childhood epilepsy with centrotemporal spikes. *Epilepsia* **30,** 564–568.

692. Russell, M.B., Iversen, H.K. & Olesen, J. (1994): Improved description of the migraine aura by a diagnostic aura diary. *Cephalalgia* **14,** 107–117.

693. Russell, M.B. & Olesen, J. (1996): A nosographic analysis of the migraine aura in a general population. *Brain* **119,** 355–361.

694. Russell, W.R. & Whitty, C.W.M. (1955). Studies in traumatic epilepsy 3. Visual fits. *J. Neurol. Neurosurg. Psychiatry* **18,** 79–96.

695. Ryan, S.G., Wiznitzer, M., Hollman, C., Torres, M.C., Szekeresova, M. & Schneider, S. (1991): Benign familial neonatal convulsions: evidence for clinical and genetic heterogeneity. *Ann.Neurol.* **29,** 469–473.

696. Sabbadini, G., Francia, A., Calandriello, L., Di Biasi, C., Trasimeni, G., Gualdi, G.F., Palladini, G., Manfredi, M. & Frontali, M. (1995): Cerebral autosomal dominant arteriopathy with subcortical infarcts and leucoencephalopathy (CADASIL). Clinical, neuroimaging, pathological and genetic study of a large Italian family. *Brain* **118,** 207–215.

697. Sacks, O. (1993): *Migraine.* London: Picador.

698. Sadeh, M., Goldhammer, Y. & Kuritsky, A. (1983): post-ictal blindness in adults. *J.Neurol.Neurosurg.Psychiatry* **46,** 566–569.

699. Saint-Hilaire, J.M., Laplante, P. & Bouvier, G. (1987): Epileptic headache:study with depth electrodes. In: *Migraine and epilepsy,* eds. F. Andermann & E. Lugaresi, pp. 265–271. Boston, MA:Butterworths.

700. Salanova, V., Andermann, F., Olivier, A., Rasmussen, T. & Quesney, L.F. (1992): Occipital lobe epilepsy: electroclinical manifestations, electrocorticography, cortical stimulation and outcome in 42 patients treated between 1930 and 1991. Surgery of occipital lobe epilepsy. *Brain* **115,** 1655–1680.

701. Salanova, V., Andermann, F. & Rasmussen, T.B. (1993): Occipital lobe epilesy. In: *The treatment of epilepsy,* ed. E. Wyllie, pp. 533–540. Philadelphia: Lee & Febiger.

702. Samson-Dollfus, D., Samson, M. & Jouvin, M. (1963): Les pointes-ondes occipitales chez l'enfant. *Electroencephalogr. Clin. Neurophysiol.* **15,** 504–507.

703. Sand, T. (1991): EEG in migraine: a review of the literature. *Functional Neurology* **6,** 7–22.

704. Santanelli, P. (1989): Idiopathic partial epilepsy with reflex visual seizures and both multifocal and generalised EEG discharges. In: *Reflex seizures and reflex epilepsies,* eds. A. Beaumanoir, H. Gastaut & R. Naquet, pp. 229–232. Geneve: Editions Medecine & Hygiene.

705. Santucci, M., Giovanardi Rossi, P., Ambrosetto, G., Sacquegna, T. & D'Alessandro, R. (1985): Migraine and benign epilepsy with Rolandic spikes in childhood: a case-control study. *Dev. Med. Child Neurol.* **27,** 60–62.

706. Sawhney, I.M., Robertson, I.J., Polkey, C.E., Binnie, C.D. & Elwes, R.D. (1995): Multiple subpial transection: a review of 21 cases. *J.Neurol.Neurosurg.Psychiatry* **58,** 344–349.

707. Schaffler, L. & Karbowski, K. (1988): Epileptic activity in the occipital lobe. Clinico-electroencephalographic contribution. *Fortschritte Neurol. Psychiatrie* **56,** 268–299.

708. Scheffer, I.E., Jones, L., Pozzebon, M., Howell, R.A., Saling, M.M. & Berkovic, S.F. (1995): Autosomal dominant Rolandic epilepsy and speech dyspraxia: a new syndrome with anticipation. *Ann. Neurol.* **38,** 633–642.

709. Schmidt, E.M., Bak, M.J., Hambrecht, F.T., Kufta, C.V., O'Rourke, D.K. & Vallabhanath, P. (1996): Feasibility of a visual prosthesis for the blind based on intracortical microstimulation of the visual cortex. *Brain* **119,** 507–522.

710. Schon, F. & Blau, J.N. (1987): Post-epileptic headache and migraine. *J.Neurol. Neurosurg. Psychiatry* **50,** 1148–1152.

711. Schwartz, R.B., Jones, K.M., Kalina, P., Bajakian, R.L., Mantello, M.T., Garada, B. & Holman, B.L. (1992): Hypertensive encephalopathy: findings on CT, MR imaging, and SPECT imaging in 14 cases. *Am. J. Roentgenol.* **159,** 379–383.

712. Scott, D.F., Moffett, A. & Swash, M. (1972): Observations on the relation of migraine and epilepsy. An electroencephalographic, psychological and clinical study using oral tyramine. *Epilepsia* **13,** 365–375.

713. Septien, L., Pelletier, J.L., Brunotte, F., Giroud, M. & Dumas, R. (1991): Migraine in patients with history of centrotemporal epilepsy in childhood: a Hm-PAO SPECT study. *Cephalalgia* **11,** 281–284.

714. Seto, H., Shimizu, M., Futatsuya, R., Kageyama, M., Wu, Y., Kamei, T., Shibata, R & Kakishita, M. (1994): Basilar artery migraine. Reversible ischemia demonstrated by Tc–99m HMPAO brain SPECT. *Clinical Nuclear Medicine* **19,** 215–218.

715. Shafrir, Y. & Prensky, A.L. (1995): Acquired epileptiform opercular syndrome: a second case report, review of the literature, and comparison to the Landau–Kleffner syndrome. *Epilepsia* **36,** 1050–1057.

716. Shahar, E., Desatnik, H., Brand, N., Straussberg, R. & Hwang, P.A. (1996): Epileptic blindness in children: a localizing sign of various epileptic disorders. *Clin. Neurol. Neurosurg.* **98,** 237–241.

717. Sharf, B. & Bental, E. (1974): Basilar artery migraine. *Harefuah* **86,** 361–362.

718. Shestakov, V.V. & Larikova, T.I. (1994): Migraine and epilepsy: clinical comparisons and the characteristics of the cerebral blood circulation. *Zhurnal Nevropatologii i Psikhiatrii Imeni S - S - Korsakova* **94,** 3–5.

719. Shevell, M.I. (1996): Acephalgic migraines of childhood. *Pediatr. Neurol.* **14,** 211–215.

720. Shevell, M.I. (1997): Acephalgic migraine or childhood occipital seizures. *Reply. Neurology* **49,** 1479–1480.

721. Shian, W.J., Chi, C.S., Mak, S.C., Chen, C.H. & Hsu, N.Y. (1994): Benign partial epilepsy with centrotemporal spikes: analysis of 94 Chinese children. *Acta Paediatr. Sinica* **35,** 108–112.

722. Shinnar, S., Berg, A.T., Moshe, S.L., O'Dell, C., Alemany, M., Newstein, D., Kang, H, Goldensohn, E.S. & Hauser, W.A. (1996): The risk of seizure recurrence after a first unprovoked afebrile seizure in childhood: an extended follow-up. *Pediatrics* **98,** 216–225.

723. Shinnar, S., Kang, H., Berg, A.T., Goldensohn, E.S., Hauser, W.A. & Moshe, S.L. (1994): EEG abnormalities in children with a first unprovoked seizure. *Epilepsia* **35,** 471–476.

724. Shirota, A., Yamane, K., Shimizu, Y., Sato, M., Nagayama, T., Takahashi, M. & Oto, T. (1991): A case of basilar artery migraine. *Nippon Naika Gakkai Zasshi – J. Japan.Soc. Int. Med.* **80,** 1297–1298.

725. Sidenvall, R., Forsgren, L., Blomquist, H.K. & Heijbel, J. (1993): A community-based prospective incidence study of epileptic seizures in children. *Acta Paediat.Scand.* **82,** 60–65.

726. Sidenvall, R., Forsgren, L. & Heijbel, J. (1996): Prevalence and characteristics of epilepsy in children in northern Sweden. *Seizure* **5,** 139–146.

727. Silberstein, S.D. & Lipton, R.B. (1997): Migraine. In: *Epilepsy: A comprehensive textbook, eds.* J.J. Engel & T.A. Pedley, pp. 2681–2691. Philadelphia: Lippincott-Raven Publishers.

728. Silva, D.F., Lima, M.M., Anghinah, R., Zanoteli, E. & Lima, J.G. (1995): Dipole reversal: an ictal feature in a patient with benign partial epilepsy of childhood with centrotemporal spike. *Arquiv. Neuro-Psiquiatria* **53,** 270–273.

729. Silvestri, R., De Domenico, P., Lombardo, N., Leuzzi, R. & Di Perri, R. (1989): Photosensitive epilepsy with occipital spikes occurring during sleep. A case report. In: *Reflex seizures and reflex epilepsies,* eds. A. Beaumanoir, H. Gastaut & R. Naquet, pp. 225–227. Geneve: Editions Medecine & Hygiene.

730. Sjaastad, O. (1986): Transitory isolated, global blindness and headache the possible relationship to migraine. *Functional Neurology* **1,** 467–471.

731. Slatter, K.H. (1968): Some clinical and EEG findings in patients with migraine. *Brain* **91,** 85–98.

732. Smith, J.M.B. & Kellaway, P. (1964): Central (Rolandic) foci in children: an analysis of 200 cases. *Electroencephalogr. Clin. Neurophysiol.* **17,** 460–461.

733. Smith, M.C. (1997): Landau-Kleffner Syndrome and Continuous Spikes and Waves During Slow Sleep. In: *Epilepsy: A Comprehensive Textbook,* eds. J.J. Engel & T.A. Pedley. Philadelphia: Lippincott-Raven Publishers.

734. Solomon, G.D. & Spaccavento, L.J. (1982): Lateral medullary syndrome after basilar migraine. *Headache* **22,** 171–172.

735. Sorel, L. & Rucquoy-Ponsar, M. (1969): L'epilepsie functionelle de maturation. Apport des montages verticaux en E.E.G. dans le diagnostic de cette forme d'epilepsie. *Rev. Neurol.* **121,** 289–297.

736. Soriani, S., Scarpa, P., Arnaldi, C., De Carlo, L., Pausini, L. & Montagna, P. (1996): Migraine aura without headache and ictal fast EEG activity in an 11-year-old boy. *Eur. J. Pediatr.* **155,** 126–129.

737. Soriani, S., Feggi, L., Battistella, P.A., Arnaldi, C., De Carlo, L. & Stipa, S. (1997): Interictal and ictal phase study with Tc 99m HMPAO brain SPECT in juvenile migraine with aura. *Headache* **37,** 31–36.

738. Sowa, M.V. & Pituck, S. (1989): Prolonged spontaneous complex visual hallucinations and illusions as ictal phenomena. *Epilepsia* **30,** 524–526.

738a. Staden, U., Isaaca, E., Boyd, S.G., Brandl, U. & Neville, B.G. (1998): Language dysfunction in children with Rolandic epilepsy. *Neuropediatrics* **29,** 242–248.

739. Steinborn, B., Junik, R., Wigowska-Sowinska, J., Galas-Zgorzalewicz, B., Sowinski, J. & Gembicki, M. (1996): The Landau–Kleffner syndrome. SPECT and EEG investigations. *Neurol.Neuroch. Polska* **30,** 771–781.

740. Steinlein, O., Schuster, V., Fischer, C. & Haussler, M. (1995): Benign familial neonatal convulsions: confirmation of genetic heterogeneity and further evidence for a second locus on chromosome 8q. *Hum.Genet.* **95,** 411–415.

741. Sturzenegger, M.H. & Meienberg, O. (1985): Basilar artery migraine: a follow-up study of 82 cases. *Headache* **25,** 408–415.

742. Sudo, K. & Tashiro, K. (1996): Psychogenic basilar migraine. *Neurology* **46,** 1786 1787.

743. Sulkava, R. & Kovanen, J. (1983): Locked-in syndrome with rapid recovery: a manifestation of basilar artery migraine? *Headache* **23,** 238–239.

744. Sumi, T. & Kohsaka, M. (1988): A study of benign epilepsy of children with centrotemporal EEG foci, with special reference to clinical course and Rolandic discharge. *No to Hattatsu [Brain Dev.]* **20,** 10–14.

745. Suwa, K., Kobayashi, S., Miyao, M., Nozaki, Y., Mori, Y., Yamagata, T. & Momoi, M.Y. (1996): Landau–Kleffner syndrome: relationship between aphasia and electroencepharographic changes. *No to Hattatsu [Brain Dev.]* **28,** 306–311.

746. Sveinbjornsdottir, S. & Duncan, J.S. (1993): Parietal and occipital lobe epilepsy: a review. *Epilepsia* **34,** 493–521.

747. Swanson, J.W. & Vick, N.A. (1978): Basilar artery migraine, 12 patients with an attack recorded electroencephalographically. *Neurology* **28,** 782–786.

748. Takahashi, K., Saito, M., Kyo, K., Gomibuchi, K., Niijima, S., Tada, H., Honda, T, Sato, Y., Takahashi, H. & Ohtsuka, C. (1990): Prognosis of benign epilepsy of children with centrotemporal EEG foci. *Jap. J. Psychiatry Neurol.* **44,** 360–361.

749. Takahashi, N. & Kawamura, M. (1996): Simple partial seizure consisting of complex visual hallucinations due to left temporo-occipital lesion. *Rinsho Shinkeigaku – Clinical Neurology* **36,** 665–669.

750. Takaishi, Y., Hashimoto, K. & Enokido, H. (1991): A study of idiopathic epilepsy of childhood with occipital electroencephalographic foci. *Nippon Ika Daigaku Zasshi – J. Nippon Med. School* **58,** 686–695.

751. Takeda, A., Bancaud, J., Talairach, J., Bonis, A. & Bordas-Ferrer, M. (1969): A propos des acces epileptiques d'origine occipitale. *Rev. Neurol.* **12,** 306–315.

752. Talwar, D., Arora, M.S. & Sher, P.K. (1994): EEG changes and seizure exacerbation in young children treated with carbamazepine. *Epilepsia* **35,** 1154–1159.

753. Talwar, D., Rask, C.A. & Torres, F. (1992): Clinical manifestations in children with occipital spike-wave paroxysms. *Epilepsia* **33,** 667–674.

754. Tapiador Sanjuan, M.J., Zuazo Zamalloa, E., Garaizar Axpe, C. & Prats Vinas, J.M. (1995): Tics and carbamazepine in benign partial epilepsy of childhood. *Neurologia* **10,** 59–60.

755. Tassinari, C.A. (1995): The problems of 'continuous spikes and waves during slow sleep' or 'electrical status epilepticus during slow sleep' today. In: *Continuous spikes and waves during slow sleep. Electrical status epilepticus during slow sleep. Acquired epileptic aphasia and related conditions,* eds. A. Beaumanoir, M. Bureau, T. Deonna, L. Mira & C.A. Tassinari, pp. 251–255. London: John Libbey & Company Ltd.

756. Tassinari, C.A., Bureau, M., Dravet, C., Dalla Bernardina, B. & Roger, J. (1985): Epilepsy with continuous spikes amd waves during slow sleep – otherwise described as ESES (epilepsy with electrical status epilepticus during slow sleep). In: *Epileptic syndromes in infancy, childhood and adolescence,* eds. J. Roger, C. Dravet, M. Bureau, F.E. Dreifuss & P. Wolf, pp. 194–204. London: John Libbey Eurotext Ltd.

757. Tassinari, C.A., Bureau, M., Dravet, C., Dalla Bernardina, B. & Roger, J. (1992): Epilepsy with continuous spikes amd waves during slow sleep – otherwise described as ESES (epilepsy with electrical status epilepticus during slow sleep). In: *Epileptic syndromes in infancy, childhood and adolescence,* eds. J. Roger, M. Bureau, C. Dravet, F.E. Dreifuss, A. Perret & P. Wolf, pp. 245–256. London: John Libbey & Company Ltd.

758. Tassinari, C.A., Bureau-Paillas, M., Dalla Bernardina, B., Picornell-Darder, I., Mouren, M.C., Dravet, C. & Roger, J. (1978): Lafora disease. *Rev. Electroencephalogr. Neurophysiol. Clin.* **8,** 107–122.

759. Tassinari, C.A. & De Marco, P. (1992): Benign partial epilepsy with extreme somato-sensory evoked potentials. In: *Epileptic syndromes in infancy, childhood and adolescense,* eds. J. Roger, M. Bureau, C. Dravet, F.E. Dreifuss, P. Wolf & A. Perret, pp. 225–229. London: John Libbey & Company Ltd.

760. Tassinari, C.A., De Marco, P., Plasmati, R., Pantieri, R., Blanco, M. & Michelucci, R. (1988): Extreme somatosensory evoked potentials (ESEPs) elicited by tapping of hands or feet in children: a somatosensory cerebral evoked potentials study. *Neurophysiol. Clin.* **18,** 123–128.

761. Tassinari, C.A., Rubboli, G., Plasmati, R., Salvi, F., Ambrosetto, G., Bianchedi, G., Forti, A. & Michelucci, R. (1989): Television-induced epilepsy with occipital seizures. In: *Reflex seizures and reflex epilepsies,* eds. A. Beaumanoir, H. Gastaut & R. Naquet, pp. 241–243. Geneve: Editions Medecine & Hygiene.

762. Tenembaum, S., Deonna, T., Fejerman, N., Medina, C., Ingvar-Maeder, M. & Gubser-Mercati, D. (1997): Continuous spike-waves and dementia in childhood epilepsy with occipital paroxysms. *J. Epilepsy* **10,** 139–145.

763. Terasaki, T., Yamatogi, Y. & Ohtahara, S. (1987): Electroclinical delineation of occipital lobe epilepsy in childhood. In: *Migraine and epilepsy,* eds. F. Andermann & E. Lugaresi, pp. 125–137. Boston, MA: Butterworths.

764. Terwindt, G.M., Ophoff, R.A., Haan, J., Frants, R.R. & Ferrari, M.D. (1996): Familial hemiplegic migraine: a clinical comparison of families linked and unlinked to chromosome 19.DMG RG. *Cephalalgia* **16,** 153–155.

765. Terzano, M.G., Manzoni, G.C. & Parrino, L. (1987): Benign epilepsy with occipital paroxysms and migraine: The question of intercalated attacks. In: *Migraine and epilepsy,* eds. F. Andermann & E. Lugaresi, pp. 83–96. Boston, MA: Butterworths.

766. Terzano, M.G., Parrino, L., Pietrini, V. & Galli, L. (1993): Migraine-epilepsy syndrome:intercalated seizures in benign occipital epilepsy. In: *Occipital seizures and epilepsies in children,* eds. F. Andermann, A. Beaumanoir, L. Mira, J. Roger & C.A. Tassinari, pp. 93–99. London: John Libbey & Company Ltd.

767. Terzano, M.G., Parrino, L., Spaggiari, M.C., Barusi, R. & Simeoni, S. (1991): Discriminatory effect of cyclic alternating pattern in focal lesional and benign Rolandic interictal spikes during sleep. *Epilepsia* **32,** 616–628.

768. Terzano, M.G., Pietrini, V., Parrino, L. & Milone, F.F. (1986): Migraine and intercalated seizures with occipital EEG paroxysms: observations on a family. *Headache* **26,** 509–512.

769. Thomas, M. & Boyle, R. (1979): A possible connection between basilar migraine and the Arnold–Chiari malformation [letter]. *Neurology* **29,** 527–528.

770. Thurston, S.E., Leigh, R.J. & Osorio, I. (1985): Epileptic gaze deviation and nystagmus. *Neurology* **35,** 1518–1521.

771. Tinuper, P., Aguglia, U., Pellissier, J.F. & Gastaut, H. (1983): Visual ictal phenomena in a case of Lafora disease proven by skin biopsy. *Epilepsia* **24,** 214–218.

772. Tinuper, P., Aguglia, U., Farnarier, G. & De Carvalho, G.V. (1983): Vomiting: symptom of an epileptic seizure. *Revue Electroencephalogr Neurophysiol Clinique* **13,** 168–173.

773. Tinuper, P., Gobbi, G., Aguglia, U., Rossi, P.G. & Lugaresi, E. (1985): Occipital seizures in Lafora disease: a further case documented by EEG. *Clin. Electroencephalogr.* **16,** 167–170.

774. Tomaiolo, S., Stiglich, F., Bonomo, F., Barbonetti, C., Di Lorenzo, I., Campani, R, Bottinelli, O. & Bottinelli, G. (1991): SPECT with 99m-TC HM PAO in the study of classical hemicrania. *Radiologia Medica* **81,** 537–541.

775. Triulzi, F. (1997): Neuroradiologial findings in coeliac disease, epilepsy and cerebral calcifications. In: *Epilepsy and other neurological disorders in coeliac disease,* eds. G. Gobbi, F. Andermann, S. Naccarato & G. Banchini, pp. 187–194. London: John Libbey & Company Ltd.

776. Trojaborg, W. (1966): Focal spike discharges in children, a longitudinal study. *Acta Paediatr. Scand.* **Suppl 168,** 1–111.

777. Tusa, R.J., Kaplan, P.W., Hain, T.C. & Naidu, S. (1990): Ipsiversive eye deviation and epileptic nystagmus. *Neurology* **40,** 662–665.

778. Vahedi, K., Chabriat, H., Joutel, A., Ducros, A., Lutz, G., Alamowitch, S. & Iba-Zizen, M.T. (1997): Analysis of symptoms in migraine with aura in CADASIL. *Cephalalgia* **17,** 236.

779. Vahedi, K., Joutel, A., Van Bogaert, P., Ducros, A., Maciazeck, J., Bach, J.F., Bousser, M.G. & Tournier-Lasserve, E. (1995): A gene for hereditary paroxysmal cerebellar ataxia maps to chromosome 19p. *Ann.Neurol.* **37,** 289–293.

780. van der Meij, W., Van der Dussen, D., van Huffelen, A.C., Wieneke, G.H. & Van Nieuwenhuizen, O. (1997): Dipole source analysis may differentiate benign focal epilepsy of childhood with occipital paroxysms from symptomatic occipital lobe epilepsy. *Brain Topogr.* **10,** 115–120.

781. van der Meij, W., van Huffelen, A.C., Wieneke, G.H. & Willemse, J. (1992): Sequential EEG mapping may differentiate 'epileptic' from 'non-epileptic' Rolandic spikes. *Electroencephalogr. Clin. Neurophysiol.* **82,** 408–414.

782. van der Meij, W., van Huffelen, A.C., Willemse, J., Schenk-Rootlieb, A.J. & Meiners, L.C. (1992): Rolandic spikes in the inter-ictal EEG of children: contribution to diagnosis, classification and prognosis of epilepsy. *Dev. Med. Child Neurol.* **34,** 893–903.

783. van der Meij, W., Wieneke, G.H. & van Huffelen, A.C. (1993): Dipole source analysis of Rolandic spikes in benign Rolandic epilepsy and other clinical syndromes. *Brain Topogr.* **5,** 203–213.

784. van der Meij, W., Wieneke, G.H., van Huffelen, A.C., Schenk-Rootlieb, A.J. & Willemse, J. (1993): Identical morphology of the Rolandic spike-and-wave complex in different clinical entities. *Epilepsia* **34,** 540–550.

785. Van Hout, A. (1997): Acquired aphasia in children. *Seminars in Pediatr. Neurol.* **4,** 102–108.

786. van Huffelen, A.C. (1989): A tribute to Martinus Rulandus. A 16th-century description of benign focal epilepsy of childhood. *Arch.Neurol.* **46,** 445–447.

787. Varma, N.K., Kushwaha, R., Beydoun, A., Williams, W.J. & Drury, I. (1997): Mutual information analysis and detection of interictal morphological differences in interictal epileptiform discharges of patients with partial epilepsies. *Electroencephalogr. Clin. Neurophysiol.* **103,** 426–433.

788. Vascotto, M. & Fois, A. (1997): Frequency of epilepsy in coeliac disease and vice versa: a collaborative study. In: *Epilepsy and other neurological disorders in coeliac disease,* eds. G. Gobbi, F. Andermann, S. Naccarato & G. Banchini, pp. 105–110. London: John Libbey & Company Ltd.

789. Verin, M., Rolland, Y., Landgraf, F., Chabriat, H., Bompais, B., Michel, A., Vahedi, K., Martinet, J.P., Tournier-Lasserve, E., Lemaitre, M.H. *et al.* (1995): New phenotype of the cerebral autosomal dominant arteriopathy mapped to chromosome 19: migraine as the prominent clinical feature. *J. Neurol. Neurosurg. Psychiatry* **59,** 579–585.

790. Verma, N.P., Chheda, R.L., Nigro, M.A. & Hart, Z.H. (1986): Electroencephalographic findings in Rett syndrome. *Electroencephalogr. Clin. Neurophysiol.* **64,** 394–401.

791. Verret, S. & Steele, J.C. (1971): Alternating hemiplegia in childhood, a report of eight patients with complicated migraine beginning in infancy. *Pediatrics* **47,** 675–680.

792. Viani, F., Romeo, A., Viri, M., Mastrangelo, M., Lalatta, F., Selicorni, A., Gobbi, G., Lanzi, G., Bettio, D. & Briscioli, V. (1995): Seizure and EEG patterns in Angelman's syndrome. *J. Child Neurol.* **10,** 467–471.

793. Vigevano, F. & Ricci, S. (1993): Benign occipital epilepsy of childhood with prolonged seizures and autonomic symptoms. In: *Occipital seizures and epilepsies in children,* eds. F. Andermann, A. Beaumanoir, L. Mira, J. Roger & C.A. Tassinari, pp. 133–140. London: John Libbey & Company Ltd.

794. Vigevano, F., Ricci, S., Di Capua, M., Claps, D. & Fusco, L. (1989): Vomito, deviazione oculare, emiconvulsione: una particolare forma di stato epilettico nel bambino. *Boll. Lega Ital. Epil,* **65–66,** 315–316.

795. Walker, M.C., Smith, S.J., Sisodiya, S.M. & Shorvon, S.D. (1995): Case of simple partial status epilepticus in occipital lobe epilepsy misdiagnosed as migraine: clinical, electrophysiological, and magnetic resonance imaging characteristics. *Epilepsia* **36,** 1233–1236.

796. Waragai, M., Takaya, Y. & Hayashi, M. (1996): Complex visual hallucinations in the hemianopic field following an ischemic lesion of the occipitotemporal base – confirmation of the lesion by MRI and speculations on the pathophysiology. *No to Shinkei – Brain & Nerve* **48,** 371–376.

797. Watanabe, K. (1996): Benign partial epilepsies. In: *Epilepsy in Children,* ed. S. Wallace, pp. 293–313. London: Chapman & Hall.

798. Watanabe, K., Negoro, T., Matsumoto, A., Inokuma, K., Takaesu, E. & Maehara, M. (1984): Epileptic nystagmus associated with typical absence seizures. *Epilepsia* **25,** 22–24.

798a. Weglage, J., Demsky, A., Pietsch, M. & Kurlemann, G. (1997): Neuropsychological, intellectual, and behavioral findings in patients with centrotemporal spikes with and without seizures. *Dev. Med. Child Neurol.* **39,** 646–651.

799. Weinberg, H., Wong, P.K., Crisp, D., Johnson, B. & Cheyne, D. (1990): Use of multiple dipole analysis for the classification of benign Rolandic epilepsy. *Brain Topogr.* **3,** 183–190.

800. Welch, K.M. (1997): Pathogenesis of migraine. *Semin. Neurol.* **17,** 335–341.

801. Westmoreland, B.F. (1998): The EEG findings in extra-temporal seizures. *Epilepsia* **99 Suppl 4,** S1–8.

802. Whitehouse, W., Diebold, U., Rees, M., Parker, K., Doose, H. & Gardiner, R.M. (1993): Exclusion of linkage of genetic focal sharp waves to the HLA region on chromosome 6p in families with benign partial epilepsy with centrotemporal sharp waves. *Neuropediatrics* **24,** 208–210.

803. Wielaard, R., Bornebroek, M., Ophoff, R.A., Winter-Warnars, H.A., Scheltens, P., Frants, R.R., Ferrari, M.D. & Haan, J. (1995): A four-generation Dutch family with cerebral autosomal dominant arteriopathy with subcortical infarcts and leukoencephalopathy (CADASIL), linked to chromosome 19p13. *Clinical Neurology & Neurosurgery* **97,** 307–313.

804. Wilder-Smith, E. & Nirkko, A.C. (1991): Contribution of concurrent Doppler and EEG in differentiating occipital epileptic discharges from migraine. *Neurology* **41,** 2005–2007.

805. Wilkins, A. (1995): Towards an understanding of reflex epilepsy and absence. In: *Typical absences and related epileptic syndromes,* eds. J.S. Duncan & C.P. Panayiotopoulos, pp. 196–205. London: Churchill Communications Europe.

806. Wilkins, A.J. (1987): Visual sensitivity and hyperexcitability in epilepsy and migraine. In: *Migraine and epilepsy,* eds. F. Andermann & E. Lugaresi, pp. 339–365. Boston, MA: Butterworths.

807. Wilkins, A.J., Binnie, C.D. & Darby, C.E. (1980): Visually-induced seizures. *Progress in Neurobiology* **15,** 85–117.

808. Williamson, P.D. (1994): Seizures with origin in the occipital or parietal lobes. In: *Epileptic seizures and syndromes,* ed. P. Wolf, pp. 383–390. London: John Libbey & Company Ltd.

809. Williamson, P.D. & Engel, J.J. (1997): Complex partial seizures. In: *Epilepsy: A comprehensive textbook,* eds. J.J. Engel & T.A. Pedley, pp. 557–566. Philadelphia: Lippincott-Raven Publishers.

810. Williamson, P.D., Engel, J.J. & Munari, C. (1997): Anatomic classification of localisation-related epilepsies. In: *Epilepsy: A comprehensive textbook,* eds. J.J. Engel & T.A. Pedley, p. 2405. Philadelphia: Lippincott-Raven Publishers.

811. Williamson, P.D., Thadani, V.M., Darcey, T.M., Spencer, D.D., Spencer, S.S. & Mattson, R.H. (1992): Occipital lobe epilepsy: clinical characteristics, seizure spread patterns, and results of surgery. *Ann.Neurol.* **31,** 3–13.

812. Wirrell, E.C. (1998): Benign epilepsy of childhood with centrotemporal spikes. *Epilepsia* **99 suppl 4,** S32–41.

813. Wirrell, E.C., Camfield, P.R., Gordon, K.E., Dooley, J.M. & Camfield, C.S. (1995): Benign Rolandic epilepsy: atypical features are very common. *J. Child Neurol.* **10,** 455–458.

814. Wolf, P. (1992): Reading epilepsy. In: *Epileptic syndromes in infancy, childhood and adolescence,* eds. J. Roger, M. Bureau, C. Dravet, F.E. Dreifuss, A. Perret & P. Wolf, pp. 281–298. London: John Libbey & Company Ltd.

815. Wolf, P. (1994): Historical aspects: the concept of idiopathy. In: *Idiopathic generalised epilepsies: clinical, experimental and genetic aspects,* eds. A. Malafose, P. Genton, E. Hirsch, C. Marescaux, D. Broglin & R. Bernasconi, pp. 3–6. London: John Libbey & Company Ltd.

816. Wong, P.K. (1990): Dynamic correlation of Rolandic spikes. *Brain Topogr.* **3,** 129–136.

817. Wong, P.K. (1991): Source modelling of the Rolandic focus. *Brain Topogr.* **4,** 105–112.

818. Wong, P.K. (1993): The importance of source behavior in distinguishing populations of epileptic foci. *J. Clin. Neurophysiol.* **10,** 314–322.

819. Wong, P.K. (1996): Quantitative analysis of epileptic discharges. *Brain Topogr.* **8,** 209–214.

820. Wong, P.K., Bencivenga, R. & Gregory, D. (1988): Statistical classification of spikes in benign Rolandic epilepsy. *Brain Topogr.* **1,** 123–129.

820a. Worster-Drought, C. (1971): An unusual form of acquired aphasia in children. *Dev. Med. Child Neurol.* **13,** 563–571.

821. Wright, D.H. (1995): The major complications of coeliac disease. *Baillieres Clinical Gastroenterology* **9,** 351–369.

822. Wu, L. (1995): A long-term follow-up of 29 cases of benign epilepsy in childhood with central-temporal electroencephalographic foci. *Chung-Hua Shen Ching Ching Shen Ko Tsa Chih [Chinese J. Neurol. & Psychiatry]* **24,** 235–236.

823. Wu, L., Hirokazu, O., Makiko, O. & Yukio, F. (1993): Fukuyama type congenital muscular dystrophy with central-temporal EEG foci (Rolandic spikes). *Chin. Med. Sci. J.* **8,** 162–166.

824. Wyllie, E. (1993): *The treatment of epilepsy. Principles and practice.* Philadelphia: Lee & Febiger.

825. Wyllie, E., Luders, H., Morris, H.H., Lesser, R.P., Dinner, D.S. & Goldstick, L. (1986): Ipsilateral forced head and eye turning at the end of the generalized tonic–clonic phase of versive seizures. *Neurology* **36,** 1212–1217.

826. Yalcin, A.D., Kaymaz, A. & Forta, H. (1997): Childhood occipital epilepsy: seizure manifestations and electroencephalographic features. *Brain Dev.* **19,** 408–413.

827. Yamagata, T., Momoi, M.Y., Miyao, M. & Kobayashi, S. (1997): Blink induced centrotemporal spikes in benign childhood epilepsy with centrotemporal spikes. *J.Neurol.Neurosurg.Psychiatry* **63,** 528–530.

828. Yamane, K., Hashimoto, S., Kobayashi, I. & Maruyama, S. (1989): Basilar artery migraine associated with transient global amnesia. *No to Shinkei – Brain & Nerve* **41,** 1103–1107.

829. Yasuda, Y., Matsuda, I., Namura, S. & Morita, T. (1993): Ophthalmoplegia, hemiparesis and cheiro-oral syndrome in basilar artery migraine. *Eur. Neurol.* **33,** 185–187.

830. Yoshikawa, H., Kaga, M., Suzuki, H., Sakuragawa, N. & Arima, M. (1991): Giant somatosensory evoked potentials in the Rett syndrome. *Brain Dev.* **13,** 36–39.

831. Yoshimura, K., Hamada, F., Morita, H. & Kurashige, T. (1993): Identical twins with atypical benign partial epilepsy. *No to Hattatsu [Brain Dev.]* **25,** 283–288.

832. Yoshinaga, H., Amano, R., Oka, E. & Ohtahara, S. (1992): Dipole tracing in childhood epilepsy with special reference to Rolandic epilepsy. *Brain Topogr.* **4,** 193–199.

833. Yoshinaga, H., Kobayashi, K., Sato, M., Mizukawa, M. & Ohtahara, S. (1993): Clinical application of spike averaging to dipole tracing method. *Brain Topogr.* **6,** 131–135.

834. Yoshinaga, H., Sato, M., Oka, E. & Ohtahara, S. (1995): Spike dipole analysis using SEP dipole as a marker. *Brain Topogr.* **8,** 7–11.

835. Young, G.B. & Blume, W.T. (1983): Painful epileptic seizures. *Brain* **106,** 537–554.

836. Zardini, G., Molteni, B., Nardocci, N., Sarti, D., Avanzini, G. & Granata, T. (1995): Linguistic development in a patient with Landau–Kleffner syndrome: a nine-year follow-up. *Neuropediatrics* **26,** 19–25.

837. Zung, A. & Margalith, D. (1993): Ictal cortical blindness: a case report and review of the literature. *Dev. Med. Child Neurol.* **35,** 921–926.

Index